PRINCIPLES AND PRACTICE OF
RENAL TRANSPLANTATION

To Jim —

With every good wish

Jerry

11-7-2000

PRINCIPLES AND PRACTICE OF
RENAL TRANSPLANTATION

BARRY D KAHAN, PhD, MD, Director of the Division of Immunology and Organ Transplantation, The University of Texas Health Science Center, Houston, Texas, USA

and

CLAUDIO PONTICELLI, MD, FRCP(Ed), Director of the Divisione di Nefrologia e Dialisi, Policlinico IRCCS, Ospedale Maggiore, Milan, Italy

Martin Dunitz

© Martin Dunitz Ltd 2000

Although every effort has been made to ensure that all owners of copyright material have been acknowledged in this publication, we would be glad to acknowledge in subsequent reprints or editions any omissions brought to our attention.

First published in the United Kingdom in 2000
by Martin Dunitz Ltd, The Livery House, 7–9 Pratt Street, London NW1 0AE

Although every effort has been made to ensure that drug doses and other information are presented accurately in this publication, the ultimate responsibility rests with the prescribing physician. Neither the publishers nor the authors can be held responsible for errors or for any consequences arising from the use of information contained herein. For detailed prescribing information or instructions on the use of any product or procedure discussed herein, please consult the prescribing information or instructional material issued by the manufacturer.

A CIP record for this book is available from the British Library.

ISBN 1 85317 819 5

Distributed in the United States by:
Blackwell Science Inc.
Commerce Place, 350 Main Street
Malden MA 02148, USA
Tel: 1-800-215-1000

Distributed in Canada by:
Login Brothers Book Company
324 Salteaux Crescent
Winnipeg, Manitoba R3J 3T2
Canada
Tel: 1-204-224-4068

Distributed in Brazil by:
Ernesto Reichmann Distribuidora de Livros, Ltda
Rua Coronel Marques 335, Tatuape 03440-000
Sao Paulo,
Brazil

Composition by Wearset, Boldon, Tyne and Wear.
Printed and bound in Singapore by Kyodo Pte Ltd.

CONTENTS

PREFACE

Over the last few years, the continued progress in basic science, clinical medicine, and immunopharmacology has engendered exciting improvements in the field of renal transplantation. Today, this procedure offers longer patient survival, improved quality of life, and reduced medical expenses compared to dialysis. Yet, despite the many advantages of renal transplantation, a number of problems remain. The transplant recipient is subject to the complications of lifelong immunosuppression, and many allografts are lost because of a poorly defined form of chronic allograft nephropathy. Moreover, immunosuppressive drugs may exacerbate morbidities that developed prior to transplantation.

This book is aimed at physicians, surgeons, and medical students who are interested in the fundamental principles and clinical problems of renal transplantation. It represents a cooperative effort that arose out of a professional collaboration and friendship spanning nearly the entire era of modern transplantation therapy. Although the seeds of a collaboration were sown 20 years ago, it was not until 1998 that we first edited a book together—*New Dimensions in Transplantation: Weaving the Future* (Elsevier Science, Philadelphia), the result of an international conference held in Florence and attended by more than a thousand delegates. With the motif of the Three Fates of Greek mythology who spun, measured, and cut the thread of life—representing the selectivity, synergy, and specificity that are the hallmarks of novel immunosuppressive drugs—the meeting presented a panoply of current results, as well as the challenges to be faced in the new millennium of organ transplantation.

Another collaboration, this time to produce the comprehensive textbook *Principles and Practice of Renal Transplantation*, seemed like a natural next step. But 'What would we have to offer that was unique?' was a question that repeatedly arose as we mulled over the concept of the present book. The answer soon emerged from the general pattern of our collaborative efforts through the years: a consistent approach to address the surgical and immunological problems by Kahan, and the etiologies for transplant and the postoperative management challenges by Ponticelli. Some of the chapters would be written individually, some in collaboration between the two of us, and still others with the assistance of our own colleagues in Houston or in Milan. As requested by the publisher, tables and figures would be used liberally to illustrate the text. Such a volume, we hoped, would be distinct from other multi-authored volumes in that it would provide consistent analyses, nomenclature, and algorithms of diagnosis and treatment.

The first two chapters of the book address the basic science of transplantation, from histocompatibility to the immunobiology of rejection. The four chapters following are devoted to clinical selection of the recipient, to cadaveric and living donors, and to the transplant operation as well as its surgical complications. Four additional chapters deal with the mechanisms of action, clinical effects, pharmacokinetics and new strategies for the design of immunosuppressive agents. The remainder of the book is dedicated to the diagnosis and treatment of rejection, recurrence of primary diseases, medical complications, and psychological and obstetrical considerations. The final chapter outlines current results and the promising technological endeavors being undertaken to meet the demands of renal transplantation in the new millennium. We hope that the joint efforts of an American immunosurgeon and a European nephrologist have produced a comprehensive and useful work, and that readers will benefit from this volume as much as we have enjoyed collaborating on it.

Barry D Kahan PhD, MD
Claudio Ponticelli MD, FRCP(Ed)

ACKNOWLEDGEMENTS

We thank publishers Mr Martin Dunitz and Mr Robert Peden, who invited us to produce this book and who enthusiastically supported us throughout its preparation.

The realization of the book would not have been possible without the invaluable efforts of our colleagues Kerman, Stepkowski, Kelly, Kara Kahan, and Allan Katz in Houston, and Aroldi, Campise, Elli, Montagnino, Zorzi, and Antonio Tarantino in Milan.

The outstanding editorial assistance of Ms Kate Ó Súilleabháin and Ms Luciana Costadoni rendered the text clear and consistent. The artwork had been prepared over the years by Mike De La Flor, Michael Cooley, and Dwavalon Young, with the addition of new figures by Peg Garrity.

Most of all, our wives Rochelle and Titti supported our efforts, not only on this project, but also throughout the years as we worked to gain the expertise required to bring this book to fruition.

1 IMMUNOGENETICS, HISTOCOMPATIBILITY, AND CROSSMATCHING FOR KIDNEY TRANSPLANTATION

*In collaboration with RH Kerman**

The success of organ transplantation is limited primarily by allograft rejection, an immune defense mechanism that differentiates self from nonself, thereby protecting the organism from foreign invaders. Two sets of cell surface antigens serve as the primary markers for transplant survival. The ABO major blood group glycolipids are the targets for naturally occurring hemagglutinin antibodies (Landsteiner 1900) that upon transfusion cause reactions of incompatible blood or deposit on the endothelium bearing incompatible antigens, thereby attracting platelets and granulocytes and leading to immediate, usually irreversible, allograft rejection (Flye 1989). The blood group antigens are widely distributed on tissues and in body fluids. The second series of transplantation antigens—the major histocompatibility complex (MHC)—is present on the cells of all mammalian species and is encoded by a single chromosomal region (Klein 1987).

The concept of the MHC evolved following experiments in murine models that showed that a series of erythrocyte antigens that provoke alloantibodies (Gorer et al 1948; Snell 1948) was linked to genes, located on chromosome 17 (the MHC), that determine an anomaly of tail development (Gorer et al 1948). Little and Johnson (1922) showed that the donor–recipient disparities at loci encoding these antigens govern acceptance of splenic implants. In fact, Snell (1948) not only coined the term 'histocompatibility genes' to describe the special class of codominant genes that determine the fate of allotransplants, but also formulated the four 'laws' of transplantation:

(1) Grafts between individuals of identical genetic composition, such as strains of inbred mice wherein father and mother are identical twins (save for the Y-chromosome), are uniformly accepted (isografts);
(2) Grafts exchanged between members of different strains are rejected (allografts);
(3) F_1 hybrids accept transplants from either parental strain;
(4) Parental hosts reject F_1 hybrid donor grafts (Figure 1.1).

*Division of Immunology and Organ Transplantation, Department of Surgery, University of Texas Medical School, Houston

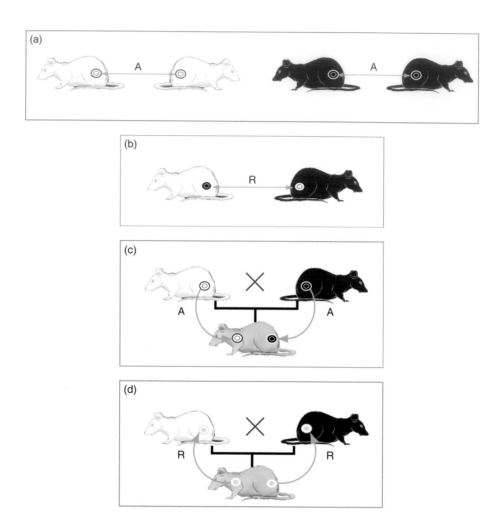

Figure 1.1. Snell's Laws of Transplantation. (a) Grafts between members of an inbred mouse strain are permanently accepted (A). (b) Grafts exchanged between members of different inbred strains are rejected (R). (c) Grafts from parental strains to their F_1 progeny are accepted. (d) Grafts from F_1 progeny to parental strains are rejected.

Pursuant to this work documenting acceptance of transplants from genetically identical animals, Murray and Thomas (1993) documented that kidney transplants between monozygotic twins are permanently accepted. Indeed, the extended survival of allografts from familial donors that are MHC-identical but otherwise genetically disparate, compared with that of grafts transplanted across MHC disparities, strongly supports the hypothesis that a major genetic system—the MHC region—determines the outcome of transplants. Moreover, the rate of failure among unrelated cadaveric grafts seems to increase as a function of the number of MHC-mismatched donor antigens (Opelz et al

1977). Thus, MHC matching is a method recognized to increase the chance of graft success.

In addition to the MHC, there are multiple systems of minor histocompatibility genes (mHC), the products of which are expressed on the cell surface and can potentially stimulate or act as targets of host immune responses. However, within the human species, most mHC molecules are highly conserved, that is, either they do not show allelic determinants or, if they do, these antigens are not highly polymorphic. Thus, relatively few mHC antigen systems are relevant to clinical transplantation. Thus, the role of these vascular endothelial cell (VEC) and human monocyte antigenic determinants remains unclear (Moraes and Stastny 1977; Cerilli et al 1985; Jager et al 1987). Other tissue-specific, nonHLA, gender-linked antigens have been suggested as targets for reactions toward bone marrow transplants, but have not been clinically linked to rejection of solid organ transplants.

One glycoprotein system implicated in the resistance of African-American patients to allografts is the Lewis (Le) blood group. Exposure to Le^a, particularly via blood transfusions from Caucasian donors, can elicit an antibody response by Le^b patients, who are primarily African-Americans. If anti-Le^a cytotoxic (as well as hemagglutinating) alloantibodies are produced, they adhere to the Le^a-positive vascular endothelium, provoking rejection of renal allografts. However, the overall importance of this rejection mechanism within the spectrum of transplantation remains unclear (Spetalnik et al 1984).

MAJOR HISTOCOMPATIBILITY COMPLEX

Anatomy of the genetic region

The MHC comprises a series of 100 closely linked genetic regions occupying 2 centromorgans (approximately 4000 kilobases) on the short arm of chromosome 6 (Figure 1.2). The centromorgan is a standard unit of map distance, representing the chromosomal equivalent of a 1% frequency of genetic recombination between linked genes. The genes within the MHC are physically grouped into three regions. The MHC genes encode cell surface proteins, as well as the human leukocyte antigens (HLA), which play a critical role in discriminating self versus nonself. The class I region encodes the heavy polypeptide chain gene products of the HLA-A, -B, and -C loci; the nonclassical class I genes HLA-E, -F, and -G; several pseudogenes, that is, DNA sequences that resemble a gene but are not expressed because of defects that impair some stage of product expression; and other genes of indeterminate function. The class II region encodes both the α- and the β-chains of HLA-DR, -DP, -DQ, -DM, and -DO molecules. In addition, the class II region contains at least four genes that encode proteins that transport peptides into the endoplasmic reticulum for loading into class I molecules (denoted TAP-1 and TAP-2) as well as genes encoding proteins that mediate antigen processing by the peptide-producing proteasomes (LMP-1 and LMP-2; Monaco 1995).

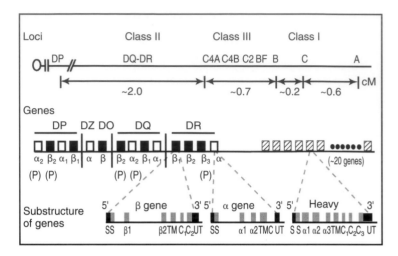

Figure 1.2. Schematic representation of the major histocompatibility complex (MHC) of chromosome 6. (Norman DJ, Suki WN, *Primer on Transplantation*, page 52. © 1998, American Society of Transplant Physicians. Reprinted with permission.)

In addition to the histocompatibility loci within the MHC, a class III region encodes the second (C2) and fourth (C4) components of the complement pathway, as well as properdin factor B (Bf) of the alternate complement pathway. The complement loci are polymorphic, with four alleles for the Bf, three for the C2, eight for the C4, and four for the C4B locus. In addition, this region contains genes encoding tumor necrosis factors α and β (TNF-α; TNF-β, now known as lymphotoxin, LT-A), heat shock protein 70 (HSP-70), and the 21-hydroxylases α and β. A lymphotoxin gene (LT-B) and an NF-κB-like gene (Browning et al 1993) are encoded in the region between the TNF and the HLA-B loci—a region that has also been suggested as a site for disease suscepti-bility genes (Marshall et al 1993).

Structural anatomy of gene products

Class I products

MHC class I antigens, which are encoded by the HLA-A, -B, and -C genes, were ini-tially identified as the targets of human alloantibody, and subsequently of cell-mediated immune, responses. Every nucleated cell displays class I antigens on its cell surface (Reis-feld and Kahan 1972; Figure 1.3). Each of the HLA-A, -B, and -C genes encodes the message for synthesis of a polymorphic glycoprotein heavy chain (45 kD), which bears a distinctive amino acid sequence (Kahan and Reisfeld 1968). Because these gene prod-ucts exhibit a high degree of homology, it is believed that they arose by duplication of an ancestral gene (Bjorkman and Parham 1990). The heavy chain forms a noncovalent complex with a 12-kD β_2-microglobulin (β_2m), which is encoded on chromosome 15 (Figure 1.4). The amino terminal portion of the heavy chain, which projects from the

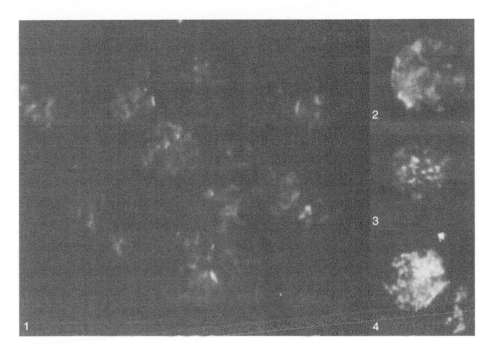

Figure 1.3. Cell surface distribution of the class I HLA-A2 antigen on lymphocytes demonstrated by the reaction of a monospecific alloantibody. Panels 2, 3, 4 show high power views of antibody coating of individual cells.

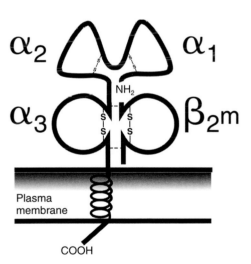

Figure 1.4. Schematic illustration of the structure of the MHC class I heterodimer. Heavy chain, including the α_1, α_2, α_3 transmembrane, and the intracytoplasmic domains, is noncovalently associated in the α_3 domain with a light chain (β_2m). (Thomas A Miller (ed.), *Modern Surgical Care: Physiologic Foundations and Clinical Applications*, 2nd edn. St Louis: Quality Medical Publishing Inc., 1998. Reprinted with permission.)

cell membrane into the extracellular space, includes three globular domains composed of amino acid residues 1–90 (α_1), 91–180 (α_2), and 181–271 (α_3). The α_3 domain contains the binding site for the $CD8^+$ T-cell marker. The $\alpha_1\alpha_2\alpha_3$ β_2m heterodimer is anchored in the cell membrane via a transmembrane portion of the heavy chain with a short intracellular cytoplasmic tail.

5

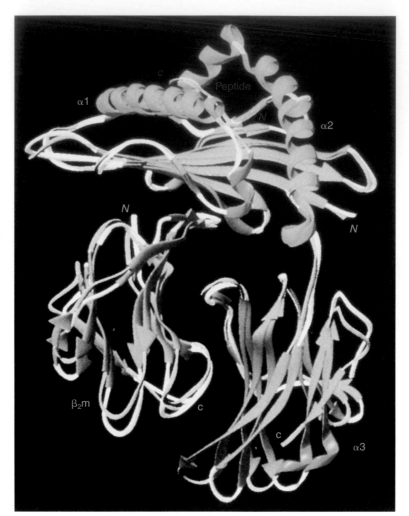

Figure 1.5. Ribbon diagram of HLA class I molecular structure as determined by X-ray crystallography, showing the three extracellular domains, α_1, α_2, α_3, in association with β_2m. The antigen-binding (peptide, shown in red) cleft lies between the helices of the α_1 and α_2 domains. N= nitrogen terminus; C= carbon terminus. (Reprinted with permission from *Nature*. Bjorkman PJ, Saper MA, Samraoui B, Bennett WS, Strominger JL, Wiley DC. Structure of the human class I histocompatibility antigen, HLA-A2. *Nature*. 1987; **329**:506–512. © 1987 Macmillan Magazines Ltd.)

The polymorphic antigenic determinants reside in the α_1 and α_2 domains; the α_3 and β_2m portions are relatively conserved, bearing amino acid sequences and structural folds that are homologous to those of immunoglobulin constant chain domains. In contrast, the polymorphic α_1 and α_2 domains are not homologous to immunoglobulin molecules, but rather show weak sequence homology among one another. The α_1 and α_2 helices sit upon a platform formed by eight antiparallel β strands. The cleft between the helices provides a binding site or groove, within which is displayed an antigenic peptide derived from either host or foreign invader intracellular proteins (Figure 1.5). The distinctive peptide binding properties of the polymorphic class I antigen are determined by the sequence of polymorphic amino acids bordering the internal surface of the groove.

Thus, only a limited spectrum of processed peptides can be presented by an individual product of a histocompatibility locus.

DNA sequence analysis has revealed several other class I HLA genes within the MHC region: HLA-F and -G lie between the telomere and the HLA-A locus, and HLA-E lies between the HLA-A and HLA-C loci. However, neither HLA-E nor HLA-F gene products are expressed on the cell surface, although their respective mRNA can be found in cells of the placenta. Because HLA-G molecules are expressed on the surface of fetal cytotrophoblasts, which lack expression of conventional HLA class I and class II products, it has been suggested that HLA-G factors protect the fetus from attack by maternal natural killer (NK) cells.

Class II products

The class II molecules—HLA-DP, -DQ, and -DR—differ from the class I molecules in cell distribution and protein structure. Whereas class I molecules are expressed on all nucleated cells, including both B and T lymphocytes, class II molecules have more limited distribution, namely, on monocytes, macrophages, endothelial cells, Langerhans cells of the skin, and activated (but not resting) T cells. In addition to B cells, HLA-DP antigens may be detected on monocytes, macrophages, and activated T cells, but the distribution of HLA-DQ on other cells is unknown.

The class II gene products, which are encoded in the MHC, form glycoprotein heterodimers by virtue of a noncovalent association between an α-chain of approximately 34 kD (229 amino acids) and a β-chain of approximately 29 kD (237 amino acids). These chains form three structural regions (Figure 1.6): namely, an extracellular membrane distal portion including polymorphic amino acids, which form a cleft similar to the α_1- and α_2-portions of class I gene products; a second membrane proximal extracellular

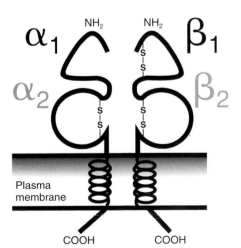

Figure 1.6. MHC class II. Schematic illustration of the α- and β-chains of the MHC class II product. Each unit contains membrane-distal α_1 and β_1 domains that form the peptide groove and membrane-proximal α_2 and β_2 domains. Each is followed by a transmembrane and an intracytoplasmic domain. (Thomas A Miller, *Modern Surgical Care: Physiologic Foundations and Clinical Applications*, 2nd edn. St Louis: Quality Medical Publishing Inc., 1998. Reprinted with permission.)

domain, which forms loop structures with significant sequence homology to immunoglobulin constant regions; and a transmembrane portion.

The genetic organization of the class II region is complex, containing both functional and defective (pseudo) genes in the DR, DQ and DP regions (Figure 1.2). Each locus includes a single gene for the α-chain and one or more loci for the β-chains. Four DR genes (DRB1, DRB3, DRB4, and DRB5) encoding β-chain antigens have been identified by the reactions of antibodies. The allelic products of the DRB1 gene include the private or allele-specific DR antigens DR1, DR2, DR3, etc. The DRB3 gene encodes a serologically defined antigen, DR52; DRB4 encodes DR53; and DRB5, DR1. A single common DR allele encodes the α-chain that completes the DR heterodimer.

Function

Although MHC molecules serve as antigens in the artificial situation of transplantation, their physiologic role is quite different: namely, to present foreign peptides to lymphocytes bearing the corresponding T cell receptor, thereby initiating the immune response of clonal activation, proliferation, and differentiation. Induction of a response by T cells toward a foreign antigen is specific for both the peptide determinant and the presence of a host-type class I or class II MHC product/MHC restriction (Zinkernagel and Doherty 1975). Thus, individual T cells recognize a complex epitope, including foreign peptide, in the context of a polymorphic domain of the appropriate MHC molecule expressed on the surface of an antigen-presenting cell (APC). The close interaction between antigen and class I MHC proteins has been described by X-ray crystallographic studies that reveal a fragment of the processed antigen within the groove of the MHC molecule (Bjorkman et al 1987; Figure 1.7).

Based upon the components of the MHC-restricted recognition unit, T cells may be grouped into subsets. $CD8^+$ (effector) T cells recognize antigen in association with class I MHC products, and $CD4^+$ (inducer/amplifier) T cells recognize antigen in association with class II MHC products (Figure 1.8). During the evolution of the alloimmune process, host T cells may directly recognize foreign antigens on donor cells or indirectly recognize determinants presented by host cells. The initial phase of these processes is a class II MHC-mediated activation of $CD4^+$ T cells, followed by class I antigen-mediated activated of $CD8^+$ T cells and B cells. Thus, the amplification of the immune response and the induction of antibodies depend upon the initial generation of antigen-activated $CD4^+$ T cells.

The peptides that are presented within the binding site (or peptide groove) of MHC molecules are derived from two distinct sources. The classical pathway of APC action depends upon the capture, processing, and presentation of exogenous antigens, which are subsequently presented in association with class II MHC molecules. These antigens are endocytosed into cells, digested by liposomes, and bound primarily to class II MHC molecules into complexes that are exported to the cell surface by lysosomes, where they serve as ligands triggering $CD4^+$ helper T cells. In contrast, endogenous antigens, which include

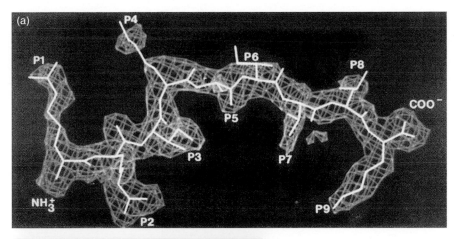

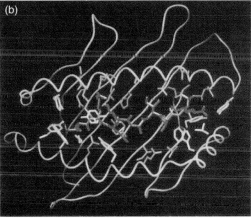

Figure 1.7. Top view of class I product-bearing peptide within the cleft between the α_1 and α_2 domains. (a) Diagram of nonapeptide with residue number indicated by P showing amino acid carboxy terminal residues. (b) Stick diagram showing van der Waals attractions between peptides and MHC class I amino acid residues on the edges of the cleft.

cytosolic peptides originating from the host or from degradation of viral proteins produced in infected cells, are transported by the action of TAP molecules into the endoplasmic reticulum. There they associate with class I MHC molecules for export to and expression on the cell surface, and for recognition by $CD8^+$ cytotoxic T lymphocytes (CTL; Dallman 1999).

Identification of MHC antigens

The HLA determinants were first identified as targets of agglutinating antibodies, which were produced by patients either afflicted with a variety of diseases, including agranulocytosis, or stimulated by blood transfusions (Goudsmit and Van Loghem 1953; Dausset

(a)

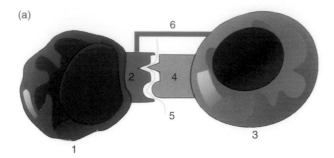

(b)

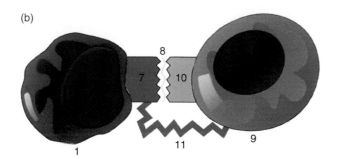

Figure 1.8. Interactions between antigen presenting cells (APCs) and T lymphocytes. (a) An APC (1) bearing class II MHC antigens (2) delivers a stimulation signal to a CD4+ T lymphocyte (3) via cognate interaction with the T cell receptor (4) recognizing a specific peptide (5) with the coreceptor CD4 (6). (b) The APC (1) via its class I MHC antigen (7) and its nonapeptide (8) activates the CD8+ T lymphocyte (9) via its T cell receptor (10) in conjunction with the coreceptor CD8 (11).

1954; Van Rood et al 1958). Because these antibodies reacted with peripheral leukocytes from some but not all individuals, they were *allo*immune rather than autoimmune in nature (Dausset 1954; Figure 1.9). Subsequently, these antileukocyte antibodies were found in the sera of multiparous women, presumably representing an immune response against foreign paternal antigens. Exploiting the cytotoxic properties of these sera (Payne and Rolfs 1958; Van Rood et al 1958), Terasaki and McClelland (1964) developed complement-dependent assays for tissue typing.

The first HLA antigens to be serologically defined with the use of alloantisera were the class I HLA-A, -B, and -C factors (Van Rood and Van Leeuen 1963; Payne et al 1964). Initially, the alleles of the (HLA-D) locus were defined based upon the degree of proliferative response when lymphocytes from two unrelated individuals were admixed in tissue culture. The magnitude of this response, termed the mixed lymphocyte culture (MLC) or mixed lymphocyte response (MLR), appeared to be proportional to the immunogenetic disparity between the two individuals (Bach and Hirschorn 1964; Bain et al 1964; Figure 1.10). HLA-D, the putative gene that regulated this response, was mapped within the MHC but outside the site of HLA-B on chromosome 6 (Eijsvoogel et al 1972). The basic assumption for assignment of HLA-D alleles was that two individuals are compatible (or identical) if the MLC test between them is negative, that is, does not elicit proliferation. Based on the patterns of reactivity, HLA-D alleles were provisionally identified (Figure 1.11). However, it is now clear that no single D locus per se

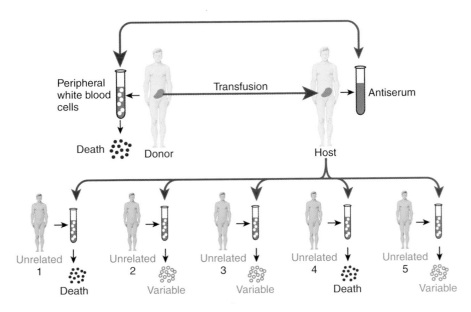

Figure 1.9. Seminal observation suggesting the HLA system. Patients sensitized by blood transfusion display alloantibodies that react with some but not all other patients. The host received a transfusion (or skin graft) from a donor, and thereafter developed antibodies that react with lymphocytes from not only the donor but patients 1 and 4 but not 2, 3, or 5.

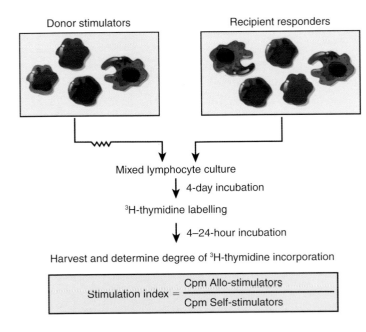

Mixed lymphocyte culture

↓ 4-day incubation

³H-thymidine labelling

↓ 4–24-hour incubation

Harvest and determine degree of ³H-thymidine incorporation

$$\text{Stimulation index} = \frac{\text{Cpm Allo-stimulators}}{\text{Cpm Self-stimulators}}$$

Figure 1.10. Performance of a one-way mixed lymphocyte culture reaction (MLC, MLR). Peripheral blood lymphocytes from a potential recipient are admixed with irradiated donor cells in vitro. After 96 hours, ³H-thymidine is added for an additional incubation. The incorporation of ³H-thymidine into DNA is assessed by harvesting the cells on fiber disks for beta scintillation counting. The results are expressed as the stimulation index by comparison of the incorporation of ³H thymidine in the presence of potential donor cells versus the recipient's own cells.

Responding cells (R)		Stimulating cells (Sm)								
HLA type	Patient	Nm	Pm	Rm	DMm	DWm	Cm	Mm	Sm	Jm
2, 14; 2, WS	N.	–	0.88	0.93	1.0	4.6	5.0	4.9	3.3	4.4
2, 14; 2, WS	P.	0.9	–							
2, 14; 2, WS	R.	0.9		–	0.93	5.2			4.1	3.4
2, 14; 2, WS	D.M.	1.1		1.3	–	4.7			4.8	6.2
2, 14; 9, WS	D.W.				7.8	–	1.7	1.3	10.0	8.0
2, 14; 9, WS	C.				4.8	0.55	–	0.88	5.2	4.4
2, 14; 9, WS	M.				4.7	1.0	1.2	–	6.3	4.8

Figure 1.11. HLA-D alleles shown by MLR results of seven siblings within members of a large family. The patients N., P., R., and D.M. form an MLR-nonstimulatory group, and D.W., C., and M. form another group. Note that cells from one group stimulate cells from the other group to proliferate to disparate HLA-D alleles. Note also two other HLA-D alleles in the family, as documented by the reactions of S. and J.

accounts for MLC results, but, rather, the results reflect the polymorphism of at least three expressed class II loci: DR (D-related), DQ, and DP.

Because the MLC method required 5–7 days of in vitro culture, a method that was only useful for living-related (but not for cadaveric) donor transplants, progress in the field demanded identification of antibodies that recognize 'HLA-D region' determinants. These antibodies were initially identified by their capacity to inhibit MLC proliferation by interacting with specific class II determinants on B, but not resting T, lymphocytes (Van Rood et al 1975; Wernet and Kunkel 1975). Furthermore, reagents specific for the B cell antigens HLA-DR, -DP, or -DQ were prepared by platelet absorption of polyspecific anticlass I and -class II HLA antisera determinants, thereby removing the antibodies directed against class I antigens. Although serologic tools provided a glimpse, the vast polymorphism of MHC products was only appreciated following development of molecular DNA typing procedures.

Although the HLA-DQ antigens are distinct from the -DR antigens, the two antigens show strong linkage disequilibrium, that is, some DQ alleles are represented more frequently among patients bearing certain DR specificities. For example, DQ1 is associated with DR1, DR2, DR6, and DR10; DQ2 with DR3 and DR7; and DQ3 with DR4, DR7, DR9, and sometimes DR6. In contrast, the DP antigens do not display linkage disequilibrium with DR or DQ alleles, a finding consistent with the greater map distances between them (Figure 1.2). In addition to these loci, the D region contains several unexpressed pseudogenes, such as DZ and DN, the functions of which are poorly understood, as well as the DO and DM genes that lie between DQ and DP in the class II region. DO encodes a chaperone molecule that carries and protects peptides destined for presentation by class II antigens, and DM, a product that catalyzes the loading of peptides onto class II antigens. For the purposes of clinical kidney transplantation, the HLA-A, -B, and -DR antigens are considered the most relevant factors.

HLA nomenclature

In 1967, the World Health Organization developed a standard HLA nomenclature; the system has been further refined by international histocompatibility workshops held every few years. Of the two nomenclature systems, one is based on epitopes defined immunologically using either serological or cellular techniques, and the other is defined biochemically by nucleotide sequences of allelic genes.

The former nomenclature utilizes the following system: HLA followed by a hyphen (-) represents the MHC; the capital letters thereafter—A, B, C, DR, DP, or DQ—designate the segregant series; and the number stipulates the specific allele, beginning with the number 1, save for the A and B loci, wherein numbers were sequentially assigned to one or the other allele (A or B) as new specificities were described (yielding A1, A2, A3, B5, B7, B8, A9, A10, A11, B12, B13, B14, etc.) As new allelic specificities were described, they were preceded by a 'w' until the identification was confirmed by multiple investigators. However, the letter 'w' is no longer used for that purpose, but rather to distinguish HLA-C locus alleles from complement components. (The 'w' prefix in all HLA-C alleles has been permanently retained.) DP and Dw alleles also retain a 'w' to indicate that both series were originally defined by the MLR cellular assay. Finally, two series of broad specificities, Bw4 and Bw6, retain the 'w' to indicate that they are physiologic, cross-reactive epitopes rather than discrete allelic products (Table 1.1).

The second nomenclature system is more complex than the first because it is based on nucleotide sequences. Furthermore, several HLA allelic variants discovered with genetic tools cannot be detected by traditional serological techniques. In the second system, as in the first, HLA followed by a hyphen (-) represents the MHC; a series of capital letters, with or without a number, designates a specific locus or 'segregant series'. In addition, specific alleles are designated by an asterisk (*) with a two-digit number indicating the most closely associated serological specificity, and thereafter a two-digit number defining the allele. Thus, the 25 molecular variants of the serologically defined HLA-A2 antigen are designated HLA-A* 0201–HLA-A* 0225. When an additional number is added to the nomenclature, for example, *02011 and *020112, it discriminates between two alleles that differ by only a single nucleotide—a difference that does not change the amino acid sequence encoded by the DNA sequence. When the product bearing a known nucleotide sequence is recognized by a new serological reagent, an extended number is used to indicate the coincidence of serologic and molecular nomenclatures of the particular allele; for example, an MHC class I serological specificity that is the gene product of the HLA-A* 0210 is known as HLA-A210 (Bodmer et al 1997). When the second nomenclature includes an 'N' designation, the allele is not expressed (null allele), whereas an 'L' designation indicates a mutation in a noncoding region that results in reduced expression of the gene product.

A	B		C	D	DR	DQ	DP
A1	B5	B50(21)	Cw1	Dw1	DR1	DQ1	DPw1
A2	B7	B51(5)	Cw2	Dw2	DR103	DQ2	DPw2
A203	B703	B5102	Cw3	Dw3	DR2	DQ3	DPw3
A210	B8	B5103	Cw4	Dw4	DR3	DQ4	DPw4
A3	B12	B52(5)	Cw5	Dw5	DR4	DQ5(1)	DPw5
A9	B13	B53	Cw6	Dw6	DR5	DQ6(1)	DPw6
A10	B14	B54(22)	Cw7	Dw7	DR6	DQ7(3)	
A11	B15	B55(22)	Cw8	Dw8	DR7	DQ8(3)	
A19	B16	B56(22)	Cw9(w3)	Dw9	DR8	DQ9(3)	
A23(9)	B17	B57(17)	Cw10(w3)	Dw10	DR9		
A24(9)	B18	B58(17)		Dw11(w7)	DR10		
A2403	B21	B59		Dw12	DR11(5)		
A25(10)	B22	B60(40)		Dw13	DR12(5)		
A26(10)	B27	B61(40)		Dw14	DR13(6)		
A28	B2708	B62(15)		Dw15	DR14(6)		
A29(19)	B35	B63(15)		Dw16	DR1403		
A30(19)	B37	B64(14)		Dw17(w7)	DR1404		
A31(19)	B38(16)	B65(14)		Dw18(w6)	DR15(2)		
A32(19)	B39(16)	B67		Dw19(w6)	DR16(2)		
A33(19)	B3901	B70		Dw20	DR17(3)		
A34(10)	B3902	B71(70)		Dw21	DR18(3)		
A36	B40	B72(70)		Dw22			
A43	B4005	B73		Dw23	DR51		
A66(10)	B41	B75(15)		Dw24	DR52		
A68(28)	B42	B76(15)		Dw25	DR53		
A69(28)	B44(12)	B77(15)		Dw26			
A74(19)	B45(12)	B78					
A80	B46	B81					
	B47	Bw4					
	B48	Bw6					
	B49(21)						

Table 1.1. Complete listing of recognized serological and cellular HLA specificities

HLA splits

An 'antigen split' of an original HLA specificity is defined by sera that react with only a limited subset of the cells that bear the original determinant. The designation of a 'split' is confirmed when one identifies other sera that react with a complementary (but not the original) subset of cells. One example of a 'split' is represented by the two antigens

HLA-B51 and -B52. The existence of new alleles or of splits of old alleles, as suggested by alloantibody reactivities, must be confirmed as structurally distinct using DNA sequencing procedures. HLA splits are now recognized to represent subtle variations in the amino acid sequence of the parent allele.

Private and public epitopes

Antigenic epitopes are defined as three-dimensional molecular conformations that induce an immune response. One type of epitope is determined by discrete structures governed by a single unique HLA allele—HLA private antigens. Most of these epitopes have been defined by the reactivity of specific alloantisera, produced after direct exposure to HLA antigens—for example, by pregnancy, organ transplantation, whole blood or platelet transfusions, and/or some types of microbial infections (Payne and Rolfs 1958; Van Rood et al 1958; Kissmeyer-Nielsen et al 1966). Other alloantisera define 'cross-reactive' specificities, that is, a structural determinant recognized by alloantibodies that show frequent cross-reactions among an array of molecules that also bear private antigens. These conformations are denoted as HLA 'public' antigens. The best-known examples of public antigens are HLA-Bw4 and HLA-Bw6. Indeed, each member of the HLA-B locus antigens bears the feature that defines it as a member of the Bw4 versus the Bw6 broad public antigen family.

Among the array of private antigens, some show a more limited degree of cross-reactivity and are denoted as CREGs (Table 1.2). For example, the B-7 CREG includes the HLA-B7, -B27, -B42, -B54, -B55, and -B56 private specificities that show cross-reactivity of specific alloantisera (Rodey and Fuller 1987).

CLINICAL TISSUE TYPING

Inheritance of HLA antigens

HLA genes display classic Mendelian inheritance, that is, each individual inherits a single chromosome (haplotype) from each parent and therefore has two HLA haplotypes (one paternal and one maternal in origin). Haplotypes are usually inherited intact, although in approximately 2% of cases recombinations between HLA-A and HLA-DR occur during meiosis, resulting in a new haplotype. Typically, a child carries one haplotype derived from each parent. Since the expression of HLA-A, -B, and -DR antigens is codominant, each person displays a phenotype that includes two specificities for each locus (two HLA-A, two -B, and two -DR antigens). In Figure 1.12, Child 1 bears the haplotype (A1, B8, DR2) derived from his father, and (A2, B7, DR4) from his mother. If Child 1 is the potential recipient, a graft from Child 2 is HLA-identical; from either parent or from Child 3, haploidentical; and one from Child 4, a double-haplotype mismatch. Occasionally, only one serological specificity is identified at an A, B, or DR

CREG	Antigens included
A01C	A1, A3, A11, A29, A30, A31, A36, A80
A10C	A10, A11, A19,* A25, A26, A32, A33, A34, A43, A66, A74
A02C	A2, A9, A23, A24, A28, A68, A69, A203, A210, A2403, B17, B57, B58
B05C	B5, B18, B35, B51, B52, B53, B78, B5102, B5103
B07C	B7, B8, B13, B22, B27, B40, B41, B42, B47, B48, B54, B55, B56, B59, B60, B61, B67, B81, B8201, B703
B08C	B8, B14, B16, B18, B38, B39, B59, B64, B65, B67, B3901, B3902
B12C	B12, B13, B21, B37, B40, B41, B44, B45, B47, B49, B50, B60, B61, B4005
B21C	B5, B15, B17, B21, B35, B46, B49, B50, B51, B52, B53, B57, B58, B62, B63, B70, B71, B72, B73, B75, B76, B77, B78, B4005, B5102, B5103
BW4	A9, A23, A24, A25, A32, B5, B13, B17, B27, B37, B38, B44, B47, B49, B51, B52, B53, B57, B58, B59, B63, B77, A2403, B5102, B5103
BW6	B7, B8, B14, B18, B22, B35, B39, B40, B41, B42, B45, B48, B50, B54, B55, B56, B60, B61, B62, B64, B65, B67, B70, B71, B72, B73, B75, B76, B78, B81, B8201, B703, B3901, B3902, B4005

*A19 is included in A10C CREG only when the donor or recipient is typed as A19 and its split A74 cannot be identified.

Table 1.2. Cross-reactive groups (CREGs) and their private serological component antigens

locus. This circumstance may be due to both parents sharing an antigen (the patient is homozygous); to the antigen not being sufficiently strongly displayed on the cell surface to be recognized by the typing sera; or to the gene product not having been identified, a circumstance that occurs at a particularly high rate among African-American patients (Hurley 1993; Zachary 1993).

The HLA phenotype is defined as the HLA antigens identified in the patient, using either serological or molecular tissue typing procedures. However, this information does not reveal the patient's genotype: namely, it does not identify which HLA-A, -B, and -C antigens are arrayed on a single haplotype. To determine the genotype, several family members must be phenotyped. For any family (in the absence of recombinations), there are four genotypic combinations of MHC inheritance: a 25% chance that two siblings are HLA-identical, that is, share both haplotypes; a 25% chance that they receive different parental haplotypes and do not share any antigens; and a 50% chance that they are HLA-haploidentical, sharing one of the two chromosomes. Therefore, when living-related donors are available, there is a high (75%) probability of finding an individual who is matched for at least one HLA haplotype (Figure 1.12). However, in the absence of family members, tissue typing procedures can only identify the HLA phenotype and

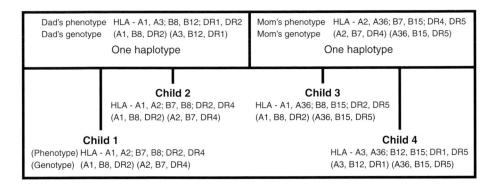

Figure 1.12. Inheritance of HLA haplotypes. Each child has inherited one haplotype from each parent. All children are HLA-haploidentical to mother and father. Children 1 and 2 are HLA-identical to each other and haploidentical to Child 3, but share no HLA antigens with Child 4. Children 3 and 4 are HLA-haploidentical.

not the haplotypes. Thus, potential recipients can only be matched with cadaveric donors based upon the phenotype, whereas genotypic matching is readily accomplished for living-related transplants (Bollinger and Sanfilippo 1989; Terasaki et al 1992; Garovoy 1998).

Because the HLA system is highly polymorphic, it would in theory be rare for two random, unrelated people to be even phenotypically HLA-identical. However, the prevalence is greater than would be predicted by chance, due to the occurrence of 'linkage disequilibrium' in the HLA system. Certain combinations of HLA alleles are encountered more frequently than would be predicted—A1, B8, DR3; A2, B7, DR1. Linkage disequilibrium increases the possibilities of obtaining individuals matched for common antigens, particularly among Caucasian patients (Bollinger and Sanfilippo 1989; Garovoy 1998). Yet despite the sharing of HLA-A, -B, and -DR phenotypes (and presumably a similar haplotype), there is no guarantee for these patients that all of the other genetic material in the MHC is identical, whereas chromosomal inheritance among family members is certain.

HLA typing procedures

Serologic detection of class I antigens

The standard procedure for serological identification of class I HLA-A, -B, and -C antigens is the complement-dependent microlymphocytotoxicity (CDC) test (Terasaki and McClelland 1964). Each well of a microtiter plate is loaded with either a monoclonal antibody or a specific alloantiserum obtained from a multiparous woman who during gestation had been sensitized toward disparate paternal antigens. To be assured of

(a)

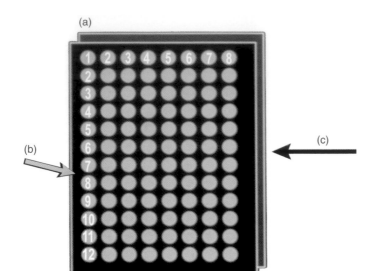

(b)

(c)

Figure 1.13. Serological HLA tissue typing procedure. (a) AntiHLA antibodies to individual class I (or class II) antigens are preloaded into 96-well microtiter trays. (b) Peripheral blood lymphocytes from individuals to be tissue typed. (c) After an initial incubation with rabbit complement, the dye eosin is added, formalin is used to fix the reactions and the trays are examined under inverted phase-contrast microscopy.

proper antigen identification, multiple reagents recognizing each of the HLA-A, -B, and -C specificities are loaded into separate compartments. The plates are frozen until needed to perform a tissue typing procedure. To each well of the thawed microtiter plate is added a 0.001 ml volume containing approximately 2000 lymphocytes that have been purified from peripheral blood, spleen, or lymph nodes. After 60 min, 0.005 ml rabbit complement is added for a further 15-min incubation. Binding of specific antibody to its HLA target on the cell surface activates the complement cascade, leading to cytotoxic injury (Figure 1.13). Thereafter, eosin is added to test whether the targets are dead and stained or are viable and able to exclude the vital dye, as ascertained by examination of the trays under phase-contrast microscopy. The binding of specific antisera to a test cell, as evidenced by a dark red, swollen appearance, indicates the presence of the corresponding antigen. In contrast, cells that do not bear the antigen remain alive, appearing as clear dots under the microscope (Figure 1.14). The percentage of cells in each well that have been lysed by the individual antiserum is estimated; the presence of a specific HLA-A, -B, or -C antigen is established by greater than 20% variable cells in wells bearing antisera that are reactive toward a single specificity.

Serologic detection of class II antigens

Since class II molecules are only present on B (but not resting T) cells, HLA-DR and -DQ antigens may be identified by a microlymphocytotoxicity assay using purified B cells. This population is isolated either by nylon-wool adherence or by antibody-specific capture into a solid phase coated with anti-CD20, a specific B cell marker. Despite the alloantisera and complement being pretested to ensure that they do not detect class I

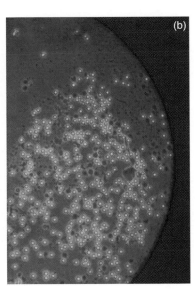

Figure 1.14. Eosin exclusion crossmatch. (a) Dark dots show dead cells (a positive test). (b) Refractile droplets are live cells (a negative test).

antigens, identification of class II antigens by serological reagents may be hard to interpret and nonreproducible. These problems have been attributed to the limited array of potent monospecific class II typing sera and to the difficulties inherent in the isolation and handling of B lymphocytes. However, the more potent class I and class II typing reagents now available routinely achieve concordant serologic results between HLA laboratories, with a degree of accuracy that is nearly comparable to that obtained with molecular typing procedures.

Molecular typing

Molecular typing procedures to identify HLA class II alleles HLA-DR, -DQ and -DP are based on recognition of specific nucleotide sequences. Because of their molecular basis, the chemical procedures reveal a much greater degree of polymorphism of the individual alleles than that detected by serologic tests. The three procedures used for molecular identification include restriction fragment length polymorphism (RFLP), an analysis of genomic DNA that has been fingerprinted after amplification by the polymerase chain reaction (PCR) and hybridized with either a sequence-specific primer (SSP) or a sequence-specific oligonucleotide probe (SSOP); single-strand conformational analysis by PCR (PCR-SSCP); and nucleotide sequence analysis (sequence-based typing, SBT) (Savage et al 1993).

Molecular procedures are commonly used to identify HLA-DR and -DQ alleles. The most commonly employed SSP method utilizes DNA primers that are specific for individual (or similar groups of) class II alleles (Figure 1.15). When the sequence corresponding to the PCR primer is present in the DNA extract from the patient,

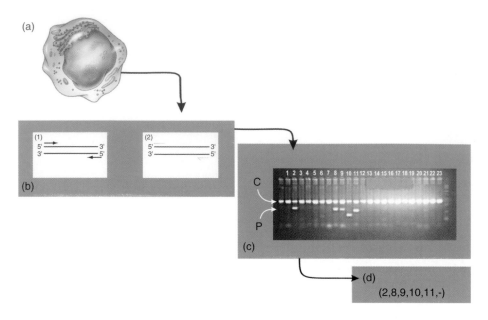

Figure 1.15. Molecular method for class II MHC typing. (a) Peripheral blood lymphocytes are lysed and DNA extracted. (b) PCR amplification of selected class II alleles is sought by addition of sequence-specific primers that generate product in (1), but do not polymerize in (2). (c) Detection of PCR products by polyacrylamide gel electrophoresis. The positive controls are shown as the row marked C, and the specific products of alleles present in the patient as row P. (d) Interpretation of the results, based on the products (P) identified in (c).

amplification occurs, generating a product of known base-pair size, which is separated on gel electrophoresis and visualized by staining. This method, which is especially useful for typing individual patients, can be performed within a 2–3-hour period and does not require radioactive materials. Sequence-specific primers not only provide an accuracy comparable to or better than serological class II typing, but can also be refined using additional amplification cycles with ever more selective primers that hybridize specific nucleotide sequences characteristic of a precise allele (Hurley et al 1997).

A second procedure, PCR-SSO, uses locus- or group-specific primers to amplify the corresponding genomic DNA, which is attached to a membrane through linking molecules. In a dot blot procedure, the specific allele is identified by the binding of a radio-labeled DNA oligonucleotide probe to the allele-specific sequence. Recently, a number of sensitive, nonradioactive labels have been developed to detect the specific allele in this system. The dot blot methodology is useful to test large numbers of samples (Hurley et al 1997), and a reverse dot blot method for allele-level typing of individual patients.

Because the number of variant HLA class I alleles is greater and because, rather than just one exon, there are two polymorphic exons, molecular typing for these gene products requires more complex methodology than does class II identification. Furthermore, the large number of class I pseudogenes may interfere with the reactions if primers or probes are poorly designed. Fortunately, the forthcoming development of semi-automated, radioisotope-free, direct nucleotide sequencing technology will provide more accessible molecular typing tools.

Impact of HLA matching in renal transplantation

Clinical outcome

Among living-related donor–recipient combinations, grafts from HLA-identical siblings display the best survival, followed by one-haplotype matches, which in turn show superior survival rates to transplants obtained from totally mismatched living-related or cadaveric donor transplants (Opelz et al 1977). Even in the cyclosporine era, HLA-identical sibling transplants display the best outcome; however, the outcomes of grafts exchanged across other HLA disparities are nearly comparable (Flechner et al 1983, 1984; Kaufman et al 1989). Therefore, most transplant units accept any suitably motivated, healthy family member as a kidney donor.

The importance of HLA matching to determine the clinical outcomes of renal transplants from cadaveric donors remains controversial. In contrast to the azathioprine era from 1978 to 1984, when there appeared to be a strong correlation between HLA matching and graft survival (Cecka 1986), opinions differ about a similar correlation in the present cyclosporine era. On the one hand, studies from large collaborative registries, including University of California—Los Angeles (UCLA), South Eastern Organ Procurement Foundation (SEOPF), United Network for Organ Sharing (UNOS), Collaborative Transplant Study (CTS), and the United States Renal Disease System (USRDS) suggest that the degree of HLA compatibility represents a significant factor determining the long-term survival of cadaveric allografts (as reviewed in Kerman 1994). Figure 1.16 shows the findings from the United States Renal Data System (Held et al 1994), indicating that increasing numbers of HLA-A, -B, or -DR mismatches are associated with higher adjusted relative risks of failure of first renal transplants performed between 1984 and 1990; a linear estimate revealed a 1.06 relative risk of graft loss for each HLA mismatch.

On the other hand, in contrast to these registry data, numerous individual and cooperative transplant center reports have failed to observe a benefit of HLA-A, -B, and -DR donor–recipient matching (Ferguson 1988; Matas et al 1989; Greenstein et al 1990; Kerman et al 1993). These reports attribute the disparity to significant differences in the immunosuppressive protocols, patient demographics, crossmatch criteria, etc., among various centers, and suggest that the large database in a registry does not overcome these differences to obtain a 'valid' trend. Thus, Matas and Fryd (1989) have suggested that the 'collective conclusions' of large registries may not apply to individual centers.

In addition to the interest in correlating HLA typing with 1-year graft survival rates, Terasaki et al (1993) reported the benefit of typing to increase allograft half-lives ($t_{1/2}$)— namely, the rate of loss after 1 year—as a measure of chronic attrition. Among patients

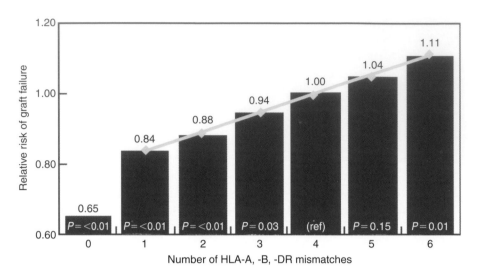

Figure 1.16. The adjusted relative risk (RR) of graft failure as a function of the number of HLA mismatches among first transplants performed in the US between 1984 and 1990 on patients 10–60 years of age under cyclosporine–prednisone immunosuppression. Cox multivariate analysis used nonlinear estimates (shown by the bars, with P values shown at their base) and linear estimates as shown by the line ($P < 0.01$). (Held PJ, Kahan BD, Hunsicker LG et al. *N Engl J Med* **331**(12):765–770. © 1994 Massachusetts Medical Society. All rights reserved.)

treated with azathioprine and prednisone, the overall half-life of primary cadaveric renal allografts across all match grades was 8.2 years, compared with 19.7 years for transplants from zero-mismatched donors. Each mismatch grade (1–6) seemed to display a progressive decrement in graft survival by 1.6 years. Although the initial results suggested that patients treated with a cyclosporine–prednisone regimen experienced less benefit of HLA matching than had been observed in the azathioprine–prednisone era (Lundgren et al 1986), some workers report that even with more intense immunosuppressive regimens, HLA mismatches cause a serial reduction in graft half-life (Cecka 1997; Opelz et al 1999). Gjerston (1997) reported that recipients of a zero-HLA-A, -B, -DR mismatched cadaveric donor kidney displayed a 12-year half-life, which was significantly longer than the 9–10-year mean graft survival among recipients of mismatched kidneys. However, the 0.6-year difference in the half-lives of grafts between donors and recipients mismatched for 1–2 versus 3–4 versus 5–6 HLA factors was significantly lower than the previously reported 1.6-year difference per match grade. While refinements in DNA molecular technology may more precisely discriminate the degree of donor–recipient mismatches, any advances may be obfuscated in the future by new immunosuppressive agents that are likely to achieve uniform 1-year cadaver kidney graft survival rates above 90% despite the HLA disparities (Halloran et al 1997).

Interestingly, data reported by 68 active transplant centers showed no correlation between the 1-year graft survival rates, ranging from 60% to 90%, and graft half-lives

(Gjerston and Terasaki 1992). Some centers with high 1-year graft survival rates reported poor half-life data; other centers with lower 1-year graft survivals reported excellent half-life data. Indeed, HLA mismatches affected only the short- or long-term survival rates in cases in which the center displayed relatively poor results during that posttransplant period. Thus, centers that achieved high rates of short- and/or long-term graft survival did not display an effect of HLA matching (Gjerston and Terasaki 1992).

Another paradox that belies the hypothesis that HLA matching determines allograft outcome is that kidneys from living, genetically unrelated donors bearing full HLA mismatches display outcomes superior to those of organs from cadaveric donors with the same degree of mismatch (Terasaki et al 1997). Furthermore, at more than 175 transplant centers, there was little difference between the graft survival rates of organs obtained from spousal compared with those from haplotype-matched living-related donors. One hypothesis to explain these unexpected results suggests that all living donor kidneys experience reduced risks of rejection due to a blunted injury response, including a muted upregulation of MHC antigen expression on vascular endothelial and renal parenchymal cells (Shoskes and Halloran 1991).

Alternate approaches

A potential alternate approach to the application of donor–recipient HLA matching seeks to avoid antigenic disparities that are likely to result in graft failure—differences denoted as 'taboo' HLA combinations. When this strategy was applied to a single HLA antigen mismatch, it did not detect any taboo factors (Maruya et al 1993; Van Rood et al 1994; Doxiadis et al 1996). Another approach to match donor organs with potential recipients utilizes the CREG concept (Table 1.2). A donor is only selected for a given recipient if the HLA mismatches occur among antigens within the same CREG, on the basis that this qualification would ensure an absent, or at most a muted, alloimmune response. By extending the range of putatively compatible antigens, CREG matching would particularly benefit minority recipients, since the highly polymorphic HLA determinants displayed by African-Americans tend to belong to a limited number of CREG groups. Although preliminary results suggested that a greater percentage of minority patients received a 'well-matched' graft compared to the historical fraction assigned based upon conventional matching by private specificities (Thompson et al 1997), there is no consensus that the CREG concept resulted in a benefit on graft outcome.

CROSSMATCH STRATEGIES

Histocompatibility testing seeks to identify donor–recipient combinations likely to yield successful transplants utilizing three principles: ABO blood group compatibility, HLA matching, and donor-specific crossmatching. The last principle seeks to exclude recipients who bear pre-existing antidonor immunity likely to cause graft failure. Beside ABO compatibility, the pretransplant crossmatch is generally regarded as representing the most important procedure performed in the histocompatibility laboratory.

The strength and nature of the recipient antidonor immune response is critical to the fate of the allograft. If preoperative exposure to donor-type antigens has resulted in sensitization, as evidenced by the development of cytotoxic antibodies and/or alloimmune memory T cells, the graft is likely to be condemned to failure. Indeed, pretransplant detection of humoral (or cellular) sensitization has markedly reduced the incidence of hyperacute and accelerated forms of rejection. Since no test is currently widely available to assess donor-specific cell-mediated allosensitization, the crossmatch relies on serological procedures. Because of their great importance in the clinical arena, crossmatch procedures have become increasingly more sensitive and accurate to detect and characterize host reactivity.

Test procedures

There are two general types of methods to detect antidonor humoral reactivity: the complement-dependent-cytotoxicity (CDC) assays, namely, the standard NIH-CDC (Terasaki and McClelland 1964), the Amos-modified CDC (Amos et al 1970) as well as the antihuman globulin-enhanced CDC (AHG) (Johnson et al 1972), and the binding assays, namely, the flow cytometric (Cicciarelli et al 1992) and enzyme-linked immunosorbent assays (ELISA) (Kao et al 1993; Buelow et al 1994). These tests differ in their sensitivity, incubation temperatures (warm versus cold), reaction times for target cells with serum and/or complement, wash steps, and use of unseparated peripheral blood lymphocytes (PBL) versus separated T and B cells as targets, as well as their distinction of IgM versus IgG antibodies. Clinical interpretation of crossmatch results demands a knowledge of the methodology, of the patient's primary renal disease, and of the preceding transfusion/transplant history, which may have provided events leading to allosensitization.

Complement-dependent assays

The standard microlymphocytotoxicity-CDC assay adds PBLs isolated from the donor as target cells to each well of a microtest tray that has been preloaded with either undiluted or diluted serum from an individual transplant candidate. The patient's serum is added either undiluted or diluted 1:2, 1:4, or 1:8 (Figure 1.17). The serum dilutions are used because of the possibility of prozone, wherein excessive amounts of antibody interfere with cytotoxic reactions. The assay methodology is similar to that previously described for class I MHC serological typing (Figures 1.13 and 1.14), except that crossmatches utilize individual patient serum samples, rather than standard HLA-typing sera preloaded into the wells. After a 30-min incubation to allow binding of potential patient antibodies to donor cell-surface membrane antigens, 0.005 ml complement is added for

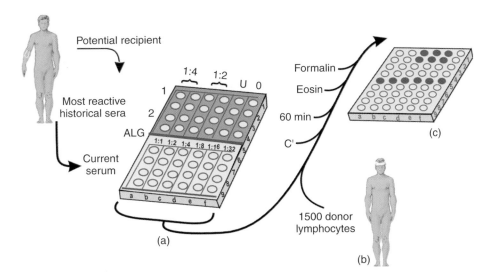

Figure 1.17. Methodology for the full visual crossmatch utilizing recipient sera preloaded into microtiter plates. (a) Plates are preloaded with duplicate wells containing no addition (O), or patient's sera undiluted (U), or diluted at 1:2 or 1:4 with culture medium for comparison of reactivity with the negative control containing no serum (0) and a positive control goat antihuman lymphocyte globulin (ALG). The stored trays are defrosted on demand. The tray shows two historical sera in the upper portion and a current surveillance serum in the lower portion. (b) Addition of donor lymphocytes and complement for a 60-min incubation, followed by evaluation of results by vital dye exclusion. (c) The tray shows positive results for the undiluted and the 1:2 dilution of historical serum 1 as well as ALG.

an additional 60-min incubation. If complement is fixed to cell surface antigen–antibody complexes, cell membrane permeability is augmented as visualized under phase-contrast microscopy using a vital dye, eosin or trypan blue. A test is considered positive when there is at least a 20% increase in the percentage of dead cells in the test well compared with the control wells (Terasaki and McClelland 1964). To display a positive test, the serum must contain a large amount of antibodies so that a sufficient number of antigen–antibody complexes are arrayed on the cell surface and complement is fixed for cell lysis.

This method detects not only alloantibodies, but also clinically irrelevant autoantibodies, namely, antibodies that are produced by the patient and capable of lysing his own cells. Therefore, an additional test examines the capacity of the serum to lyse the recipient's own PBLs as targets (Cross et al 1976). Autolymphocytotoxic antibodies, which are mostly of the IgM class (Chapman et al 1986), are encountered in many conditions that do not involve alloimmunization, such as infectious mononucleosis; autoimmune diseases; viral diseases; and reactions to medications, for example, the antiarrhythmia drug procainamide or the antihypertensive agent hydralazine.

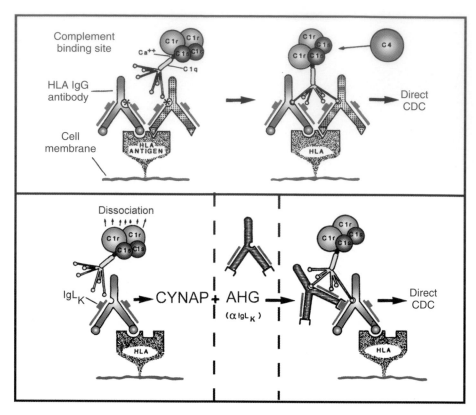

Figure 1.18. Illustration of the mechanism of CYNAP and AHG-CDC reactions. (From Mayer 1973 with permission.)

Amos et al (1970) described a wash step modification of the standard assay—the Amos-modified CDC. The wash step is added after the cells and serum have been incubated, but before the addition of complement. The wash step seeks to eliminate auto- or alloantibodies that are only weakly bound to target cells and thus capable of producing false-positive reactions. These antibodies are unlikely to be clinically relevant in vivo.

However, the standard microlymphocytotoxicity CDC is relatively insensitive; a negative test may signify not only the absence of antibodies, but also the presence of antibodies unable to fix complement (although able to mediate graft destruction by other pathways) or the adhesion of too few antibodies to trigger cell-membrane lysis. The presence of a subliminal amount versus an absence of antibody may be distinguished by adsorption tests. The cytotoxicity negative-absorption positive (CYNAP) phenomenon (Yunis et al 1971) occurs when a negative cytotoxicity reaction is shown by a patient's serum, while antibodies therein are able to adsorb to donor targets (Figure 1.18). There are several alternate approaches to detect these antibodies using modifications of the microlymphocytotoxicity crossmatch. One approach uses an extension of

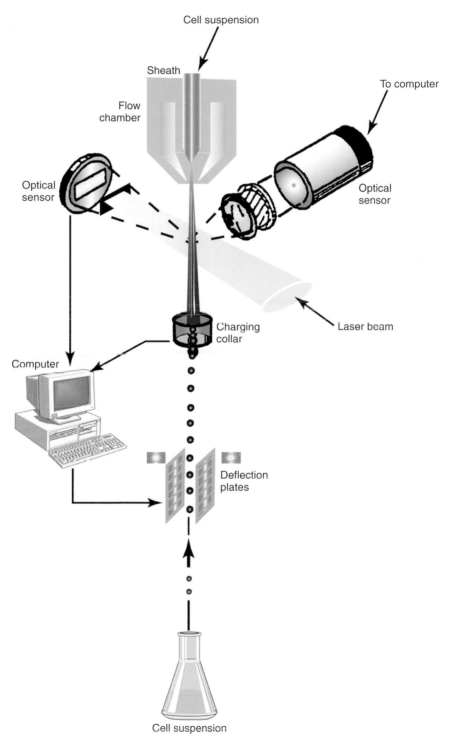

Figure 1.19. Schematic diagram of a typical unilaser flow cytometer. (Adapted from Becton Dickinson Immunocytometry Systems.)

the incubation time for cells and serum to 60 min and then for complement to 120 min—the extended crossmatch. This technique enhances the binding of low avidity antibodies as well as the fixation of complement.

However, other antibodies that bind relatively avidly to the target cell surface, yet are of an isotype that poorly fixes complement, are relevant in transplantation, since they can execute cell damage via other immune processes in collaboration with lymphocytes (antibody-mediated cell-dependent lysis) or by binding to monocytes or macrophages. To detect these antibodies, a second step may be added to the crossmatch procedure: an antihuman kappa light chain antibody is used to amplify the binding of patient antibodies to donor target cells—the antihuman globulin-enhanced cytotoxicity assay (AHG) (Johnson et al 1972). The AHG crosslinks IgM or IgG antibodies, thereby increasing the efficiency of binding of C1q and initiation of complement-mediated lympholysis by two- to three-fold (Fuller et al 1982, 1997; Figure 1.19). In addition, before the addition of AHG and complement, this technique incorporates wash steps to rid the test wells of weakly bound serum factors that might cause false-positive reactivity.

Binding techniques

Garovoy et al (1983) introduced a flow cytometry assay, which sensitively detects antidonor antibodies since it does not rely on complement fixation. Flow cytometry measures the fluorescence of stained cells within a fluid stream passing a set of fixed detectors (Figure 1.20). A flow cytometer provides information on the size (forward scatter), granularity or internal complexity (side scatter), and relative fluorescence intensity of the cells (Garovoy 1988). By combining the two light scatter parameters to assess size and granularity, it is possible to discern three distinct populations: lymphocytes, monocytes, and granulocytes.

Donor cells are incubated with potential recipient serum followed by addition of a goat antihuman IgG or IgM reagent that has been linked to fluorescein isothiocyanate (FITC). In addition, a phycoerythrin (PE)-labeled anti-CD20 monoclonal antibody is used to discriminate B cells from T cells that have been stained with a peridinin chlorophyll protein (PerCP)-conjugated monoclonal antibody directed against the surface marker CD3 (Figure 1.21). This three-color combination simultaneously discerns alloantibodies that react with T cells versus B cells, yet ignores background antibody binding due to reactions with natural killer cells or monocytes. The results of flow cytometry are expressed as 'positive' if, compared with a negative control or an autologous donor serum, the patient's serum shifts the median channel fluorescence intensity by 20 fluorescence units for T cells and 30 units for B cells, suggesting binding of antibody to the target cell (Figure 1.22).

Antigen-specificity studies must be performed to confirm that the observed reaction is due to antiHLA antibodies, since CDC, AHG-CDC, and flow cytometry assays may also detect immunoglobulins directed against other lymphocyte surface receptors (Chapman et al 1986). To expeditiously address the question of immunoglobulin specificity, sera may be tested in ELISA using microtest trays with wells coated with soluble

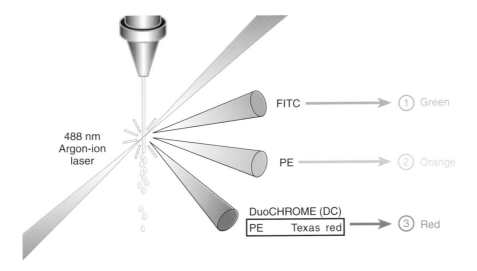

Figure 1.20. Depiction of simultaneous three-color analysis with a single Argon-ion laser using the fluorochromes FITC, PE, and DuoCHROME. (Adapted from Becton Dickinson Immunocytometry Systems.)

HLA antigens, or in flow cytometry using a suspension of polystyrene (flow) beads bearing antigen-immobilized HLA antigens (Buelow et al 1994; Pei et al 1998). These methods not only offer greater objectivity and reproducibility, but also require neither viable targets nor separations of T versus B cells. More importantly, these methods have the potential to identify the exact HLA specificity toward which the patient is reactive and thereby define that person's 'taboo' incompatibilities.

Serum screening procedures

Because patients may display an anamnestic (memory) response leading to hyperacute rejection and/or early graft loss despite a negative pretransplant crossmatch result using a current serum (Braun 1989), current practice assesses the presence of antiHLA reactivity in serial monthly or bimonthly patient serum samples. Before it is concluded that the crossmatch is negative, the historical sample displaying the greatest degree of antiHLA reactivity should be tested along with the current sample. Furthermore, continued surveillance of patient sera is necessary due to the changes over time as circulating antibody levels fluctuate and/or the patient receives a blood transfusion or other form of alloimmune sensitization. Thus, serial serum samples are tested against a panel of cells using the lymphocyte-based cytotoxicity technique (Figure 1.22), a soluble HLA antigen ELISA, or a flow beads method (Table 1.3). The results of the serum screening test are reported as the percentage of donors among a panel of unrelated individuals (or of soluble HLA antigens among a battery of protein products) to which the recipient shows a reaction: namely,

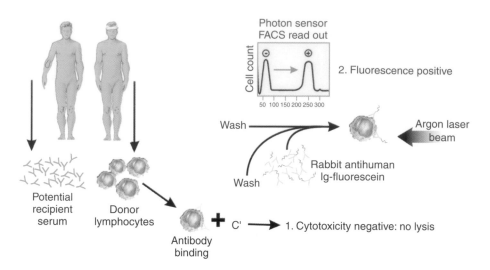

Figure 1.21. Performance of the flow crossmatch. Pathway 1: addition of complement to the mixture of patient serum and donor targets fails to cause cell lysis. Pathway 2: to the mixture is added a rabbit antihuman immunoglobulin that is fluorescein-tagged, and placed into a FACS detection system that records a channel shift on the photon sensor showing a positive result.

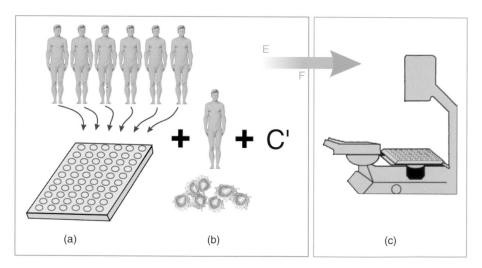

Figure 1.22. The serum screening procedure using the microlymphocytotoxicity method. (a) Each well of a microtiter plate is loaded with a monthly serum from an individual transplant candidate and frozen. (b) When a cell sample is received by the laboratory, the tray is thawed, and the lymphocytes (and subsequently complement) are added. (c) The reactions in individual wells are read under inverted phase-contrast microscopy after addition of the vital dye eosin (E) and fixation with formalin (F). The content of antibody in a particular patient's serum sample is expressed as the percentage of tested lymphocytes toward which the serum was cytotoxic, that is, the fraction of donors whose cells showed lysis on the eosin exclusion assay.

NIH-complement dependent cytotoxicity (CDC)*

Amos-modified CDC[†]

Antihuman globulin enhanced (AHG) CDC[‡]

Flow cytometry[§]

ELISA-based soluble HLA assays[¶,**]

---

*Terasaki and McClelland 1964

[†]Amos et al 1970

[‡]Johnson et al 1972

[§]Cicciarelli et al 1992

[¶]Kao et al 1993

**Buelow et al 1994

Table 1.3. Assays determining percent PRA

the percent panel reactive antibody (% PRA). In addition to the historical serum that displays the highest reactivity, crossmatch tests against specific donor targets generally include the most recent shipped sample (current), and, if both of these tests are negative, a fresh, immediately pretransplant serum obtained on the day of the planned operation.

Only half of the studies in the literature suggest a correlation between the % PRA of a recipient and his clinical outcome (Kerman et al 1996). Since historic sera may display a broad spectrum of antiHLA reactivity, it is important to focus on the critical IgG antidonor antibodies that clearly mediate rejection, in contradistinction to IgM alloantibodies that seem either to be irrelevant to or to have a beneficial impact on the outcome of primary renal allografts (Chapman et al 1986; McCalmon et al 1997; Przybylowski et al 1999). Thus, crossmatch techniques have been modified by the addition of dithioerythrethrelol (DTE) or dithiothreitol (DTT), reagents that reduce the disulfide bonds that link the pentameric complexes of immunoglobulin chains in IgM antibodies without affecting IgG molecules (Barger et al 1989; McCalmon et al 1997). A positive IgG antibody crossmatch detected by either the CDC or the ELISA technique forecasts an adverse prognosis for graft outcome (Kerman et al 1996).

Clinical implications of crossmatch tests

When it was documented that a positive crossmatch predicted early graft rejection, the standard microlymphocytotoxicity crossmatch was introduced into routine renal transplant practice (Kissmeyer-Nielsen et al 1966; Williams et al 1968; Patel and Terasaki 1969). Certain patients were recognized to be at high risk for a positive crossmatch, including multiparous females, retransplants, and recipients of blood transfusions. Implementation of the practice that patients may *not* receive a transplant from a donor toward whom *any one* of their sera displays a positive cytotoxic reaction significantly reduced the incidence of hyperacute rejection.

The next refinement in crossmatching was the discrimination of the significance of the target of antibody reactivity, be it T cells or B cells. The presence of antibodies that lysed T cells (a positive T cell crossmatch) contraindicates transplantation, whereas B cell positive reactions were *not* associated with graft failure in some (Ettenger et al 1979; Ayoub et al 1980) but not other (Braun 1989; Noreen et al 1989) reports. This discrepancy was probably due to the failure to discriminate whether the B cell reactivity was due to IgG or IgM antibodies in the patient's serum. For example, if the antiB cell antibody is an IgG immunoglobulin, the graft outcome is likely to be poor. Using the Amos-modified and the antiglobulin techniques, Phelan et al (1989) reported the presence of IgG (DTT-resistant but platelet-absorbed) anticlass I antibodies reactive with B cells but not T cells in 10 patients. Although two recipients displayed uneventful clinical courses, four lost their grafts within 3 months and the remaining four experienced significant but partially reversible rejection episodes. Another seven sera displayed cytotoxic reactions toward B cells that were due to IgG antiHLA class II activity ($N = 4$) or IgM immunoglobulins ($N = 3$). Among the last group, two patients displayed uneventful clinical courses, and one, a reversible rejection episode. Therefore, 14/17 (82%) patients whose sera displayed T cell-negative, B cell-positive reactions due to IgG anticlass I antigens experienced poor graft outcomes. Ten Hoor et al (1993) also reported that both primary and retransplant renal recipients who displayed positive IgG antiB cell crossmatches (detected by standard NIH-CDC) experienced poor graft survivals, in contrast to patients with IgM antiB-cell-positive crossmatches, who showed excellent outcomes. Furthermore, these investigators found that only IgG antiHLA antibodies were deleterious to the allograft; two-thirds of patients bearing high titers of IgG antibodies directed toward nonHLA antigens displayed good allograft function at 1 year posttransplant. Similarly, Shroyer et al (1993) observed that three retransplant recipients whose sera displayed positive T cell crossmatches against nonHLA determinants experienced better graft survival than patients with positive flow crossmatch reactions toward HLA antigens. Therefore, IgG antibodies directed toward HLA determinants on T or B cells are clinically relevant, representing an exclusion for transplantation.

The next development, the antihuman globulin (AHG) crossmatch, enhanced the sensitivity of the tests beyond that achieved with the standard CDC technique. An AHG-positive result represented an absolute exclusion of a recipient from transplants from that donor. This policy decreased the rates of accelerated and acute rejection episodes, even when alloreactivity could not be detected by standard CDC techniques (Johnson et al 1972). For retransplant recipients, AHG-negative results with both the historical high PRA and the pretransplant sera increased the 1-year graft survival rate from 64%, using only a negative NIH-CDC crossmatch, to 84% (Kerman et al 1990). However, our studies showed that an AHG-positive crossmatch should not be considered a contraindication to a first transplant if the antibody is of the IgM class (Kerman et al 1991).

Recently, there has been interest in the significance of a positive historical crossmatch when the result with the current or pretransplant serum is negative. Whereas a positive crossmatch result using a historical positive serum represents a contraindication for retransplantation, it does not seem to have the same adverse prognostic significance for a candidate for primary renal transplant (Cardella et al 1982; Kerman et al 1985). This important finding has allowed many primary transplant recipients, who were previously excluded due to the presence of cytotoxic reactivity in historical sera, to be transplanted. Among a cohort of 320 cyclosporine–prednisone-treated primary renal allograft recipients, 17 (5%) displayed an historic-positive, current-negative AHG crossmatch. The reactivity of 10 sera was abrogated by DTE reduction, suggesting the presence of IgM antibodies. Among the seven IgG-reactive patients whose antibody activity was insensitive to DTE treatment, five recipients have functioning renal allografts at 2–4 years posttransplant. The four patients whose donor cells were available underwent repeat crossmatches posttransplant, revealing IgG antiT (but not antiB) cell antibodies, suggesting that the alloreactivity was not directed against HLA. The two other recipients among the seven IgG-reactive patients showed positive tests against both donor B and T cells, suggesting antiHLA activity. Both lost their grafts due to hyperacute or accelerated rejections. Therefore, tests with separated B and T cell targets help to discriminate antibody specificity toward HLA (both positive) versus nonHLA (one cell type negative) determinants on donor cells.

The most recent and sensitive assay for pretransplant crossmatch testing utilizes the flow cytometer. This test does not rely on complement fixation, but rather measures the binding of immunoglobulin molecules onto target cells. Garovoy (1988) found an 18% lower 1-year graft survival rate among renal recipients who displayed a positive versus a negative T cell flow crossmatch. A subsequent study not only confirmed the reduced graft survival, but also discovered a poorer quality of early graft function among patients, particularly retransplant recipients, who had displayed T cell positive flow crossmatches (Cook et al 1987). Iwaki et al (1987) subsequently reported a 22% rate of nonfunction of renal allografts among T cell flow-positive versus 4% for flow-negative primary recipients. However, this finding was not confirmed in a subsequent study (Cook et al 1989). Indeed, the correlation of flow crossmatches with clinical outcome is controversial. One study claimed similar 1-year graft survival rates: namely, 82% for T cell flow-positive and 75% for flow-negative crossmatches (Ogura et al 1993). In contrast, we found a significant difference in graft survival rates between retransplant recipients whose sera displayed flow-positive versus -negative crossmatch results (Kerman et al 1990).

Indeed, Ogura et al (1993) reported a greater incidence (39%) of positive T-cell flow crossmatches among sensitized compared to 8% among unsensitized patients. However, these workers compared the flow procedure with the two least sensitive procedures (the standard CDC or Amos-modified CDC), but not the AHG crossmatch test, which may have actually detected the antibodies. Future studies must compare the utility of the flow with the AHG-crossmatch procedures to assess whether antibodies solely detected by flow cytometry reflect a form of presensitization that forecasts an adverse outcome. Our studies suggest that, regardless of the pretransplant flow cytometry crossmatch result with peak PRA and the pretransplant sera, first but not repeat transplant patients who are AHG crossmatch-negative show similar renal graft survival rates (Kerman et al 1991).

Of some interest is the difference for heart allograft recipients: it has been our policy to transplant these patients following a negative AHG crossmatch, using the highest PRA historical and the pretransplant sera. It was, therefore, of great interest (and surprise) when we found that among 140 cardiac transplants, patients who were AHG crossmatch-negative but IgG flow crossmatch-positive displayed a significantly poorer 1-year graft survival than flow cytometry crossmatch-negative recipients (68% versus 86%, $P < 0.02$; Przybylowski et al 1999). Moreover, 50% of the IgG-positive flow crossmatch recipients experienced early rejection episodes, compared with only 16% of negative recipients ($P < 0.01$). The most provocative finding was an improved rate of graft survival among IgM-positive versus either the IgM-negative ($P < 0.05$) or the IgG-positive ($P < 0.02$) flow crossmatch recipients, suggesting that the presence of IgM antibodies confers a beneficial effect.

Despite these provocative findings in cardiac recipients, we believe that one can rely on the results of an AHG crossmatch utilizing historic high PRA sera for renal recipients, particularly since the flow crossmatch is a technically difficult and expensive procedure. However, if an historic high PRA serum is not available, flow crossmatching may be useful for retransplant candidates to reliably detect low levels of alloantibody reactivity. We nevertheless believe that accepting only flow cytometry crossmatch-negative recipients results in a policy of transplanting nonreactive recipients, thereby denying grafts to some alloreactive patients. Thus, it is our policy that among primary graft recipients, only an AHG-detected, IgG-antiHLA alloreactive antibody represents a contraindication to transplantation. This policy demands that alloreactivity be documented by positive IgG reactions against donor B or both B and T cell targets. Save for immunologically high-risk patients, such as retransplants, polytransfused African-Americans, or multiparous polytransfused females, IgG alloantibodies are encountered among less than 2% of primary recipients. Indeed, most candidates for renal transplants present with *no* reactivity, with a clinically irrelevant IgM antibody, or with an IgG antibody directed toward nonHLA antigen(s).

CONCLUSION

The outcome of renal transplantation depends upon multiple factors: the efficacy of the immunosuppressive regimen, the HLA antigen matching, ethnicity, gender, degree of presensitization, and transfusion history, as well as the recipient's immune responder status. A prerequisite for transplantation is that the graft is ABO-compatible and that the recipient displays a negative crossmatch against donor lymphocyte targets. The role of HLA matching in organ allocation for transplantation remains controversial, except in the case of donors matched for 6 HLA antigens. In this era of new immunosuppressants, many recipients are disadvantaged by allocation schemes based upon intermediate degrees of HLA match with the donor. The advent of sensitive crossmatch techniques, such as those exploiting an antihuman globulin as a second, crosslinking reagent to facilitate complement-mediated lysis, provides a sensitive and specific tool, particularly when applied in conjunction with maneuvers to eliminate IgM reactivity using dithiothreitol, and with detection of selective reactions against B and T cells. Exploiting these strategies, one can detect the presence of IgG antibodies directed toward HLA class I antigens—an absolute contraindication to transplantation.

REFERENCES

Amos DB, Bashir H, Bogle W (1970) A simple microcytotoxicity test. *Transplantation* 7:220–224.

Ayoub G, Park MS, Terasaki PI et al (1980) B cell antibodies and crossmatching. *Transplantation* 29:227–229.

Bach F, Hirschorn K (1964) Lymphocytic interaction: a potential histocompatibility test in-vitro. *Science* 143:813–814.

Bain B, Vas MR, Lowenstein L (1964) The development of large immature mononuclear cells in mixed leucocyte cultures. *Blood* 23:108–113.

Barger BO, Shroyer TW, Hudson SL et al (1989) Successful renal transplantation in recipients with a positive standard, DTE negative, crossmatch. *Transplant Proc* 21:746–747.

Bjorkman PF, Parham P (1990) Structure, function and diversity of class I major histocompatibility complex molecules. *Ann Rev Biochem* 59:253–281.

Bjorkman PJ, Saper MA, Samraoui B et al (1987) Structure of the human class I histocompatibility antigen, HLA-A2. *Nature* 329:502–512.

Bodmer JG, Marsh SGE, Ekkehard AD et al (1997) Nomenclature for factors of the HLA system. *Hum Immunol* 53:98–128.

Bollinger RR, Sanfilippo F (1989) Immunogenetics of transplantation. In: Flye MW (ed.). *Principles of Organ Transplantation*, Philadelphia: WB Saunders, pp. 47–71.

Braun WE (1989) Laboratory and clinical management of the highly sensitized organ recipient. *Hum Immunol* 26:245–260.

Browning JL, Ngam-ek A, Lawton P et al (1993) Lymphotoxin-B, a novel member of the TNF family that forms a heteromeric complex with lymphotoxin on the cell surface. *Cell* 72:847–856.

Buelow R, Monteiro F, Chiang TR et al (1994) Soluble HLA antigens and ELISA: a new technology for panel reactive antibody and crossmatch testing. *Hum Immunol* 40(Suppl 1):62.

Cardella CJ, Falk JA, Nicholson MJ et al (1982) Successful renal transplantation in patients with T-cell reactivity to donor. *Lancet* ii:1240–1243.

Cecka JM (1986) The changing role of HLA matching. In: Terasaki PI (ed.). *Clinical Transplants*, Los Angeles: UCLA Tissue Typing Laboratory, pp. 141–155.

Cecka JM (1997) The role of HLA in renal transplantation. *Hum Immunol* 56:6–16.

Cerilli J, Brasile L, Galouzis T et al (1985) The vascular endothelial cell antigen system. *Transplantation* 39:286–289.

Chapman JR, Taylor CJ, Ting A, Morris PJ (1986) Immunoglobulin class and specificity of antibodies causing positive T cell crossmatches. *Transplantation* 42:608–613.

Cicciarelli J, Helstab K, Mendez (1992) Flow cytometry PRA, a new test that is highly correlated with graft survival. *Clin Transplant* 6:159–164.

Cook DJ, Terasaki PI, Iwaki Y et al (1987) An approach to reducing early kidney transplant failure by flow cytometry crossmatching. *Clin Transplant* 1:253–256.

Cook DJ, Terasaki PI, Iwaki Y et al (1989) Flow cytometry crossmatching for kidney transplantation. In: Terasaki PI (ed.). *Clinical Transplants 1988*, Los Angeles: UCLA Tissue Typing Laboratory, pp. 375–380.

Cross DE, Greiner R, Whittier RC (1976) Importance of the autocontrol crossmatch in human renal transplantation. *Transplantation* 21:307–311.

Dallman MJ (1999) Immunobiology of graft rejection. In: Ginns LC, Cosimi AB, Morris PJ (eds). *Transplantation*, Malden: Blackwell Science, pp. 23–42.

Dausset J (1954) Leuco-agglutinins and blood transfusions. *Vox Sang* 4:190–198.

Doxiadis IN, Smits JA, Schreuder GMTh et al (1996) Association between specific HLA combinations and probability of graft loss: the taboo concept. *Lancet* 348:850–852.

Eijsvogel VP, Bois MJGJ, du Melief CMJ et al (1972) Position of a locus determining MLR distinct from the known HLA-A loci and its relation to cell mediated lympholysis (CML). In: Kissmeyer-Nielsen F (ed.). *Histocompatibility Testing*, Copenhagen: Munksgaard, pp. 501–508.

Ettenger RB, Uittenbogaart CH, Pennisi AJ et al (1979) Long-term cadaver allograft survival in the recipient with a positive B lymphocyte crossmatch. *Transplantation* 27:315–318.

Ferguson RM (1988) A multicenter experience with sequential ALG-cyclosporine therapy in renal transplantation. *Clin Transplant* 2:285–294.

Flechner SM, Kerman RH, Van Buren CT et al (1983) The use of cyclosporine and prednisone for high MLC haploidentical living related renal transplants. *Transplant Proc* 15:442–445.

Flechner SM, Kerman RH, Van Buren CT, Kahan BD (1984) Successful transplantation of cyclosporine-treated haploidentical living related recipients without blood transfusions. *Transplantation* 37:73–76.

Flye MW (1989) Immunohematology. In: Flye MW (ed.). *Principles of Organ Transplantation*, Philadelphia: WB Saunders, pp. 236–252.

Fuller TC, Phelan D, Gebel HM, Rodey GE (1982) Antigenic specificity of antibody reactive in the antiglobulin augmented lymphocytotoxicity test. *Transplantation* 34:24–28.

Fuller TC, Fuller AA, Golden M, Rodey GE (1997) HLA alloantibodies and the mechanism of the antiglobulin-augmented lymphocytotoxicity procedure. *Hum Immunol* 56:94–105.

Garovoy MR (1988) Flow cytometry crossmatch testing in renal transplantation. *Transplant Immunol Lett* 5:1–2.

Garovoy MR (1998) Basic immunogenetics. In: Norman DJ, Suki WN (eds). *ASTP Primer in Transplantation*, New Jersey: American Society of Transplantation, pp. 51–59.

Garovoy MR, Rheinschmidt MA, Bigos M et al (1983) Flow cytometry analysis: a high technology crossmatch technique facilitating transplantation. *Transplant Proc* 15:1939–1944.

Gjerston DW (1997) Look up survival tables for renal transplantation. In: Cecka JM, Terasaki PI (eds). *Clinical Transplants 1997*, Los Angeles: UCLA Tissue Typing Laboratory, pp. 337–383.

Gjerston DW, Terasaki PI (1992) The large center variation in half-lives of kidney transplants. *Transplantation* 53:357–362.

Gorer PA, Lyman S, Snell GD (1948) Studies on the genetic and antigenic basis of tumor transplantation. Linkage between a histocompatibility gene and 'fused' in mice. *Proc R Soc Lond* 135:499–505.

Goudsmit R, Van Loghem JJ (1953) Studies on the occurrence of leucocyte antibodies. *Vox Sang* 3:58–67.

Greenstein SM, Schnecter RS, Louis P et al (1990) Evidence that zero antigen matched cyclosporine treated renal transplant recipients have graft survival equal to that of matched recipients. *Transplantation* 49:332–336.

Halloran PF, Lui SL, Miller LW (1997) Review of transplantation. In: Cecka JM, Terasaki PI (eds). *Clinical Transplants 1996*, Los Angeles: UCLA Tissue Typing Laboratory, pp. 291–319.

Held PJ, Kahan BD, Hunsicker LG et al (1994) The impact of HLA mismatches on first cadaver kidney graft survival. *N Engl J Med* 331:765–770.

Hurley CK (1993) HLA diversity in African Americans. *Transplant Proc* 25:2399–2401.

Hurley CK, Tang T, Ng J, Hartzman R (1997) HLA typing by molecular methods. In: Rose NR, deMacario EC, Folds JD, Lane HC, Nakamura RM (eds). *Manual of Clinical Laboratory Immunology*, Washington, DC: ASM Press, pp. 1098–1111.

Iwaki Y, Cook CJ, Terasaki PI (1987) Flow cytometry crossmatching in human cadaver kidney transplantation. *Transplant Proc* 19:764–766.

Jager MJ, Claas FHJ, D'Amaro J (1987) Two alloantigens on human monocytes. A diallelic system? *Hum Immunol* 19:215–224.

Johnson AH, Rossen RD, Butler WT (1972) Detection of alloantibodies using a sensitive antiglobulin microcytotoxicity test: identification of low levels of preformed antibodies in accelerated allograft rejection. *Tissue Antigens* 2:215–220.

Kahan BD, Reisfeld RA (1968) Differences in the amino acid compositions of allogeneic guinea pig transplantation antigens. *J Immunol* 101:237–241.

Kao KS, Scornik JC, Small SJ (1993) Enzyme-linked immunoassay for anti-HLA antibodies: an alternative to panel studies by lymphocytotoxicity. *Transplantation* 55:192–196.

Kaufman DB, Sutherland DER, Noreen H et al (1989) Renal transplantation between living related sibling pairs matched for zero-HLA haplotypes. *Transplantation* 47:113–119.

Kerman RH (1994) The major histocompatibility complex in human transplantation. In: Tejani A, Fine R (eds). *Pediatric Renal Transplantation*, New York: John Wiley-Liss, pp. 51–67.

Kerman RH, Van Buren CT, Flechner SM et al (1985) Successful transplantation of cyclosporine treated allograft recipients with serologically positive historical but negative preoperative donor crossmatches. *Transplantation* 40:615–619.

Kerman RH, Van Buren CT, Lewis RM et al (1990) Improved graft survival for flow cytometry and anti-human globulin negative retransplant recipients *Transplantation* 49:52–56.

Kerman RH, Kimball PM, Van Buren CT et al (1991) AHG and DTE/AHG procedures identify crossmatch-appropriate donor–recipient pairings which result in improved graft survival. *Transplantation* 51:316–320.

Kerman RH, Kimball PM, Lindholm A et al (1993) Influence of HLA matching on rejections and short and long term primary cadaveric allograft survival. *Transplantation* 56:1242–1247.

Kerman RH, Susskind B, Buelow R et al (1996) Correlation of ELISA-detected IgG and IgA anti-HLA antibodies in pretransplant sera with renal allograft rejection. *Transplantation* 62:201–205.

Kissmeyer-Nielsen F, Olson S, Peterson VP, Fjeldborg O (1966) Hyperacute rejection of kidney allografts associated with pre-existing humoral antibodies against donor cells. *Lancet* i:662–665.

Klein J (1987) *Natural History of the Major Histocompatibility Complex*, New York: John Wiley.

Landsteiner K (1900) Zur kenntnis der antifermentativen, lytischen und agghitinierenden wirkungen des blut-serums und der lymphe. *Zentralbl Bacteriol* 27:357–571.

Little CC, Johnson BW (1922) Inheritance of susceptibility to implants of splenic tissue in mice: 1. Japanese waltzing mice, albinos and their F1 generation hybrids. *Proc Soc Exp Biol Med* 19:163.

Lundgren G, Albrectson D, Flatmark A (1986) HLA matching and pretransplant transfusion in cadaveric transplantation: a changing picture with cyclosporine, *Lancet* i:66–69.

Marshall B, Leelayuwat C, Degli-Eposti A et al (1993) New major histocompatibility complex genes. *Hum Immunol* 38:24–29.

Maruya E, Takemoto S, Terasaki PI (1993) HLA matching: identification of permissible HLA mismatches. In: Terasaki PI, Cecka JM (eds). *Clinical Transplants 1993*, Los Angeles: UCLA Tissue Typing Laboratory, pp. 521–531.

Matas AJ, Fryd DS (1989) Renal transplantation: the importance of well designed single institution and multicenter studies. *Clin Transplant* 3:63–65.

Matas AJ, Tellis VA, Quinn T et al (1989) Short and long term graft survival with 0-antigen matched first cadaver renal transplants. *Clin Transplant* 3:22–26.

Mayer MM (1973) The complement system. *Sci Am* 229:54–66.

McCalmon RT, Tardif GN, Sheeham MA et al (1997) IgM antibodies in renal transplantation. *Clin Transplant* 11:558–564.

Monaco JJ (1995) Pathways for the processing and presentation of antigens to T cells. *J Leukoc Biol* 57:543–547.

Moraes JR, Statsny P (1977) A new antigen system expressed in human endothelial cells. *J Clin Invest* 60:449–454.

Murray JE, Thomas ED (1993) Discoveries concerning organ and cell transplantation in the treatment of human disease. In: Lindsten J (ed.). *Nobel Lectures in Physiology or Medicine 1981–1990*, Stockholm: World Scientific Publishing Company.

Noreen HJ, van der Hagen E, Bach FH et al (1989) Renal allograft survival in CsA-treated patients with positive donor-specific B lymphocyte crossmatches. *Transplant Proc* 21:691–692.

Ogura K, Terasaki PI, Johnson C et al (1993) The significance of a positive flow cytometry cross-match test in primary kidney transplantation. *Transplantation* 56:294–298.

Opelz G, Mickey MR, Terasaki PI (1977) Calculations on long-term graft and patient survival in human kidney transplantation. *Transplant Proc* 9:27–30.

Opelz G, Wujciak T, Dohler B for The Collaborative Transplant Study (1999) Is HLA matching worth the effort? *Transplant Proc* 31:717–720.

Patel R, Terasaki PI (1969) Significance of the positive crossmatch test in kidney transplantation. *N Engl J Med* 280:735–739.

Payne R, Rolfs MR (1958) Feto-maternal leucocyte incompatibility. *J Clin Invest* 37:1756–1763.

Payne R, Tripp M, Weigle J (1964) A new leucoisoantigen system in man. *Cold Spring Harb Symp Quant Biol* 29:285–298.

Pei R, Wang G, Tarsitanic C et al (1998) Simultaneous HLA class I and class II antibodies screening with flow cytometry. *Hum Immunol* 59:313–322.

Phelan DC, Rodey GE, Flye MW et al (1989) Positive B cell crossmatches: specificity of antibody and graft outcome. *Transplant Proc* 21:687–688.

Przybylowski P, Balogna M, Radovancevic B et al (1999) The role of flow cytometry detected IgG and IgM anti-donor antibodies in cardiac allograft recipients. *Transplantation* 67:258–262.

Reisfeld RA, Kahan BD (1972) Markers of biological individuality. *Sci Am* 226:28–37.

Rodey GE, Fuller TC (1987) Public epitopes and the antigenic structure of the HLA molecules. *CRC Crit Rev Immunol* 7:229–243.

Savage D, Baxter-Lowe LA, Gorski J, Middleton D (1993) Molecular methods of HLA typing. In: Dyer P, Middleton D (eds). *Histocompatibility Testing: A Practical Approach,* Oxford: Oxford University Press, pp. 107–142.

Shoskes DA, Halloran PF (1991) Ischemic injury induces altered MHC gene expression in kidney by an interferon-gamma-dependent pathway. *Transplant Proc* 23:599–601.

Shroyer TW, Deirhoi MH, Hudson SL, Diethelm AG (1993) The importance of B cell flow cytometry crossmatching in interpretation of positive T cell flow crossmatches in renal retrans-plantation. *Hum Immunol* 37(Suppl 1):76.

Snell D (1948) Methods for the study of histocompatibility genes. *J Genet* 49:87–108.

Spetainik S, Pfaff W, Cowles J et al (1984) Correlation of humoral immunity to Lewis blood group antigens with renal transplant rejection. *Transplantation* 37:265–268.

Ten Hoor GM, Coopmans M, Allebes WA (1993) Specificity and Ig class of preformed alloanti-bodies causing a positive crossmatch in renal transplantation. *Transplantation* 56:298–304.

Terasaki PI, McClelland JD (1964) Microdroplet assay of human serum cytotoxins. *Nature* 204:998–1000.

Terasaki PI, Park MS, Danovitch GM (1992) Histocompatibility testing, crossmatching and allo-cation of cadaveric kidney transplants. In: Danovitch GM (ed.). *Handbook of Kidney Transplanta-*

tion, Boston: Little Brown, pp. 43–58.

Terasaki PI, Cecka JM, Gjerston DW et al (1993) A ten-year prediction for kidney transplant survival. In: Terasaki PI, Cecka JM (eds). *Clinical Transplants 1992*, Los Angeles: UCLA Tissue Typing Laboratory, pp. 502–512.

Terasaki PI, Cecka JM, Gjerston DW, Cho YW (1997) Spousal and other living renal donor transplants. In: Terasaki PI, Cecka JM (eds). *Clinical Transplants 1997*, Los Angeles: UCLA Tissue Typing Laboratory, pp. 269–283.

Thompson J, Thacker L, Takemoto S (1997) CREG matching for first kidney transplants performed by SEOPF Centers between 1987 and 1995: an analysis of outcome and benefit. *Transplant Proc* 29:1435–1438.

Van Rood JJ, Van Leeuen A (1963) Leucocyte grouping: a method and its application. *J Clin Invest* 42:1382–1387.

Van Rood JJ, Van Leeuen A, Eerniss JG (1958) Leucocyte antibodies in sera of pregnant women. *Nature* 181:1735–1736.

Van Rood JJ, Van Leeuen A, Parvliet J (1975) LD typing by serology. Description of a new locus with three alleles. In: Kissmeyer-Nielsen F (ed.). *Histocompatibility Testing*, Copenhagen: Munksgaard, pp. 629–639.

Van Rood JJ, Lagaaij EL, Doxiadis IN et al (1994) Permissible mismatches, acceptable mismatches and tolerance. New trends in decision making. In: Terasaki PI, Cecka JM (eds). *Clinical Transplants 1993*, Los Angeles: UCLA Tissue Typing Laboratory, pp. 285–292.

Wernet P, Kunkel HG (1975) Demonstration of specific T-lymphocyte membrane antigen associated with antibodies inhibiting the MLC in man. *Transplant Proc* 5:1875–1878.

Williams GM, Hume DM, Hudson RP et al (1968) Hyperacute renal homograft rejection in man. *N Engl J Med* 279:611–618.

Yunis EJ, Ward FE, Amos DB (1971) Observations of the CYNAP phenomenon. In: Terasaki PI (ed.). *Histocompatibility Testing 1970*, Baltimore: William & Wilkins, pp. 351–356.

Zachary AA (1993) The genetics of race. *Transplant Proc* 25:2397–2398.

Zinkernagel RM, Doherty PC (1975) H-2 compatibility requirement for T-cell mediated lysis of target infected with lymphocytic choriomeningitis virus: different cytotoxic T cell specificities are associated with structures coded in H-2K of H-2D. *J Exp Med* 141:1427–1436.

2 IMMUNOBIOLOGY OF ALLOGRAFT REJECTION

In collaboration with SM Stepkowski*

Save for the circumstances of identical twins (Murray et al 1958) or of the use of intervention to disrupt the immune response, transplanted allografts—organs, tissues, and living cells exchanged between members of the same species—are destined to destruction. Despite the administration of immunosuppressants, allograft rejection remains the primary cause of human renal transplant failure (Table 2.1). This alloaggression, while harmful in the situation of transplantation, reflects a natural response to protect the integrity of the organism against microorganisms and neoplasms. It also represents a manifestation of the immune system's function to distinguish 'self' from 'nonself' and reflects recognition of foreign antigens, including products of the major histocompatibility complex (MHC) and minor histocompatibility (mH) genes. Because an understanding of the mechanisms of graft rejection is necessary to optimize clinical results, this chapter describes the immunobiological principles of alloimmunity, including the molecular features and modes of recognition of alloantigenic and adhesion molecules; the cellular populations that mediate these events; and the clinical manifestations of the responses to foreign tissues.

Cause of graft failure*	N(%)[†]
Rejection	4545 (66.4)
Surgical complications	638 (9.3)
Sepsis	541 (7.9)
Arterial thrombosis	113 (1.7)
Primary non-function	104 (1.5)

*Causes of allograft failure, excluding patients who died with a functioning graft.

[†]N = number of transplants (and percentage of total).

Table 2.1. Incidence of various causes of allograft failure among 6845 renal transplants

* Division of Immunology and Organ Transplantation, Department of Surgery, University of Texas Medical School, Houston

TRANSPLANTATION ANTIGENS

Endothelial glycoproteins

Blood group glycolipids—the A, B, and H substances—are ubiquitously expressed on many cell types, and humans display natural antibodies (Abs) against the carbohydrate determinants that are foreign to them. Because these determinants are present on cells lining blood vessels, ABH group mismatches trigger immediate Ab deposition and early allograft thrombosis. The antigenic specificity of the glycolipid antigens is determined by the action of glycosylation enzymes A (or B) that catalyze the addition of epitopes distinctive for glycolipid A (or glycolipid B, respectively) determinants to the H structure backbone. Individuals of blood type A or B express the respective antigens; patients of the AB type, both antigens; and subjects of the O type, neither A nor B antigen. Consequently, O type individuals display Abs against both A and B substances; individuals of blood type A, Abs against B (and vice versa); and AB individuals, neither. Thus, the O recipient is only compatible with O donor tissues; A or B recipients, with grafts from O donors or from donors sharing the same blood group; and AB recipients, with donors of any blood group (Szulman 1962). The blood group glycolipids do not elicit cellular immune responses.

Major histocompatibility complex antigens

Another group of foreign structures that provoke a potent immune response comprises the class I, II, and III MHC antigens. Not only are these structures the most immunogenic cell surface markers, but they also exhibit extremely high degrees of polymorphism; indeed, they show the largest number of allelic forms among all genes sequenced to date (Takaki et al 1993).

The MHC complex is encoded on human chromosome 6. The class I MHC encodes three highly polymorphic (and immunogenic) glycoproteins HLA-A, -B, and -C, as well as five less polymorphic (and less immunogenic) molecules HLA-E, -F, -G, -H, and -J (Hedrick et al 1991; Powis and Trowsdale 1993). The human class II MHC genes include the highly polymorphic HLA-DP and -DQ, as well as the less polymorphic HLA-DR and -DZ loci (see Chapter 1). Whereas class I MHC molecules are present on all nucleated cells, class II MHC proteins are constitutively expressed on macrophages, dendritic cells, and B cells, and are upregulated on activated T cells (Glimcher and Kara 1992).

Experiments in mice document that class I and/or class II MHC alloantigens display a variable potential to induce allograft rejection (Table 2.2). Mouse strains that are genetically identical except for a single class I and/or class II MHC allele—termed congenic mice—display a spectrum of graft survival rates. Multiple MHC disparities tend to provoke early graft rejection, whereas nonMHC differences often elicit a slowly paced rejection reaction (Klein 1986; Peugh et al 1986; Stepkowski et al 1987). In addition,

Donor	Recipient	Disparity	Median survival (days)	Reference
C57 BL/10	B10.D1	MHC	9	Peugh et al 1986
C57 BL/10	B10.H	MHC	>100	Peugh et al 1986
Balb/c	B10.D2	NonMHC	11	Peugh et al 1986
Balb/c	DBA/2	NonMHC	>100	Peugh et al 1986
A.SW	A.TH	Class I MHC	19	Stepkowski et al 1987
BID.AKM	B10.BR	Class I MHC	>100	Stepkowski et al 1987
A.TH	A.TL	Class II MHC	19	Stepkowski et al 1987
B10.T (6R)	B10.AQR	Class II MHC	>100	Stepkowski et al 1987
C3H	Balb/c	MHC/nonMHC	11	Tu et al 1995
C56 BL/6	C3H	MHC/nonMHC	36	Tu et al 1995

*Transplantation of the vascularized heterotopic heart allografts was performed between donors and recipients selected to differ at MHC and/or nonMHC, as indicated in the third column. Heart function was evaluated daily, and the last day of beating was considered the rejection day. Results are presented as median values ($N = 5$–6).

Table 2.2. Impact of disparity on survival of heart allografts in mice*

different species seem to display various forms of rejection; whereas pigs, monkeys, and humans display prominent vascular responses, rodents show only a modest vascular component, possibly due to the lack of class II MHC proteins on their endothelial cells (Pescovitz et al 1984).

Although human renal allografts matched for MHC antigens tend to display a better outcome than mismatched transplants (Opelz et al 1999), they are not uniformly successful, particularly if environmental antigen exposure or pretransplant blood transfusions prime host antidonor T cells (Heeger et al 1999). In contrast, some recipients of poorly matched grafts never show rejection. The factors that determine host immunoresponsiveness are poorly understood, but at least some seem to be encoded within the MHC on chromosome 6. Indeed, using nonspecific immune assays, one can distinguish patients that display high reactivity pretransplant as more likely to experience rejection episodes. For example, patients who bear a high frequency of interferon (IFN)-γ-producing, donor-specific T cells pretransplant display a greater risk for developing acute rejection episodes posttransplant, regardless of the degree of donor–recipient mismatch (Heeger et al 1999).

Minor histocompatibility antigens

Kidney allograft rejection may also be incited by mH antigen disparities, as shown by the occurrence of rejection episodes in transplants exchanged between HLA-identical human donor and recipient pairs, and mouse strains congenic save for mH disparities (Peugh et al 1986). Among the more than 80 mH loci implicated in alloimmune responses in inbred mice, the male antigen (mapped to the Y-chromosome) has been shown to induce acute skin allograft rejection in female mice (Coons and Goldberg 1978). Although some mH antigens do not elicit rejection (Table 2.2), the allograft is destined to destruction when mH differences are combined with MHC disparities. Although virtually every human allograft displays multiple disparities compared to the recipient, it is widely believed that the immune responses to mH antigens are generally vitiated by immunosuppressive treatment.

EVENTS IN REJECTION: THE INITIAL VASCULAR CONTACT

Adhesion molecules contribute to nonspecific reperfusion injuries, participate in the process of specific alloactivation of T and B cells, and mediate the effector phase of graft destruction. The ischemic period consequent to organ procurement and storage triggers an inflammatory response, which dramatically increases the expression of adhesion molecules on both endothelial cells and leukocytes. The enhanced cell-to-cell contact facilitates diapedesis of antigen-specific and nonspecific effector cells, leading to allorecognition and activation (Bevilacqua 1993; Bonventre 1993; Land and Messmer 1996).

Three overlapping steps of rolling, chemoattraction, and strong adhesion of leukocytes to endothelial cells involve the sequential expression of unique surface markers, as well as the production of distinctive cytokines (Figure 2.1). Within minutes of endothelial cell activation, histamine and thrombin are released from storage granules and appear on the cell surface. Similarly, leukocytes activated by the presence of ischemic tissue generate interleukin-1 (IL-1) and tumor necrosis factors (TNFs), which stimulate the synthesis and increase the expression of adhesion molecules—selectins—on both the leukocytes and the endothelium. Selectins bear carbohydrate ligands that mediate the transient interactions, producing rolling of leukocytes over the vascular lining. In addition, endothelial cells produce IL-8 and platelet activation factor (PAF), both of which stimulate leukocyte adhesion (Wu et al 1993). In the presence of these mediators, resting platelets (Weibel–Palade bodies) and endothelial cells release platelet activation-dependent granule-external membrane protein (PADEGEM) and P-selectin molecules from their granules (McEver et al 1989) for rapid redistribution within minutes on the surface of cells. Endothelial–leukocyte adhesion molecules (E-selectins), which are upregulated on activated endothelial cells by IL-1, TNFs, and endotoxin, display maximum expression at 4–6 hours after reperfusion, followed by a gradual decline over 48 hours. Leukocytes constitutively express L-selectin, previously called murine lymph node receptor substance MEL-14. Interestingly, L-selectin may be shed from the surface

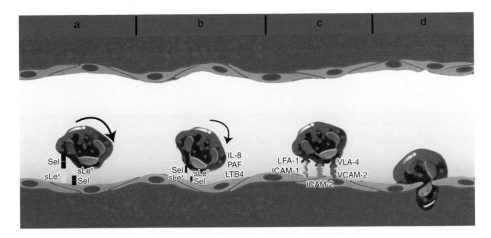

Figure 2.1. Leukocyte adhesion events prior to cell migration into the graft. Cells migrate in three major steps: rolling (a); chemoattraction (b); and strong adhesion (c). Selectins (Sel) bind to the carbohydrate ligand sialylated Lewis^x (sLe^x), mediating rolling. (b) The presence of mediators, such as IL-8, leukotriene B4 (LTB4), and platelet activating factor (PAF), cause tethering of flowing leukocytes. (c) Firm attachment of leukocytes to endothelial cells is achieved by interaction of ICAM-1 with LFA-1, MAC-1, or p150, and ICAM-2 with LFA-1, and VLA-4 with VCAM-1 molecules. (d) Transendothelial migration facilitates entry of leukocytes into the graft.

of lymphocytes and neutrophils, thus permitting the detachment of cells prior to extravasation into the allograft.

The lectin domains of P-, E-, and L-selectins display identical unique amino acid compositions. L-selectins bind sialylated Lewis^a (sLe^a) and sLe^x (fucosylated lactosamine) oligosaccharide structures, which are expressed on neutrophils and monocytes. In addition to binding sLe^x-related structures, selectins bind with varying affinity to a variety of other carbohydrate ligands, including sulfated polysaccharides (heparin, fucoidan), phosphorylated monosaccharides (mannose-6-phosphate), and polysaccharides (Tiemeyer et al 1991).

The rolling phenomenon slows the motion of leukocytes, enhancing their chance to be exposed to local chemoattractants, including N-formyl peptides, IL-8, C5a, leukotriene B4, PAF, c-x-c chemokines, monocyte chemotactic protein-1 (MCP-1), and macrophage inflammatory protein-1 (MIP-1) $\alpha\beta$. These attractants encourage firmer tethering and attachment to endothelial cells.

These firm adhesions are mediated by interactions between β_2-integrins on lymphocytes and cell adhesion molecules of the immunoglobulin (Ig) superfamily (Ig-CAM) on endothelial cells. The β_2-integrin family includes three members: molecules that share the β_2 subunit CD18 that is noncovalently linked to different α-chains—α_1 (CD11a), α_2 (CD11b), or α_3 (CD11c)—to form lymphocyte function associated antigen-1 (LFA-1; CD11a/CD18), macrophage antigen-1 (MAC-1; CD11b/CD18), and p150

(CD11c/CD18), respectively. The endothelial surface Ig-CAM family of molecules—intracellular adhesion molecule-1 (ICAM-1), ICAM-2, ICAM-3, and vascular cell adhesion molecule-1 (VCAM-1)—share Ig-like domains. ICAM-1 (CD54), which contains five extracellular Ig-like domains, is constitutively expressed at low levels by nonstimulated endothelial cells and lymphocytes; IFN-γ or TNF production markedly increases its surface expression. ICAM-2 (CD102), which contains two extracellular domains, is constitutively expressed on endothelial cells and therefore always available to bind β_2-integrins (Springer 1990). ICAM-3 (CD50), which contains five domains, is expressed on granulocytes, but not on endothelial cells (Campanero et al 1993). The expression on endothelial cells of VCAM-1, which contains seven domains, is upregulated by IL-1 and IFN-γ, or (unlike other Ig-CAM molecules) by IL-4. VCAM-1 is also expressed on dendritic cells present in lymph nodes and bone marrow. Although ICAM-1, ICAM-2, and ICAM-3 bind to LFA-1, only ICAM-1 also binds to MAC-1 and p150, while VCAM-1 binds to the molecule very late antigen-4 (VLA-4; integrin α_4/β_1 CD49d/CD29).

In addition to these structures, the three other major families of adhesion molecules include: (1) the Ig-CAM family, namely, LFA-2, LFA-3, CD4, CD8, CD28, CD22, B7, and class I and class II MHC molecules; (2) the β_1-integrins, namely, VLA-1 (CD49a/CD29), VLA-2 (CD49b/CD29), VLA-3 (CD49c/CD29), VLA-5 (CD49e/CD29), and VLA-6 (CD49f/CD29) (Shimizu et al 1990); and (3) the β_2-integrins (α_{IIb}/β_3, α_v/β_3, α_R/β_3, α_6/β_4, α_v/β_5, α_v/β_6, and α_4/β_7). The $\alpha_4\beta_7$-integrins are expressed on leukocytes and nonhematopoietic cells, and bind to extracellular matrix components, including fibronectin, laminin, and collagen.

ALLOANTIGEN RECOGNITION

T cells recognize donor alloantigens in the form of peptides, either displayed on the surface of the graft (direct recognition; Figure 2.2a), or processed and presented by host cells (indirect recognition; Figure 2.2b). Because hosts bear 10–100-fold higher frequencies of T cells that are capable of recognizing alloantigens as opposed to cells that respond to other antigens (Sherman and Chattopadhyay 1993; Shoskes and Wood 1994), the direct recognition pathway induces a strong immune response. In contrast, alloantigens shed by the graft may be processed by and presented as allopeptides on host-type, 'self' antigen presenting cells (APCs), thereby activating CD4$^+$ T cells (Liu et al 1992). The indirect presentation pathway may provide an especially important mechanism of allosensitization, particularly in long-term-surviving allografts in which the majority of interstitial dendritic cells are of recipient origin (Sherman and Chattopadhyay 1993). This mechanism has been documented using cloned human T cells to recognize a foreign HLA-DR peptide presented by syngeneic MHC antigens on host-type cells (Harris et al 1992).

In addition to presentation of foreign antigens, host APCs bear 'self' peptides that

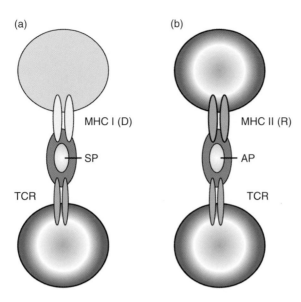

(a) (b)

MHC I (D)

SP

TCR

MHC II (R)

AP

TCR

Figure 2.2. Modes of alloantigen presentation. (a) Alloantigens are recognized directly as foreign markers expressed on donor cells or (b) indirectly after processing and presentation by host-type APCs. In direct recognition, donor MHC class I antigens on donor tissue (MHC I (D)) with donor 'self' peptide (SP) are recognized by recipient T cells via their T cell receptor (TCR). In indirect recognition, donor allopeptide (AP) has been processed by host APC and presented on host class II MHC antigen (MHC II (R)) to stimulate host T cells via TCR. (Brown represents donor; blue, recipient.)

may be eluted from their surface HLA-DR1 or class I molecules, suggesting that direct and indirect presentation are natural processes (Rammensee et al 1993). However, during the allorecognition process, there appears to be a selection of a dominant foreign allopeptide, namely, a single peptide (or at least a limited number of peptides) contributes the primary stimulus for heart allograft rejection (Tugulea et al 1997). In the event that the graft survives for a prolonged period, particularly with recurring acute and/or chronic rejection processes, the spectrum of antigens that trigger reactive T-cell clones broadens to involve new epitopes, a process known as intramolecular epitope 'spreading'. Although the spreading phenomenon is not fully understood, it has been suggested that it is due to APC-mediated, indirect presentation of a variety of polymorphic sequences, which thereby increases the frequency of T cells directed against *sub*dominant epitopes (Suciu-Foca et al 1998). Thus, the processing and presentation of allopeptides play important, dynamic roles in allograft rejection.

Administration of synthetic polypeptides triggers indirect presentation, thereby sensitizing mice to display accelerated rejection of skin (Fangmann et al 1992a) or kidney (Rammensee et al 1989) allografts. T cells harvested from mice that have been presensitized by skin allografts undergo proliferation in vitro upon exposure to synthetic allopeptides that bear polymorphic class I MHC amino acid sequences corresponding to a foreign antigenic epitope on donor skin (Fangmann et al 1992b). Similarly, allopeptides bearing sequences representing polymorphic regions of donor class II MHC induce faster rejection of heart allografts (Watschinger et al 1994).

In summary, experiments in rodents (Benichou et al 1992; Wang et al 1997) and circumstantial evidence in patients (Harris et al 1992; Liu et al 1993) suggest that, during allograft rejection, the T cell response is directed against dominant determinant(s) within the polymorphic regions of class I or class II MHC alloantigens. During recurrent episodes of acute or chronic rejection, T cell responses are also directed toward secondary (subdominant) epitopes (Suciu-Foca et al 1998).

Processing and presentation of allopeptides

During the induction of alloimmune responses against alloantigens (Germain and Margulies 1993), 'self' peptides derived from endogenous proteins through the processes of intracellular degradation and turnover are loaded onto class I MHC antigens (Sherman and Chattopadhyay 1993). The 'self' class I MHC antigens on the surface of normal cells naturally display a variety of self peptides that do not provoke immune responses, because host T cells have been 'educated' in the thymus to accept these determinants. In addition, altered self peptides present in neoplastic cells or intracellular microbial invaders may be loaded onto class I MHC antigens. The process of peptide loading is influenced by characteristics of the peptide: concentration, efficiency of transport through the endoplasmic reticulum (ER), and presence of specific motif residues that are able to bind to residues on the adjoining cleft of class I MHC antigens.

Class I and class II MHC molecules bind distinctive peptides (Shoskes and Wood 1994). For class I molecules, the peptide must be eight or nine amino acid residues in length (Table 2.3); for class II MHC antigens, 12–20 residues. The peptide motifs must be complementary to the amino acids lining the cleft, as well as bear specific molecular requirements termed 'anchors'. For example, the structure of the mouse class I MHC antigen H-2K^d stipulates that the nine-residue peptide bear the amino acid Tyr at position 2 and an aliphatic residue (Ile, Leu, or Val) at the C-terminus. Individual cells may display only a few to almost 10^4 peptides on its 10^5 class I MHC molecules, including as many as 200 different peptides.

The process of direct presentation by peptide binding to class I MHC proteins begins with an initial degradation of the antigen by endopeptidase(s). Cytosolic proteasomes, which are multicomponent units equipped with proteolytic enzymes, degrade proteins into peptides by scission of the residue at the C-terminus of a hydrophobic residue (Met, Ile, Val, or Phe; Goldberg and Rock 1992; Rammensee et al 1993; Figure 2.3). These peptides, generally longer than nine amino acid residues, are moved into the ER by two transporters associated with antigen processing, TAP1 and TAP2. In the ER, the peptides are loaded onto class I (α/β_2-microglobulin; m) MHC molecules (Schumacher et al 1994). The C-terminal amino acid of the precursor peptide initially shows only low affinity for the positively charged, conserved portion of the groove within the peptide-binding site of the class I MHC molecule. However, after the N-terminal amino acids are trimmed by proteolysis to a sequence of eight or nine amino acid residues by an unknown peptidase, the resulting peptide binds with high affinity, forming a trimolecular complex (peptide/class I heavy-chain/β_2m) that is transported from the Golgi apparatus to the surface membrane (Figure 2.3a). The assembly process in the ER is facilitated by calnexin, a protein that preferentially binds to misfolded or incompletely

	Anchor residues								
	1	2	3	4	5	6	7	8	9
Human MHC									
HLA-A2.1 (0201)		Leu							Val
HLA-A2.1 (0205)									Leu
HLA-B27 (2705)		Arg							
Mouse MHC									
H-2K^d		Tyr							Leu
									Ile
H-2K^b					Phe				Leu
					Tyr				
H-2K^k		Glu							Ile
H-2K^{km1}								Ile	
H-2D^b					Asn				Met

*Amino acid residues representing motif sequences (anchors) for peptide binding to different class I MHC markers. Amino acid code: Arg, arginine; Asn, aspartic acid; Glu, glutamic acid; Ile, isoleucine; Leu, leucine; Met, methionine; Phe, phenylalanine; Tyr, tyrosine; Val, valine.

Table 2.3. Anchor residues for peptides binding to the groove of class I MHC molecules*

assembled glycoproteins (Hansen and Lee 1997). Calnexin associates with the class I MHC heavy chain prior to noncovalently binding β_2-microglobulin as well as after formation of the class I MHC/β_2 complexes.

Exogenous proteins are endocytosed and degraded by endosomal proteolysis to allopeptides bearing 12–22 amino acid residues (Figure 2.3b). To increase the stability of the class II molecule for intercellular transport, these peptides are loaded onto class II MHC molecules after dissociation of an invariant chain (Ii), which is initially assembled with the α- and β-chains and calnexin in the ER (Blum and Cresswell 1988; Cresswell et al 1990; Viville et al 1993). The trimolecular class II MHC α/β-peptide complex is then transported to and expressed on the cell membrane (Figure 2.3b). Nonpolymorphic MHC molecules may, in the fashion of class I and II MHC molecules, bind to and display a wide array of self peptides (Joyce et al 1994).

Antigen-presenting cells

The elements that process and present foreign materials, APCs, include macrophages and B cells, and most importantly dendritic cells (Steinman 1991; Murase et al 1996).

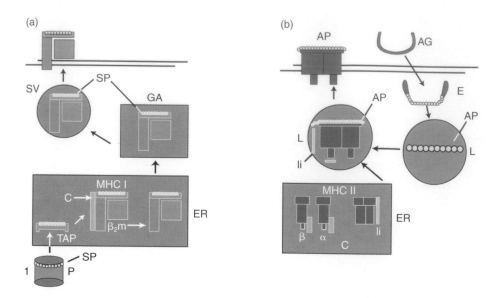

Figure 2.3. Processing and presentation of allopeptides by MHC molecules. (a) Endogenous proteins are degraded to 'self' peptides (SP) in the cytosol as part of the housekeeping function of the proteasome (P)—a multicomponent unit equipped with multicatalytic proteases—for transfer by the transporters of antigen peptides, TAP1 and TAP2 (TAP), to bind into the groove of the class I MHC molecule (MHC I) in association with a calnexin molecule (C), which provides a Ca^{2+}-sensitive sequence-translocation mechanism. The 'self' peptide/class I MHC/C complex binds β_2-microglobulin (β_2m) and releases calnexin prior to transport of the peptide/class I MHC complex into the Golgi apparatus (GA), and then into a secretory vesicle (SV) to the cell membrane. (b) Exogenous alloantigens (AG) are engulfed in endosomes (E) and processed in lysosomes (L) to produce allopeptides (AP), which are then attached to the groove of a host-type class II MHC molecule. These latter molecules are generated as single α- and β-chains stabilized by calnexin (C) in the endoplasmic reticulum (ER) and heterodimerized with an attached invariant chain (Ii), thereby increasing the stability of the complex for more efficient transport to lysosomes, where the allopeptide is loaded onto class II MHC molecules displacing the Ii. Subsequently, the complex is transported to the cell membrane for presentation of allopeptides.

APCs are derived from hematopoietic stem cell progenitors that either have migrated from the bone marrow, or have been generated in the interstitial connective tissue of the graft (Kaissling and Le Hir 1994). Dendritic cells and their precursors reside near the termini of afferent lymphatics, in the arterial adventitia, and in the epithelial lining of mucosa-associated lymphoid tissue (Gong et al 1992). Although immature dendritic cells display phagocytic activity, they express only small amounts of class II MHC or of B7–1 and -2 costimulatory molecules (Austyn et al 1994). In contrast, mature dendritic cells have no phagocytic function, but express large quantities of the costimulatory molecules.

Transplanted organs carry intragraft donor-type hematopoietic cells, including dendritic cells, that represent 'passenger cells' capable of providing a potent immunogenic stimulus (Steinmuller 1967). Replacement of donor-type passenger cells with recipient-type (syngeneic) passengers by transplantation into immunocompromised recipients greatly reduces the immunogenicity of organs (Guttmann et al 1969) and prolongs graft survival upon retransplantation into a fully immunocompetent recipient (Lechler and Batchelor 1982). Furthermore, the injection of 10^4 fresh donor dendritic (but not purified donor T or B) cells restores the immunogenicity of an organ. Even in the absence of passenger cells, however, the rejection process does continue, albeit at a slower pace (Larsen et al 1990).

CELLULAR MECHANISMS OF MEDIATING ALLOGRAFT REJECTION

The immune system is a dynamic network of hematolymphoid cells that continuously survey the interstitial spaces of all solid organs. T and B cells traffic from the blood circulation through the fluid interstitium, and then enter afferent lymphatics to lymph nodes.

T cells

First signal activation

To regulate the events that trigger T cell proliferation upon exposure to specific alloantigen, the army of mature T cells is tightly controlled. Full T cell activation requires at least three sequential signals, each of which must be delivered above the minimum threshold to trigger the cascade of signal transduction events necessary to promote an immune response as opposed to progression toward programmed cell death (apoptosis). Unchecked division of a single T cell every 4–5 hours may theoretically produce a clone of 10^{12} daughter cells in 7 days. Because of this potential for a rapid increase in T cell numbers, and because allograft donors bear multiple antigenic disparities, tight control is necessary to prevent adventitiously selected T cell clones from hijacking the immune response.

The first signal for full T cell activation is delivered by the contact of alloantigen with its specific T cell receptor (TCR; Figure 2.4). T cell receptor structures are heterodimers bearing covalently linked α- and β- (or γ- and δ-) chains. Each TCR chain contains variable (v) and constant (c) regions. Through an embryonal process of hypermutation, the TCR v regions display diversity. Following a sojourn in the thymus, T cells are selected based upon their capacity to bind only self antigen with low affinity (positive selection), with elimination of T cells that bind self with high affinity (negative selection). The TCR stipulates the antigens to which a given cell can respond; the range of

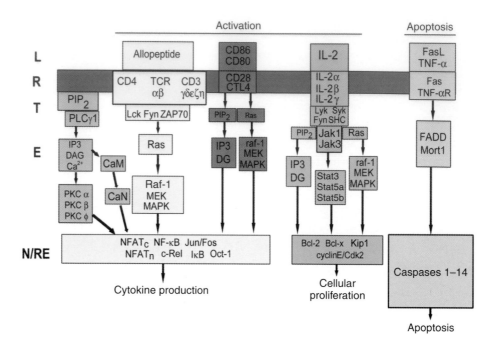

Figure 2.4. Sequential activation signals 1, 2, and 3 that control activation versus apoptosis of T cells. As shown from top to bottom, the exogenous ligands (L) initiate the response through the cell surface receptors (R), followed by the signal transducers (T), and their associated enzymes (E) that generate regulators (RE) of the nuclear transcription factors (N) necessary for cytokine production, cellular proliferation, or apoptosis. The first signal is delivered by allopeptide through the TCR/CD3 complex via immediate phosphorylation of ITAM, followed by activation of Lck, Fyn, and ZAP70 kinases. Following TCR activation, signaling involves engagement of multiple molecules, including the PLC pathway and the Ras/Raf-1/MEK/MAPK pathway, leading to activation of multiple transcription factors (NF-AT, NF-κB, AP-1, c-Rel, IκB, Oct-1 and others). The second signal is delivered by B7-2/B7-1 (CD86/CD80) interaction with CD28/CTL4 receptors. The cytokine third signal is delivered by the Jaks/Stats system to complete T-cell activation. Limitation of the T-cell response is achieved by apoptotic mechanisms through FasL and TNF-α receptor (TNF-αR).

TCRs in a person constitutes his T cell repertoire. Because the interaction between presented peptide and TCR is weak, the TCR signal is strengthened by coreceptors that link APCs to T cells, including β_2-integrins with CD2, which is present on all T cells, and either CD4 on one T cell subset with class II MHC molecules, or CD8 on a second subset with class I MHC molecules.

The TCR recognition complex is associated with a pentameric signal transduction CD3 complex, which includes γδεζη- or ζζ-chains that couple the membrane signal reception to intracellular activation (Weiss and Littman 1994). Within seconds to minutes after engagement of an antigenic peptide, the CD3ζ chain is phosphorylated and in turn associates with and phosphorylates the ZAP70, Lck, and Fyn protein kinases.

The cytoplasmic domain of the CD3ζ chain bears three conserved consensus sequences of immunoreceptor tyrosine-based activation motif (ITAM; Reth 1989), and each of the other CD3 chains contains a single ITAM copy. The pattern of phosphorylation of tyrosine residues on CD3-associated ITAMs increases both the sensitivity and rate of amplification of the TCR signal (Irving 1993) by regulating the activation program of Fyn, Lck, and ZAP70 intermediates. Complete TCR engagement produces full activation of ZAP70, resulting in T cell differentiation into IL-2- and IFN-γ-producing (T helper 1 (Th$_1$)) cells. In contrast, partial TCR activation, with consequent incomplete ZAP70 activation, seems to result in differentiation into IL-4- and IL-10-producing T (Th$_2$) cells (Boutin et al 1997).

Three intermediary kinases, Fyn, Lck, and ZAP70, initiate TCR signal transduction (Figure 2.4). Whereas Fyn-deficient mice show strikingly impaired TCR signal amplification (Appleby et al 1992), increased Fyn expression in transgenic mice augments the response (Cooke et al 1991). Similarly, Lck-deficient T cells display marked impairment of protein tyrosine phosphorylation, of generation of the downstream cytoplasmic cascade, and of thymic development (Straus and Weiss 1992). Deficiency of ZAP70, a kinase that is expressed exclusively in T and natural killer (NK) cells, is associated with severe immunodeficiency syndrome (SCID; Chan et al 1994).

A second but independent pathway of activation after TCR signaling is the generation of phosphatidylinositol intermediates such as Cγ1 (PLCγ1), which cannot be activated in either Lck- or ZAP70-deficient T cells (Wiest et al 1997). Within seconds after TCR engagement (Imboden and Stobo 1985), phosphorylation of PLCγ1 generates the second messengers, phosphatidylinositol 4,5-bisphosphate (PIP$_2$), inositol 1,4,-bisphosphate (IP$_2$), and thereafter inositol 1,4,5-trisphosphate (1,4,5-IP$_3$) and 1,2-diacylglycerol (DAG). These events increase the cytoplasmic Ca^{2+} content by opening surface membrane calcium channels and mobilizing the ion from intracellular membranes (Figure 2.4). The increased intracellular content of 1,4,5-IP$_3$, DAG, and Ca^{2+} has two effects: it activates the protein kinase C (PKC) family, which includes a series of closely related enzymes (PKCα, PKCβ, and PKCθ), and it activates calmodulin (CaM), to which it complexes and in turn activates calcineurin (CaN), a phosphatase that displays only low activity levels constitutively in T cells. Calcineurin dephosphorylates and translocates nuclear factor of activated T cells (NF-AT) from the cytoplasm into the nucleus, where NF-AT binds as the first regulatory factor in the promoter region of many lymphokine genes, including IL-2 (Rao et al 1997).

Another TCR-initiated cascade is Ras activation, which causes hydrolysis of guanine nucleotide triphosphate (GTP; Downward et al 1992), an event that is regulated by intermediary molecules such as Sos (Polakis and McCormick 1993). Ras activation generates Raf-1 and the mitogen activated protein (MAP) kinases (MEK and MAPK; Cantrell 1975). This process is necessary for the production of the transcription factors NF-AT, NF-κB, AP-1, c-Rel, IκB, Oct-1, etc., which are required for the transcription of IL-2 and other cytokines.

Second signal activation

The second T cell activation signal is delivered independent of TCR events by costimulatory molecules such as B7/CD28 (Freeman et al 1993; Figure 2.4). One set of molecules, B7-2 (CD86), is present at all times at low concentration (constitutive expression) and rapidly upregulated after APC activation, thus delivering an early signal. In contrast, the B7-1 (CD80) molecules are not expressed until 24 hours after activation, thus mediating continued T cell clonal proliferation. The B7-1 and B7-2 molecules interact with CD28 on the surface of lymphocytes. Reception of this second signal strengthens the activation of both the PIP_2 and the Raf-1/MEK/MAPK pathways, thereby augmenting the activation of the transcription factors NF-AT, NF-κB, AP-1, c-Rel, IκB, Oct-1, etc. In fact, timely delivery of the B7/CD28 signal spares clones from TCR-induced apoptosis.

Third signal activation

The third signal required for progression of T cells toward division is delivered via specific receptors for cytokines, local hormones produced by activated $CD4^+$ cells (Figure 2.4). The IL-2 receptor (IL-2R) is frequently used as an example of receptor function. This receptor includes three noncovalently associated polypeptides, namely, the α- (55 kD), β- (70 kD), and γ- (64 kD) chains. Formation of the heterotrimeric α,β,γ-chain complex enhances the avidity of binding of IL-2 over that displayed by single- or double-chain complexes. Indeed, one of the earliest events following initial T cell activation is upregulated transcription of CD25, which is expressed on the cell surface and rapidly associates with the β- and γ-chains. Within minutes of engagement of IL-2 ligand by IL-2R, Lyk, Syk, and Fyn become activated, followed by phosphorylation and consequent activation of Janus (Jak1 and Jak3) tyrosine kinases. The phosphorylated JAKs reciprocally phosphorylate the signal transducers and activators of transcription (Stat5a, Stat5b, and Stat3), which then dimerize and serve as transcriptional regulatory proteins. In addition, the third signal activates the Ras/Raf-1/MEK/MAPK pathway, thereby amplifying the earlier activation triggered by the first two signals. As shown in Table 2.4, various combinations of Jaks and Stats are utilized to generate the unique cellular profiles observed after T cells receive triggering signals delivered by various cytokines.

Apoptosis

Balancing these activation events is programmed cell death, or apoptosis, a process that serves to limit the immune response (Figure 2.4). After reception of only one of the three activation signals, or after one or more cycles of cell division, T cells are susceptible to passive or active mechanisms of apoptosis (Boehme and Leonardo 1993). Active apoptosis, which occurs even in the presence of cytokines that induce T cell proliferation (Kung et al 1998), depends upon a death signal upon engagement of the Fas receptor on T cells by Fas ligand (FasL) presented by other T cells. The Fas–FasL interaction

	Jaks	Stats
Type I cytokine receptors		
Sharing γ-chain		
IL-2, IL-7, IL-9, IL-15	Jak1, Jak3	Stat5a, Stat5b, Stat3
IL-4	Jak1, Jak3	Stat6
IL-13*	Jak1, Jak2, Tyk2	Stat6
Sharing β-chain		
IL-3, IL-5, GM-CSF	Jak2	Stat5a, Stat5b
Sharing gp130		
IL-6, IL-11, OSM, CNTF	Jak1, Jak2, Tyk2	Stat3
IL-12[†]	Jak2, Tyk2	Stat4
Leptin[†]		Stat3
Homodimeric receptors		
Growth hormone	Jak2	Stat5a, Stat5b, Stat3
Prolactin	Jak2	Stat5a, Stat5b
Erythropoietin	Jak2	Stat5a, Stat5b
Thrombopoietin	Jak2	Stat5a, Stat5b
Type II cytokine receptors		
Interferons		
IFN-α, IFN-β	Jak1, Tyk2	Stat1, Stat2
IFN-γ	Jak1, Jak2	Stat1
IL-10[‡]	Jak1, Tyk2	Stat3

*IL-13 does not share γ_c, but uses IL-4Rα.

[†]IL-12 and leptin do not share gp130, but their receptors are related to gp130.

[‡]IL-10 is not an interferon, but its receptor is a type II cytokine receptor.

Table 2.4. Utilization of Jaks and Stats by various cytokine receptors

produces aggregation of adapter proteins bearing the Fas-associated death domain (FADD), with consequent activation of caspase proteolytic enzymes present in the cytoplasmic tail of Fas (Muzio et al 1996). The caspase family bears a conserved cysteine within the active protease site, which is necessary for cleavage of cellular substrates at a point downstream of an aspartate residue, causing the cytoskeletal and the chromatin damage that leads to apoptosis (Nicholson and Thornberry 1997). The IL-1β-converting enzyme (ICE), which is designated as caspase 1 (Zou et al 1997), is only one of 14 caspase family members, each of which contains three domains, namely, an N-terminal prodomain followed by large and small subdomains. Cleavage of the prodomain releases the large and small subdomains, which associate as enzymatically active heterodimers (Walker et al 1994).

In contrast to active apoptosis, which does not require protein synthesis—in fact, inhibitors of DNA transcription and mRNA translation enhance the process by preventing generation of proteins that block apoptosis (Itoh et al 1991)—the passive form of apoptosis requires new protein synthesis. Passive apoptosis is mediated through a mitochondrial mechanism that does not involve FasL or the death intermediates. Passive apoptosis is prevented by the presence of the cytokines IL-2, IL-4, IL-7, or IL-15, and is strongly inhibited by Bcl-2, Bcl-X, and other related antiapoptotic proteins (Lenardo et al 1999). The fraction of T cells that undergoes sequential activation after reception of the three signals (and thereby escapes apoptosis) represents the effectors of allograft rejection. The small number of these effector cells that eventually escape both the passive and active processes of apoptosis become memory T cells (Murali-Krishna et al 1998).

B cells

Activation

Similar to T cells, activation of B cells depends upon three sequential signals, with many B cells undergoing apoptosis to limit the number of responsive elements. Binding of the corresponding antigen to membrane Ig, which serves as the specific B cell receptor (BCR), produces the initial activation signal (Figure 2.5). The diversity of BCRs is determined by the heterogenicity of the v regions of their Ig molecules: namely, the Fab portions of the light and heavy chains distal to the cleavage point of the papain, in contradistinction to the Fc tail, which bears constant regions of the heavy chains. However, unlike the T cell response, the B cell response is not MHC-restricted; that is, it does not require that the APCs bearing peptide bar the same MHC antigens (Reth 1992).

Overall, the processes of activation and signal transduction are remarkably similar for B and T cells (Figure 2.5). The BCR is associated with signal transducing elements, invariant, disulfide-linked Igα (mb-1) and Igβ (B29; Reth 1992), which bear more extensive cytoplasmic domains than the antigen-binding Ig-chain, as well as ITAM sequences that undergo phosphorylation and within minutes trigger downstream activation of the tyrosine kinases Lyn, Fyn, Syc, Blc, and Btk (Samelson and Klausner 1992). For example, phosphorylation of Syk, the B cell equivalent to the T cell enzyme ZAP70, on two adjacent tyrosines within its kinase domain upregulates its activity by 10-fold (Rowley et al 1995; Kurosaki 1997). The variety of B cell functional defects in Lyn-deficient mutant mice suggests the important role of the Lyn tyrosine kinase (Hibbs et al 1995). Similarly, expression of a defective form of the tyrosine kinase Btk, as observed in X-linked human immunodeficiency syndrome, may represent the cause of impaired Ab production (Tarakhovsky 1997).

Other tyrosine-phosphorylated signaling components following BCR engagement include Vav (Bustelo and Barbacid 1992), Cbl (Cory et al 1995), and HS1 (Yamanashi et al 1993). The activity of Ras is upregulated by the critical intermediate proto-oncogene

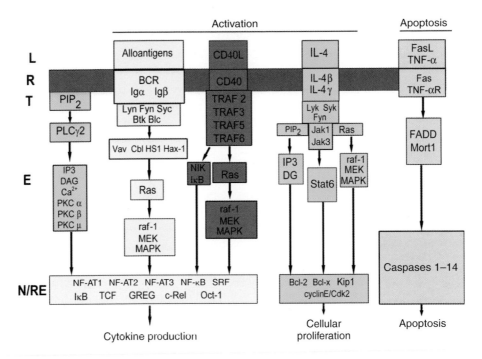

Figure 2.5. Sequential activation signals 1, 2, and 3 that control activation versus apoptosis of B cells. The exogenous ligands (L) initiate the response through the cell surface receptors (R), followed by the signal transducers (T) and their associated enzymes (E), affecting regulators (RE) of the nuclear transcription factors (N), which control Ab class switching and cytokine production, cellular proliferation, or apoptosis. Full B-cell activation requires BCR engagement by alloantigen, followed by phosphorylation of Lck, Fyn, Syc, and Btk kinases. Engagement of PLC and Ras/MAPK pathways leads to activation of multiple transcription factors, such as NF-AT, NF-κB, and AP-1. The second signal is delivered by the CD40/CD40L interaction. The third cytokine (IL-4) signal is delivered by the Jak/Stat system to complete B cell activation. Apoptotic mechanisms similar to those in T cells are observed in B cells.

product Vav (Bonnefoy-Berard et al 1996) and downregulated by another proto-oncogene product, Cbl (Yoon et al 1995). After phosphorylation, HS1, which is widely expressed in hematopoietic cells, is translocated to the nucleus (Yamanashi et al 1997). Interestingly, phosphorylated HS1 interacts with the HAX-1 protein, which is localized in mitochondria and associates with and upregulates the Bcl-2/BAX antiapoptotic proteins (Suzuki et al 1997). Thus, BCR engagement also activates the transduction of the Ras/MAP/MAPK pathways. Like T cells, B cells use NF-AT, NF-κB, and other transcription factors to upregulate transcription of functional genes that are necessary for Ab production.

B cell receptor engagement also leads to rapid hydrolysis of PIP_2 by phospholipase Cγ. Whereas T cell activation causes phosphorylation of PLCγ1, in B cells there is predominant appearance of the tyrosine phosphoprotein PLCγ2. However, the 1,4,5-IP3 and DAG second messengers after PIP_2 hydrolysis are identical among T and B cells. In B cells, the consequent activation of PKCβ appears to upregulate the transcription factor CREB (the cyclic monophosphate (cAMP) response element; Xie and Rothstein 1995—a critical event, since PKCβ-deficient mice display decreased Ab production (Tarakhovsky 1997). Another B cell isoform, PKCμ, may exert a negative regulatory function, since its activation prevents phosphorylation of PLCγ1.

T cells deliver a second signal to B cells via CD40 ligand (CD40L; CD154) interacting with CD40 (CD150), a marker that is constitutively expressed on the surface of B cells (Weiss 1991; Figure 2.5). Within 4–8 hours after T cell activation, CD40L expression on T cells peaks. Patients with X-linked immunodeficiency, who display a mutation in the CD40L gene, are unable to produce any Abs other than IgM (Vitetta et al 1989; Allen et al 1993). The importance of the CD40/CD40L interaction for B cell activation has also been documented by the immunologic properties of mice displaying γ-chain-linked hyper-IgM syndrome. These mice exhibit normal IgM levels, but essentially are incapable of producing IgG, IgA, or IgE (Tamura et al 1993). Although the mechanism of CD40 signal transduction is not fully understood, TNF-receptor-associated factors (TRAF2, TRAF3, TRAF5, and TRAF6) have been implicated as potential mediators (Hostager and Bishop 1999; Lee et al 1999). In particular, oligomerization of CD40 leads to engagement of TRAF3, which promotes isotype class switch recombination. TRAF2 and TRAF6 bind to distinct sites on the CD40 cytoplasmic tail linking the serine/threonine kinase NIK, which then phosphorylates and activates a large, multi-component complex called IκB. An IκB kinase autophosphorylates two neighboring serine residues, leading to degradation of IκB units and thus releasing NF-κB for translocation to the nucleus and binding to DNA target sites. Furthermore, CD40/CD40L engagement in the presence of IL-4 activates c-Rel and Stat6 (Schaffer et al 1999). In addition to the CD40/CD40L second signal, B cell growth and differentiation requires a third signal delivered by any of a variety of cytokines, including IL-4, IL-5, IL-6, IL-10, or IL-13 (Finkelman et al 1990).

Apoptosis

As is the case for T cells, the size of the B cell peripheral pool is tightly regulated by similar apoptotic processes (Figure 2.5; Craxton et al 1999). Although on a daily basis the bone marrow produces precursors that account for 20% of the total number of peripheral B cells, only a very small number of these precursors become mature B cells, while the rest die at different developmental stages (Osmond 1991). B cell precursors released from bone marrow migrate to the marginal zone of the sinus regions in the spleen on their way to the outer zone of the peripheral lymphoid sheath (PALS), the primary site of B-cell proliferation after contact with antigens (including alloantigens). On the one hand, BCR ligation on immature B cells always initiates apoptosis, whereas BCR engagement on mature B cells induces death unless they are rescued by the second CD40/CD40L and eventually by a third cytokine signal. On the other hand, even fully activated mature B cells may succumb to apoptosis through a Fas/FasL signal. Thus, only a small fraction of activated B cells eventually become memory B cells capable of producing high-affinity Ab.

CYTOKINES

Cytokines are small proteins produced by a variety of activated cells. They serve as autocrine or paracrine mediators of inflammatory responses, producing a wide range of effects on various tissues and cells, often in redundant fashion (Paul and Seder 1994). These proteins act by binding to high-affinity target cell receptors that are expressed either constitutively or after activation (Figure 2.6). The effects of cytokines are regu-

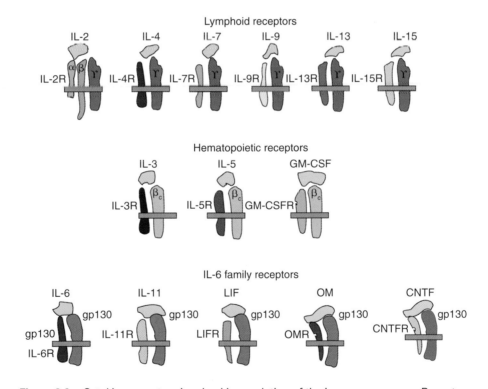

Figure 2.6. Cytokine receptors involved in regulation of the immune response. Receptors consist of public (group-specific) and private (specific for each cytokine) chains. The public chains define three groups of receptors: lymphoid receptors share the γ-chain, including IL-2R, IL-4R, IL-7R, IL-9R, IL-13R, and IL-15R; hematopoietic receptors share a β-chain, including IL-3R, IL-5R, and granulocyte/macrophage colony stimulating factor (GM-CSF) receptor; and the IL-6 family of receptors share a gp130 chain, including IL-6R, IL-11R, leukemia inhibitory factor (LIF) receptor, oncostatin M receptor (OMR), and ciliary neurotrophic factor (CNTF).

lated by antagonists that block their binding, including circulating soluble forms of receptors that absorb free cytokines. Recently, it has been suggested that the types and concentrations of cytokines determine whether the host displays a rejection versus an acceptance or even a tolerance response to a transplant (Bushell et al 1999). This hypothesis suggests that manipulation of cytokine production at the initial stage of transplantation can redirect the immune response from alloaggression to tolerance. Based on their cellular origin and location on the genome, cytokines have been divided into five families: ILs, IFNs, TNFs, colony-stimulating factors (CSFs), and TGFs (Tables 2.5 and 2.6).

Interleukin family

Among the members of the first family, IL-1α and IL-1β are produced primarily by activated macrophages, by T and B lymphocytes, as well as by other cells (Table 2.5). Production of IL-1 causes fever, prostaglandin synthesis, and induction of synthesis of other proinflammatory cytokines, including IFN-γ, TNFs, and IL-6. IL-1 augments the production of IL-2 and IL-2R proteins, and complements the actions of IL-4 to increase proliferation of and Ig production by B lymphocytes.

A second member of this family is IL-2, a product of activated T cells, particularly the Th_1 population. IL-2 stimulates the proliferation and differentiation of T cells, including the generation of T cytotoxic cells (Tc). It also contributes to the activation of NK and lymphokine-activated killer (LAK) cells. However, IL-2 is not the exclusive mediator of these effects. IL-2-gene knockout mice not only retain normal development of thymocytes and peripheral T lymphocytes, but also display prompt allograft rejection (Schonrich et al 1992; Steiger et al 1995). Even IL-2/IL-4 double-knockout mice are able to destroy pancreatic islet allografts, suggesting that other members of the IL family—such as IL-7 and/or IL-15—play an active role in allograft rejection (Li et al 1998). Indeed, blockade of the public γ-chain that is common to the receptors for IL-2, IL-4, IL-7, and IL-15 has been shown to prolong the survival of islet allografts in IL-2/IL-4 double-knockout mice.

Among the other cytokines of the family, IL-3, produced by activated T cells, causes proliferation of pluripotent hematopoietic progenitor cells (Sonoda et al 1988) and augments production of granulocyte-CSF (G-CSF)-dependent neutrophils and of erythropoietin-dependent red blood cells. The IL cytokines also regulate Ab production by B cells. In particular, IL-4 induces the switch from Bμ(IgM)- to Bγ_1(IgG$_1$)- and B$_\epsilon$(IgE)-producing cells (Vitetta et al 1985). Mice displaying an IL-4 gene mutation not only fail to produce IgE, but also display strikingly reduced levels of IgG$_1$ (Kühn et al 1993). At the same time, the presence of IL-4 increases expression of class I MHC antigens on cells, and preferentially stimulates the proliferation of IL-4-producing Th_2 cells while inhibiting the function of IL-2- and IFN-γ–producing Th_1 cells.

IL-5, a cytokine produced by activated Th_2 cells, activates eosinophils and induces proliferation of and Ig production by B cells. IL-6, which is produced by macrophages,

Interleukin	Produced by	Effect on
IL-1α IL-1β	Macrophages, T and B cells, NK cells, neutrophils, keratinocytes, fibroblasts, endothelial cells	Production of: prostaglandins $\uparrow$; IFN-γ $\uparrow$, TNFs $\uparrow$, IL-6 $\uparrow$, IL-2 $\uparrow$, IL-4 $\uparrow$, Ab $\uparrow$
IL-2	Th$_1$ cells	Tc $\uparrow$; NK $\uparrow$; LAK $\uparrow$; T and B cell growth $\uparrow$; macrophage activity $\uparrow$; expression of IL-2β and IL-2γ receptor chains $\uparrow$; allograft rejection $\uparrow$; Th$_1$ differentiation $\uparrow$
IL-3	T cells	Hematopoietic progenitor cells $\uparrow$; G-CSF $\uparrow$; neutrophils $\uparrow$; erythropoietin $\uparrow$; RBC $\uparrow$
IL-4	Th$_2$ cells	MHC class II $\uparrow$; IL-2 $\downarrow$; IFN-γ $\downarrow$; Ab production $\uparrow$; expression of IL-2β and IL-4α receptor chains $\uparrow$; Th$_2$ differentiation $\uparrow$
IL-5	Th$_2$ cells	Eosinophils $\uparrow$; Ab production $\uparrow$
IL-6	Macrophages, fibroblasts, endothelial cells, mast cells, keratinocytes	Ig $\uparrow$; IL-2 $\uparrow$; IL-4 $\uparrow$
IL-7	Stromal cells, thymic epithelium	Thymocyte growth $\uparrow$; TCR gene rearrangement $\uparrow$; allograft rejection $\uparrow$; IL-2 production $\uparrow$
IL-8	Monocytes, T, B endothelial cells, neutrophils	Adhesion of cells $\uparrow$
IL-9	T cells	T cell growth $\uparrow$; mast cell growth $\uparrow$; erythropoiesis $\uparrow$; allograft rejection $\uparrow$
IL-10	Th$_2$, mast cells, macrophages, keratinocytes	IL-2 $\downarrow$; IFN-γ $\downarrow$; T cell growth $\downarrow$; Th$_1$ $\downarrow$; MHC class II $\uparrow$; CTL $\uparrow$
IL-12	Macrophages, B cells	IFN-γ $\uparrow$; NK $\uparrow$; T cell proliferation $\uparrow$
IL-13	Th$_2$ cells	Monocytes $\uparrow$; B cells $\uparrow$; VLA-5 $\uparrow$, MHC class II $\uparrow$; F$_{c\gamma}$I $\downarrow$; F$_{c\gamma}$II $\downarrow$; F$_{c\gamma}$III $\downarrow$; Ig production $\uparrow$; ADCC $\downarrow$; Bμ(IgM)$\rightarrow$ I$_{gE}$ (IgE) $\uparrow$
IL-15	Monocytes, muscle cells, keratinocytes, renal epithelial cells, endothelial cells	Tc $\uparrow$; T$_{DFH}$ $\uparrow$; NU $\uparrow$; rejection $\uparrow$; Th$_1$ $\uparrow$
IL-17	Activated T cells	Osteoclastic resorption $\uparrow$; IL-6 $\uparrow$; IL-8 $\uparrow$; nitric oxide $\uparrow$; stromal cells $\uparrow$; macrophages $\uparrow$; dendritic cell maturation $\uparrow$; keratinocyte activation $\uparrow$; G-CSF $\uparrow$; ICAM-1 $\uparrow$; neutrophil differentiation $\uparrow$; allograft rejection $\uparrow$

Table 2.5. Function of cytokines (ILs) in allograft rejection

	Produced by	Effect on
Interferons (IFNs)		
IFN-α	Macrophages	T cell activation $\uparrow$; Ig production $\uparrow$
IFN-β	Fibroblasts	Proliferation of cells $\downarrow$
IFN-γ	Th$_1$	Macrophages $\uparrow$; NK cells $\uparrow$; MHC class I and II $\uparrow$; adhesion molecules $\uparrow$; Th$_2$ $\downarrow$
Tumor necrosis factors (TNFs)		
TNF-α	Macrophages, T cells,	MHC class I and II $\uparrow$; adhesion molecules $\uparrow$;
TNF-β	neutrophils	IL-1 $\uparrow$; proliferation and differentiation of T and B cells $\uparrow$
Colony stimulating factors (CSFs)		
GM-CSF	T cells, fibroblasts, macrophages, endothelial cells	Macrophages $\uparrow$; activation $\uparrow$; neutrophil differentiation $\uparrow$; eosinophils $\uparrow$
M-CSF	Fibroblasts	Macrophage differentiation $\uparrow$; granulocyte differentiation $\uparrow$
G-CSF	Macrophages, fibroblasts, endothelial cells	Granulocyte differentiation $\uparrow$
Transforming growth factors (TGFs)		
TGF-β1	Macrophages, platelets, B	Wound healing $\uparrow$; fibroblast growth $\uparrow$;
TGF-β2	cells, T cells, fibroblasts,	angiogenesis $\uparrow$; Igμ (IgM) and Igα (IgA);
TGF-β3	endothelial cells, osteoblasts, astrocytes, microglial cells	class switching; chronic rejection $\uparrow$; tolerance $\uparrow$; memory T cells $\uparrow$; Th$_1$ differentiation $\uparrow$; hematopoiesis $\downarrow$; lymphopoiesis $\downarrow$; Ig production $\downarrow$; CTL $\downarrow$; Nμ $\downarrow$; Lau $\downarrow$; local inflammation and fibrosis $\uparrow$

Table 2.6.   Function of cytokines (IFNs, TNFs, CSFs, and TGFs) in allograft rejection

fibroblasts, endothelial cells, mast cells, keratinocytes, and T cells, increases Ig production and enhances IL-2- and IL-4-driven proliferation of thymocytes (Akira and Kishimoto 1992). IL-7, a cytokine produced by the stromal cells of bone marrow, thymic epithelium, and spleen, regulates the gene rearrangement of TCRs in stem cells, leading to the polymorphic repertoire of T cells, and increases IL-2 production by activated T cells. IL-8, produced by activated lymphocytes, monocytes, and endothelial cells, activates neutrophils, but in some circumstances may inhibit neutrophil adhesion to endothelial cells (Gimbrone et al 1989). IL-9, a multifunctional growth factor produced by T cells, promotes the proliferation of T cells, mast cells, and megakaryocytes, as well as the erythroid burst of hematopoietic progenitor cells. IL-10, produced by activated Th$_2$ cells, mast cells, macrophages, and keratinocytes, inhibits production of IL-2 and IFN-γ by Th$_1$ cells (de Waal et al 1991). T lymphocytes from immunodeficient (SCID) patients transplanted with allogeneic fetal liver stem cells display unusually high levels of IL-10 and low amounts of IL-2 (Bacchetta et al 1994). Thus, increased IL-10 production in vivo has been associated with downregulation of the immune response. IL-12, which is produced by activated macrophages and B cells, enhances by 10-fold the production of IFN-γ by Th$_1$ (Gubler et al 1991), and thereby amplifies the T cell response.

IL-13, the most recently described cytokine of the IL family, is produced by activated Th$_2$ cells and modulates the in vitro activity of human monocytes and B cells. IL-13 shares many biological activities with IL-4, and their genes are closely related. Like IL-4, IL-13 enhances expression of integrin VLA-5, but not VLA-2, VLA-3, or VLA-4. In addition, IL-13 upregulates expression of class II MHC, but downregulates expression of the constant Ig fragment (F$_{c\gamma}$) type I (F$_{c\gamma}$I), type II (F$_{c\gamma}$II), and type III (F$_{c\gamma}$III) receptors used by the cells to selectively bind Abs with different F$_{c\gamma}$ fragments. In contrast to IL-10 and IFN-γ, IL-13 inhibits the effects of IL-10 and IFN-γ on Ab-dependent cell-mediated cytotoxicity, but enhances Ig production and triggers the switch from Bμ(IgM) to Bε(IgE). Whereas IL-4 activates T cells, IL-13 downregulates the inflammatory response (Moore et al 1993).

IL-15, which is produced by activated macrophages, muscle cells, keratinocytes, renal epithelial cells, and endothelial cells (Tagaya et al 1996), exerts IL-2-like activities, namely, stimulation of the proliferation and differentiation of T and NK cells. Both IL-15 and IL-7 can deliver costimulatory signals to induce Th$_1$ cells, particularly in the absence of a robust B7/CD28 interaction (Borger et al 1999). IL-15 mRNA transcripts, as well as those of IL-2, IL-4, and IL-10, have been identified in the renal transplant biopsies of apparently quiescent patients, suggesting the presence of borderline allograft rejection (Lipman et al 1998). Thus, IL-15 may contribute to the subclinical progression of allograft rejection.

IL-17, a homodimeric cytokine produced by activated T cells, induces production of IL-6, IL-8, and G-CSF by fibroblasts, keratinocytes, and epithelial and endothelial cells (Fossiez et al 1998). In addition, IL-17 promotes ICAM-1 surface expression, proliferation of T cells, and differentiation of neutrophils. Antagonist-mediated inhibition of IL-17 activity prolongs the survival of heart allografts in mice (Antonysamy et al 1999).

Interferon family

Among the IFN family, IFN-α and IFN-β genes are located in close proximity, and their gene products display similar activities (Friedman 1988; Table 2.6). Fibroblasts produce mainly IFN-β, whereas macrophages produce mainly IFN-α. Although both proteins display strong antiviral and antiproliferative effects, they also enhance T cell activation, as well as B-cell production of Ig. However, their in vivo activities are complex, producing either stimulatory or inhibitory effects on the immune system. Interferon-γ, produced by activated Th_1 cells, stimulates macrophages, lymphocytes, NK cells, and leukocytes, in part by increasing their cell surface content of class I MHC, class II MHC, and adhesion molecules. On the other hand, IFN-γ inhibits the activity of IL-4-producing T cells (Th_2).

Tumor necrosis factor family

TNFs (TNF-α and TNF-β) are primarily produced by macrophages (Carswell et al 1975), and to a lesser extent by lymphocytes and neutrophils (Table 2.6). TNFs increase the expression of MHC antigens and adhesion molecules on endothelial cells, induce IL-1 production, and promote B and T cell proliferation and differentiation. Granulocyte/macrophage-CSF (GM-CSF), which is produced by activated T cells, fibroblasts, macrophages, and endothelial cells, activates macrophages and supports the differentiation of neutrophils and eosinophils (Burgess and Metcalf 1980). Macrophage-CSF (M-CSF), produced by fibroblasts, promotes the differentiation of monocytes, macrophages, and granulocytes; G-CSF, produced by macrophages, fibroblasts, and endothelial cells, promotes differentiation of granulocytes.

Transforming growth factor family

TGF-β is a multifunctional cytokine that regulates the growth and differentiation of many cells (Table 2.6). Macrophages, platelets, fibroblasts, endothelial cells, osteoclasts, astrocytes, and microglial cells all produce TGF-β. Of the five identified isoforms, three (namely, TGF-β1, TGF-β2, and TGF-β3) are expressed in mammals. TGF-β may display either a pro- or an anti-inflammatory effect, depending on the type and maturational state of the responding cell type, as well as on the local environment. The opposing effects of TGF-β are based on the site of administration: systemic delivery induces an inhibitory effect on the immune system, whereas local release produces a stimulatory effect (McCartney-Francis and Wahl 1994). It seems that increased systemic TGF-β levels correlate on the one hand with the state of oral tolerance, and on the other hand with increased local levels, increased fibrosis in the graft, and the development of chronic rejection.

CYTOKINE RECEPTORS

The redundant patterns of cytokine action may be explained at least in part by the similar structures of the surface membrane receptors that mediate their effects by triggering signal transduction (Figure 2.6). Most cytokine receptors consist of a private (ligand-specific) component and a public (group-specific) signal transducer (Miyajima et al 1992; Kishimoto et al 1994). For example, the receptors for IL-2, IL-4, IL-7, IL-9, IL-13, and IL-15 utilize the same γ-chain (Takeshita et al 1992; Russell et al 1993). The IL-2 receptor includes three polypeptide chains: α (55 kD), β (70 kD), and γ (64 kD). The heterotrimer αβγ displays greater avidity for ligand than the βγ heterodimer, which is constitutively expressed on cells. Although they share the same γ-chain, the unique actions of IL-4, IL-7, IL-9, IL-13, or IL-15 are mediated by their private chains, which seem to direct specific patterns of signal transduction by utilizing a distinct combination of Jaks, together with Stats (Table 2.4). Similarly, the regulators of hematopoietic cell development—IL-3, IL-5, and GM-CSF receptors—all share a common β-chain (Takahata et al 1992). Finally, the IL-6 family of receptors—IL-6, IL-11, IL-12, leukemia inhibitory factor (LIF), oncostatin M (OM), and ciliary neurotrophic factor (CNTF)—use a common gp130 signal transducer (Taga et al 1989).

A single Jak/Stat pathway tends to determine the selective effect of each group of cytokines (Leonard and O'Shea 1998). The Jaks (Jak1, Jak2, Jak3, and Tyk2) are relatively large (120–130 kD) kinases. In contrast to the relatively ubiquitous expression of Jak1, Jak2, and Tyk2 tyrosine kinases, Jak3 is expressed constitutively in thymocytes and NK cells, and is only upregulated in activated T and B cells. The gp130 subunit binds Jak1, Jak2, and Tyk2 (Stahl et al 1994); the β-chain, only Jak2 (Quelle et al 1994); and the γ-chain, Jak3 (Boussiotis et al 1994). However, except for one molecular target, the Stat family of transcription factors, understanding of the relevant downstream Jak substrates is limited.

The seven known Stat proteins (Stat1, Stat2, Stat3, Stat4, Stat5a, Stat5b, and Stat6) range from 750 to 850 amino acids in length, with molecular weights of 89–100 kD. Table 2.4 shows the pattern of associations between Jaks and Stats during signal transduction cascades of various cytokines. For example, the γ-chains of IL-2, IL-7, IL-9, and IL-15 cytokine receptors utilize Jak3, Stat5a, and Stat5b; the γ-chains of IL-4, Jak1, Jak3, and Stat6; and the γ-chains of IL-13, Jak1, Jak2, Tyk2, and Stat6.

The IL-2 signaling pathway is one of the best understood receptor transduction cascades (Figure 2.7). Binding of IL-2 to its receptor rapidly triggers tyrosine phosphorylation of the β- and γ-chains, and subsequent binding of Jak1 to the β-chain and Jak3 to the γ-chain, leading to phosphorylation of their tyrosine-based docking sites for Stat3 and Stat5a and Stat5b, respectively, which are in turn phosphorylated. Thereafter, the Stats detach from their docking sites, form dimers, and are translocated to the nucleus, where they modulate the transcription of target genes. Although the gene targets regulated by the Jak/Stat system are little understood, they do include oncostatin and perforin DNA sequences.

Figure 2.8 presents a schematic representation of the variety of functions mediating the acute allograft rejection of differentiated T cells. In particular, activated $CD4^+$ Th_0 cells become either Th_1 clones that predominantly produce IL-2, IFN-γ, and TNF, or Th_2 clones that predominantly produce IL-4, IL-5, IL-6, IL-10, and IL-13. In the cytokine environment, $CD4^+$ and $CD8^+$ T cells differentiate into either T delayed-type

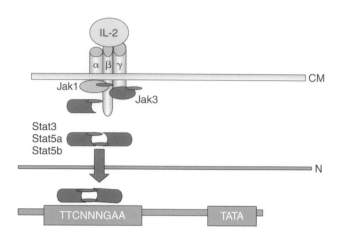

Figure 2.7. Model of IL-2 receptor-induced activation of Jak/Stat signal transduction. After IL-2 binds to the IL-2 receptor in the cell membrane (CM), Jak1 binds to the β-chain and Jak3 to the γ-chain, thereby allowing phosphorylation of tyrosine-based docking sites for Stat3, Stat5a, and Stat5b. After docking, Stats are phosphorylated and detach from the β- or γ-chains to form heterodimers, which are translocated to the nucleus (N), thereby modulating transcription of target genes.

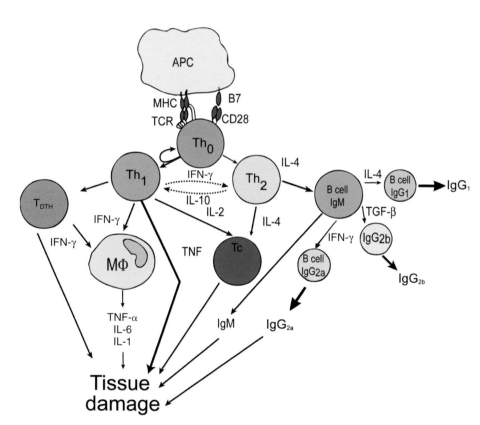

Figure 2.8. Mechanisms of acute allograft rejection. Acute allograft rejection is initiated by activation of Th_1 and Th_2 cells, which mutually regulate generation of Tc and T_{DTH} effector cells. Th_2 cells may downregulate Th_1 cells; conversely, Th_1 cells may downregulate Th_2 cells. Tc cells directly lyse donor cells, whereas T_{DTH} cells activate macrophages (MΦ) to destroy donor cells. Cytokines also regulate maturation and immunoglobulin (Ig) class switching in B cells: IL-4 to IgG_1, IFN-γ to IgG_{2a}, and TGF-β to IgG_{2b}.

hypersensitivity (T_{DTH}) effector cells or Tc elements, respectively. Although the two cell types are believed to act cooperatively, either is capable of mediating allograft destruction. In addition, the humoral immune response leads to alloantibody production.

TYPES OF REJECTION

Hyperacute

Clinical graft rejection is classified based upon its timing as hyperacute, accelerated, acute, or chronic. Hyperacute rejection is characterized by the sudden, irreversible cessation of graft function minutes to hours after revascularization (Table 2.7). This form of rejection is mediated by the presence of preformed Abs against donor antigens present on the endothelium.

One setting for hyperacute rejection is ABO incompatibility, wherein circulating antidonor ABO blood group hemagglutinins bind to glycolipid determinants on endothelial cells. A second setting is the attachment of preformed recipient antidonor HLA Abs to the vascular lining of the graft. The Ab attachment activates a rapid response that includes both complement (C') endothelial type I activation and coagulation cascades, thereby resulting in the destruction of the transplanted organ (Figure 2.9). The histopathologic consequence of these events is extensive glomerular and vascular thrombosis (Myburgh et al 1969). The activation of C' is restrained at the endothelial cell level by production of several regulatory proteins, including C' receptor-1, decay accelerating factor (DAF; CD55), and CD59. Although these regulatory proteins can prevent graft damage by small amounts of low-affinity Abs, such as those directed against minor blood group antigens, the regulatory proteins are much less effective at blocking damage mediated by high-affinity Abs, such as those directed against MHC determinants. Whereas these events produce rapid destruction of kidney grafts, liver transplants have been reported to survive despite pre-existing antidonor Abs (Gordon et al 1986), although their eventual fate seems to be compromised (Katz et al 1994).

Time of onset	<48 hours
Response	Secondary
Mechanism	Preformed C' binding Ab
Histopathology	Ab, platelet, granulocyte/depot
Therapy	None
Success	0%

Table 2.7. Characteristics of hyperacute rejection

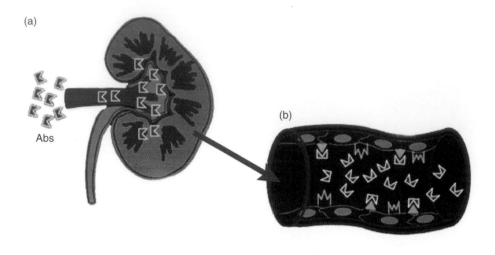

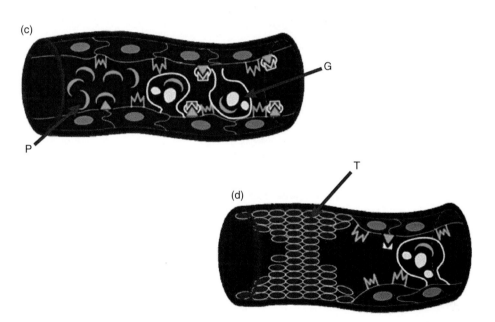

Figure 2.9. Mechanism of hyperacute allograft rejection. (a) Donor-specific Abs enter the graft. (b) Abs bind to class I MHC alloantigens or to A or B blood group glycolipids expressed on the surface of endothelial cells. (c) Fc tails of Ab molecules project into the lumen, attracting deposition of granulocytes (G) and platelets (P). (d) These events trigger thrombosis (T).

While studies in experimental animals suggest that hyperacute rejection may be delayed by host treatment with cobra venom factor, which depletes C' (Diefenbeck et al 1998), this therapy is too toxic for human use. In clinical practice, the risk of hyperacute rejection of kidney and heart transplants is minimized by routine pretransplant cross-match testing (see Chapter 1), which is fortunate, since this condition is not amenable to pharmacological intervention.

Accelerated

Accelerated rejection is characterized by anamnestic responses that occur within 5 days posttransplant (Figure 2.10). These responses may include the production of generally low-affinity antidonor Abs by presensitized B cells or the generation of cytotoxic T cells from memory elements (Table 2.8). The immune elements bind to the donor endothelium without involvement of C' (type II endothelial activation), leading to disruption of the vascular layer and interstitial hemorrhage. On gross examination, the kidney is tense due to the hemorrhage (Figure 2.11). In cases in which the reaction is extensive or not controlled by therapy, parenchymal tears or fracture may produce not only acute pain, tenderness, and swelling, but also life-threatening hemorrhage. Histologic examination of kidney transplant confirms extensive intraparenchymal hemorrhage caused by accelerated rejection (Figure 2.12). Accelerated rejection, which occurred not-infrequently in the azathioprine era, may often be reversed by a combination of three therapies. First, rigorous treatment with xenogenic polyclonal antilymphocyte Abs, which lyse lymphocytes, removes the intermediates that are either directly executing or acting as intermediates with Abs to destroy the graft. Second, plasmapheresis seeks to immediately remove antidonor Abs from the circulation. Third, pharmacotherapy with cyclophosphamide seeks to dampen Ab production (Browne and Kahan 1994).

Acute

In clinical practice, the most common type of allograft rejection, affecting up to 40% of patients, is acute rejection (Table 2.9). This type usually occurs between 7 and 90 days postgrafting, but may only be clinically evident after 12 months. In the early postgrafting period, kidney transplants induce activation of alloantigen-specific T cells, which may initiate acute rejection or subclinical graft injury (Tullius et al 1994a). Although acute rejection is generally initiated by alloantigen-specific T cells, in which case it is generally responsive to steroid therapy, the response in some patients may include an Ab component, a form of rejection that tends to be refractory to steroids and only partially controllable by antilymphocyte Abs.

The primary role of lymphocytes in acute rejection was documented by a seminal series of animal experiments. First, histologic examination of allografts showed an abundant mononuclear infiltrate, suggesting a delayed-type hypersensitivity (DTH) reaction

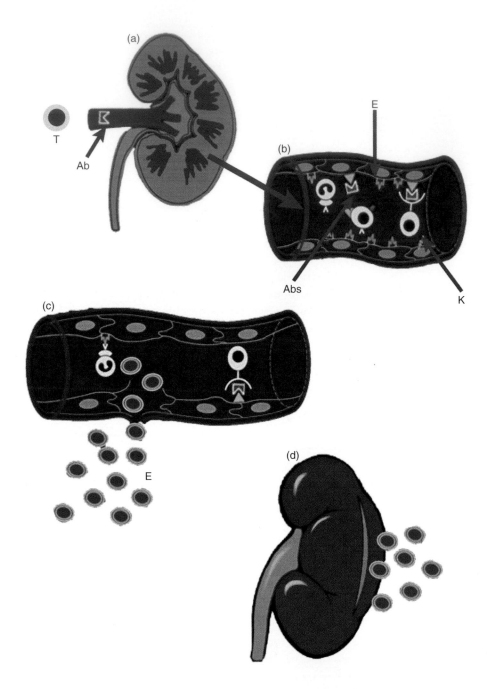

Figure 2.10. Mechanism of accelerated allograft rejection. (a) Presensitized T cells are capable of recognizing specific donor alloantigens via their TCR, whereas B cells produce Abs, albeit of low affinity. (b) Activated T cells and/or antibodies (Abs) attach to endothelium (E) of the graft. (c) Low-affinity antibodies attract lymphocytes (K cells) bearing Fc receptors (FcR). Cellular activation disrupts the vascular layer leading to extravasation of erythrocytes (E) and rupture of the kidney capsule (d).

Time of onset	3–5 days
Response	Secondary
Mechanism	Preformed non-C' binding Ab, cellular immunity
Histopathology	Hemorrhage
Therapy	Polyclonal antilymphocyte globulin/plasmapheresis/cyclophosphamide
Success	60%

Table 2.8. Characteristics of accelerated rejection

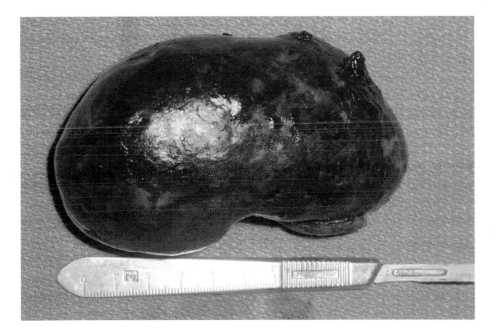

Figure 2.11. Gross appearance of a kidney transplant removed due to accelerated rejection showing extensive intraparenchymal hemorrhage.

(Figure 2.13). Second, intradermal injection of semisoluble extracts of donor tissue into hosts that had rejected grafts provoked a tuberculin (DTH) cutaneous response. Third, transfer of lymphocytes from a host that had rejected an allograft to another member of the same inbred strain adoptively conferred resistance (accelerated rejection) toward donor tissue. Fourth, lymphocytes primed in vitro against donor lymphocytes were able to passively confer alloresistance toward donor tissue.

Figure 2.14 shows the events at the level of the tissue undergoing acute rejection. DTH effector cells produce cytokines that attract the intragraft migration of macrophages, uncommitted lymphocytes, and granulocytes, all of which can contribute to allograft destruction. In addition, Tc cells recognize and lyse graft cells by injecting

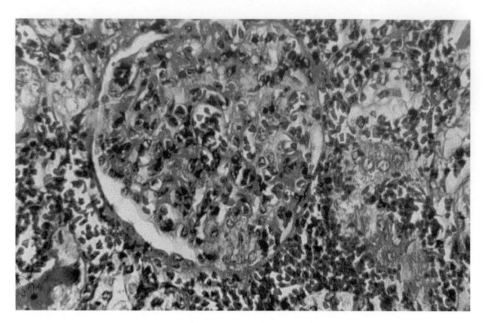

Figure 2.12.   Histologic appearance of a renal allograft showing interstitial hemorrhage due to accelerated rejection (hematoxylin and eosin (H&E ×25).

Time of onset	>6 days	
Response	Primary	
Mechanism	Cellular immunity	Humoral immunity
Histopathology	Lymphocyte infiltrate	Endovasculitis
Therapy	Steroids/OKT3	Steroids/OKT3
Success	80–90%	60–85%

Table 2.9.   Characteristics of acute rejection

into target cells potent lytic enzymes, such as serine proteases, esterases, and perforins. Interestingly, a single Tc cell can engage in several rounds of lysis of different target cells, and the Tc cell itself is not destroyed in the course of killing of target cells. Abs may also contribute to acute rejection. In particular, Abs capable of fixing C' can directly lyse cells, whereas Abs incapable of fixing C' adhere to macrophages/monocytes and direct these phagocytic cells to contact alloantigens on the graft.

Two types of histopathologic changes are associated with acute rejection. The most characteristic appearance of cellular rejection is 'tubulitis', wherein lymphocytes infiltrate below the basement membrane and attack the tubule cells (Figure 2.15). This

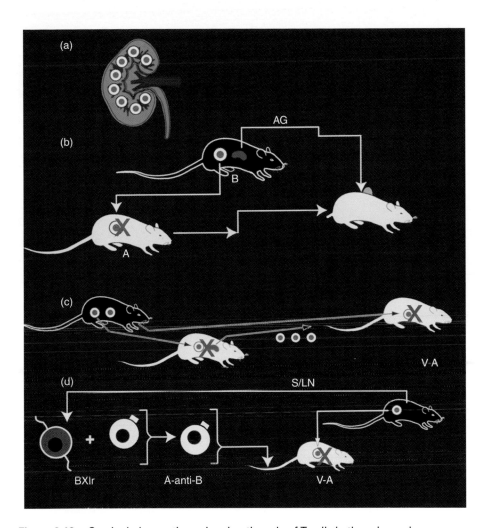

Figure 2.13. Seminal observations showing the role of T cells in the primary immune response. (a) Presence of lymphocyte infiltrate in the graft. (b) Host A that has rejected a skin allograft from donor B is challenged interdermally 4 weeks later with donor antigen (AG) extracted from B-strain spleen cells, leading to a delayed-type hypersensitivity reaction (shown by brown bump). (c) Spleen and lymph node cells (S/LN) from host A (which had rejected a skin graft from B) are transferred to a virgin syngeneic host A (V-A). Due to the adoptive transfer, V-A rejects the graft in accelerated fashion. (d) Coculture of irradiated donor B cells (BXIr) with normal host (A) cells leads to specific sensitization (A anti-B). Upon intravenous transfer (I.V.) of these sensitized A cells to a virgin host A (V-A), accelerated rejection of donor tissue is evident.

pattern of rejection is generally mild (Banff grade I; Solez et al 1993) and responds to steroid therapy. Although chronic rejection may be accompanied by infiltration of the tissue with mononuclear cells, the mere presence of interstitial cells is rarely diagnostic except for the presence of eosinophils, a harbinger of a B-cell response that is likely to be

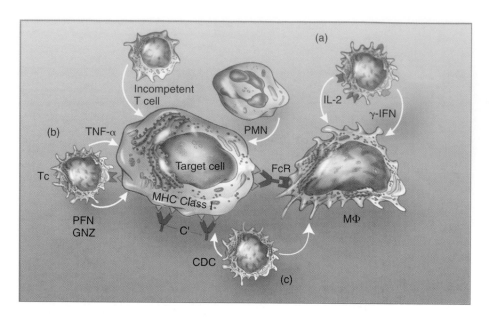

Figure 2.14. Mechanisms of target cell destruction during acute rejection. (a) Cytokines produced by delayed-type hypersensitivity T cells (T_{DTH}) recruit incompetent T cells, granulocytes (PMN) and macrophages (MΦ) to attack graft. (b) Specific Tc cells directly kill targets via TNF-α, granzyme (GNZ), and perforin (PFN). (c) Humoral response includes Abs that directly fix C' (CDC) or attach to MΦ to attack graft cells (Ab-dependent cell-mediated cytotoxicity).

pernicious. The second form of acute rejection is a vascular response, which can present as a spectrum spanning from extensive lymphocyte adhesion, to marked endothelial cell swelling, to endothelial cell proliferation with moderate-to-severe narrowing of the arterial bed and a predisposition for thrombosis (Banff grades II and III; Figure 2.16). The result of the uncontrolled acute rejection is kidney swelling, vascular occlusion, and necrosis (Figure 2.17).

Chronic

At least half of all heart and kidney organ allografts eventually succumb to chronic rejection within 10 years. After the first year of allograft survival, chronic rejection causes a continuous, 3–5% per year attrition of renal grafts (Cecka 1998). In contrast to acute rejection, chronic rejection is refractory to immunosuppressive therapy (Table 2.10).

The histologic appearance of kidney transplants undergoing chronic rejection (depicted schematically in Figure 2.18) reveals immuno-obliterative processes of arterial

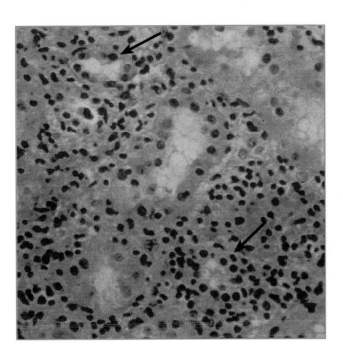

Figure 2.15. Histopathologic stigma of acute rejection: tubulitis. Arrows show lymphocytes infiltrating below basement membranes to destroy tubule cells (H&E ×40).

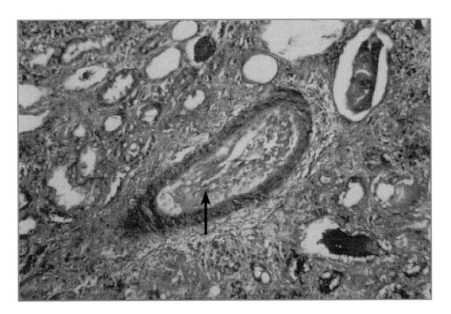

Figure 2.16. Histopathologic stigma of acute rejection: endovasculitis. Arrow shows swollen and damaged endothelium and intimal layer (Banff grade IIB; Mallory trichrome stain ×40).

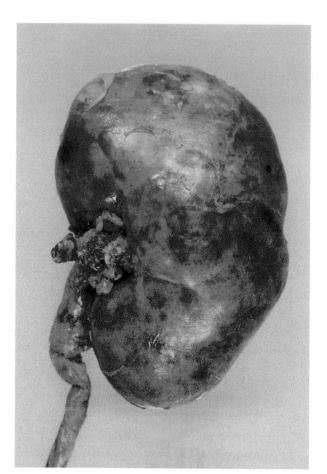

Figure 2.17. Gross appearance of an acutely rejected kidney. Note the swelling of the graft with areas of hemorrhage (deep red) and necrosis (gray).

narrowing and hyalinization, which in turn result in interstitial fibrosis, a process associated with increased expression of vascular endothelial growth factor (VEGF; Pilmore et al 1999). Initial insults are inflicted directly by alloantigen-specific T cells or by alloantigen-specific Abs, or indirectly by Abs bound through Fc receptors on macrophages or granulocytes (Figure 2.18a). Damaged endothelial cells and local macrophages initiate remodeling of the intima, which is infiltrated with smooth muscle cells (SMCs), macrophages, granulocytes, and T and B cells (Figure 2.18b). Intraintimal migration of SMCs and their proliferation upon cytokine stimulation produce the characteristic change of 'onion-skinning' (Figure 2.18b; Russell et al 1994). The cells infiltrating human kidney allografts showing histological evidence of chronic rejection display CD40/CD40L molecules, suggesting the vital role of B cells in chronic rejection (Gaweco et al 1999). Thickening and eventual disruption of the internal elastic lamina leads to intramural infiltration with T cells producing cytokines and macrophages, including vascular endothelial growth factor (VEGF).

Time of onset	>60 days
Response	Primary
Mechanism	Humoral antibody/nonantigen-dependent mechanisms
Histopathology	Vascular smooth muscle cell proliferation
Therapy	None
Success	0%

Table 2.10. Chronic rejection

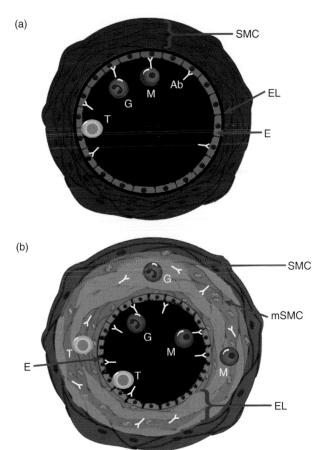

Figure 2.18. Schematic representation of mechanisms of chronic allograft rejection. (a) Chronic rejection is initiated by a continuous subclinical insult delivered to graft vessels by: antidonor Abs alone (white Y); Abs attached through the Fc receptors to monocytes/macrophages (M) or granulocytes (G); and alloantigen-specific T cells (T). Initially there are no changes observed in the internal elastic lamina (EL), endothelium (E), or in smooth muscle cells (SMCs). (b) The progressive damage induces thickening of the internal elastic lamina (EL). The underlying intima is infiltrated by migrating smooth muscle cells (mSMC), macrophages (M), granulocytes (G), alloantigen-specific T cells (T) and Abs (white Y), producing significant narrowing of the lumen. Infiltrating and local cells produce cytokine and growth factors, intensifying remodeling changes that lead to vessel obstruction, ischemia, and fibrosis.

While subclinical rejection episodes may be identified by the presence of mild histopathologic changes on surveillance biopsies, their implication for graft loss remains controversial. Activated T cells produce cytokines, which attract other cells, including macrophages. Subendothelial plaques containing macrophages are found in kidney allografts with chronic rejection (Dimeny et al 1993; Tullius et al 1994b). Macrophages are also associated with intragraft expression of fibrosis-inducing products, including IL-1, IL-6, and TNFs, as well as growth factors, basic fibroblast growth factor (bFGF), and TGF-β (Nadeau et al 1995). All these changes contribute to progressive vascular hypertrophy and glomerulosclerosis (Figure 2.19). In addition, the glomerular capillary endothelium and other renal structures exhibit increased expression of ICAM-1 and of VCAM-1 adhesion molecules (Heemann et al 1994). The vascular changes compromise arterial inflow, leading to tubular atrophy, interstitial fibrosis, and nephron scarring that

(a)

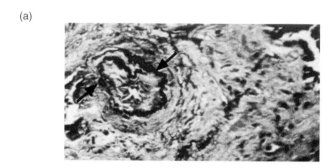

Figure 2.19. Histopathologic changes of chronic rejection in renal allografts. (a) Thickening of intima and internal elastic lamina, with breakdown of lamina producing an obliterative arterial lesion (arrowed). (b) Progression of glomerular lesion with abnormalities of the basement membrane. (c) Fibrosis and tubular atrophy due to ischemic changes (H&E ×40).

(b)

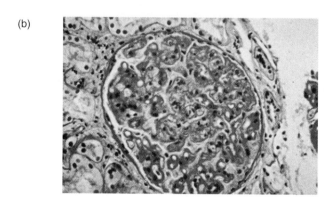

(c)

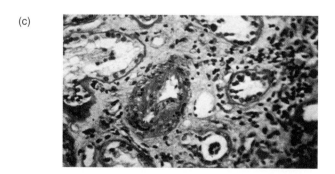

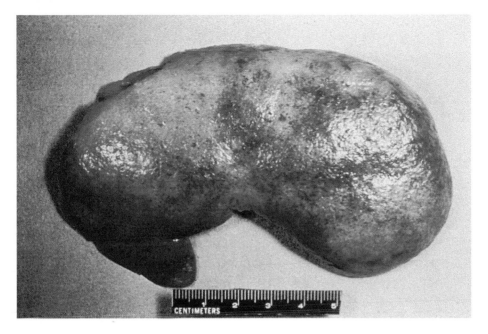

Figure 2.20. Gross appearance of a chronically rejected renal allograft.

progressively reduce renal function. The chronically rejected renal allograft appears pale at the time of nephrectomy (Figure 2.20).

Chronic kidney rejection is often associated with the presence of antidonor Abs, which correlates with histopathologic findings of arterial hyalinization (Petersen et al 1975). Patients bearing long-term kidney allografts infrequently reveal chronic rejection in the absence of HLA-specific Abs (Martin et al 1987; Barr et al 1993; Christiaans et al 1998). The 5-year graft survival of patients with antiHLA Abs was only 12%, in comparison to 76% among patients without Abs (Barr et al 1993). The most compelling evidence for the involvement of Abs in chronic rejection was the six-fold higher incidence of chronic rejection among living-related donor recipients whose sera contained antidonor HLA Abs (Abe et al 1997). In heart transplants, diffuse myointimal hyperplasia precedes the appearance of fibrosis of the coronary arteries. Although liver transplants are relatively resistant to chronic rejection, progressive destruction of bile ducts—a condition known as vanishing bile syndrome—often occurs.

In addition to these antigen-dependent factors, the development of chronic rejection seems to be influenced by nonimmunological factors, including evidence of cardiovascular compromise in the donor, prolonged cold ischemia time prior to transplantation, and impaired kidney blood flow in the recipient, all of which contribute to the ischemic/reperfusion injury (Tullius and Tilney 1995). Interestingly, reduced expression of class I or II MHC antigens in kidney allografts does not seem to diminish the severity of chronic rejection (Mannon et al 1999), suggesting that chronic antigen-independent changes result in ischemia and fibrosis of the graft (Tilney et al 1991). Results from isograft models in rats and autografts in humans (Glassock et al 1968; Tullius et al 1994b) suggest that these adverse conditions lead to progressive renal changes similar to those observed in chronic rejection. Thus, a variety of complex but independent mechanisms are capable of predisposing to, initiating, and compounding the as-yet-unidentified trigger for chronic rejection of renal allografts.

CONCLUSION

Our understanding of allograft rejection depends upon advances in basic immunologic research. Although the critical events of T cell recognition are beginning to be elucidated, the complex intracellular cascades producing T and B cell activation have been only partially defined. Substantial gaps in our knowledge remain, particularly about events that determine the type of immune response initiated by a given patient toward his allograft, and about how to redirect the mechanisms from alloaggression to allotolerance. Due to the redundancy of the cytokine mediators and cellular products, it is difficult or impossible to predict a single pathway or even multiple pathways that might mediate rejection reactions. Furthermore, to date, it has not been possible to link specific immune processes with distinct histopathologic appearances to understand the clinical impact of molecular cascades. Yet, although our knowledge of the precise events of antigen recognition is indeed limited, an understanding of the signal transduction, differentiation, and effector function properties of immune cells provides the clinician with a robust foundation to understand the mechanisms of action of immunosuppressive drugs.

REFERENCES

Abe M, Kawai T, Futatsuyama K et al (1997) Postoperative production of anti-donor antibody and chronic rejection in renal transplantation. *Transplantation* **63**:1616–1619.

Akira S, Kishimoto T (1992) IL-6 and NF-IL-6 in acute-phase response and viral infection. *Immunol Rev* **127**:25–50.

Allen RC, Armitage RJ, Conley ME et al (1993) CD40 ligand gene defects responsible for x-linked hyper-IgM syndrome. *Science* **259**:990–993.

Antonysamy MA, Fanslow WC, Fu F et al (1999) Evidence for a role of IL-17 in alloimmunity: a novel IL-17 antagonist promotes heart graft survival. *Transplant Proc* **31**:93.

Appleby MW, Gross JA, Cooke MP et al (1992) Defective T cell receptor signaling in mice lacking the thymic isoform of p59fyn. *Cell* **70**:751–763.

Austyn JM, Hankins DF, Larsen CP et al (1994) Isolation and characterization of dendritic cells from mouse heart and kidney. *J Immunol* 152:2401–2410.

Bacchetta R, Bigler M, Touraine JL et al (1994) High levels of interleukin-10 production in vivo are associated with tolerance in SCID patients transplanted with HLA mismatched hematopoietic stem cells. *J Exp Med* 179:493–502.

Barr ML, Cohen DJ, Benvenisty AI et al (1993) Effect of anti-HLA antibodies on the long-term survival of heart and kidney allografts. *Transplant Proc* 25:262–264.

Benichou G, Takizawa PA, Olson CA et al (1992) Donor major histocompatibility complex (MHC) peptides are presented by recipient MHC molecules during graft rejection, *J Exp Med* 175:305–308.

Bevilacqua MP (1993) Endothelial-leukocyte adhesion molecules. *Ann Rev Immunol* 11:767–804.

Blum JS, Cresswell P (1988) Role of intracellular proteases in the processing and transport of class II HLA antigen. *Proc Natl Acad Sci USA* 85:3975–3979.

Boehme SA, Leonardo MJ (1993) Propriocidal apoptosis of mature T lymphocytes occurs at S phase of the cell cycle. *Eur J Immunol* 23:1552–1560.

Bonnefoy-Berard N, Munshi A, Yron I et al (1996) Vav: function and regulation in hematopoietic cell signaling. *Stem Cells* 14:250–268.

Bonventre JV (1993) Mechanisms of ischemic acute renal failure. *Kidney Int* 43:1160–1178.

Borger P, Kauffman HF, Postma DS et al (1999) Interleukin-15 differentially enhances the expression of interferon-gamma and interleukin-4 in activated human (CD4$^+$) T lymphocytes. *Immunology* 96:207–214.

Boussiotis VA, Barber DL, Nakarai T et al (1994) Prevention of T cell anergy by signaling through the gamma c chain of the IL-2 receptor. *Science* 266:1039–1042.

Boutin Y, Leitenberg D, Tao X, Bottomly K (1997) Distinct biochemical signals characterize agonist- and altered peptide ligand-induced differentiation of naive CD4$^+$ T cells into Th$_1$ and Th$_2$ subsets. *J Immunol* 159:5802–5809.

Browne B, Kahan BD (1994) Renal transplantation. *Surg Clin North Am* 74:1097–1116.

Burgess AW, Metcalf D (1980) The nature and action of granulocyte-macrophage colony stimulating factors. *Blood* 56:947–958.

Bushell A, Niimi M, Morris PJ, Wood KJ (1999) Evidence for immune regulation in the induction of transplantation tolerance: a conditional but limited role for IL-4. *J Immunol* 162:1359–1366.

Bustelo XR, Barbacid M (1992) Tyrosine phosphorylation of the vav proto-oncogene product in activated B cells. *Science* 256:1196–1199.

Campanero MR, del Pozo MA, Arroyo AG et al (1993) ICAM-3 interacts with LFA-1 and regulates the LFA-1/ICAM-1 cell adhesion pathway. *J Cell Biol* 123:1007–1016.

Cantrell RW (1975) Current concepts, head and neck cancer surgery. *AORN J* 22:253–254.

Carswell EA, Old LJ, Kassell RL et al (1975) An endotoxin induced serum factor that causes necrosis of tumors. *Proc Natl Acad Sci USA* 72:3666–3670.

Cecka JM (1998) The UNOS scientific transplant registry. In Cecka JM, Terasaki PI (eds). *Clinical Transplants 1998*, Los Angeles: UCLA Tissue Typing Laboratory, pp. 1–17.

Chan AC, Kadlecek TA, Elder ME et al (1994) ZAP-70 deficiency in an autosomal recessive form of severe combined immunodeficiency. *Science* 1994 264:1599–1601.

Christiaans MH, Overhof-de Roos R, Nieman F et al (1998) Donor-specific antibodies after transplantation by flow cytometry: relative change in fluorescence ratio most sensitive risk factor for graft survival. *Transplantation* 65:427–433.

Cooke MP, Abraham KM, Forbush KA, Perlmutter RM (1991) Regulation of T cell receptor signaling by a src family protein-tyrosine kinase (p59fyn). *Cell* 65:281–291.

Coons TA, Goldberg EH (1978) Rejection of male skin grafts by splenectomized female mice. *Science* 200:320–321.

Cory GO, Lovering RC, Hinshelwood S et al (1995) The protein product of the c-cbl protooncogene is phosphorylated after B cell receptor stimulation and binds the SH3 domain of Bruton's tyrosine kinase. *J Exp Med* **182**:611–615.

Craxton A, Otipoby KL, Jiang A, Clark EA (1999) Signal transduction pathways that regulate the fate of B lymphocytes. *Adv Immunol* **73**:79–152.

Cresswell P, Avva RR, Davis JE et al (1990) Intracellular transport and peptide binding properties of HLA class II glycoproteins. *Semin Immunol* **2**:273–280.

de Waal Malefyt R, Aabrams J, Bennett B et al (1991) IL-10 inhibits cytokine synthesis by human monocytes: an autoregulatory role of IL-10 produced by monocytes. *J Exp Med* **174**:1209–1220.

Diefenbeck M, Linke R, Seehofer D et al (1998) Intravital microscopic investigation of xenogeneic microcirculation and impact of complement depletion by cobra venom factor. *Xenotransplantation* **5**:262–273.

Dimeny E, Fellstrom B, Larsson E et al (1993) Hyperlipoproteinemia in renal transplant recipients: is there a linkage with chronic vascular rejection? *Transplant Proc* **25**:2065–2066.

Downward J, Graves J, Cantrell D (1992) The regulation and function of p21ras in T cells. *Immunol Today* **13**:89–92.

Fangmann J, Dalchau R, Fabre JW (1992a) Rejection of skin allografts by indirect allorecognition of donor class I major histocompatibility complex peptides. *J Exp Med* **175**:1521–1529.

Fangmann J, Dalchau R, Sawyer GJ et al (1992b) T cell recognition of donor major histocompatibility complex class I peptides during allograft rejection. *Eur J Immunol* **22**:1525–1530.

Finkelman FD, Holmes J, Katana IM et al (1990) Lymphokine control of in vivo immunoglobulin isotype selection. *Ann Rev Immunol* **8**:303–333.

Fossiez F, Banchereau J, Murray R et al (1998) Interleukin-17. *Int Rev Immunol* **16**:541–551.

Freeman GJ, Gribben JG, Boussiotis VA et al (1993) Cloning of B7-2: a CTLA-4 counter-receptor that costimulates human T cell proliferation. *Science* **262**:909–911.

Friedman RM (1988) Interferons. In: Oppenheimer JJ, Shevach EM (eds). *Textbook of Immunophysiology*, New York: Oxford Press.

Gaweco AS, Mitchell BL, Lucas BA et al (1999) CD40 expression on graft infiltrates and parenchymal CD154 (CD40L) induction in human chronic renal allograft rejection. *Kidney Int* **55**:1543–1552.

Germain RN, Margulies DH (1993) The biochemistry and cell biology and antigen processing and presentation. *Ann Rev Immunol* **11**:403–450.

Gimbrone MA, Obin MS, Brock AF et al (1989) Endothelial interleukin 8. A novel inhibitor of leukocyte-endothelial interactions. *Science* **246**:1601–1603.

Glassock RJ, Feldman D, Reynolds ES et al (1968) Human renal isografts: a clinical and pathologic analysis. *Medicine (Baltimore)* **47**:411–454.

Glimcher LH, Kara CJ (1992) Sequences and factors: a guide to MHC class-II transcription. *Ann Rev Immunol* **10**:13–49.

Goldberg AL, Rock KL (1992) Proteolysis, proteasomes and antigen presentation. *Nature* **357**:375–379.

Gong JL, McCarthy KM, Telford J et al (1992) Intraepithelial airway dendritic cells: a distinct subset of pulmonary dendritic cells obtained by microdissection. *J Exp Med* **175**:797–807.

Gordon RD, Iwatsuki S, Esquivel CO et al (1986) Liver transplantation across ABO blood groups. *Surgery* **100**:342–348.

Gubler V, Chua AD, Schoenhaut DS et al (1991) Coexpression of two distinct genes is required to generate secreted bioactive cytotoxic lymphocyte activation factor. *Proc Natl Acad Sci USA* **88**:4143–4147.

Guttmann RD, Lindquist RR, Ockner SA (1969) Renal transplantation in the inbred rat. IX. Hematopoietic origin of an immunogenic stimulus of rejection. *Transplantation* **8**:472–484.

Hansen TH, Lee DR (1997) Mechanism of class I assembly with β_2 microglobulin and loading with peptide. *Adv Immunol* **64**:105–137.

Harris PE, Liu Z, Suciu-Foca N (1992) MHC class II binding of peptides derived from HLA-DR 1. *J Immunol* **148**:2169–2174.

Hedrick PW, Whittam TS, Parham P (1991) Heterozygosity at individual amino acid sites. Extremely high levels for HLA-A and -B genes. *Proc Natl Acad Sci USA* **88**:5897–5901.

Heeger PS, Greenspan NS, Kuhlenschmidt S et al (1999) Pretransplant frequency of donor-specific, IFN-gamma-producing lymphocytes is a manifestation of immunologic memory and correlates with the risk of posttransplant rejection episodes. *J Immunol* **163**:2267–2275.

Heemann UW, Tullius SG, Tamatami T et al (1994) Infiltration patterns of macrophages and lymphocytes in chronically rejecting rat kidney allografts. *Transpl Int* **7**:349–355.

Hibbs ML, Tarlinton DM, Armes J et al (1995) Multiple defects in the immune system of Lyn-deficient mice, culminating in autoimmune disease. *Cell* **83**:301–311.

Hostager BS, Bishop GA (1999) Cutting edge: contrasting roles of TNF receptor-associated factor 2 (TRAF2) and TRAF3 in CD40-activated B lymphocyte differentiation. *J Immunol* **162**:6307–6311.

Imboden JB, Stobo JD (1985) Transmembrane signalling by the T cell antigen receptor. Perturbation of the T3-antigen receptor complex generates inositol phosphates and releases calcium ions from intracellular stores,. *J Exp Med* **161**:446–456.

Irving BA, Chan AC, Weiss A (1993) Functional characterization of a signal transducing motif present in the T cell antigen receptor zeta chain. *J Exp Med* **177**:1093–1103.

Itoh N, Yonehara S, Ishii A et al (1991) The polypeptide encoded by the cDNA for human cell surface antigen Fas can mediate apoptosis. *Cell* 1991 **66**:233–243.

Joyce S, Tabaczewski P, Angeletti RH et al (1994) A nonpolymophic major histocompatibility complex class Ib molecule binds a large array of diverse self-peptides. *J Exp Med* **179**:579–588.

Kaissling B, Le Hir M (1994) Characterization and distribution of interstitial cell types in the renal cortex of rats. *Kidney Int* **45**:709–720.

Katz SM, Kimball PM, Ozaki C et al (1994) Positive pretransplant crossmatches predict early graft loss in liver allograft recipients. *Transplantation* **57**:616–620.

Kishimoto T, Taga T, Akira S (1994) Cytokine signal transduction. *Cell* **76**:253–262.

Klein J (1986) The gene: molecular approach (the protein). In: *Natural History of the Major Histocompatibility Complex*, New York: John Wiley, pp. 87–228.

Kühn R, Löhler J, Rennick D et al (1993) Interleukin-10 deficient mice develop chronic enterocolitis. *Cell* **75**:263–274.

Kung JT, Beller D, Ju ST (1998) Lymphokine regulation of activation-induced apoptosis in T cells of IL-2 and IL-2R beta knockout mice. *Cell Immunol* **185**:158–163.

Kurosaki T (1997) Molecular mechanisms in B cell antigen receptor signaling. *Curr Opin Immunol* **9**:309–318.

Land W, Messmer K (1996) The impact of ischemia/reperfusion injury on specific and non-specific early and late chronic events after organ transplantation. *Transplant Rev* **10**: 99–110.

Larsen CP, Morris PJ, Austyn JM (1990) Migration of dendritic leukocytes from cardiac allografts into host spleens. A novel pathway for initiation of rejection. *J Exp Med* **171**:307–314.

Lechler RI, Batchelor JR (1982) Restoration of immunogenicity to passenger cell-depleted kidney allografts by the addition of donor strain dendritic cells. *J Exp Med* **155**:31–41.

Lee HH, Dempsey PW, Parks TP et al (1999) Specificities of CD40 signaling: involvement of TRAF2 in CD40-induced NF-κB activation and intercellular adhesion molecule-1 up-regulation. *Proc Natl Acad Sci USA* **96**:1421–1426.

Lenardo M, Chan KM, Hornung F et al (1999) Mature T lymphocyte apoptosis: immune regulation in a dynamic and unpredictable antigenic environment. *Annu Rev Immunol* **17**:221–253.

Leonard WJ, O'Shea JJ (1998) Jaks and STATs: biological implications. *Ann Rev Immunol* **16**:293–322.

Li XC, Roy-Chaudhury P, Hancock WW et al (1998) IL-2 and IL-4 double knockout mice reject islet allografts: a role for novel T cell growth factors in allograft rejection. *J Immunol* **161**:890–896.

Lipman ML, Shen Y, Jeffery JR et al (1998) Immune-activation gene expression in clinically stable renal allograft biopsies: molecular evidence for subclinical rejection. *Transplantation* **66**:1673–1681.

Liu Z, Braunstein NS, Suciu-Foca N (1992) T cell recognition of allopeptides in context of syngeneic MHC. *J Immunol* **148**:35–40.

Liu Z, Sun YK, Xi YP et al (1993) Limited usage of T cell receptor V beta genes by allopeptide-specific T cells. *J Immunol* **150**:3180–3186.

Mannon RB, Kopp JB, Ruiz P et al (1999) Chronic rejection of mouse kidney allografts. *Kidney Int* **55**:1935–1944.

Martin S, Dyer PA, Mallick NP et al (1987) Posttransplant antidonor lymphocytotoxic antibody production in relation to graft outcome. *Transplantation* **44**:50–53.

McCartney-Francis NL, Wahl SM (1994) Transforming growth factor beta: a matter of life and death. *J Leukoc Biol* **55**:401–409.

McEver RP, Beckstead JH, Moore KL et al (1989) GMP-140, a platelet alpha-granule membrane protein, is also synthesized by vascular endothelial cells and is localized in Weibel–Palade bodies. *J Clin Invest* **84**:92–99.

Miyajima A, Kitamura T, Harada N et al (1992) Cytokine receptors and signal transduction. *Ann Rev Immunol* **10**:295–331.

Moore KW, O'Garra A, de Waal Malefyt R et al (1993) Interleukin-10. *Ann Rev Immunol* **11**:165–190.

Murali-Krishna K, Altman JD, Suresh M et al (1998) Counting antigen-specific CD8 T cells: a reevaluation of bystander activation during viral infection. *Immunity* **8**:177–187.

Murase N, Starzl TE, Ye Q et al (1996) Multilineage hematopoietic reconstitution of supralethally irradiated rats by syngeneic whole organ transplantation. With particular reference to the liver. *Transplantation* **61**:1–4.

Murray JE, Merrill JP, Harrison JH (1958) Kidney transplantation between seven pairs of identical twins. *Ann Surg* **148**:343–357.

Muzio M, Chinnaiyan AM, Kischkel FC et al (1996) FLICE, a novel FADD-homologous ICE/CED-3-like protease, is recruited to the CD95 (Fas/APO-1) death-inducing signaling complex. *Cell 1996* **85**:817–827.

Myburgh JA, Cohen I, Gecelter L et al (1969) Hyperacute rejection in human-kidney allografts—shwartzman or arthus reaction? *N Engl J Med* **281**:131–135.

Nadeau KC, Azuma H, Tilney NL (1995) Sequential cytokine dynamics in chronic rejection of rat renal allografts: roles for cytokines RANTES and MCP-1. *Proc Natl Acad Sci USA* **92**:8729–8733.

Nicholson DW, Thornberry NA (1997) Caspases: killer proteases. *Trends Biochem Sci* **22**:299–306.

Opelz G, Wujciak T, Dohler B (1999) Is HLA matching worth the effort? Collaborative Transplant Study. *Transplant Proc* **31**:717–720.

Osmond DG (1991) Proliferation kinetics and the lifespan of B cells in central and peripheral lymphoid organs. *Curr Opin Immunol* **3**:179–185.

Paul WE, Seder RA (1994) Lymphocyte responses and cytokines. *Cell 76*:241–251.

Pescovitz MD, Sachs DH, Lunney JK, Hsu SM (1984) Localization of class II MHC antigens on porcine renal vascular endothelium. *Transplantation* **37**:627–630.

Petersen VP, Olsen TS, Kissmeyer-Nielsen F et al (1975) Late failure of human renal transplants. An analysis of transplant disease and graft failure among 125 recipients surviving for one to eight years. *Medicine (Baltimore)* **54**:45–71.

Peugh WN, Suprina RA, Wood KJ, Morris PJ (1986) The role of H-2 and non-H-2 antigens and genes in the rejection of murine cardiac allografts. *Immunogenetics* 23:30–37.

Pilmore HL, Eris JM, Painter DM et al (1999) Vascular endothelial growth factor expression in human chronic renal allograft rejection. *Transplantation* 67:929–933

Polakis P, McCormick F (1993) Structural requirements for the interaction of p21ras with GAP, exchange factors, and its biological effector target. *J Biol Chem* 68:9157–9160.

Powis SM, Trowsdale J (1993) Major and minor histocompatibility antigens. In: Thomson AW, Catto GRD (eds). *Immunology of Renal Transplantation*, London: Edward Arnold, pp. 3–26.

Quelle FW, Sato N, Witthuhn BA et al (1994) JAK2 associates with the beta c chain of the receptor for granulocyte-macrophage colony-stimulating factor, and its activation requires the membrane-proximal region. *Mol Cell Biol* 14:4335–4341

Rammensee HG, Kroschewski R, Frangoulis B (1989) Clonal anergy induced in mature V beta 6+ T lymphocytes on immunizing Mls-1b mice with Mls-1a expressing cells. *Nature* 339:541–544.

Rammensee HG, Falk K, Rotzschke (1993) Peptides naturally presented by MHC class I molecules. *Ann Rev Immunol* 11:213–244.

Rao A, Luo C, Hogan PG (1997) Transcription factors of the NFAT family: regulation and function. *Ann Rev Immunol* 15:707–747.

Reth M (1989) Antigen receptor tail clue. *Nature* 338:383–384.

Reth M (1992) Antigen receptors on B lymphocytes. *Ann Rev Immunol* 10:97–121.

Rowley RB, Burkhardt AL, Chao HG et al (1995) Syk protein-tyrosine kinase is regulated by tyrosine-phosphorylated Ig alpha/Ig beta immunoreceptor tyrosine activation motif binding and autophosphorylation. *J Biol Chem* 270:11590–11594.

Russell SM, Keegan AD, Harada N et al (1993) Interleukin-2 receptor chain: a functional component of the interleukin-4 receptor. *Science* 262:1880–1883.

Russell PS, Chase CM, Winn HJ, Colvin RB (1994) Coronary atherosclerosis in transplanted mouse hearts. II. Importance of humoral immunity. *J Immunol* 152:5135–5141.

Samelson LE, Klausner RD (1992) Tyrosine kinases and tyrosine-based activation motifs. Current research on activation via the T cell antigen receptor. *J Biol Chem* 267:24913–24916.

Schaffer A, Cerutti A, Shah S et al (1999) The evolutionarily conserved sequence upstream of the human Ig heavy chain S gamma 3 region is an inducible promoter: synergistic activation by CD40 ligand and IL-4 via cooperative NF-κB and STAT-6 binding sites. *J Immunol* 162:5327–5336

Schonrich G, Momburg F, Malissen M et al (1992) Distinct mechanisms of extra thymic T cell tolerance due to differential expression of self antigen. *Int Immunol* 4:581–590.

Schumacher TN, Kantesaria DV, Heemels MT et al (1994) Peptide length and sequence specificity of the mouse TAP-1/TAP-2 translocator. *J Exp Med* 179:533–540.

Sherman LA, Chattopadhyay S (1993) The molecular basis of allorecognition. *Ann Rev Immunol* 11:385–402.

Shimizu Y, Van Seventer GA, Horgran KJ, Shaw S (1990) Roles of adhesion molecules in T cell recognition. Fundamental similarities between four integrins on resting human T cells (LFA-1, VLA-4, VLA-5, VLA-6) in expression, binding and co-stimulation. *Immunol Rev* 114:109–143.

Shoskes DA, Wood JR (1994) Indirect presentation of MHC antigens in transplantation. *Immunol Today* 15:32–38.

Solez K, Axelsen RA, Benediktsson H et al (1993) International standardization of criteria for the histologic diagnosis of renal allograft rejection: the Banff working classification of kidney transplant pathology. *Kidney Int* 44:411–422.

Sonoda Y, Yang YC, Wong GG et al (1988) Analysis in serum-free culture of the targets of recombinant human hemopoietic growth factors. Interleukin-3 and granulocyte/macrophage-colony-stimulating factor are specific for early development stages. *Proc Natl Acad Sci USA* 85:4360–4364.

Springer TA (1990) Adhesion receptors of the immune system. *Nature* 346:425–434.

Stahl N, Boulton TG, Farruggella T et al (1994) Association and activation of Jak-Tyk kinases by CNTF-LIF-OSM-IL-6 beta receptor components. *Science* 263:92–95.

Steiger J, Nickerson PW, Steurer W et al (1995) IL-2 knockout recipient mice reject islet cell allografts. *J Immunol* 155:489–498.

Steinman RM (1991) The dendritic cell system and its role in immunogenicity. *Ann Rev Immunol* 9:271–296.

Steinmuller D (1967) Immunization with skin isografts taken from tolerant mice. *Science* 158:127–129.

Stepkowski SM, Razo-Ahmad A, Duncan WR (1987) The role of class I and class II MHC antigens in the rejection of vascular red heart allografts in mice. *Transplantation* 44:753–759.

Straus DB, Weiss A (1992) Genetic evidence for the involvement of the lck tyrosine kinase in signal transduction through the T cell antigen receptor. *Cell* 70:585–593.

Suciu-Foca N, Harris PE, Cortesini R (1998) Intramolecular and intermolecular spreading during the course of organ allograft rejection. *Immunol Rev* 164:241–246.

Suzuki Y, Demoliere C, Kitamura D et al (1997) HAX-1, a novel intracellular protein, localized on mitochondria, directly associates with HS1, a substrate of Src family tyrosine kinases. *J Immunol* 158:2736–2744.

Szulman AE (1962) The histological distribution of blood group substances A and B in man. *J Exp Med* 115:977.

Taga T, Hibi M, Hirata Y et al (1989) Interleukin-6 triggers the association of its receptor with a possible signal transducer, gp 130. *Cell* 58:573–581.

Takahata N, Satta Y, Klein J (1992) Polymorphism and balancing selection at major histocompatibility complex loci. *Genetics* 130:925–938.

Takaki S, Murata Y, Kitamura T et al (1993) Reconstitution of the functional receptors for murine and human interleukin-5. *J Exp Med* 177:1523–1529.

Tagaya Y, Bamford RN, DeFilippis AP, Waldmann TA (1996) IL-15: a pleiotropic cytokine with diverse receptor/signaling pathways whose expression is controlled at multiple levels. *Immunity* 4:329–336.

Takeshita T, Asao H, Ohtani K et al (1992) Cloning of the γ chain of the human IL-2 receptor. *Science* 257:379–382.

Tamura T, Yamagida T, Nariuchi H (1993) Difference in signal transduction pathway for IL-2 and IL-4 production in T helper 1 and T helper 2 cell clones in response to anti-CD3. *J Immunol* 151:6051–6061.

Tarakhovsky A (1997) Xid and Xid-like immunodeficiencies from a signaling point of view. *Curr Opin Immunol* 9:319–323.

Tiemeyer M, Swiedler SJ, Ishihara M et al (1991) Carbohydrate ligands for endothelial-leukocyte adhesion molecule. *Proc Natl Acad Sci USA* 88:1138–1142.

Tilney NL, Whitley WD, Diamond JR et al (1991) Chronic rejection—an undefined conundrum. *Transplantation* 52:389–398.

Tu Y, Stepkowski SM, Chou T-C, Kahan BD (1985) The synergistic effects of cyclosporine, sirolimus, and brequinar on heart allograft survival in mice. *Transplantation* 59:177–183.

Tugulea S, Ciubotariu R, Colovai AI et al (1997) New strategies for early diagnosis of heart allograft rejection. *Transplantation* 64:842–847.

Tullius SG, Tilney NL (1995) Both alloantigen-dependent and -independent factors influence chronic allograft rejection. *Transplantation* 59:313–318.

Tullius SG, Heemann U, Azuma H et al (1994a) Early ischemic injury leads to long-term functional and morphologic deterioration of naive rat kidneys and may contribute to changes of chronic allograft rejection. *Transplant Proc* 26:2041–2042.

Tullius SG, Heemann U, Hancock WW et al (1994b) Long-term kidney isografts develop functional and morphologic changes that mimic those of chronic allograft rejection. *Ann Surg*

220:425–432.

Vitetta ES, Ohara J, Myers CD et al (1985) Serological, biochemical and functional identify of B cell-stimulatory factor-1 and B cell differentiation factor for IgG_1. *J Exp Med* 162:1726–1731.

Vitetta ES, Fernandez-Botran R, Myers CD, Sanders VM (1989) Cellular interactions in the humoral immune response. *Adv Immunol* 45:1–105.

Viville S, Neefjes Y, Lotteau V et al (1993) Mice lacking the MHC class II-associated invariant chain. *Cell* 72:635–648.

Walker NP, Talanian RV, Brady KD et al (1994) Crystal structure of the cysteine protease interleukin-1 beta-converting enzyme: a (p20/p10)2 homodimer. *Cell* 78:343–352

Wang M, Stepkowski SM, Yu J et al (1997) Localization of cryptic tolerogenic epitopes in the alpha1-helical region of the RT1.Au alloantigen. *Transplantation* 63:1373–1379.

Watschinger B, Gallon L, Carpenter CB, Sayegh MH (1994) Mechanism of allorecognition. *Transplantation* 57:572–576.

Weiss A (1991) Molecular and genetic insights into T cell antigen receptor structure and function. *Ann Rev Genet* 25:487–510.

Weiss A, Littman DR (1994) Signal transduction by lymphocyte antigen receptors. *Cell* 76:263–274.

Wiest DL, Ashe JM, Howcroft TK et al (1997). A spontaneously arising mutation in the DLAARN motif of murine ZAP-70 abrogates kinase activity and arrests thymocyte development. *Immunity* 6:663–671.

Wu D, LaRosa GJ, Simon MI (1993) G protein-coupled signal transduction pathways for interleukin-8. *Science* 261:101–103.

Xie H, Rothstein TL (1995) Protein kinase C mediates activation of nuclear cAMP response element-binding protein (CREB) in B lymphocytes stimulated through surface Ig. *J Immunol* 154:1717–1723.

Yamanashi Y, Okada M, Semba T et al (1993) Identification of HS1 protein as a major substrate of protein-tyrosine kinase(s) upon B-cell antigen receptor-mediated signaling. *Proc Natl Acad Sci USA* 90:3631–3635.

Yamanashi Y, Fukuda T, Nishizumi H et al (1997) Role of tyrosine phosphorylation of HS1 in B cell antigen receptor-mediated apoptosis. *J Exp Med* 185:1387–1392.

Yoon CH, Lee J, Jongeward GD, Sternberg PW (1995) Similarity of sli-1, a regulator of vulval development in *C. elegans*, to the mammalian proto-oncogene c-cbl. *Science* 269:1102–1105.

Zou H, Henzel WJ, Liu X et al (1997) Apaf-1, a human protein homologous to *C. elegans* CED-4, participates in cytochrome c-dependent activation of caspase-3. *Cell* 1997 90:405–413.

3 SELECTION AND PREPARATION OF THE RECIPIENT

In collaboration with M Campise*

Evaluating chronic renal failure patients as candidates for kidney transplantation is among the most difficult aspects of the transplantation enterprise. Although today very few conditions represent absolute contraindications to renal transplantation, the increasing shortage of organs and the potential risks associated with immunosuppressive therapy necessitate careful selection and preparation of the recipient (Table 3.1).

Absolute contraindications	Relative contraindications
Unresolved malignancy	Lipoprotein glomerulopathy
Ongoing metabolic disorders (oxalosis)	Sickle cell disease
Active tuberculosis	Obesity or malnutrition
Active AIDS or hepatitis	Recurrent, intractable urinary tract infection
Severe vascular disease	Peripheral vascular disease
Active intravenous drug abuse	Poorly controlled diabetes
Life expectancy <5 years	Prior malignancy
Recent myocardial infarction	Severe amyloidosis
Other end-stage organ disease (cardiac, pulmonary, hepatic)	History of noncompliance
Insufficient financial resources (for post transplant medications)	Inadequate social support
	Primary renal disease with high postoperative recurrence rate
	Severe chronic obstructive lung disease
	Walderström's macroglobulinemia
	Extremes of age
	Emotional instability, particularly psychosis
	Decreased mental capacity

Table 3.1. Exclusion criteria for renal transplantation

* Division of Nephrology and Dialysis, Ospedale Maggiore, Milan

HISTORY

The screening of candidates for renal transplantation should include a careful and complete medical history. The history may be useful to ascertain whether the renal disease has a hereditary or familial origin, information that is particularly important in cases of living-related donation. Patients with a high familial incidence of diabetes mellitus, cardiovascular disease, or neoplasia may be at increased risk for developing these complications after transplantation (Table 3.2). The history of the transplantation candidate should also include inquiries about any chronic or recurrent infections, malignancy, gastrointestinal complications, or viral hepatitis. Myocardial infarction and/or lower limb arteriopathy does not always represent a formal contraindication to transplantation, but necessitates a particularly careful evaluation. A long duration of dialysis is an independent variable associated with poorer long-term results (Montagnino et al 1997) and with an increased mortality rate (Cosio et al 1998).

The renal history should focus on the nature and duration of the original renal disease, the correct diagnosis of which is extremely important to estimate the possible risk of recurrence. Whenever possible, the transplant specialist should re-examine clinical documents and the results of the renal biopsy of the native kidneys. The severity and duration of hypertension, a condition that is usually associated with renal disease, must

---

Familial history

- Are members of the family affected by renal disease?
- Is there a strong familial history of diabetes, cardiovascular disease, neoplasia?

Candidate

- Are there possible contraindications to transplantation?
- Are there infections; neoplasia; gastrointestinal disorders; viral hepatitis; cardiac infarction; claudication; long duration and complications of dialysis?

Renal history

- What was the nature of the original renal disease (indicating risk of recurrence)?
- Were there any previous steroid or immunosuppressive treatments (drug tolerance, potential risk for overimmunosuppression)?
- In cases of previous transplant, what were the cause and the timing of allograft failure (indicating risk of loss of a retransplant)?

Compliance

- Has the patient been compliant to dietetic and therapeutic prescriptions, and does the patient have a history of smoking, or alcohol or drug abuse?

Table 3.2. Information to be obtained when taking the history of the candidate for renal transplantation

also be carefully described, since patients with a long history of poor blood pressure control are at greater risk of cardiovascular disease. The therapeutic results of and adverse reactions to vigorous or prolonged prior immunosuppressive therapy for vasculitis, lupus, rapidly progressive nephritis, or a previous transplant may forecast the events after the planned allograft. To avoid the risk of severe toxicity due to the residual effects of prior immunosuppressants and to permit recovery from a catabolic state induced by steroids, it may be necessary to postpone a planned transplantation for several months with initiation of interim maintenance dialysis.

Metabolic diseases

Diabetes mellitus

Diabetes mellitus is among the most frequent causes of end-stage renal disease (ESRD) in Western countries. Transplantation poses several additional problems in these patients: (1) an increased risk of infection, above that already engendered by immunosuppressive therapy; (2) exacerbation of the metabolic disorder as well as its common complications of hypertension and hyperlipemia, which augment the risk of cardiovascular disease, by calcineurin inhibitor and steroid immunosuppressive drugs; (3) recurrence of nephropathy in the transplanted allograft (Figure 3.1), a risk that remains

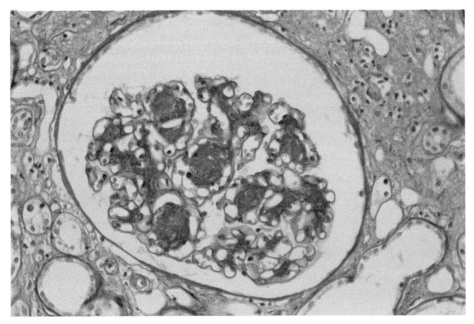

Figure 3.1. Recurrence of diabetic nephropathy in a renal transplant patient. Biopsy was performed 10 years after transplantation.

Disease	Risk of recurrence
Diabetic nephropathy	Recurrence is frequent. Progressive renal disease develops only 15–20 years after transplantation
Primary hyperoxaluria type 1	Early and constant recurrence that usually leads to allograft loss; 20–30% of patients respond to pyridoxine
Cystinosis	Possible recurrence that does not affect graft function or survival
Fabry's disease	Possible recurrence. Slow progression to graft failure
Polycystic kidney disease	No recurrence
Alport's syndrome	No recurrence. Possible development of anti-GBM antibodies (usually without clinical consequences)

Table 3.3. Risk of recurrence of metabolic or hereditary disease of the renal allograft.

relatively low until 10 years after transplantation (Najarian et al 1989) but progressively increases thereafter; and (4) hazards of reduced quality and length of life due to extrarenal complications, such as retinopathy, peripheral vascular disease, and neuropathy, even in the presence of a well-functioning kidney allograft (Table 3.3).

Despite these potential problems, renal transplantation is considered the treatment of choice for many diabetics with end-stage renal failure. However, the pretransplant investigations, particularly cardiovascular examinations of these patients, must be particularly thorough. Since atherosclerotic complications are more common and severe among diabetics (Raine et al 1992), a careful evaluation of the cardiovascular system is vital. Patients with an ejection fraction below 30% (Weinrauch et al 1992) or severe peripheral arteriopathy (Rischen-Vos et al 1992) should be excluded from consideration for transplantation, since the risk of mortality is exceedingly high.

No controlled trials have yet been performed to assess whether simultaneous pancreas and kidney transplantation reduces the long-term complications of diabetes compared with kidney transplantation alone. Simultaneous pancreas and kidney transplantation is associated with longer hospitalization times and increased morbidity rates, due at least in part to the increased risk of infection concomitant with the need for stronger immunosuppression (Rosen et al 1991; Douzdyian et al 1994). However, excellent results with a good quality of life and a high degree of rehabilitation have been reported in large series, leading some physicians to suggest that this procedure is the treatment of choice for many diabetics with end-stage renal failure (Sutherland et al 1998).

Type 1 primary hyperoxaluria

Type 1 primary hyperoxaluria is a rare autosomal recessive error of oxalate metabolism, caused by the partial or complete deficiency of alanine glycoxalate-aminotransferase (AGT) in liver cells. Lack of AGT leads to accumulation of glyoxalate, which is then oxidized to oxalate or reduced to glycolate, resulting in hyperglycolic hyperoxaluria. In infancy, the increased oxalate load leads to nephrocalcinosis and ultimately to renal failure. The disease is usually characterized by progressive nephrolithiasis resulting in renal failure within the first two decades or, in milder cases, even later in life (Marangella 1999).

The initial experience with kidney transplantation for patients afflicted with this disorder was extremely disappointing, due to the almost invariable recurrence of the disease leading to early graft loss (Figure 3.2). Therefore, oxalosis was considered an absolute contraindication to transplantation. Today, the attitude has changed, because it has been recognized that more than 20% of cases show pyridoxine sensitivity. In these patients, pyridoxine supplementation during the early posttransplant period may prevent or delay progression to renal failure. Thus, before deciding whether a patient should be considered for liver plus kidney transplantation or for kidney transplantation alone, the candidate should undergo a challenge with pyridoxine supplementation (5–10 mg/kg per day). If this treatment restores oxalate and glycolate levels to normal within a few weeks, the patient is deemed pyridoxine-sensitive. Measurement of plasma

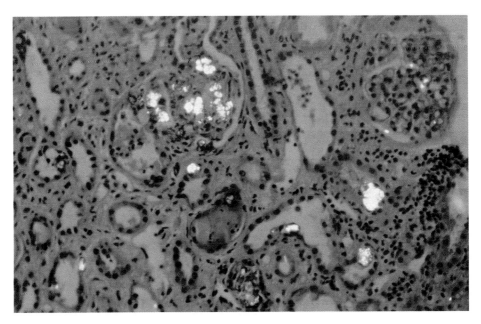

Figure 3.2. Renal biopsy taken 10 days after transplantation, showing recurrence of oxalosis in an 11-year-old child with primary oxalosis.

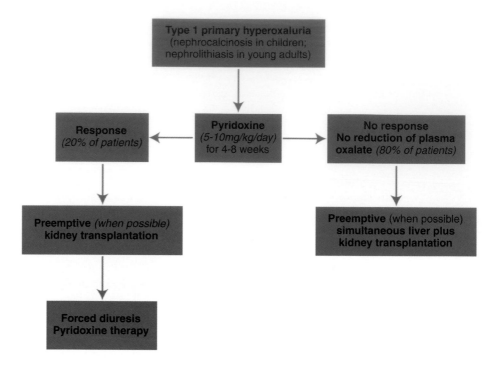

Figure 3.3. Indications to kidney transplantation or simultaneous liver and kidney transplantation in patients with type 1 primary hyperoxaluria.

oxalate concentrations per se may also indicate whether liver plus kidney transplantation is necessary. Plasma oxalate levels exceeding 50 μmol/l are usually associated with an elevated risk of calcium oxalate accumulation (Marangella 1999).

Thus, renal transplantation alone may be indicated for the few patients with pyridoxine sensitivity and relatively low plasma levels of oxalate, since the 3-year graft survival rate of these patients is about 60% (Mehls et al 1994). The best results tend to be obtained when transplantation is performed with a forced diuresis and with early administration of pyridoxine to convert glyoxalate to glycine to reduce the degree of oxalate deposition in the allograft (Scheinman 1991). For patients with more severe disease, preemptive liver–kidney transplantation is the treatment of choice. In fact, in contrast to dialysis treatments, which do not prevent accumulation of oxalate crystals in other organs, such as heart, or in bone, liver transplantation corrects the enzyme defect and facilitates excellent graft survival (Figure 3.3).

Cystinosis

Cystinosis is a rare, autosomal-recessive, metabolic defect affecting the specific lysosomal system that transports cystine outside of cells. Early administration of cysteamine may delay the onset of end-stage renal failure (Markello et al 1993). The results with kidney transplantation in cystinosis are similar to those observed with other primary renal diseases (Raine et al 1992). However, after successful transplantation, cystine continues to accumulate in other organs, including the eye and brain, as well as in muscle tissue. To prevent or limit the deleterious consequences of cystine accumulation, early and continuous administration of cysteamine is recommended.

Fabry's disease

Fabry's disease is an X-linked recessive glycosphingolipidosis characterized by accumulation of glycosphingolipids in most tissues. Hypertension and renal failure are late complications, generally occurring during the fourth or fifth decade. There are few reports of the results of renal transplantation among patients with Fabry's disease. In a review of the European experience with 12 patients, the longest survival was 66 months after a second transplant (Donati et al 1987). Infections were common and severe. A more recent report suggested that histological recurrence had no clinically relevant effect on transplant function (Mosnier et al 1991). Based on these limited experiences, Fabry's disease is not considered an absolute contraindication to renal transplantation.

Lipoprotein glomerulopathy

Lipoprotein glomerulopathy (LPG) is a newly described glomerular disease reported by Saito et al (1989). The disorder is characterized by intracapillary deposition of lipoproteins producing proteinuria, ranging from mild degrees to nephrotic range, and eventually leading to chronic renal failure, hypercholesterolemia, coronary artery disease, and Alzheimer's disease. The affected patients display a mutant phenotype due to a genetic increase in apolipoprotein E (apoE). The gene coding for this protein is located on chromosome 19; its polymorphism can result in six possible phenotypes. Of the 23 cases described to date, 21 have occurred among Japanese patients (Saito et al 1995). The four patients who underwent kidney transplant experienced disease recurrence within 7 months after transplantation, and in two cases, the recurrence was associated with a poor outcome of the allograft. Treatment with ACE-inhibitors and lipid-lowering agents has been advised to slow the progression to renal failure (Mourad et al 1998).

Inherited diseases

Alagille syndrome

Alagille syndrome, also known as arteriohepatic dysplasia (Alagille et al 1987), is the leading cause of cholestatic icterus neonatorum. It is an autosomal-dominant disease with a variable expression and a random inheritance of a deletion of the short arm of chromosome 20. A characteristic triangular-shaped face with a prominent forehead, straight nose, and pointed chin is the most common feature. The clinical findings include butterfly vertebrae, posterior embryotoxon, pulmonary artery stenosis, and a paucity of intrahepatic ducts. Liver transplantation for hepatic failure is often required in adults with Alagille syndrome. Isolated instances of renal and urinary tract involvement have been reported, such as agenesis of kidney, vesicoureteral reflux, tubulointerstitial nephritis, or IgA nephritis, although none of these disorders is diagnostic for the disease. Progression to renal failure is common in children with a full expression of the gene (Dommergues et al 1994). In contrast, underdiagnosis is possible in adult patients. Patients with Alagille syndrome who are referred for transplantation require a careful evaluation of liver function and of the vascular system, with particular attention to the pulmonic valve and the iliac arteries.

Alport's syndrome

Alport's syndrome is an X-linked hereditary disease transmitted in a dominant pattern resulting from the mutation of the COL4A5 gene, which codes for the protein α_5-chain of type IV collagen. This protein is a major and a tissue-specific constituent of glomerular basement membranes (GBM). Following transplantation, the new kidney, bearing a normal glomerular basement membrane, may elicit production of tissue-specific antibodies directed against the normal collagen chain. Although these antibodies occur in about one-third of cases, they generally have no clinical effect on the graft (Peten et al 1991; Ding et al 1994); however, rare cases of rapidly progressive glomerulonephritis have been reported. The overall outcome of renal transplants in patients afflicted with Alport's does not differ from that of recipients not affected by the disease. Thus, patients with Alport's syndrome are generally considered good candidates for renal transplantation.

Autosomal polycystic kidney disease

The outcomes of renal transplants in adult recipients afflicted with autosomal polycystic kidney disease are excellent. Because most of the patients are older than 50 years, they must be carefully screened for cardiac and neoplastic diseases. When the family history indicates intracranial bleeding, the potential recipient should undergo magnetic resonance imaging for a possible berry aneurysm, which must be treated prior to transplant. Due to the possibilities of intracystic hemorrhage, infections, stone formation, and severe hypertension (Sanfilippo et al 1984; Ben Hamida et al 1993), bilateral native nephrectomy is often indicated, preferably before rather than after transplantation. Among patients with polycystic kidney disease, the presence of diverticulosis has been associated with an increased risk of colon perforation in the early posttransplant period and during phases of increased steroid doses to treat rejection episodes (Dominguez Fernández et al 1998).

Primary glomerulonephritis

All forms of glomerulonephritis may recur after transplantation and may lead to graft failure, but the risks of disease recurrence and its consequences differ among the various subtypes of glomerulonephritis (Table 3.4).

Focal and segmental glomerulosclerosis

Of all the forms of glomerulonephritis, focal and segmental glomerulosclerosis (FSGS) is associated with the highest rate of graft failure, particularly in children. The rate of recurrence varies from 15% to 50% in different series (Ponticelli and Banfi 1997) and is even higher among children (Tejani and Stablein 1992). The risk of FSGS recurrence is particularly increased among recipients of second renal transplants (Senguttuvan et al 1990). Many patients with recurrent disease display massive proteinuria within a few days after transplantation, generally progressing to end-stage renal failure within 2 years. Unfortunately, it is difficult to predict which patients will show recurrent FSGS. Onset in childhood (Tejani and Stablein 1992), rapid progression to uremia, and the presence of diffuse mesangial expansion in the native kidneys (Cameron 1991) have been considered potential risk factors for recurrence. Other investigators failed to find an association between these parameters and FSGS recurrence (Müller et al 1998). Even more uncertain are the predisposing roles to recurrence of HLA donor–recipient haploidentity and a short duration of dialysis. The risk of recurrence in cadaveric-donor transplants is similar to that in living-donor grafts (Raine et al 1992).

Despite the risk of recurrence, FSGS is not considered a contraindication to cadaveric renal transplantation, although the use of a living donor may raise some reservations. The

Glomerular disease	Histological (%)	Clinical (%)	Graft loss (%)
Focal glomerulosclerosis	20–50	15–50	10–40
Membranous nephropathy	5–10	5–10	1–5
Membranoproliferative I	15–30 (adults)	20–25 (adults)	10 (adults)
	20–60 (children)	10–60 (children)	10 (children)
Membranoproliferative II	85 (adults)	15 (adults)	10 (adults)
	95–100 (children)	25 (children)	20 (children)
IgA nephropathy	100 (long-term)	30–50	15–30 (after 5 years)
Anti-GBM nephritis	10–30	<10	Rare

Table 3.4. Recurrence of primary glomerulonephritidies following renal transplantation

possibility of FSGS recurrence, which could destroy the allograft, must be extensively discussed with both the donor and the recipient. Early implementation of aggressive plasmapheresis or heme-adsorption with protein A columns has been suggested to reduce the degree of proteinuria and to protect renal function among a small fraction of patients afflicted with FSGS recurrence. In some cases, the prolonged use of plasmapheresis may be necessary.

Membranous nephropathy

Membranous nephropathy (MN) recurs after renal transplantation in about 20% of cases (Odorico et al 1996). No clinical or histological findings are available to allow prediction of which patients will show recurrence. Recurrence of MN has been reported to occur earlier and more frequently among living-related than cadaveric-donor recipients (Josephson et al 1994). The prognosis of recurrent MN is difficult to assess: cases of spontaneous remission of the proteinuria have occurred (Marcen et al 1996), while other workers report progressive deterioration in the majority of patients afflicted with recurrence (Josephson et al 1994). The issue is obfuscated by the observation that some transplant patients develop de novo MN, a condition that is now considered an expression of chronic rejection (Truong et al 1989) and is almost indistinguishable from recurrent MN. At present, the renal failure etiology of MN is not considered a contraindication to renal transplantation.

Membranoproliferative glomerulonephritis

An analysis of the ERA-EDTA Registry database reported a 6% rate of recurrence for type I membranoproliferative glomerulonephritis (MPGN) (Briggs and Jones 1999). Some single-center series have, however, reported higher rates of recurrence, namely, 67% (7/11) of children (Habib et al 1987) and 48% of adults (Andresdottir et al 1997). Most likely, the risk of recurrence of MPGN increases with the time of observation after transplantation. No clinical features seem to predict recurrence of type I MPGN, save for ethnicity: recurrence of MPGN is exceptional in Japanese patients (Shimizu et al 1998). Although in most cases histopathologic evaluations of kidneys displaying recurrence of type II MPGN show intramembranous dense deposits (Cameron 1991; Mathew 1991), clinical evidence of recurrent disease is much less frequent. Publications on the consequences of recurrent MPGN report quite different outcomes: the European experience suggests that 86% of patients retain graft function at 2 years after onset of recurrence—an even better rate than that seen among patients without recurrence (Briggs and Jones 1999)—while Andresdottir et al (1997) report a mean graft survival of only 40 months following the diagnosis of recurrence. At present, neither type I nor type II MPGN is considered a contraindication to renal transplantation.

IgA nephropathy

Recurrence of mesangial deposits of IgA in the renal allograft is common among patients with IgA nephropathy (IgAGN). The prevalence of recurrence depends largely on the time of transplant biopsy, being around 50% at 2–5 years and almost 100% at 10–20 years (Lee and Glassock 1997). As is the case for other primary glomerulonephritidies, no clinical or histological factors have been identified that predict the risk of posttransplant recurrence of IgAGN. However, patients with IgAGN are generally considered good candidates for renal transplantation. Some series reported no difference in graft survival rates between patients with and without IgAGN (Kim et al 1996; Bumgardner et al 1998); others reported even better graft survival rates among patients with IgAGN (Alamartine et al 1994).

Anti-GBM glomerulonephritis

Linear glomerular deposits of IgG may occur in 10–30% of transplant patients with anti-GBM glomerulonephritis (anti-GBM GN; Glassock 1997). Clinical disease is rare and usually mild, but graft failure does occur in at least a small fraction of patients. Among patients who do not display circulating anti-GBM antibodies at the time of transplantation, recurrence of anti-GBM GN has never been reported (Senguttuvan et al 1990). Thus, it is recommended that the blood of the potential recipients be tested for anti-GBM antibodies, and that renal transplantation be delayed until they have completely disappeared—a process that usually takes 6–12 months.

Systemic diseases

Systemic lupus erythematosus

Patient and graft survival rates of patients with lupus nephritis are similar to those of patients with other primary renal diseases (Clark and Jevnikar 1999). However, centers report wide variations in the outcome of allografts, probably due to differing criteria for the selection of transplant recipients. The risk of recurrent lupus nephritis is extremely low (Stone et al 1997), and the histological lesions in transplant patients with recurrent disease tend to be mild (Nyberg et al 1992).

The major posttransplant problems in lupus patients are not caused by recurrence of SLE in the graft, but by extrarenal complications related either to the disease itself or to previous steroid and/or other immunosuppressive drug treatments. Cardiovascular disease frequently occurs, and represents a leading cause of morbidity and mortality. The persistence of circulating immune complexes, hyperlipidemia, hypoalbuminemia, arterial hypertension (Moroni et al 1992), antiphospholipid antibodies (Lockshin 1992), and hyperhomocysteinemia (Petri et al 1996)—frequent complications of SLE—may be responsible for the increased risk of accelerated atherogenesis after transplantation. Pretransplant corticosteroid therapy may further exacerbate cardiovascular complications (Ettinger et al 1987), as well as produce severe osteoporosis, diabetes mellitus, myopathy, and cataracts, which impair the quality of life of these patients. Finally, both lupus per se (Abu-Sharka et al 1996) and previous immunosuppressive therapy may expose transplant recipients to an increased risk of malignancy, particularly non-Hodgkin's lymphoma. For these reasons, the evaluation of transplant candidates must accurately describe the disease and complications, particularly the cardiovascular conditions, possible existence of an underlying cancer, and bone mineral density, of patients with a long history of SLE. While the activity of lupus quenches under dialysis therapy, frequently allowing complete cessation of steroid treatment, other patients stabilize only when treated with daily doses of 5–10 mg prednisone. For more frail patients, we recommend a 1–2-year waiting period before transplantation for stabilization and recovery from the metabolic and toxic effects of steroids and other immunosuppressive agents (Ponticelli et al 1998).

Henoch–Schönlein purpura

The short-term results of patients transplanted after a primary renal disease of Henoch–Schönlein purpura are similar to those obtained with other diseases (Briggs and Jones 1999). While histologic evidence of recurrence of the mesangial deposits containing IgA may occur in about half these patients, clinical recurrence has been reported in less than 20% of cases (Meulders et al 1994). Clinical recurrence is more likely in children, as well as in patients with active disease at the time of transplantation (Nast et al 1987). To reduce the risk of recurrence, it may be safer to postpone renal transplantation for at least 18 months after the last manifestation of activity.

Amyloidosis

Amyloidosis is a systemic disease that may involve several organs (Figure 3.4) and may lead to death due to infections, cardiovascular disease, or progressive cachexia. Moreover, the risk of recurrence of disease in the kidney transplant is approximately 10–40% (Heering et al 1989; Hartman et al 1992). Although transplantation should be discouraged for patients with severe sequelae of amyloidosis (Kasiske et al 1995), individuals affected by familial Mediterranean fever may be exempted from this exclusion, since early and regular administration of colchicine can prevent intrarenal deposits of amyloid substances (Livneh et al 1992). In addition, acceptable results of renal transplantation have also been obtained in young patients with concomitant rheumatoid arthritis.

Hemolytic uremic syndrome

The risk of recurrence of hemolytic uremic syndrome (HUS) ranges between 2% (Gagnadoux et al 1999) and 45% (Hebert et al 1991). The risk is higher among children and among patients who display a rapidly progressive course of their primary disease. While HUS presents no formal contraindication to renal transplantation once the candidate has achieved hematological quiescence as evidenced by an absence of ongoing hemolysis

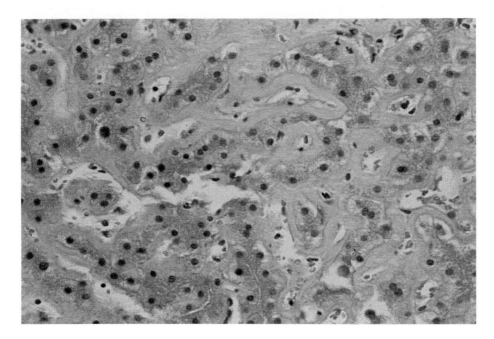

Figure 3.4. Hepatic amyloidosis. Perisinusoidal deposition of amyloid in the space of Disse. Hematoxylin and eosin stain (H&E) ×75. (Courtesy of Dr MF Donato, Ospedale Maggiore, Milan, Italy.)

and thrombocytopenia, some measures have been suggested to prevent recurrent disease. Hypertension must be treated vigorously, and bilateral nephrectomy should be considered in cases of primary disease refractory to treatment. It has been suggested that the use of cyclosporine, tacrolimus, or antilymphocyte antibodies should be avoided after transplantation, since these agents have been associated with recurrent or de novo HUS (Hebert et al 1986; Doutrelepont et al 1992). However, a large series reported only one case of recurrent HUS among 44 cyclosporine-treated renal transplant children (Gagnadoux et al 1999). No association has been found between HUS and sirolimus therapy.

Vasculitis

Polyarteritis

After transplantation, patients with polyarteritis display lower 3-year patient (77% versus 91%) and graft survival rates (60% versus 69%) compared to patients with other primary renal diseases (Briggs and Jones 1999). Cardiovascular complications accounted for 54% of the deaths. Since only three of 112 patients lost their allograft due to recurrent disease, the inferior outcomes have been attributed to the older mean age, longer period of pretransplant immunosuppressive therapy, and widespread small-vessel involvement among patients with polyarteritis. Thus, renal transplantation may be successful for well-selected recipients affected with polyarteritis. However, patients who have received vigorous immunosuppression prior to the onset of ESRD should wait several months before being transplanted, and must be carefully evaluated for concomitant cardiovascular disorders.

Wegener's granulomatosis

Neither patient nor graft survival rates at 3 years differed significantly between 115 transplant patients with Wegener's granulomatosis compared to transplant patients with other primary renal diseases (Briggs and Jones 1999). The recurrence rate of this disease is low (Wrenger et al 1997). Good results were obtained even among patients with short intervals between clinical onset and transplantation, as well as among antineutrophil cytoplasmic antibody (ANCA)-positive patients with symptoms of acute disease (Schmitt et al 1994). Despite these good results, however, caution is required, since Wegener's is a multisystem disease that can cause severe involvement of various organs, particularly the lungs. Moreover, most of these patients have received intensive steroid and immunosuppressive therapy before dialysis, rendering them more susceptible to infections, cardiovascular disease, and neoplasia after transplantation. Therefore, a thorough evaluation must be performed before accepting a patient with Wegener's vasculitis as a transplant candidate.

Cryoglobulinemia nephritis

Little information is available about the outcome of cryoglobulinemia nephritis after transplantation. Although there was a high rate of recurrence among a few patients transplanted because of this disease, this recurrence did not seem to jeopardize the outcome of the allograft (Tarantino et al 1994). Since most patients who develop the disease due to hepatitis C virus-related cryoglobulinemia die from vascular complications, liver failure, or infections, a careful evaluation of these systems must be performed and hypertension strictly controlled prior to transplantation.

Analgesic nephropathy

A recent European review reported the results of renal transplantation among 798 patients with analgesic nephropathy (Briggs and Jones 1999). Although the mean age of patients affected by this disease was slightly older—53 years compared to 39 years for patients with other primary renal diseases—the 8-year graft survival rates were similar, namely, 51% versus 47%, and the patient survival rates, 61% versus 77%, respectively. Death from neoplasia was three times more frequent among patients with analgesic nephropathy, particularly urothelial tumors, which accounted for most of the cancers (Kliem et al 1996a).

This disorder does not represent a contraindication to transplantation, provided that the patient stops taking analgesic drugs. During the evaluation, the patient should undergo cystoscopy and retrograde ureteropyeloscopy. A bilateral nephroureterectomy should be considered prior to transplantation to prevent the development of urothelioma in the native upper tracts, and the transplant procedure should be performed using the Leadbetter–Politano antireflux technique to reduce the risk of colonization of malignant cells in the allograft. After transplantation, the urine should be regularly examined for the presence of malignant cells.

Waldenström's macroglobulinemia

Very few patients with Waldenström's macroglobulinemia have undergone renal transplantation (Bradley et al 1988), due to a major risk of death from sepsis. Recurrences have been reported, and about half of the grafts are lost. Thus, patients with Waldenström's macroglobulinemia are poor candidates for renal transplantation.

Light-chain deposition disease/myeloma

Only a few patients afflicted with light-chain deposition disease/myeloma have been transplanted, because it is generally recognized that the rates of disease recurrence as well as death caused by the original disease or its treatment are high. The rare cases who experienced prolonged graft survival were patients who were in remission after intensive therapy with melphalan and corticosteroids prior to transplantation (Gerlag et al 1986). At present, patients with this disease should not be considered for transplantation.

Sickle-cell disease

The experience with renal transplantation for patients with sickle-cell disease is limited. A recent publication reported that although the incidences of delayed graft function and acute rejection were similar to those observed for other renal diseases, the 3-year patient (59%) and graft (47%) survival rates were poor (Ojo et al 1999). Even among the few successful cases, patients experience persistence of painful crises that may produce erythrocyte sickling in the allograft (Montgomery et al 1994); thus, renal transplantation must be undertaken with great caution and only in the absence of recent sickling crises (Barber et al 1987). In the rare case of an available HLA-identical sibling donor free of sickle-cell disease, consideration should be given to combining bone marrow or stem cell transplantation with kidney transplantation (Ribot 1999). Special preparation prior to the transplant procedure must include transfusion of 4–6 units of hemoglobin AA blood (with recipient phlebotomy as necessary) and liberal use of sodium bicarbonate to maintain the blood at an alkaline pH and thus reduce the proclivity to sickling.

Paroxysmal hemoglobinuria

Paroxysmal hemoglobinuria is characterized by nocturnal hemoglobinuria, hemolytic anemia, and thrombosis. Renal failure may develop due to vascular thrombosis or iron overload. Although a successful case of renal transplantation has been recently reported (Vanwalleghem et al 1998), the long-term risks of malignancy or of allograft deterioration remain unknown.

Medullary cystic disease/nephronophthisis

Medullary cystic disease or nephronophthisis does not pose any particular problem for transplant candidacy.

Scleroderma

The overall results of renal transplantation for patients with scleroderma are considerably worse than those observed in other renal diseases (Nissenson and Port 1990). In particular, patients afflicted with cardiac, pulmonary, or gastrointestinal involvement should not be considered for transplantation. Since many affected patients have severe hypertension, pretransplant bilateral nephrectomy is generally recommended for suitable candidates.

Fibrillary glomerulopathy

Fibrillary-immunotactoid glomerulopathy is an ultrastructural entity characterized by extracellular deposition of nonbranching microfibrils or microtubules within the mesangium and capillary walls of renal glomeruly. Since the initial description by Rosenmann and Eliakim in 1977 more than 200 cases have been reported (Rosenmann and Eliakim 1977). Patients with fibrillary-immunotactoid glomerulopathy present with nephrotic range proteinuria, microscopic hematuria, hypertension, and renal insufficiency in about 50% of cases. The progression to end-stage renal failure occurs within 4 years after diagnosis. Little information is available on the results of renal transplantation for this rare disease. Fibrillary deposits can recur in about 50% of cases after renal transplantation. However, the decline of glomerular filtration rate in transplanted is slower than in native kidneys so that a satisfactory renal function can be maintained for at least 5 years (Pronovost et al 1996; Brady 1998). Thus transplantation has to be considered as a possible option for these patients.

PHYSICAL EXAMINATION

Following the interview in which a full medical history is obtained, a general screening examination should be conducted. This screening should give special attention to the exit wound of the peritoneal dialysis catheter or the site of the arteriovenous fistula/graft, either of which represents a potential site of infection. In patients with adult polycystic kidney disease, the size of the kidneys should be evaluated to determine whether nephrectomy is required to afford adequate space for the placement of a renal allograft. In addition to cardiac auscultation, the physician should search for bruits in the carotid arteries, the aorta, and the lower limb vessels as evidence of arteriosclerotic disease. Evaluation of the dorsalis pedis and posterior tibial pulses may help to discern the better side to place the allograft with less risk of vascular steal from the distal arterial circulation. To complete the physical examination, men should undergo a rectal examination to detect polypoid neoplasms as well as a prostate palpation, and women, a gynecological examination.

PSYCHOLOGICAL EVALUATION

Although many candidates exhibit active symptoms of or a predisposition to psychiatric disorders or have a history of substance abuse, a psychiatric evaluation is generally not an integral part of the screening procedure for transplantation (De Geest et al 1995). However, the physician should use his own skills of psychological evaluation during the initial examination to assess the patient's motivation for and likelihood of compliance with the posttransplant regimen. Poor patient compliance to the posttransplant medical regimen represents one of the most frequent causes of graft loss (Didlake et al 1988). Although only a small number of patients display complete noncompliance, which almost inevitably results in graft failure, about 22% of patients will admit on intense inquiry posttransplant that they take some but not all the prescribed drugs. These cases of occasional noncompliance may eventuate in late rejection episodes, leading to graft loss (Kiley et al 1993). Thus, patients who in the past have not followed therapeutic or dietetic prescriptions as evidenced by sporadic attendance for dialytic treatments, who have refused to stop smoking, or who have an ongoing saga of alcohol or drug abuse are not good candidates for transplantation.

LABORATORY INVESTIGATIONS

A series of laboratory investigations should be performed to complete the evaluation process (Table 3.5). Prior to transplantation, some investigations should be repeated,

Immunologic evaluation

- Blood group
- HLA tissue typing (A, B, DR)
- Preformed anti-HLA antibodies

Hematology

- Complete blood count with leukocyte differential
- Platelet counts
- Bleeding time
- Prothrombin time
- Partial thromboplastin time

Renal evaluation

- Serum creatinine
- Serum electrolytes
- Urine culture
- Parathormone level

Metabolic evaluation

- Blood sugar (basal and postprandial)
- Glycosylated hemoglobin (for diabetics)
- Plasma (serum) triglycerides and cholesterol
- Homocysteine

Infections

- Hepatitis markers (A, B, C)
- HBV DNA if HBV-positive
- HCV RNA if HCV-positive
- anti-HIV antibodies
- Epstein–Barr virus titer
- Herpes virus titer
- Toxotest
- Purified protein-derived (PPD) skin test

Gastrointestinal evaluation

- Stool guaiac
- Serum amylase, lipase
- Serum transaminases, bilirubin, cholinesterase

Table 3.5. Primary laboratory investigations for the renal transplant candidate

particularly serum potassium, erythrocyte and leukocyte counts, serum calcemia, blood glucose, liver function tests, and, in selected cases, serum cholinesterase (to avoid the risk of curarization in the case of low levels).

Splenectomy

Indications

Splenectomy was initially advocated as a maneuver to modify the immune response, since the spleen is a major site of antibody production from its germinal centers. Indeed, Hume (1972) recommended splenectomy for immunomodulation to facilitate acceptance of repeat renal transplants. Although this indication for splenectomy is poorly understood and not widely accepted, the usual reason for pretransplant splenectomy is clinical hypersplenism. Many patients with leukopenia and/or thrombocytopenia have an associated degree of splenomegaly. Once the physician has excluded a diagnosis of primary bone marrow aplasia, excess destructive activity represents the logical cause of the cytopenia, and the spleen, a likely site. Persistent cytopenia posttransplant may limit the doses of the antiproliferative purine synthesis antagonists (azathioprine or mycophenolate mofetil), or G_1 build-up inhibitors (sirolimus or SDZ RAD).

Procedure

With the patient in a 30° left-rotated position, a midline, subcostal, or left paramedian incision represents a convenient approach for the procedure. Once the retroperitoneum has been incised, a rolled towel is inserted posteriorly to elevate the spleen. Injuries to the adjacent pancreatic tail during control of the splenic vein or to the greater curvature of the stomach during control of the short gastric vessels pose higher morbidities in ESRD patients than in other individuals. For the initial 24 hours postoperatively, nasogastric suction is preferable; thereafter, alimentation is progressively introduced over a variable time course, but rarely requiring more than 72 hours to return to the preoperative diet. Fortunately, transplant candidates rarely display thrombocytosis requiring long-term aspirin therapy, since their bone marrow tends to be quiescent or only mildly hyperreactive prior to the procedure. Administration of Pneumovax prior to splenectomy has been recommended to minimize the risk of pneumococcal bacteremia posttransplant, although in many cases the vaccine fails to elicit neutralizing immunoglobulin production in ESRD patients and poses the theoretical possibility of antibody cross-reactivity with histocompatibility antigens.

Subtotal parathyroidectomy

Indications

Pretransplant parathyroidectomy may be considered in cases of severe osteodystrophy accompanied by hypercalcemia as well as elevated parathormone and alkaline phosphatase levels (see below). Although renal failure is frequently associated with secondary hyperparathyroidism, the severity and rate of progression of the disorder can generally be controlled by vigorous medical and dialytic therapy. In some patients, the parathyroid glands gain autonomous function, acting independently of the serum calcium concentration.

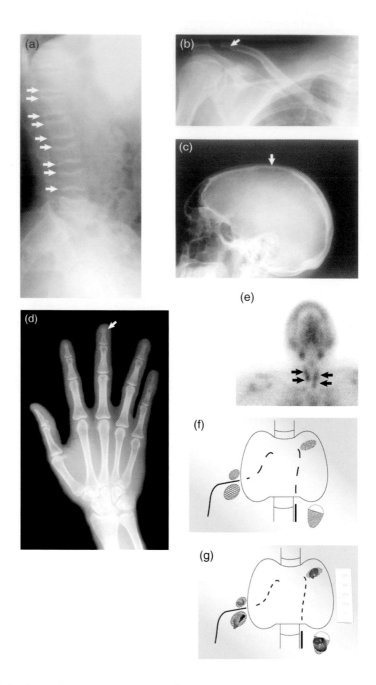

Figure 3.5. Bone changes characteristic of the osteodystrophy caused by hyperparathyroidism. (a) 'Rugger jersey' appearance of lumbar spine. (b) Resorption of distal clavicle. (c) Salt-and-pepper appearance of the calvarium. (d) Resorption of subungual tufts. (e) Sestamibi parathyroid scan showing glands as areas of uptake indicated by the arrows. (f) Diagrammatic representation of location of glands visualized at surgery. (g) Onlay of surgical specimens of hyperplastic parathyroid tissue onto diagram.

These patients display evidence of severe osteodystrophy, including a 'salt-and-pepper' configuration of the bones of calvarium; resorption of the lamina dura of the teeth, of the subungual tufts of the distal phalanges, and/or of the distal end of the clavicle; rib fractures; and/or vertebral body decalcification leading to a 'rugger jersey' appearance, particularly of the lower lumbar vertebrae (Figure 3.5). If not detected prior to the transplant, the condition is likely to progress thereafter to tertiary hyperparathyroidism requiring parathyroidectomy. Furthermore, there must be a suspicion that the hyperparathyroidism represents the primary etiology of ESRD, particularly when there is evidence of associated kidney stone disease or nephrocalcinosis. An additional indication for an aggressive approach to subtotal parathyroidectomy prior to transplantation is the proclivity of immunosuppressive agents—particularly steroids—to exert osteopenic effects that exacerbate the hyperparathyroidism, predisposing to accelerated bone loss and fracture. Furthermore, hyperparathyroidism is not infrequently associated with tissue calcification; for example, skin lesions producing pustules as foci of infection, or coronary arterial deposition predisposing to the progression of arteriosclerotic disease. Thus, subtotal parathyroidectomy permits at least stabilization of the osteolytic disorder, and possibly partial recalcification of the skeleton, prior to transplantation.

Procedure

A transverse neck incision is placed one finger's breadth above the suprasternal notch, exploiting a natural crease in the neck and extending 1 cm lateral to the edge of each sternocleidomastoid muscle (Figure 3.6a). After incision of the platysma muscle, which is then used for retraction, a plane is developed superior to the level of the hyoid bone and inferior to the clavicles (Figure 3.6b). A midline incision then separates the strap muscles (Figure 3.6c), which are either divided in their distal third or left intact and retracted laterally. The superior parathyroid gland is usually identified at the inferior cornu of the thyroid cartilage, the site where the recurrent laryngeal nerve penetrates the tracheal membrane. The inferior glands have a more variable location, tending to be anterior and adjacent to the inferior thyroid artery, but not infrequently lying within the thymic tongue, the carotid sheath, or even the thyroid gland (Figure 3.6d).

After identification of the four parathyroid glands, three and three-quarters of the glands are resected (Figure 3.6e), leaving a remnant of one-quarter of one gland. It is generally convenient to leave a specific gland remnant—for example, a piece of the left inferior parathyroid. It must be ensured that the remnant is adequately vascularized before the other glands are removed. It is most convenient to control bleeding from the gland fragment using a piece of sternocleidomastoid muscle, which releases tissue thromboplastin and thus provides hemostasis in the fashion described by Cushing using a flap of temporalis muscle to control bleeding from the brain surface.

A difficult issue arises when only three parathyroid glands are identified despite an intensive search from the hyoid bone to the thymic tongue in the cephalocaudad plane, across from one carotid sheath to the other, and posterior to the esophagovertebral space. In this instance, a total parathyroidectomy may be performed, and four or five thin slices, which in toto represent about the size of one-third of one gland, are implanted in the sternocleidomastoid muscle using metal sutures for subsequent identification (Figure 3.7). Since the fragments require more than 5 days to gain a blood supply, determination of the serum parathormone level on day 4 provides a diagnostic tool to assess the presence of a missing gland. If the parathormone level is low, it is likely that all parathyroid tissue has been identified. If the level is above normal, the patient is likely to have an unidentified gland. If the clinical laboratory has the capacity to perform parathormone levels on a short time line, this tool can be used to direct a parathyroid exploration; alternatively, samples may be obtained to assist a future exploration to find the errant gland (Reitz et al 1969).

While radionuclide scans to identify the locations of the parathyroids seem to be neither necessary nor valuable as a routine tool, radionuclide scanning may be useful in the case of an unidentified gland. Re-exploration of the neck at an interval of 3–6 months after the first procedure must include not only the area within the previous field,

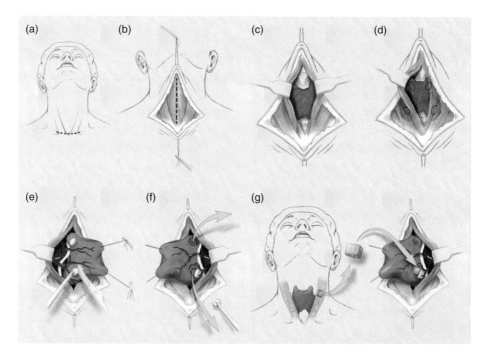

Figure 3.6. Procedure for subtotal parathyroidectomy. (a) Low transverse neck incision—a wry smile. (b) Development of subplatysmal superior and inferior flaps. Dotted line shows incision in midline with (c) retraction of strap muscles. (d) Exposure of thyroid gland. The positions of parathyroid glands are indicated by dotted ovals. (e) Exposure of glands on right side with excision of lower gland; note that the recurrent nerve crosses lateral to medial on the right. (f) Dissection of glands on left (note that the recurrent nerve lies medial along the trachea), with excision of two-thirds of the left lower gland. (g) Harvest of a fragment of sternocleidomastoid muscle, which is placed onto the remaining fragment for hemostasis.

but also, if this survey is unsuccessful, sternal splitting to gain access to the upper mediastinum. The latter measure is necessary because the aberrant parathyroid gland may lie as low as the aortic valve, as it did in the classic case of Captain Martel described by Cope (1966).

Postoperative management

Particularly in instances of high serum alkaline phosphatase values, the patient may display profound 'bone hunger'. Although the parathyroid hormone level generally reaches its nadir at 48–72 hours, supplemental intravenous delivery of calcium may be required as soon as 6 hours postoperatively. During the first 24 hours, the patient receives nothing by mouth, to avoid friction of the mobile esophagus against the paratracheal sutures. During this period, calcium must be delivered intravenously as 1–2 g of the gluconate formulation every 1, 2, or 4 hours, depending on the extent of the downward trend of serum calcium values. Once alimentation has begun, oral calcium (1–2 g four times daily) and vitamin D (0.25–0.5 µg twice daily) supplementation are initiated and continued for several months in conjunction with the use of high calcium content

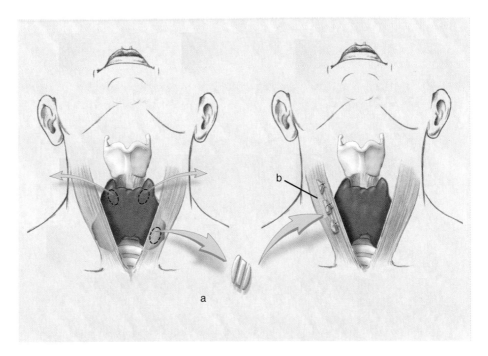

Figure 3.7. Procedure for cases in which only three parathyroid glands are identified. (a) Schematic representation of resection of three glands, one of which is sliced into 2-mm segments (for diagrammatic purposes, the figure suggests that the slices are much thicker). (b) Implantation of gland fragments in sternocleidomastoid muscle, with each fragment fixed with a metal suture.

dialysis bath fluids, until there is evidence of recalcification of the skeleton and stabilized serum calcium values within the normal range. Calcium absorption and recalcification are promoted by avoiding an acidotic state in the recipient. In some instances, magnesium supplementation may also be required by the oral route to facilitate skeletal reossification.

Immunological aspects

The ABO blood group as well as HLA-A, -B, and -DR antigens should be determined once the individual is deemed a transplant candidate. Even in the era of modern immunosuppression, increasing numbers of HLA mismatches appear to correlate with a stepwise decrease in the rate of cadaveric graft survival (Opelz 1997). In addition to estimating the extent of preformed cytotoxic antibodies at the time of acceptance for transplantation, sera should be collected at least every 2 months thereafter, both to ascertain the state of sensitization and to have materials on hand for crossmatch testing against a potential donor. The extent of presensitization may afford an index to predict the risk of graft failure: the risk is minimal if the patient bears antibodies against less than 10% of unrelated individuals in a panel, intermediate if the fraction is between 11 and 50%, and high if the fraction exceeds 50% (Feucht and Opelz 1996). Presently, the extent of sensitization among renal transplant candidates is declining, because fewer patients are receiving multiple random or donor-specific blood transfusions. In the past, this approach seemed to have a beneficial effect on allograft survival (Opelz and Terasaki 1978), but carried the risk of induction of cytotoxic antibodies or of infection with hepatitis viruses (Kahan 1984). After the advent of cyclosporine, the policy of deliberate pretransplant transfusions was almost abandoned (Flechner et al 1984). However, a recent study suggests that even cyclosporine-treated patients may experience an additional beneficial effect on cadaveric organ allograft survival by the administration of blood transfusions before transplantation (Opelz et al 1997), provided that they do not experience sensitization or viral infections therefrom. However, in view of the excellent results that are obtained with modern immunosuppressive therapy, most transplant units do not recommend deliberate pretransplant transfusions for immune conditioning.

EVALUATION OF INFECTIONS

Candidates for renal transplant must be screened for the presence of infection. Obviously, the discovery of a potentially life-threatening infection represents a formal contraindication to transplantation. One important occult site of infection is the teeth: poor dental hygiene presents an immediate and ongoing risk; repair of dental caries and necessary tooth extractions should be completed prior to transplantation. While Panorex views of the jaws are useful, they seem to be unnecessary when the patient has undergone a thorough examination by a dentist. Active infections at access sites for hemodialysis are also considered exclusions from transplantation, pending completion of at least a 2-week course of antibiotics and, in resistant cases, removal of the infected graft. Although it is generally recommended that immunosuppression be withheld from dialysis patients who have experienced peritonitis within the previous 3–4 weeks (Kasiske 1998), candidates for well-matched organs have been successfully transplanted despite recent episodes of cured peritonitis. HIV-positive patients should be disqualified from transplantation, since immunosuppressive therapy places them at elevated risk of disease progression. Patients with a previous history of tuberculosis and/or a positive reaction to purified protein-derived (PPD) mycobacterial skin tests should be considered for specific prophylaxis with isoniazid for 6 months pre- and at least the same interval posttransplant. It is useful to know whether the patient bears antibodies directed against cytomegalo-, Epstein–Barr, or varicella-zoster virus.

GASTROINTESTINAL EVALUATION

An abdominal ultrasound is recommended for patients who are symptomatic, diabetic, or aged more than 45 years. In view of the risk of posttransplant peptic ulcer disease, a gastroscopy is routinely conducted by many, but not all, centers. Patients with colonic disease or aged above 60 years should be evaluated by barium enema and, if indicated, by colonoscopy. In the case of repeated or severe bouts of diverticulitis, preemptive surgical resection may be indicated. Although little information is available about strategies for candidates who have previously experienced pancreatitis, problems due to lipid disorders or to alcohol abuse should be corrected prior to transplantation. Exclusion, by endoscopic retrograde cholangiopancreatography, of a precipitating disease within the biliary tree or of abnormalities of the pancreatic ductal tree may be necessary prior to acceptance for transplantation.

Cholecystectomy

Indications

Similar to the indications for cholecystectomy in surgical practice on non-ESRD patients, the presence of gallstones per se is usually not a sufficient cause for operative intervention. However, in transplant candidates or posttransplant patients, the occurrence of just one bout of acute cholecystitis represents a sufficient indication for operative intervention, particularly if accompanied by cholangitis, biliary colic, and/or gallstone pancreatitis. In contradistinction to most other medical conditions in ESRD patients, gallstone disease is likely to be exacerbated posttransplant, since both the endecapeptide cyclosporine and the macrocyclic lactones tacrolimus and sirolimus, as well as their metabolites, are excreted in, and increase the lithogenicity of, bile. Whereas in the

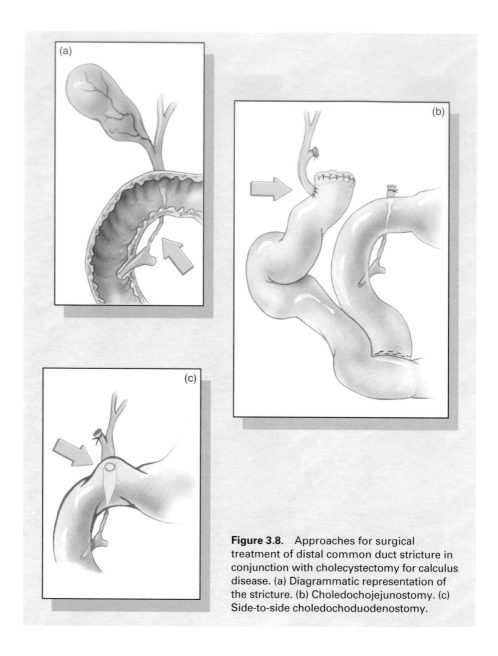

Figure 3.8. Approaches for surgical treatment of distal common duct stricture in conjunction with cholecystectomy for calculus disease. (a) Diagrammatic representation of the stricture. (b) Choledochojejunostomy. (c) Side-to-side choledochoduodenostomy.

pretransplant period the gallstones tend to be large and solitary or, at most, modest in number and readily visualized by abdominal ultrasonography, in the posttransplant period new stones tend to be formed as small fragments of mixed composition. While many ESRD patients display elevated serum amylase levels or lipase values, it is rare to document pancreatic lesions either by computerized tomography (CT) scan or by endoscopic retrograde pancreatography in the absence of a history of acute or chronic pancreatitis or polycystic pancreatic disease.

Procedure

Isolated gall bladder disease without another indication for laparotomy may be approached laparoscopically; also, the procedure can be utilized electively if the patient has been on a stable immunosuppressive regimen with steroid doses less than 10 mg for at least 6 months. While operative approaches may be necessary for adjunctive choledochotomy and common duct exploration, transendoscopic papillotomy, due to its lower rate of morbidity, is generally preferred to open procedures for sphincterotomy. Among patients who experience unsuccessful papillotomy or display a distal fibrous common duct stricture (Figure 3.8a), choledochojejunostomy (Figure 3.8b) has been recommended because it offers the advantage of less reflux of acidic content into the biliary tree. However, choledochoduodenostomy (Figure 3.8c) has been associated with excellent results in our experience, without incurring the adverse sequelae of a stagnant bowel segment.

Colectomy

Indications

Diverticular disease and/or colonic perforations frequently represented lethal concurrent complications of the intense immunosuppressive regimens required in the azathioprine–prednisone era, probably due to the massive doses of steroids generally required to reverse rejection crises. In contrast, these colonic complications do not carry the high risk of a morbid outcome in the cyclosporine era (Rigotti et al 1986). Thus, the presence of colonic diverticula associated with a previous bout of diverticulitis no longer represents an absolute indication for colectomy; a more conservative approach, usually based on an expectant philosophy, now guides the surgeon. In planning the transplant procedure in an aged patient with extensive sigmoid diverticulosis, it may be judicious to implant the allograft on the right side so as not to steal blood supply that normally collateralizes from the internal iliac artery via the middle hemorrhoidal vessel to interanastomose with the superior hemorrhoid artery at the critical point of Sudeck in the sigmoid colon (Figure 3.9).

The occurrence of diverticulitis or, particularly, a colonic perforation during the early postoperative period may represent a surgical emergency. Transplant patients with known diverticular disease who experience inflammation that fails to respond significantly within 48 hours, as evidenced by clinical signs and laboratory tests despite treatment with vancomycin, fortaz, and clindamycin, should be considered to have a presumptive abscess and probably a perforation. As with other surgical patients, instillation of barium must be avoided, but an abdominal CT examination (without contrast) can provide information on the location, size, and presence of perforation, adherent small bowel, and/or peritoneal exudation. A history of diverticulitis refractory to antibiotic therapy may also represent an indication for intervention pretransplant. Another colonic problem frequently encountered is polyposis. Indeed, the extensive screening procedures within the pretransplant evaluation have decreased the rate of colon cancer among transplant recipients to an incidence lower than that seen among normal adult populations.

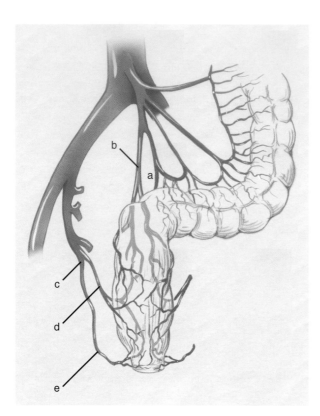

Figure 3.9. Collateral blood supply to the left colon. (a) Critical point of Sudeck. (b) Superior hemorrhoidal artery from inferior mesenteric artery. (c) Internal pudendal artery termination of left internal iliac artery. (d) Middle hemorrhoidal artery. (e) Inferior hemorrhoidal artery.

Procedure

The usual site of complications is the sigmoid colon. In the elective setting, colectomy with end-to-end colo-colostomy is performed in the usual fashion. In the emergent setting, a conservative approach is preferable: exteriorization of the site of perforation, combined with construction of a diverting transverse colostomy, accompanied by intense antibiotic therapy. In the three-stage procedure, the diverting colostomy is followed at a 6-week interval by a sigmoid colectomy with colo-colostomy, and in the third stage (6 weeks later), by closure of the colostomy. When less inflammation is present or when, due to a short mesentery, the colon cannot be delivered to the skin surface, it may be necessary at the initial operation to perform a sigmoid colectomy with an end colostomy of the descending colon and a Hartman turn-in of the rectosigmoid segment, preferably below the peritoneal shelf (Figure 3.10). Closure of the colostomy by side-to-end anastomosis to the turn-in is generally delayed until 3–6 months after the event, depending upon the degree of immunosuppression. For example, patients receiving intense antirejection therapy, particularly with steroids, should have a delayed approach to the colo-colostomy

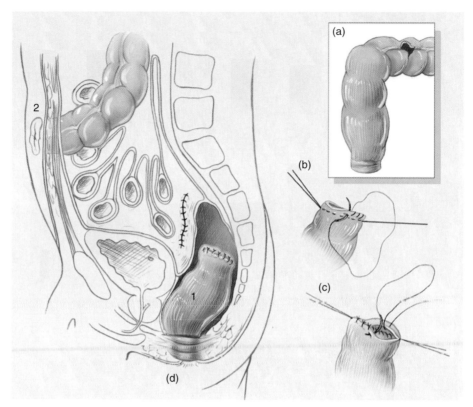

Figure 3.10. Surgical treatment of sigmoid colon perforation. (a) Frequent site of perforation corresponding to point of Sudeck. (b) First layer turn-in of Hartman pouch with a basting stitch to oppose the bowel walls, followed by an over-and-over continuous suture. (c) Second layer of interrupted nonabsorbable sutures placed in Lambert fashion. (d) Sagittal section showing the retroperitoneal position of (1) the Hartman turn-in and (2) the end colostomy.

anastomosis or to the closure of the colostomy. A gravity Gastrografin barium enema may be useful to assure adequate patency of the colo-colostomy, since recipient vascular disease may predispose to an anastomotic stricture. The operative procedure associated with the greatest morbidity is a subtotal colectomy, usually performed due to massive gastrointestinal bleeding from extensive diverticular or cytomegalovirus disease. The approach associated with the least morbidity is a total colectomy with an end ileostomy and a Hartman turn-in of the rectosigmoid segment. Closure of the ileostomy as an ileoproctostomy may be fraught with complications, due not only to the tenuous blood supply, but also to the possibilities of chronic low-grade infection and poor nutrition.

Cardiovascular investigations

- Repeated measurements of blood pressure
- Chest X-ray
- Electrocardiogram (at rest, after effort or chemical stress)
- Echocardiography
- Myocardial scintigraphy (particular cases)
- Coronary angiography (particular cases)
- Abdominal aorta echography
- Carotid echo color Doppler ($>$50 years)
- Lower limb echo color Doppler (heavy smokers, older patients)

Nephrourological investigations

- Echography (kidney, bladder, prostate)
- Cystography (when appropriate)
- Urodynamic tests (when appropriate)

Gastroenterologic investigations

- Upper abdomen echography
- Gastroscopy
- Barium enema or colonoscopy

Gynecological investigations

- Pelvic and annexal echography
- Mammography ($>$40 years)
- Pap test

Table 3.6. Primary investigations in renal transplant candidates

UROLOGICAL INVESTIGATIONS

While the patient history generally guides investigations of the urinary apparatus, several diagnostic tools can be exploited to assess risks in transplant candidates (Table 3.6). An abdominal CT or an ultrasonographic investigation may reveal nephrolithiasis versus abnormal renal masses or acquired cystic disease. Although the utility of routine voiding cystourethrograms has been challenged due to the cost and the potential morbidity of the procedure, it does afford useful information about the presence and extent of vesicoureteral reflux, the size of the bladder (and anomalies such as trabeculations or diverticula of its surface), as well as post-void residua. In some cases, this study may provide the information that guides a pretransplant bilateral nephroureterectomy, bladder augmentation, bladder neck revision, prostrate resection, or intermittent self-catheterization programs, respectively. Cystography has been recommended by some workers only for patients with pyuria, massive crystalluria, a positive urine culture, or previously diagnosed urologic abnormalities (Shandera et al 1993).

Nephroureterectomy

Indications

Probably the most frequent pretransplant surgical consideration is the patient's need for nephrectomy without or with ureterectomy (Table 3.7). Pretransplant nephrectomy is *mandatory* in some instances: clear evidence of a nidus for infection, including staghorn calculi, renal cortical abscess, or the presence of resistant organisms on urine culture; evidence of malignant renovascular hypertension, particularly by renal vein renin determinations; or the presence of a mass suggestive of malignancy, the incidence of which is increased among ESRD patients. The goals of nephrectomy for these indications are to clear a potential nidus for septicemia, to ameliorate hypertension, and to eliminate a neoplastic focus. Preoperative bilateral nephrectomy is preferable but not mandatory in other cases: the diagnosis of chronic pyelonephritis with an ongoing or a recent history of

Indication	Rationale	Etiology
Mandatory	Ongoing infection	Staghorn calculus
		Renal cortical abscess
		Resistant organisms by urine culture
	Malignant hypertension	Renovascular disease
		Idiopathic unresponsive to medical therapy
	Renal mass	Rule out malignancy
Preferable	Eliminate potentially infective site	History of pyelonephritis
		Ureteral reflux: grade 3
	Renal hemorrhage requiring transfusion	Polycystic kidney disease

Table 3.7. Indications for nephrectomy

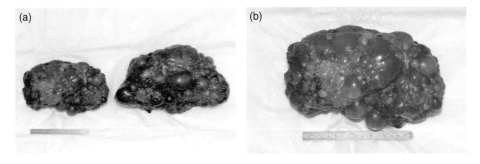

Figure 3.11. Adult polycystic renal disease. (a) Anterior surface of kidneys removed from a 50-year-old patient showing evidence of hemorrhage (dark cysts). (b) Posterior surface of right kidney showing cysts filled with turbid infected fluid.

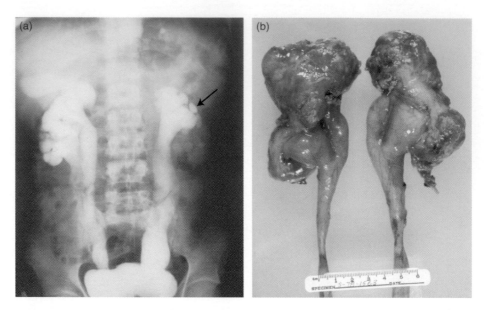

Figure 3.12. Ureterovesicle reflux. (a) Voiding cystourethrogram showing bilateral reflux with hydroureter, hydronephrosis, and caliectasis (shown by the arrow). (b) Operative specimen after bilateral nephroureterectomy.

infection, of ureteral reflux into the renal calyces, or of polycystic kidney disease with a history of intrarenal hemorrhage requiring blood transfusions and/or recurrent infections (Figure 3.11). In these cases, it is possible (but not preferable) to delay the nephrectomy procedure to 3 months posttransplant, using a cover of antibiotics during the early post-transplant period. When patients display chronic infections with organisms that are relatively resistant to antibiotics, such as *Citrobacter freundii* and *Acinetobacter calcoaceticus*, nephrectomy should not be delayed. Whenever possible, the procedure should be limited to a unilateral nephrectomy to allow continued production of erythropoietin and of urine by the remaining kidney, at least during the waiting interval before transplantation.

A second set of considerations is the need for ureterectomy as indicated by the presence of vesicoureteral reflux on voiding cystourethrogram (Figure 3.12). Some degree of urinary reflux is not infrequently observed among ESRD patients, since bladder disuse may alter the anatomic relation of the ureter to the bladder. The decision to perform ureterectomy demands evidence of grade 3 reflux into the renal pelvis, accompanied by evidence of ureteral or calyceal dilation, or the presence of urinary tract infection, particularly with an organism other than those frequently associated with primary infections such as β-hemolytic streptococci, *Escherichia coli*, or *Enterococcus faecium*. If ureterectomy is indicated, the entire ureter must be extirpated to the level of the bladder. The decision to perform ureterectomy should not be made lightly; postoperative complications of necrosis or stenosis of the donor ureter are most easily addressed using a host ureter.

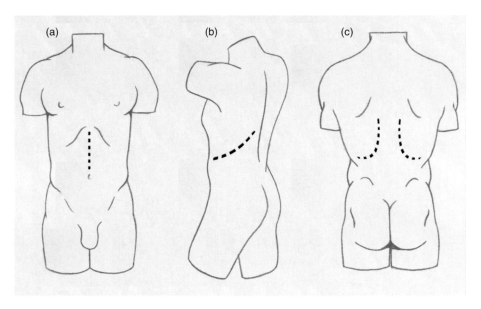

Figure 3.13. Approaches for protransplant nephrectomy. (a) Transperitoneal approach via a midline incision. (b) Flank approach. (c) Translumbar approach.

Procedure

The usual approach for bilateral nephrectomy is transperitoneal via an upper midline incision (Figure 3.13a). This approach offers the opportunity to explore the peritoneal cavity for unsuspected disease, to perform adjunctive procedures such as cholecystectomy, as well as to gain adequate access for total ureterectomy. The transperitoneal approach (Figure 3.13a) may be contraindicated in patients receiving maintenance peritoneal dialysis, since the procedure will disrupt the therapy and thus necessitate institution of hemodialysis. Alternative approaches include individual nephrectomies via a costal approach (Figure 3.13b)—for example, in patients with a colostomy or an ileostomy—or via a bilateral nephrectomy by translumbar approaches (Figure 3.13c). However, the last approach does not offer adequate exposure for either ureterectomy or the removal of large kidneys (Table 3.8).

Preoperative antibiotics must be instituted based upon bacterial sensitivities from urine cultures; if no bacterial identification is available, cephalosporins are usually used as a prophylactic measure. The patient is admitted to the hospital on the day of surgery. Using the transperitoneal approach, the left nephrectomy requires incision of the white line of Toldt, followed by medial retraction of the splenic flexure of the colon after division of the lienocolic and lienorenal ligaments. In many ESRD patients, the kidneys are small and difficult to identify, since they may only be the size of a walnut. Gerota's fascia is incised and the renal surface exposed (as shown for the living-donor nephrec-

Approach	Disadvantage	Advantage
Transperitoneal	Intestinal ileus Increased risk of pneumonia and deep venous thrombosis	Opportunity for full exploration Ready approach for bilateral nephrectomy Permits extirpation of entire ureter to bladder
Costal	Limited visualization of ureter at bladder Requires two incisions to perform bilaterally	Reduced incidence of intestinal ileus
Translumbar	Cannot remove large kidneys or perform ureterectomy	Least possibility of intestinal ileus May continue peritoneal dialysis

Table 3.8. Relative advantages of various approaches for nephrectomy.

tomy, Figure 4.11. Thereafter, serial ligation and division of the ureter, renal artery, and renal vein facilitate extirpation. Surgical misadventures that damage the spleen or the pancreas may cause serious postoperative complications. The right nephrectomy is performed in similar fashion, exerting care to gain hemostatic control of the short renal vein and to avoid traction on the hepatorenal ligament that strips the liver capsule from the hepatic surface. Postoperatively, nasogastric suction is used for the first day, with progressive alimentation thereafter. The extirpated kidneys must be cultured for bacteria and fungi; the presence of infection demands a course of at least 14 days of antibiotic therapy rather than the usual 5-day prophylactic course.

Bladder augmentation or replacement

While agenesis is rare, many ESRD patients have defunctionalized bladders. The stigma of this condition is a small bladder volume as visualized on voiding cystourethrogram. Urodynamic evaluation can determine the distensibility of the bladder, as well as its nervous and/or muscular responses to volume expansion. A small, nondistensible fibrotic bladder is unlikely to become an adequate reservoir posttransplant. Bladder augmentation may employ detubularized segments of cecum, dilated distended ureters, or ileum (Figure 3.14). These procedures are successful if coordinated contraction can be achieved. When the defunctionalized bladder displays excess irritability, the use of Ditropan can facilitate the return to more normal contractile function.

In some cases, the bladder is deemed an unsuitable reservoir. Although the initial approach to this problem was the anastomosis of native ureters to the sigmoid colon (Coffey 1911), this procedure has been abandoned due to the development of metabolic

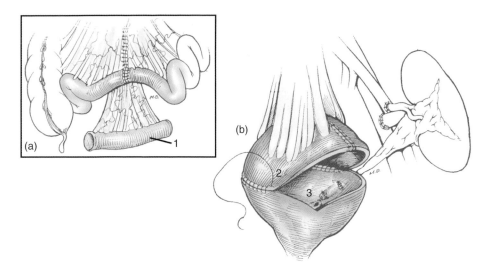

Figure 3.14. Augmentation of the bladder by a detubularized segment of ileum. (a) Isolation of an ileal segment (1). (b) Detubularized segments (2) sewn onto dome of bladder. Also shown is the implantation of transplant ureter into native bladder (3) below the augmentation site.

and other complications. Simple intestinal conduits, particularly from the ileum, have become the more widely utilized procedures (Bricker 1950). (The initial construction of the conduit and its use are described in Chapter 5. However, 20% of patients develop stomal complications, and 30% of the renal units become dilated.

Thus, there has been growing interest in continent urinary diversion, particularly utilizing vascularized, detubularized bowel. These reservoirs store urine at low pressure while preserving continence, but do not afford coordinated contraction and require catheterization to empty their contents. The construction of a continent, catheterizable conduit between the skin and the reservoir would seem to be the ideal procedure; however, 30% of patients experience problems with the continence mechanism, which is a sphincter constructed with periumbilical muscle. Other workers have explored orthotopic replacement of the bladder utilizing the membranous urethra and the distal sphincter to achieve continence. Although this procedure is performed most frequently for patients who have undergone cystectomy for cancer, it requires a wide dissection with disruption of neurovascular bundles and results in a 10–15% rate of incontinence with nocturnal leakage (Wenderoth et al 1990). Voiding is achieved by abdominal straining and pelvic floor relaxation, although 10–30% of patients require intermittent self-catheterization and 15% experience recurrent urinary infections. The secretion of mucus in the neo-bladder constructed of intestinal tissue produces not only difficulties in catheterization due to urethral and bladder neck strictures, but also the formation of bladder stones with consequent urinary tract infections. Therefore, compared with ileal diversion, orthotopic bladder replacement has been associated with higher rates of mortality and morbidity. In addition, the induction of hyperchloremic acidosis due to bicarbonate loss from the small intestinal mucosa (Nurse and Mundy 1989) may inhibit renal resorption of calcium and production of 1,25-hydroxycholecalciferol, leading to bone demineralization, which may in turn exacerbate the clinical bone disease either in ESRD patients or in transplant recipients treated with steroids and calcineurin inhibitors. Generally, deprivation of the amount of ileum used to construct the reservoir is not sufficient (namely, less than 50 cm) to produce vitamin B12 deficiency and consequent impairment of bile acid absorption mediating uptake of fats and fat-soluble vitamins. A cryptic form of diarrhea is also not infrequently encountered (N'Dow et al 1998). Because the overall results of these procedures are not entirely satisfactory, it is to be hoped that in the future tissue engineering using expanded populations of urothelial and smooth muscle cells can reconstruct a urinary bladder, as has been accomplished in the dog (Oberpenning et al 1999).

Prostatic resection

As the age of transplant recipients increases, more male patients display evidence of benign prostatic hypertrophy. Since most transplant candidates have a small urine output, it is probably premature to address the bladder outlet obstruction problem prior to successful transplantation unless a percutaneous cystostomy is created to fill the bladder intermittently. The lack of a transurethral urine output tends to predispose patients to urethral stricture formation. In general, it is preferable to perform transurethral resections after successful transplantation.

CARDIOVASCULAR EVALUATION

Indications

Since cardiovascular disease is one of the leading causes of mortality in renal transplant recipients, efforts should be made to assess the cardiac status of each potential candidate (Figure 3.15). Well-known risk factors for cardiovascular disease include diabetes, a smoking habit, elderly age, prior myocardial infarction, congestive heart failure, angina pectoris, a long history of dialysis, and/or poorly controlled hypertension. Exercise (or sestamibi-induced stress) electrocardiograms, echocardiography (with exercise or dobutamine), and thallium scintigraphy (with exercise or dipyridamole) have been performed to assess the cardiovascular risk after transplantation. Unfortunately, these tests, whether used alone or in combination, display insufficient sensitivity and specificity.

Thus, in diabetic patients, in all candidates over the age of 60 years, or in the pres-

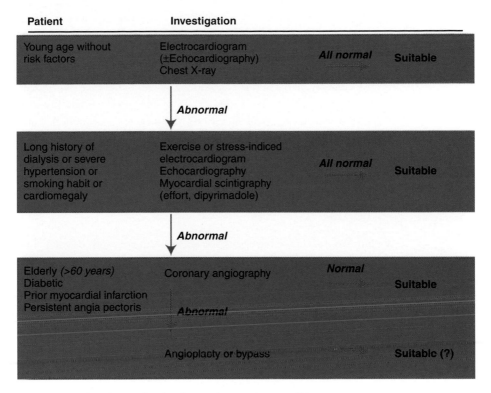

Figure 3.15. Cardiac evaluation in renal transplant candidates

ence of abnormal results on screening examinations, coronary angiography remains the best tool to evaluate the cardiovascular risk and the need for revascularization (Lorber et al 1987). Although placement of a well-functioning allograft may improve fluid status and thereby partially reverse functional impairment—such as an ejection fraction as low as 20% due to persistent uremic or congestive causes—the possibility of such a benefit is unpredictable. A more judicious approach is to address significant coronary obstruction pretransplant by performance of aortocoronary bypass grafts. Manske et al (1992) reported that more than 80% of diabetics who were submitted to coronary revascularization for transplantation remained free of cardiac events for 2 years, compared with 20% of patients who were given medical treatment. Because even a patient who undergoes surgical intervention may not sufficiently improve to be a suitable candidate, we recommend repeat echocardiography 6 months after the procedure in order to assess its benefits.

A peripheral vascular examination helps to determine the site for and the technical feasibility of transplantation. Placement of the allograft constitutes an appreciable vascular 'steal' from the extremity, particularly in the presence of an ipsilateral arteriovenous graft (Bloss et al 1979). Additionally, color Doppler studies of the carotid are recommended for symptomatic patients, as well as for asymptomatic patients who display either a bruit or risk factors for atherogenic complications. Patients with a previous history of hypercoagulability, as evidenced by repeated bouts of thrombophlebitis or recurrent occlusions of arteriovenous fistulas should be screened for antibodies directed toward clotting factors and/or phospholipids, and stabilized on anticoagulant therapy prior to the transplant. The abdominal X-ray may show calcifications in the iliac vessel, a condition that may pose challenges for the vascular anastomoses. Echography may be useful to exclude aortic aneurysms as well as abdominal masses or abnormal liver parenchyma (Table 3.6).

Surgical procedures

With the overall advancing age of transplant recipients and the general recognition of an increased degree of vascular disease severity among ESRD patients, arterial reconstructions are becoming more frequent preoperative procedures. Virtually every transplant center requires, on the same occasion as a coronary angiography, a contrast examination of the distal abdominal aorta, iliac arteries, and distal leg arterial trees. This screening procedure has generally been extended to most patients over the age of 60 years. Among patients who do not have an indication for coronary angiography, a useful screening tool is a noninvasive Doppler examination comparing ankle to brachial compression ratios.

Isolated disease in one or two coronary arteries is usually managed with percutaneous transarterial catheter dilatation with placement of intravascular stents, reserving coronary artery bypass surgery for patients with more extensive disease. Since the outcome of stenting or bypass procedures cannot be reliably predicted, it is important to estimate the cardiac ejection fraction following convalescence, as early as 4 and usually at 6 months postoperatively, but prior to the transplant. If the patient remains on the waiting list for more than 1 year thereafter, followup studies are needed to assure preservation of adequate cardiac performance.

Peripheral vascular approaches seek to assure adequate blood inflow to the renal transplant, as well as to the leg, via the iliac system. Preoperative correction of aortoiliac occlusions is performed using aortoiliac or aortofemoral bypass, femoral artery (particularly adductor canal) occlusions by femoropopliteal bypass (or percutaneous transluminal stenting), and more distal lesions by femorotibial bypass. While there may be isolated areas of stenosis in the common or proximal iliac vessels that are theoretically amenable to the placement of stents, most surgeons prefer to replace (or, rarely, to endarterectomize) these segments. Aortoiliac bypass grafts are more useful than aortofemoral grafts, because the former allow retention of a segment of host iliac artery for construction of the anastomosis to the transplant (Figure 3.16). Preservation of the native artery overcomes the intimal proliferative response when the renal artery is sewn to a prosthetic graft. Generally, it is preferable to wait at least 6 weeks between the vascular reconstruction and the transplant procedure.

Treatment of vascular disease distal to the iliofemoral arterial junction must be indi-

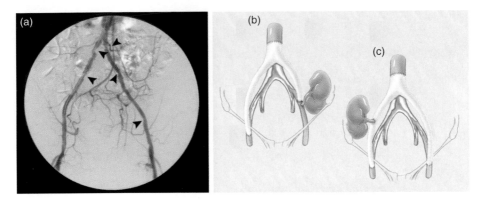

Figure 3.16. Aortoiliac vascular disease. (a) Contrast angiogram showing multiple areas of atherosclerotic disease (with arrowheads). (b) Aorto-right femoral and left iliac y-graft for vascular bypass (allowing placement of the kidney to the distal left external iliac artery). (c) Anastomosis of the transplant to the distal portion of an aortobifemoral bypass.

vidualized, depending on the presumed impact of the blood steal through the graft. One condition that can exacerbate any vascular insufficiency is the presence of an arteriovenous graft for hemodialysis access (Bloss et al 1979). A second condition that affects the physician's judgment in this situation is the diagnosis of diabetes mellitus, particularly with a history of ischemic vascular disease. The presence of skin breakdown, ulceration, rubor, or claudication represents contraindication to immediate transplant, necessitating intervention in the presence of large vessel disease or prophylactic amputation in the presence of small vessel disease.

PULMONARY EVALUATION

The risk of postoperative respiratory complications has markedly decreased since the introduction of cyclosporine immunosuppression for renal transplantation. However, pneumonia is a not-uncommon complication in the postoperative period and may become life threatening. To reduce the incidence and severity of pneumonitis, patients who smoke should be advised to stop prior to transplantation. Patients with bronchiectasis or repeated pulmonary infections are at high risk of severe pneumonia and should be excluded from transplantation unless a complete and prolonged sterilization can be obtained with antibiotic prophylaxis, frequently combined with either segmentectomy or lobectomy of a particularly virulent nidus of lung parenchyma.

PRETRANSPLANT EVALUATION IN SPECIAL SETTINGS

Pediatric recipients

Very young children have a high incidence of perioperative problems that result in increased mortality rates (Tejani et al 1994). Moreover, transplant complications are more frequent; for example, the incidence of renal vessel thrombosis is higher among children weighing less than 10 kg (Arbus et al 1986). Therefore, some pediatricians prefer to maintain infants on a regular dialysis program and to postpone the transplant by 1–2 years until the size of the recipient offers a better chance of success. The results are usually good among recipients above 5 years of age, although inferior to those observed among patients aged 16–38 years (Raine et al 1992). Two main factors may explain the lower rate of graft survival in children: a higher immunoreactivity, leading to an elevated risk of irreversible acute rejection, and a poorer rate of compliance, which has often been associated at least in part with the loss of self-esteem due to the metabolic side effects of corticosteroids and to the cosmetic toxicities of cyclosporine.

Growth represents a particular problem in children. Despite good renal function, some children do not experience growth catch-up; they remain at the tenth percentile of height compared to their peers. The problem is due to a large extent to administration of steroids, which inhibit growth hormone receptors. Indeed, reduction in the dose of or complete withdrawal from steroids may facilitate normal growth among children whose epiphyses have not yet closed (Ghio et al 1992). Administration of growth hormones may also be helpful. Growth rates generally increase by two- to three-fold during the first year of hormonal therapy, subsequently declining but remaining above the baseline. While one small study suggests that treated patients experience an increased risk of acute or chronic rejection associated with a decline in creatinine clearance levels (Fine 1997), there are no long-term data on adverse allograft outcomes or on the oncogenic risk of growth hormone therapy among transplant patients.

Aged recipients

Until recently, patients over 60 years of age were not considered suitable candidates for transplantation, due to the increased risk of cardiovascular complications (Le et al 1994). However, as the mean age of the dialysis population has progressively increased (EDTA Registry 1996) and the results of transplantation have improved, many centers are tending to accept transplantation candidates in their eighth decade. However, this policy must be tempered with an aggressive diagnostic approach to discover underlying heart disease among elderly candidates, since cardiovascular disease represents the leading cause of death and since it has been reported that about half the elderly patients who died of a cardiovascular event following transplantation were asymptomatic at the time of their inclusion on the waiting list (Cantarovich et al 1994). Moreover, screening of elderly patients must include an exhaustive search for and correction of infective foci.

While the risks of cardiovascular and infectious complications are higher among elderly patients, the incidence and the severity of acute rejection episodes among this group are lower than in younger patients (Terasaki et al 1988). Immunosuppressive therapy should be tailored to a less vigorous approach, for example, by prompt and expeditious withdrawal of steroids from a calcineurin-inhibitor-based regimen.

Although overall life expectancy is obviously lower among elderly than among younger transplant recipients, graft survival times among well-selected elderly recipients are comparable to those of young adults (Cantarovich et al 1994; Ismail et al 1994; Tesi et al 1994). Furthermore, elderly patients who fulfill the eligibility criteria for transplantation display 5-year patient survival rates that are significantly higher than those of individuals maintained on dialysis (Segoloni et al 1998). A recent paper suggests that the improving results of transplantation outweigh the risks of elderly age. For example, the success rates among 20-year-old patients who underwent transplantation between 1983 and 1990 were equal to those of 70-year-old patients undergoing transplantation between 1991 and 1993 (Roodnat et al 1999). Some transplant surgeons prefer to use cadaveric donor kidneys from aged donors for transplants to older recipients, a strategy that was initially claimed to result in inferior survival rates (Basar et al 1999). However, the pure graft survival rates, namely, the graft survival rates after deaths have been excluded, appear to be similar among older versus younger recipients of a kidney from a donor aged above 60 years (Solà et al 1998). Again, improved survival rates appear to outweigh the increased risk of the donor age: the relative risk of graft failure was lower for a patient transplanted between 1994 and 1997 with a kidney from a donor aged 75 years than for a patient engrafted between 1983 and 1990 with an organ from a donor aged 30 years (Roodnat et al 1999).

Obesity

Both patient and graft survival rates are significantly poorer in obese than in nonobese patients (Holley et al 1990; Halme et al 1997), mainly due to cardiovascular complications and to the proclivity of morbidly overweight patients to develop infective complications, not only in the wound, but also systemically, resulting in life-threatening sepsis that may lead to patient death or graft loss (Pirsch et al 1995). Special attention should be paid to preoperative weight-loss programs and to rapid steroid withdrawal from the immunosuppressive regimens of obese candidates.

Liver disease

Over the past four decades, chronic liver disease (CLD) has been a frequent cause of late morbidity and mortality in renal transplant recipients. Most cases of CLD are due to hepatitis B (HBV) or hepatitis C virus (HCV) infection. While liver cirrhosis and clinically active hepatitis are obvious contraindications to transplantation, even patients with clinically quiescent HBV and HCV infections or other evidence of hepatic impairment require careful investigation.

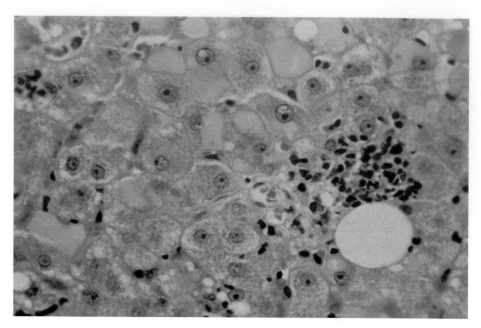

Figure 3.17. A 30-year-old male carrier of HBV. Liver biopsy shows a mild lobular hepatitis, with foci of spotty necrosis and several ground-glass hepatocytes. H&E ×75. (Courtesy of Dr MF Donato, Ospedale Maggiore, Milan, Italy.)

Hepatitis B virus infection

After transplantation, HBV-positive patients may remain asymptomatic for years, but serial liver biopsies reveal that most individuals show a progression of their histological lesions (Fornairon et al 1996), leading in the long term to death from cirrhosis or extrahepatic sepsis (Chan et al 1992b; Aroldi et al 1998; Younossi et al 1999). A few patients may even develop fibrosing cholestatic hepatitis and terminal liver failure within a few months after transplant (Tóth et al 1998).

It is generally agreed that HbsAg-positive patients with biochemically active hepatitis and serological evidence of active viral replication (positive HBV DNA and e antigen) are at high risk for the development of cirrhosis (Rao et al 1993) and should be rejected as candidates for transplantation (Parfrey et al 1985). Patients free of evidence of viral replication (HBV-DNA-negative) but displaying increased levels of liver transaminases require a liver biopsy to determine their status. While some centers do not recommend a liver biopsy for patients with normal transaminase values, a negative HbsAg, and a negative HBV DNA despite a long history of HBV infection (Morales 1998), other authorities (Rao et al 1993; Vosnides 1997) believe that biopsy must be performed regardless of blood chemistries, since liver enzymes offer poor markers of disease activity in uremic patients. Only if the liver biopsy discloses a picture of low-activity hepatitis (Figure 3.17) should the patient be accepted for renal transplantation (Kasiske 1998); otherwise, the patient should be considered a poor candidate, and renal transplantation, discouraged. To reduce the risk of liver disease, it has been recommended that HBV-infected patients receive lamivudine for at least 18–24 months after transplantation (Roth 1999).

Hepatitis C virus infection

HCV infection is growing increasingly common among dialysis patients (Pereira and Levey 1997). After renal transplantation, many HCV-positive patients remain asymptomatic for 5 years or more (Roth 1995), but repeated biopsies reveal that more than 50% of these transplant recipients display chronic liver disease within 10 years (Vosnides 1997). Although an HCV-positive status of the recipient does not seem to affect graft survival (Kliem et al 1996b; Vosnides 1997; Aroldi et al 1998), it does, in the very long term, reduce the patient survival rate (Stempel et al 1993; Roth 1995; Kliem et al 1996b; Aroldi et al 1998). Cirrhosis, extrahepatic sepsis, and cardiovascular disease are the most frequent causes of death.

In a recent multicenter study, Pereira and Levey (1997) compared the effect of anti-HCV status (positive versus negative) and treatment modality (dialysis versus transplantation) on the long-term survival of 496 patients followed for a median period of 73 months (range: 1–110 months). During this period, 302 patients underwent renal transplantation and 154 died. The presence of a positive serologic test for HCV was associated with a 1.41-fold increased risk of mortality within the first 6 months among transplant versus dialysis patients. Thereafter, the risk of death was lower among transplanted patients.

It is difficult to draw firm conclusions concerning the choice between dialysis and transplantation therapies for HCV-positive patients. Since the data of Pereira and Levey (1997) suggest that transplant patients display a better long-term survival rate, we recommend that HCV-positive patients who do not have evidence of severe liver disease be considered good candidates for transplantation. Because the histologic severity of liver disease is the best predictor of hepatic failure and death after renal transplantation, all HCV-positive patients, including those with normal liver enzymes, should undergo a hepatic biopsy to assess disease severity before acceptance as a renal transplant candidate. Patients with mild activity may be considered good candidates (Figure 3.18), while the presence of chronic active hepatitis or cirrhosis should be considered a formal contraindication to isolated kidney transplantation. To reduce the risk of liver failure after transplantation, it has been suggested that even the patients with little evidence of disease undergo therapy with interferon-α. While this treatment may be useful in some patients (Duarte et al 1995), most individuals tend to relapse after cessation of therapy, requiring ribavirin treatment. Furthermore, there is the risk that interferon-α as an immunostimulatory cytokine may provoke allograft rejection.

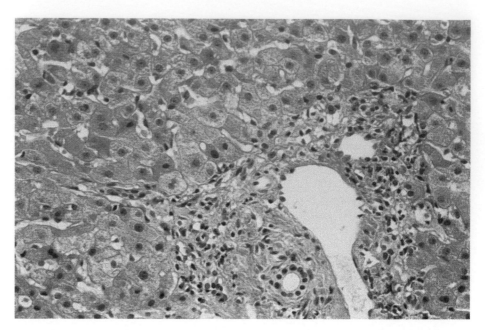

Figure 3.18. A 51-year-old man with HCV-positive hepatitis, showing no signs of activity; mild enlarged portal tract with fibrosis and scanty inflammatory cells; no evidence of periportal necrosis; and pleiomorphic hepatocytes. H&E ×75. (Courtesy of Dr MF Donato, Ospedale Maggiore, Milan, Italy.)

Hepatitis G virus infection

HGV is caused by GBV-C virus, which is closely related to HCV. HGV virus is highly prevalent among dialysis patients (Sampietro et al 1997). However, the association of HGV with liver disease has not yet been established (Murthy et al 1998). Until further studies determine whether HGV can cause an adverse outcome, renal transplantation should not be discouraged solely on the basis of a positive test for GBV-C virus.

Hemosiderosis

Patients with liver biopsy-proved hemosiderosis are at high risk of death due to liver failure (Rao and Anderson 1985). These patients should be treated with phlebotomy and erythropoietin. CT or nuclear magnetic resonance studies (Figure 3.19) may be useful in monitoring the status of iron stores in dialysis patients affected with hemosiderosis (Chan et al 1992a).

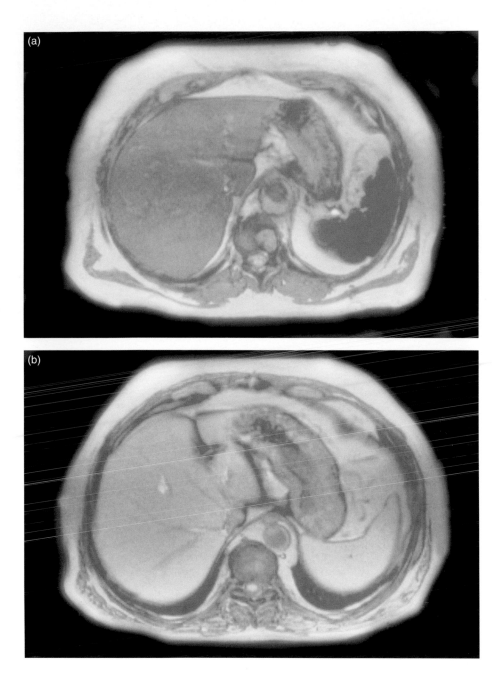

Figure 3.19. (a) Magnetic resonance imaging showing the 'black' appearance of spleen and liver of an uremic patient on chronic hemodialysis with iron overload (serum ferritin = 1990 ng/ml); liver/muscle and spleen/muscle ratios as evaluated by the Gradient Echo and Protonic Density techniques were <5, as compared to the values = 1. (b) Magnetic resonance imaging in an uremic patient on chronic hemodialysis with iron depletion (serum ferritin = 39 ng/ml) (courtesy of Dr C. Canavese, Ospedale Molinette, Turin, Italy).

Previous kidney transplant

In the case of a previous kidney transplant, the timing and cause of graft failure must be ascertained. Patients who lost their prior graft within the first 46 days have only a 40% probability of maintaining a functional second cadaveric transplant at 5 years. Conversely, patients whose first graft functioned for more than 4 years have an 84% probability of greater than a 3-year graft survival following a second transplant (Rigden et al 1999). The cause of graft failure may also predict the outcome of a retransplant; for example, patients who lost their first transplant due to an early episode of irreversible rejection display poor rates of graft survival after retransplantation (Hirata and Terasaki 1995). Similarly, patients who experienced graft failure due to recurrent primary glomerulonephritis or metabolic disease are at extremely high risk of recurrence after a second transplant. Finally, the source of the donor kidney may influence the outcome of the second transplant. In the case of retransplantation, a living donor should be sought whenever possible, since these transplants yield results far superior to those obtained using cadaveric grafts (Rigden et al 1999).

Cancer

The initial evaluation of the transplant candidate should include an exhaustive history and physical examination, with particular attention to a history or present stigmata of cancer. In addition to the aforementioned radiological and echographic investigations, the pretransplant screening should include guaiac (Hemoccult) testing of the stool and neoplasia markers, particularly prostate-specific antigen in elderly men. Women over 40 years of age or with a family history of breast carcinoma should undergo mammography. Female candidates of all ages must undergo a pelvic examination and a pap cervical smear; men over the age of 50 years should be screened for prostate carcinoma.

The decision whether to consider transplantation for a candidate with a previous history of malignancy but without current evidence of active disease is difficult. Patients may be readily accepted if their neoplasm was a noninvasive basal cell carcinoma, fully excised squamous cell carcinoma, or in situ bladder neoplasia. In other instances, particularly invasive diseases, it is difficult to determine the risk with certainty, since immunosuppressive therapy produces a variable degree of reduction of immunosurveillance, possibly favoring the development and certainly favoring the progression of occult cancer (Klein and Klein 1977). Penn (1993) has estimated the risk of recurrence of neoplastic disease as 53% of patients if the transplant is performed within 2 years, 34% if performed at 25–60 months, and 13% if performed more than 5 years after apparent recovery from neoplasia (Table 3.9).

Renal cell carcinoma

About one-quarter of renal cell carcinomas are discovered incidentally during medical evaluation for other disorders, during nephrectomy, or during surgery for other reasons

Type of cancer	Suggested waiting time (years)
Renal tumors	
• Clear cells, Wilms' tumor, urothelioma	2
Uterus carcinoma	
• In situ	2
• Non-in situ	5
Skin tumors	
• Basal cell or squamous cell carcinoma	2
• Melanoma	5
Breast carcinoma	5
Bladder carcinoma	
• Focal	1
• Diffuse	5
Prostrate carcinoma	
• Isolated nodule	1-2
• Diffuse	Transplant contraindicated
Colon-rectal carcinoma	5

Table 3.9. Suggested waiting time before transplantation after apparent cure of the tumor (data from Penn 1993)

(Penn 1998). Small, nonmetastasized, incidentally discovered carcinomas usually do not recur (Marple et al 1993). The search for renal carcinomas should be particularly intensive for patients with analgesic nephropathy. This disorder is frequently associated with malignancies, mostly transitional cell carcinoma (Kliem et al 1996a). Another frequent cause of cancer in the native kidneys is acquired cystic disease, a condition that may occur in 30–95% of long-term dialysis recipients (Penn 1998).

Although the precise incidence of carcinomas that are caused by acquired cystic disease is unknown, it is recommended that long-term dialysis recipients be screened by kidney ultrasonography and/or CT prior to their acceptance as candidates for transplantation.

Carcinomas of the uterus

In situ carcinomas display a low risk of recurrence after excision either by cone biopsy or by hysterectomy. However, a waiting time of 2 years from cancer treatment to transplant is recommended to minimize the risk of disseminated disease. In contrast, women with non-in situ (that is, invasive) carcinomas should wait at least 4–5 years before becoming a transplant candidate (Penn 1993).

Other cancers

It is difficult to decide whether and when to accept women who have had breast cancer; in most cases the cancer recurs after more than 3 years. For patients with in situ bladder cancer, a 1-year wait prior to transplantation may be sufficient, but at least 5 years should pass before considering apparently disease-free patients with a history of diffuse or invasive bladder cancers. In cases of an isolated malignant nodule of prostate, a wait of 1–2 years may be sufficient, while transplantation should be avoided in cases of diffuse prostatic cancer. A waiting time of at least 5 years is recommended in cases of carcinomas of the colon or rectum, while a 2-year wait is usually sufficient for patients with other cancers (Penn 1993).

IMMEDIATE PREOPERATIVE PREPARATION

Although preoperative hemodialysis seems to be a logical maneuver to assure chemical balance and improve fluid status, it may pose some problems. Excessive dehydration can expose the recipient to the risk of delayed graft function. Some patients with postdialysis hypokalemia may develop cardiac arrhythmias. In other instances, anticoagulation may increase the risk of hemorrhagic complications. Unless the recipient has hyperkalemia (more than 5.5 mEq/l) or severe fluid overload, we prefer not to subject the recipient to hemodialysis in the 12–24-hour period before transplantation.

Transfusions are rarely necessary either before or during the transplant operation. It has been demonstrated that the higher the levels of hematocrit before transplantation, the greater the risk of delayed graft function (Tóth et al 1998). The deleterious effect is probably related to sludge formation in the small vessels. Since the optimum level of hematocrit for a kidney transplant recipient has been estimated to be about 30% (Schmidt et al 1993), it may be recommended that this level not be exceeded in patients awaiting a transplant. Some workers advocate that patients with elevated levels of hematocrit, with positive antiphospholipid antibodies, and/or with circulating lupus anticoagulant undergo a small phlebotomy prior to transplant and administration of low-dose subcutaneous heparin (5000 Units every 8–12 hours) thereafter.

To obtain prompt recovery of allograft function after surgery, adequate intraoperative hydration of the recipient is recommended. Some centers use Swan–Ganz catheters to monitor fluid replacement, maintaining pulmonary artery pressures above 20 mmHg, while other groups use only central venous pressure measurements. The choice between the two monitoring techniques is best guided by the cardiac status of the patient, as evidenced by previous bouts of heart failure and/or cardiomegaly. Fluid is mobilized from extravascular compartments by administration of hypertonic mannitol, which significantly reduces the risk of acute tubular necrosis (van Valenberg et al 1987). Furthermore, renal vasodilation is induced by infusion of low-dose dopamine (1–3 µg/kg per min; Sandberg et al 1992). Some surgeons favor intra-arterial delivery of calcium channel blockers (Ladefoged and Anderson 1994) to relieve arterial spasm, although the results are controversial.

CONCLUSION

Although few conditions represent absolute contraindications to renal transplantation, careful selection and preparation of the recipient is necessitated by the growing shortage of donor organs and the risks associated with immunosuppressive therapy. Although the evaluation of candidates for kidney transplantation is a difficult and sometimes subjective process, a thorough investigation of the medical history of the candidate, as well as complete clinical assessment, can alert the transplant team to potential complications, and increased risks of poor clinical outcome. The presence of immunological, infectious, gastrointestinal, pulmonary, and urological conditions must be identified before a patient is considered for transplant. Other factors to be evaluated prior to transplant include elderly or pediatric age; obesity; the presence or a history of cancer; liver, metabolic, inherited, or systemic diseases; and a variety of other disorders. These indications may either suggest poor candidacy for transplantation, or necessitate that special measures be taken to prepare the recipient prior to transplantation and provide appropriate followup treatment.

The range of complicating conditions seen in patients desiring renal transplantation necessitates a broad evaluation of urologic, gastrointestinal, and vascular conditions to assess the risk of concomitant conditions and formulate therapeutic strategies to optimally prepare the patient not only for the operation, but also for the consequences of immunosuppressive therapy. An aggressive surgical approach to serious problems enhances the chance of an excellent outcome of transplantation; a delay in surgical intervention until the postoperative period may increase the risks of morbidity and/or graft loss. Among the surgical interventions frequently required are nephrectomy (and ureterectomy) in cases of infection, malignant hypertension, and neoplastic disease; parathyroidectomy in patients with hypercalcemia and serious bone disease; biliary procedures in patients with cholangitis; splenectomy to raise cell counts and thereby increase tolerability for immunosuppressive drugs; aortocoronary bypasses for serious coronary artery disease; and/or aortoiliac vascular grafts for arterial insufficiency. Owing to the advent of hemodialysis without anticoagulation, complex surgical procedures can now be performed with an added degree of safety in ESRD patients.

REFERENCES

Abu-Sharka M, Gladmann DD, Urowitz MB (1996) Malignancy in systemic lupus erythematosus. *Arthritis Rheum* 6:1050–1054.

Alagille D, Estrada A, Hadchouel M et al (1987) Syndromic paucity of intralobular bile ducts (Alagille syndrome or arteriohepatic dysplasia): review of 80 cases. *J Pediatr* 110:195–200.

Alamartine E, Boulharouz J, Berthoux F (1996) Actuarial survival rate of kidney transplants in patients with IgA glomerulonephritis: a one-center study. *Transplant Proc* 26:272–274.

Andresdottir MB, Assman KJ, Hoitsma AJ et al (1997) Recurrence of type I membranoproliferative glomerulonephritis after renal transplantation: analysis of the incidence, risk factors and impact on graft survival. *Transplantation* **63**:1628–1633.

Arbus GS, Geary DF, McLorie GA et al (1986) Pediatric renal transplants: a Canadian perspective. *Kidney Int* **19**:S31–S34.

Aroldi A, Lampertico P, Elli A et al (1998) Long-term evolution of anti-HCV positive renal transplant recipients. *Transplant Proc* **30**:2076–2078.

Barber WH, Deierhoi MH, Julian BA et al (1987) Renal transplantation in sickle cell anemia and sickle cell disease. *Clin Transplant* **1**:169–172.

Basar H, Soran A, Shapiro R et al (1999) Renal transplantation in recipients over the age of 60. *Transplantation* **67**:1191–1193.

Ben Hamida M, Bedrossian J, Duboust A et al (1993) Renal transplantation and autosomal dominant polycystic kidney disease: 20 years' experience. *Transplant Proc* **25**:2162–2163.

Bloss RS, McConnell RW, McConnell BG et al (1979) Demonstration by radionuclide imaging of possible vascular steal from a renal transplant. *J Nucl Med* **20**:1053–1054.

Bradley JR, Thiru S, Balallan N, Evans DB (1988) Renal transplantation in Waldenström's macroglobulinemia. *Nephrol Dial Transplant* **3**:214–216.

Brady HR (1998) Fibrillary glomerulopathy. *Kidney Int* **53**:1421–1429.

Bricker EM (1950) Bladder substitution after pelvis evisceration. *Surg Clin North Am* **30**:1511–1521.

Briggs JD, Jones E (1999) Renal transplantation for uncommon diseases. *Nephrol Dial Transplant* **14**:570–575.

Bumgardner GL, Amend WC, Ascher NL, Vincenti FG (1998) Single-center long-term results of renal transplantation for IgA nephropathy. *Transplantation* **65**:1053–1060.

Cameron JS (1991) Recurrence of primary disease and de novo nephritis following renal transplantation. *Pediatr Nephrol* **5**:412–421.

Cantarovich D, Baatard R, Baranger T et al (1994) Cadaver renal transplantation after 60 years of age. *Transplant Int* **7**:33–38.

Chan PC, Liu P, Cronin C et al (1992a) The use of nuclear magnetic resonance imaging in monitoring total body iron in hemodialysis patients with hemosiderosis treated with erythropoietin and phlebotomy. *Am J Kidney Dis* **19**:484–489.

Chan PC, Lok AS, Cheng IK, Chan MK (1992b) The impact of donor and recipient hepatitis B surface antigen status on liver disease and survival in renal transplant recipients. *Transplantation* **53**:128–131.

Clark WF, Jevnikar AM (1999) Renal transplantation for end-stage renal disease caused by systemic lupus erythematosus nephritis. *Semin Nephrol* **19**:77–85.

Coffey RC (1911) Physiologic implantation of the severed ureter or common bile-duct into the intestine. *JAMA* **56**:397–403.

Cope O (1966) The study of hyperparathyroidism at the Massachusetts General Hospital. *N Engl J Med* **27**:1174–1182.

Cosio FG, Alamir A, Yim S et al (1998) Patient survival after renal transplantation. I. The impact of dialysis pre-transplant, *Kidney Int* **53**:767–772.

De Geest S, Borgermans L, Gemoets H et al (1995) Incidence, determinants, and consequences of subclinical noncompliance with immunosuppressive therapy in renal transplant recipients. *Transplantation* **59**:340–347.

Didlake RH, Dreyfus K, Kerman RH (1988) Patients' noncompliance—a major cause of late graft failure in cyclosporine treated renal transplants. *Transplant Proc* **20**(Suppl 3):63–69.

Ding J, Zhou J, Tryggvason K, Kashtan CE (1994) COL4A5 deletions in three patients with Alport syndrome and post transplant antiglomerular basement membrane nephritis. *J Am Soc Nephrol* **5**:161–168.

Dominguez Fernández E, Albrecht KH, Heemann U et al (1998) Prevalence of diverticulosis and incidence of bowel perforation after kidney transplantation in patients with polycystic kidney disease. *Transplant Int* 11:28–31.

Dommergues JP, Guber MC, Habib R et al (1987) Renal involvement in Alagille syndrome. *Arch Pediatr* 110:195–200.

Donati D, Novario R, Gastaldi L (1987) Natural history and treatment of uremia secondary to Fabry's disease: a European experience. *Nephron* 46:353–359.

Doutrelepont JM, Abramowicz D, Florquin S et al (1992) Early recurrence of hemolytic uremic syndrome in a renal transplant recipient during prophylactic OKT3 therapy. *Transplantation* 53:1378–1383.

Douzdjian V, Abecassis MM, Corry RJ, Hunsicker LG (1994) Simultaneous pancreas–kidney transplantation versus kidney-alone transplants in diabetics: increased risk of early cardiac death and acute rejection following pancreas transplants. *Clin Transplant* 8:246–251.

Duarte R, Huraib S, Said R et al (1995) Interferon-alpha facilitates renal transplantation in hemodialysis patients with chronic viral hepatitis. *Am J Kidney Dis* 25:40–45.

EDTA Registry (1996) *Annual Report on Management of Renal Failure in Europe.* EDTA/ERA XXVII.

Ettinger WH, Godberg ATP, Applebaum-Bowder D, Hazzard WR (1987) Dyslipoproteinemia in systemic lupus erythematosus. Effects of corticosteroids. *Am J Med* 83:503–508.

Feucht HF, Opelz G (1996) The humoral response towards HLA class II determinants in renal transplantation. *Kidney Int* 50:1464–1475.

Fine RN (1997) Growth hormone treatment of children with chronic renal insufficiency, end-stage renal disease and following renal transplantation. Update 1997. *J Pediatr Endocrinol Metab* 10:361–370.

Flechner SM, Kerman RH, Van Buren C, Kahan BD (1984) Successful transplantation of cyclosporine-treated haploidentical living-related renal recipients without blood transfusions. *Transplantation* 37:73–76.

Fornairon S, Pol S, Legendre C et al (1996) The long-term virologic and pathologic impact of renal transplantation on chronic hepatitis B infection. *Transplantation* 62:297–299.

Gagnadoux MF, Niaudet P, Droz D et al (1999) Risk of primary disease recurrence in pediatric renal transplantation. *Transplant Proc* 31:235.

Gerlag PG, Koene RA, Berden JH (1986) Renal transplantation in light chain nephropathy: case report and review of the literature. *Clin Nephrol* 25:101–104.

Ghio L, Tarantino A, Edefonti A et al (1992) Advantages of cyclosporine as sole immunosuppressive agent in children with transplanted kidneys. *Transplantation* 54:834–838.

Glassock RJ (1997) Optimizing disease management in the next 25 years. *Semin Nephrol* 17:387–390.

Habib R, Gagnadoux M, Broyer M (1987) Recurrent glomerulonephritis in renal transplanted children. *Contrib Nephrol* 55:123–125.

Halme L, Eklund B, Kyllönen L, Salmela K (1997) Is obesity still a risk factor in renal transplantation? *Transplant Int* 10:284–288.

Hartmann A, Holdaast H, Fauchald P et al (1992) Fifteen years' experience with renal transplantation in systemic amyloidosis. *Transplant Int* 5:15–19.

Hebert D, Kim EM, Sibley RK, Mauer SM (1986) Recurrence of hemolytic uremic syndrome in renal transplant recipients. *Kidney Int* Suppl 19:S51–S58.

Hebert D, Kim EM, Sibley RK, Mauer MS (1991) Post-transplantation outcome of patients with hemolytic-uremic syndrome: update. *Pediatr Nephrol* 5:162–167.

Heering P, Kutkulum B, Brenzel H et al (1989) Renal transplantation in amyloid nephropathy. *Int Urol Nephrol* 21:339–347.

Hirata M, Terasaki PI (1995) Renal retransplantation. In: Terasaki PI, Cecka JM (eds). *Clinical Transplants 1994.* Los Angeles: UCLA Tissue Typing Laboratory, pp.419–433.

Holley JL, Shapiro R, Lopatin WB et al (1990) Obesity as a risk factor following cadaveric renal transplantation. *Transplantation* **49**:387–389.

Hume DM (1972) The operation. *Transplant Proc* **4**:625–628.

Ismail N, Hakim RM, Helderman JH (1994) Renal replacement therapies in the elderly: Part II. Renal transplantation. *Am J Kidney Dis* **23**:1–15.

Josephson MA, Spargo B, Hollandsworth DO, Thistlewait MD (1994) The recurrence of membranous glomerulopathy in a renal transplant recipient: a case report and literature review. *Am J Kidney Dis* **24**:873–878.

Kahan BD (1984) Donor-specific transfusions—a balanced view. In: Morris P, Tilney N (eds). *Progress in Organ Transplantation*, Vol 1. Boston: Little Brown, pp. 111–148.

Kasiske BL (1998) The evaluation of prospective renal transplant recipients and living donors. *Surg Clin North Am* **78**:27–39.

Kasiske BL, Ramos EL, Gaston RS et al (1995) The evaluation of renal transplant candidates: clinical practice guidelines, Patient Care and Education Committee of the American Society of Transplant Physicians. *J Am Soc Nephrol* **6**:1–34.

Kiley DJ, Lam CS, Pollak R (1993) A study of treatment compliance following kidney transplantation. *Transplantation* **55**:51–56.

Kim YS, Jeong HJ, Choi KH et al (1996) Renal transplantation in patients with IgA nephropathy. *Transplant Proc* **28**:1543–1544.

Klein G, Klein E (1977) Immune surveillance against virus-induced tumors and non-rejectability of spontaneous tumors: contrasting consequences of host-versus-tumor evolution. *Proc Natl Acad Sci USA* **74**:2121–2125.

Kliem V, Thon W, Krautzig S et al (1996a) High mortality from urothelial carcinoma despite regular tumor screening in patients with analgesic nephropathy after renal transplantation. *Transplant Int* **9**:231–235.

Kliem V, Van den Hoff U, Brunkhost R et al (1996b) The long term course of hepatitis C after kidney transplantation. *Transplantation* **62**:1417–1421.

Ladefoged SD, Anderson SB (1994) Calcium channel blockers in kidney transplantation. *Clin Transplantation* **8**:128–133.

Le A, Wilson R, Douek K et al (1994) Prospective risk stratification in renal transplant candidates for cardiac death. *Am J Kidney Dis* **24**:65–71.

Lee G, Glassok RJ (1997) Immunoglobulin A nephropathy. In: Ponticelli C, Glassock RJ (eds). *Treatment of Primary Glomerulonephritis*. Oxford: Oxford Medical Publications, pp. 186–217.

Livneh A, Zemer D, Siegal B et al (1992) Colchicine prevents kidney transplant amyloidosis in familial Mediterranean fever. *Nephron* **60**:418–442.

Lockshin MD (1992) Antiphospholipid antibody syndrome. *JAMA* **268**:1451–1453.

Lorber MI, Van Buren CT, Flechner SM et al (1987) Pretransplant coronary arteriography for diabetic renal transplant recipients. *Transplant Proc* **19**:1539–1541.

Manske CL, Wong Y, Rector T et al (1992) Coronary revascularisation in insulin-dependent diabetic patients with chronic renal failure. *Lancet* **340**:998–1002.

Marangella M (1999) Transplantation strategies in type 1 primary hyperoxaluria: the issue of pyridoxine responsiveness. *Nephrol Dial Transplant* **14**:301–303.

Marcen R, Mampso F, Tervel JL et al (1996) Membranous nephropathy: recurrence after kidney transplantation. *Nephrol Dial Transplant* **11**:1129–1133.

Markello TC, Bernardini IM, Gahl WA (1993) Improved renal function in children with cystinosis treated with cysteamine. *N Engl J Med* **328**:1157–1162.

Marple JT, MacDougall M, Chonko AM (1993) Renal cancer complicating acquired cystic kidney disease. *J Am Soc Nephrol* **12**:1951–1956.

Mathew TH (1991) Recurrent disease after renal transplantation. *Transplant Rev* **51**:1–15.

Mehls O, Tonshoff B, Haffner D et al (1994) The use of recombinant human growth hormone in short children with chronic renal failure. *J Pediatr Endocrinol* 7:107–113.

Meulders Q, Pirson Y, Cosyns JP et al (1994) Course of Henoch–Schönlein nephritis after renal transplantation. *Transplantation* 58:1172–1186.

Montagnino G, Tarantino A, Cesana B et al (1997) Prognostic factors of long-term allograft survival in 632 CyA-treated recipients of a primary renal transplant. *Transpl Int* 10:268–275.

Montgomery R, Zibari G, Hill GS, Ratner RE (1994) Renal transplantation in patients with sickle cell nephropathy. *Transplantation* 58:618–620.

Morales JM (1998) Renal transplantation in patients positive for hepatitis B or C (pro). *Transplant Proc* 5:2064–2069.

Moroni G, Banfi G, Ponticelli C (1992) Clinical status of patients after 10 years of lupus nephritis. *Q J Med* 84:681–689.

Mosnier JF, Degott C, Bedrossian J et al (1991) Recurrence of Fabry's disease in a renal allograft eleven years after successful renal transplantation. *Transplantation* 51:759–762.

Mourad G, Djamali A, Turc-Baron Cristol J-P (1998) Lipoprotein glomerulopathy: a new case of nephrotic syndrome after transplantation. *Nephrol Dial Transplant* 13:1292–1294.

Müller T, Sikora P, Offner G et al (1998) Recurrence of renal disease after kidney transplantation in children: 24 years of experience in a single center. *Clin Nephrol* 49:82–90.

Murthy BVR, Muerhoff AS, Desai SM et al (1998) Predictors of GBV-C infection among patients referred for renal transplantation. *Kidney Int* 53:1769–1774.

N'Dow J, Leung HY, Marshall C, Neal DE (1998) Bowel dysfunction after bladder reconstruction. *J Urol* 159:1470–1474.

Najarian JS, Kaufmann DB, Fryd DS et al (1989) Long-term survival following kidney transplantation in 100 type 1 diabetic patients. *Transplantation* 47:106–113.

Nast CC, Ward HJ, Koyle MA, Cohen AH (1987) Recurrent Henoch–Schöenlein purpura following renal transplantation. *Am J Kidney Dis* 9:39–43.

Nissenson AR, Port FK (1990) Outcome of end-stage renal disease in patients with rare cause of renal failure III. Systemic/vascular disorders. *Q J Med* 74:63–71.

Nurse DE, Mundy AR (1989) Metabolic complications of cystoplasty. *Br J Urol* 63:165–170.

Nyberg G, Blohmé I, Persson H et al (1992) Recurrence of SLE in transplanted kidneys: a follow-up transplant biopsy study. *Nephrol Dial Transplant* 7:1116–1123.

Oberpenning F, Meng J, Yoo JJ, Atala A (1999) De novo reconstitution of a functional mammalian urinary bladder by tissue engineering. *Nat Biotechnol* 17:149–155.

Odorico JS, Knechtle SJ, Rayhill SC et al (1996) The influence of native nephrectomy on the incidence of recurrent disease following renal transplantation for primary glomerulonephritis. *Transplantation* 61:228–234.

Ojo AO, Govaerts TC, Schmouder RL et al (1999) Renal transplantation in end-stage sickle cell nephropathy. *Transplantation* 67:291–295.

Opelz G (1997) *CTS Newsl* 3.

Opelz G, Terasaki PI (1978) Improvement of kidney-graft survival with increased numbers of blood transfusions. *N Engl J Med* 299:799–803.

Opelz G, Vanrenterghem Y, Kirste G et al (1997) Prospective evaluation of pretransplant blood transfusions in cadaver kidney recipients. *Transplantation* 63:964–967.

Parfrey PS, Farge D, Forbes RD et al (1985) Chronic hepatitis in end-stage renal disease: comparison of HBsAg negative and HBsAg positive patients. *Kidney Int* 28:959–967.

Penn I (1993) The effect of immunosuppression on pre-existing cancers. *Transplantation* 55:742–747.

Penn I (1998) De novo malignances in pediatric organ transplant recipients. *Pediatr Transplant* 2:56–63.

Pereira BJG, Levey AS (1997) Hepatitis C virus infection in dialysis and renal transplantation. *Kidney Int* 51:981–999.

Peten E, Pirson Y, Cosyns JP et al (1991) Outcome of thirty patients with Alport's Syndrome after renal transplantation. *Transplantation* 52:823–826.

Petri M, Roubenoff R, Dallal GE et al (1996) Plasma homocysteine as a risk factor for atherothrombotic events in systemic lupus erythematosus. *Lancet* 348:1120–1125.

Pirsch JD, Armbrust MJ, Knechtle ST et al (1995) Obesity as a risk factor following renal transplantation. *Transplantation* 59:631–633.

Ponticelli C, Banfi G (1997) Focal and segmental glomerulosclerosis. In: Ponticelli C, Glassock RJ (eds). *Treatment of Primary Glomerulonephritis*. Oxford: Oxford Medical Publications, pp. 108–145.

Ponticelli C, Banfi G, Moroni G (1998) Systemic lupus erythematosus (clinical). In: Davison AM, Cameron JS, Grünfeld JP, Kerr DNS, Ritz E, Winearls CG (eds). *Oxford Textbook of Clinical Nephrology*, Vol 2, 2nd edn. Oxford: Oxford Medical Publications, pp. 935–959.

Pronovost PH, Brady HR, Gunning ME et al (1996) Clinical features, predictors of disease progression and results of renal transplantation in fibrillary/immunotactoid glomerulopathy. *Nephrol Dial Transpl* 11:837–842.

Raine AE, Margreiter R, Brunner PF et al (1992) Report on management of renal failure in Europe XII. *Nephrol Dial Transpl* 7(Suppl 2):7–35.

Rao KV, Anderson WR (1985) Hemosiderosis and hemochromatosis in renal transplant recipients. *Am J Nephrol* 5:419–424.

Rao KV, Anderson WR, Kasiske BL, Dahl DC (1993) Value of liver biopsy in the evaluation and management of chronic liver disease in renal transplant recipients. *Am J Med* 94:241–250.

Reitz RE, Pollard JJ, Wang CA et al (1969) Localization of parathyroid adenomas by selective venous catheterization and radioimmunoassay. *N Engl J Med* 281:348–351.

Ribot S (1999) Kidney transplant in sickle cell nephropathy. *Int J Artif Organs* 22:61–63.

Rigden S, Mehls O, Gellert R, on behalf of the Scientific Advisory Board of the ERA-EDTA Registry (1999) Factors influencing second renal allograft survival. *Nephrol Dial Transpl* 14:566–569.

Rigotti P, Van Buren CT, Payne WT et al (1986) Gastrointestinal perforations in renal transplant recipients immunosuppressed with cyclosporine. *World J Surg* 10:137–141.

Rischen-Vos J, Van der Woude FJ, Tegzess AM et al (1992) Increased morbidity and mortality in patients with diabetes mellitus after kidney transplantation as compared with non-diabetic patients. *Nephrol Dial Transpl* 7:433–437.

Roodnat JJ, Zietse R, Mulder PGH et al (1999) The vanishing importance of age in renal transplantation. *Transplantation* 67:576–580.

Rosen CB, Fronhnert PP, Velosa JA et al (1991) Morbidity of pancreas transplantation during cadaveric renal transplantation. *Transplantation* 51:123–127.

Rosenmann E, Eliakim M (1997) Nephrotic syndrome associated with amyloid-like glomerular deposits. *Nephron* 18:301–308.

Roth D (1995) Hepatitis C virus: the nephrologists' view. *Am J Kidney Dis* 25:3–16.

Roth D (1999) Hepatitis in non-hepatic transplantation. *Graft* 2(Suppl II):S104–S107.

Saito T, Sato H, Kudo K et al (1989) Lipoprotein glomerulopathy: glomerular lipoprotein thrombi in a patient with hyperlipidemia. *Am J Kidney Dis* 13:148–153.

Saito T, Sato H, Oikawa S (1995) Lipoprotein glomerulopathy: a new aspect of lipid-induced glomerular injury. *Nephrology* 1:17–24.

Sampietro M, Badalamenti S, Graziani G et al (1997) Hepatitis G virus in hemodialysis patients. *Kidney Int* 51:348–352.

Sandberg J, Tyden G, Groth CG (1992) Low-dose dopamine infusion following cadaveric renal transplantation: no effect on the incidence of ATN. *Transplant Proc* 24:357.

Sanfilippo FP, Vaughn WK, Spees EK (1984) The association of pretransplant native nephrectomy with decreased renal allograft rejection. *Transplantation* 37:256–260.

Scheinman JI (1991) Primary hyperoxaluria: therapeutic strategies for the nineties. *Kidney Int* 40:389–399.

Schmidt R, Kupin W, Dumler F (1993) Influence of the pre-transplant hematocrit level on early graft function in primary cadaveric renal transplantation. *Transplantation* 55:1034–1040.

Schmitt WH, Haubitz M, Mistry N et al (1994) Renal transplantation in Wegener granulomatosis. *Lancet* ii:860 (letter).

Segoloni GP, Messina M, Tognarelli G et al (1998) Survival probabilities for renal transplant recipients and dialytic patients: a single center prospective study. *Transplant Proc* 30:1739–1741.

Senguttuvan P, Cameron JS, Hartley RB et al (1990) Recurrence of focal segmental glomerulosclerosis in transplanted kidneys: analysis of incidence and risk factors in 59 allografts. *Pediatr Nephrol* 4:21–28.

Shandera K, Sago A, Angstadt J et al (1993) An assessment of the need for voiding cystourethrogram for urologic screening prior to renal transplantation. *Clin Transplant* 7:299–301.

Shimizu T, Tanabe K, Oshima T et al (1998) Recurrence of membranoproliferative glomerulonephritis in renal allografts. *Transplant Proc* 30:3910–3913.

Solà R, Guirado L, López-Navidad A et al (1998) Renal transplantation with limit donors. *Transplantation* 66:1159–1163.

Stempel CA, Lake J, Kuo G, Vincenti F (1993) Hepatitis C: its prevalence in end-stage renal failure patients and clinical course after kidney transplantation. *Transplantation* 55:273–276.

Stone JH, Amend WJ, Criswell LA (1997) Outcome of renal transplantation in systemic lupus erythematosus. *Semin Arthritis Rheum* 1:17–26.

Sutherland DER, Gruessner AC, Gruessner RWG (1998) Pancreas transplantation: a review. *Transplant Proc* 30:1940–1943.

Tarantino A, Moroni G, Banfi G et al (1994) Renal replacement therapy in cryoglobulinemic nephritis. *Nephrol Dial Transpl* 9:1426–1430.

Tejani A, Stablein DH (1992) Recurrence of focal segmental glomerulosclerosis post-transplantation: a special report of the North America Pediatric Renal Transplant Cooperative Study. *J Am Soc Nephrol* 2(Suppl):S258–S261.

Tejani A, Sullivan EK, Alexander S et al (1994) Posttransplant deaths and factors that influence the mortality rate in North American children. *Transplantation* 57:547–553.

Terasaki PI, Cecka JM, Takemoto S et al (1988) Overview. In: Terasaki PI (ed.). *Clinical Transplants 1988*. Los Angeles: UCLA Tissue Typing Laboratory, pp. 409–434.

Tesi RJ, Elkhammas EA, Davies EA et al (1994) Renal transplantation in older people. *Lancet* i:461–464.

Tóth M, Réti V, Gondos T (1998) Effects of recipients' peri-operative parameters on the outcome of kidney transplantation. *Clin Transplant* 12:511–517.

Truong L, Gelfand J, D'Agati V et al (1989) De novo membranous glomerulonephropathy in renal allografts: a report of ten cases and review of the literature. *Am J Kidney Dis* 14:131–144.

van Valenberg PLJ, Hoitsma AJ, Tiggeler RG et al (1987) Mannitol as an indispensable constituent of an intraoperative protocol for the prevention of acute renal failure after renal transplantation. *Transplantation* 44:784–788.

Vanwalleghem J, Zachée P, Kuypers D et al (1998) Renal transplantation for end-stage renal disease due to paroxysmal nocturnal hemoglobinuria. *Nephrol Dial Transplant* 13:3250–3252.

Vosnides GG (1997) Hepatitis C in renal transplantation. *Kidney Int* 3:843–861.

Weinrauch LA, D'Elia JA, Monaco AP et al (1992) Preoperative evaluation for diabetic renal transplantation. Impact of clinical, laboratory and echocardiographic parameters on patient and allograft survival. *Am J Med* 93:19–28.

Wenderoth UK, Bachor R, Egghart G et al (1990) The ileal neobladder: experience and results of more than 100 consecutive cases. *J Urol* 143:492–496.

Wrenger E, Pirsch JD, Cangro CB (1997) Single-center experience with renal transplantation in patients with Wegener's granulomatosis. *Transplant Int* 10:152–156.

Younossi ZM, Braun WE, Protiva DE et al (1999) Chronic viral hepatitis in renal transplant recipients with allograft functioning for more than 20 years. *Transplantation* 67:272–275.

4 SELECTION AND OPERATIVE APPROACHES FOR CADAVERIC AND LIVING DONORS

For several years after the pioneering success of identical-twin transplantations in the 1950s (Merrill et al 1956), living-related donors represented the most frequent source of kidneys for renal transplantation. Following the acceptance of the concept of brain death (Mollaret and Goulon 1959; Ad Hoc Committee of the Harvard Medical School 1968), improvements in immunosuppressive therapy, and progress in addressing many transplant-related clinical, biological, and immunological problems, cadaveric organ transplantation has become the predominant mode of treatment for end-stage renal disease (ESRD) since the late 1960s. Today, the majority of kidneys for transplantation are obtained from heart-beating cadaveric donors.

As kidney transplantation becomes more successful, however, the supply of organ donors (Randall 1991) must be expanded to address the rapidly and continuously growing demand from the large number of patients on the waiting list—currently, more than 40 000 Western European and more than 56 000 American patients. The list grows by several hundred patients each month. The consequences of this imbalance are heavy: an increased number of deaths (Edwards et al 1997; Schnuelle et al 1998), lower quality of life (Hailbrands et al 1995; Laupacis et al 1996; Dew et al 1997), poorer rehabilitation (Matas et al 1996), and increasing costs of renal replacement therapy (Laupacis et al 1996) among patients awaiting a kidney, compared to those of transplant recipients.

Owing to the limited number of cadaveric kidneys available for transplant, living donors represent a valuable resource. The proportion of living donors currently fluctuates around 12% in Europe (Donnelly et al 1997), 35% in the United States (Hauptman and O'Connor 1997), 50% in Latin America, and 90% in Asia (Cohen et al 1998). Although living donors are in most cases parents or siblings of the recipients, the number of living-unrelated donors has increased over the last few years. The utilization of such 'unconventional' donors, including spouses, distant relatives, and even friends (Terasaki et al 1995), has produced a three-fold increase in the number of living-unrelated donor transplants. The survival of allografts from unconventional living-donors appears to be equivalent to that displayed by one-haplotype-matched living-related donors. This chapter examines the social, practical, and ethical implications of both cadaveric- and living-donor renal transplantation; it outlines some important considerations for evaluating donors; and it recommends surgical approaches to maximize success from both sources.

CADAVERIC-DONOR EVALUATION AND RENAL TRANSPLANT

Heart-beating cadaveric donors

Cadaveric donors represent the largest source of vascularized organ transplants. In the United States, as in most Western countries, the majority of transplanted kidneys are removed from brain-dead donors with a functional circulation. It has been estimated

Country/organization	Cadaveric-donor kidney transplants (per million population)
Spain	46.4
Czech Republic	42.0
Portugal	38.2
Austria	36.1
United States (UNOS)	33.6
Hungary	30.0
France	27.5
Switzerland	26.2
United Kingdom	26.0
Eurotransplant	25.6
Scandiatransplant	24.7
Canada	23.4
Italy	20.7
Australia	19.3
Poland	13.3
Greece	5.5

* Adapted from Transplantation Committee of the Council of Europe 1998

Table 4.1. International data on cadaveric-kidney transplantation per million population in 1997*

that the annual number of potential heart-beating, cadaveric organ donors in the United States may be as high as 43.7–55.2 per million population (Nathan et al 1991; Evans et al 1992). However, organ procurement efforts are only 37–59% efficient. The numbers of cadaveric donors per million population vary throughout the world, but no country seems to realize its full potential number of cadaveric renal donors (Table 4.1). The problems lie in the failure not only to identify potential donors, but also to convert potential donors into actual donors. Family consent for organ donation, limitations of medical organizations, the societal environment and strict (albeit recently more relaxed) criteria for accepting cadaveric donors constitute the most important variables influencing the success of the organ procurement enterprise.

Permission for organ donation

The now widely accepted concept of brain death is usually defined as the total and irreversible cessation of cerebral function, as manifested by apnea, unresponsiveness to all stimuli, and lack of cranial nerve reflexes in the absence of either hypothermia or drug intoxication. Objective confirmatory evidence of brain death includes the absence of cerebral flow on a nuclear perfusion study or silence on electroencephalography. Although many countries have specific laws regulating permission for harvesting organs from brain-dead donors, the criteria for the certification of brain death vary from one country to another, as do, more importantly, attitudes about the permission for organ donation. Some national transplant laws recognize the concept of presumed consent, which allows organs to be harvested from any individual who has not, prior to death, certified his or her refusal to donate organs. In Europe, presumed consent is admitted in Austria, Belgium, France, Italy, Portugal, and Sweden. Most countries, however, consider presumed consent an abuse of authority or a limit to the individual authority, and thus require an informed consent by the deceased during life or by relatives after the death.

The need to obtain family consent may represent a major barrier to organ procurement. After the death of their loved one, the family is often devastated and in shock, and may be emotionally unable to make such a decision. The need to request permission is also stressful for hospital personnel. Consequently, the rate of family consent is low (Siminoff et al 1995), in contrast to public opinion polls that show widespread support for organ donation. To overcome the obstacle of family refusal, it has been suggested that all adults should record their wishes about post-mortem organ donation, and that these wishes should be honored (Spital 1996a). Another attempt to increase the consent rate is to optimize the manner in which the family is approached. The timing and wording of the request, as well as the background of the requester, may strongly influence the decision of the family of a potential donor. Several organizations dedicate a well-trained physician or nurse to approach the donor family in an attempt to minimize the rate of refusal (Miranda and González-Posada 1998). Also relevant is the role of religious authorities; while some faiths prohibit mutilation after death, religious representatives are increasingly relenting and accepting the concept of organ donation.

Medical organization

One of the most effective models of medical organization for organ procurement has been developed in Spain, currently the country with the highest rate of cadaveric organ donation. The Spanish organization has three levels: national, regional, and local (Miranda and González-Posada 1998). The local coordinator is the key individual, identifying the potential donor, aiding in contact with the relatives, and helping to solve bureaucratic and organizational problems. Local coordinating teams have been developed in all Spanish hospitals with intensive-care facilities. A similar model is being adopted by other European countries.

The United Network for Organ Sharing (UNOS), a private, nonprofit corporation, acts as the governmental contractor for organ procurement in the United States. All potential cadaveric-kidney transplant recipients are registered on the UNOS computer system waiting list. Within 6 hours of cadaveric kidney organ retrieval, the transplant center must notify UNOS. Except for organs that are either perfectly matched or show no mismatches in human leukocyte antigen (HLA) typing, kidneys are allocated, in turn, within local, regional, and national distribution regions. Each distribution region has its own point system based on recipient waiting time, quality of HLA match, and evidence of presensitization (content of panel reactive antibodies; Table 4.2). Additional

Criterion	Level	Points
Time waiting	First year	Proportional fraction (0.5)
Quality of match	0 ABDR mismatch	10
	0 BDR mismatch	7
	0 AB mismatch	6
	1 BDR mismatch	3
	2 BDR mismatch	2
	3 BDR mismatch	1
	More mismatches	0
Panel reactive antibody	>80% and negative preliminary crossmatch	4
	<80% and/or positive preliminary crossmatch	0
Patient age	<11 years	3
	11–18 years	2
	>18 years	0

Table 4.2. Allocation of kidneys in the United States (in effect August 1995)

points are granted for pediatric patients, since it is well recognized that renal failure adversely affects the growth and development of children.

Donor Action is an international initiative that provides tools, resources, and guidelines for hospitals to assess their own potential for donation and to develop a protocol to improve their donation practices. Data from a pilot study showed that only 31% of potential donors became actual donors. According to a recent study, problems with donor identification and/or management (42%) and family or coroner refusals (26%) account for most cases of unrealized donors (Wight et al 1998). Based on these results, attempts are being made to overcome all local problems and inefficiencies that impede optimal organ procurement.

Social environment

Another issue critical to the implementation of the recruitment of cadaveric donors is social sensitivity to the problems of organ transplantation. Educational programs for students and the general population, as well as specific training courses for physicians and nurses, may help in circulating information. However, mass media, national programs of education, and religious authorities play key roles in determining social sensitivity.

Criteria for acceptance

Until recently, the majority of cadaveric donors were young patients who had died from brain trauma. However, the pressure to enlarge the donor pool has recently prompted the inclusion of cadaveric donors that have died from cerebral hemorrhage. Moreover, there is a growing tendency to accept donors who would have been previously excluded due to anatomical abnormalities, arterial hypertension, renal dysfunction, prolonged cold ischemia time, old or young age, infections, or poisoning.

Flexibility in accepting kidneys from 'marginal' donors is increasing. On the one hand, it is possible that, compared with ideal cadaveric donors, the acceptance of marginal donors might reduce the 1-year graft survival by 10–20% and increase the economic cost (Jacobbi et al 1995; Whiting et al 1998). On the other hand, expanding the criteria for donor selection could increase the number of cadaveric renal transplants by 20–50% (Light et al 1996). A study performed in the United States showed that 70% of patients awaiting a renal transplantation would accept a less-than-ideal kidney if it meant a shorter waiting time (Slakey et al 1997).

Nonheart-beating cadaveric donors

One of the most promising ways to increase the actual number of kidneys for transplantation is to expand the donor pool to include nonheart-beating donors. It has been estimated that 123 kidneys per million population could be recruited each year from nonheart-beating donors in the United States (Nathan et al 1991). A careful analysis by the Maastrich group estimated a range of 4.5–9.2 potential nonheart-beating donors per 100 in-hospital deaths. Including rates of refusal to consent, as well as technical failures, the projected number of kidneys available from cadavers after irreversible cardiac arrest would be 2–4.5 times the number of kidneys from heart-beating cadavers (Daemen et al 1997).

The initial results with asystolic cadaveric donors were poor, due to severe renal injury after cardiac arrest (Garvin et al 1980). Moreover, this source of kidney grafts has been used only rarely because of legal and logistic problems. To minimize the ischemic injury, some groups declared death after only 2 min of ineffective cardiac function. This protocol raised concerns about the adequacy of criteria for declaring death and about the fear of negative public reaction to this approach (Youngner and Arnold 1993). Less concern has been raised over the protocol used by the Maastricht group, which considers patients with irreversible circulatory arrest as potential donors if circulatory arrest lasts more than 30 min, excluding the time of effective resuscitation. After a resuscitation team declares the patient dead, cardiac massage and ventilation are restarted while relatives are informed of the death. Once the consent for donation has been obtained, femoral artery and vein catheters are introduced, phentolamine and heparin are administered, and the kidneys are perfused with preservation solution chilled to 4°C (Booster et al 1993).

Using this protocol and excluding hypertensive or diabetic donors as well as patients aged more than 60 years, Wijnen et al (1995) reported a 5-year patient survival rate of 75% and a graft survival rate of 54% among 57 recipients of kidneys from asystolic donors, compared with 77% and 55%, respectively, among 114 matched controls that received a kidney from heart-beating donors. However, kidneys from nonheart-beating donors had a significantly higher rate of delayed graft function, compared to those from heart-beating donors (60% versus 35%, respectively). Since these results are clearly inferior to those obtained using heart-beating cadaveric donors, it would seem most prudent to confine efforts with nonheart-beating donors to selected institutions seeking to develop new protocols that increase success rates.

Cadaveric donor evaluation

Medical evaluation

Once the diagnosis of irreversible brain death has been established for the potential heart-beating cadaveric donor, a general clinical evaluation is performed to identify underlying medical conditions that might contraindicate organ procurement (Table 4.3), particularly sepsis or malignancies other than basal cell skin cancers or neoplasms confined above the tentorium. The evaluation of a cadaveric organ donor includes a medical history, physical examination, and laboratory studies. The two main goals of donor evaluation are, first, to exclude donors with severe diseases that can be transmitted to the recipient, and, second, to exclude kidneys with severe anatomical or functional changes that could compromise the allograft function. The presence of any of several factors may result in the designation of a donor as 'marginal' (Alexander and Vaughn 1991), exacerbating the adverse recipient risk factors of arteriosclerotic vascular disease, long anastomosis time, hypertension, and/or acidosis. Although there is today a tendency to be more flexible than in the past in accepting suboptimal cadaveric donors, in many instances, the decision whether to accept kidneys from a marginal donor can be difficult (Table 4.4).

Presence of cancer

Since the ability to transmit cancer from donor to recipient through a transplanted kidney is well documented (Penn 1991), donors with cancer should be excluded. Exceptions may be made for donors with cutaneous basal cell carcinoma or primary brain

Absolute contraindications	Relative contraindications
Prolonged hypothermia	Prolonged hypotension
Systemic lupus erythematosus and other collagen vascular diseases with renal involvement	Diabetes mellitus
	Age over 70 years
Congenital/acquired metabolic disorders	History or evidence of renal disease
Sickle cell anemia and related hemoglobinopathies	Poorly treated or untreated pre-existent hypertension
Malignancy other than confined to the CNS or basal cell carcinoma of the skin	Pathologic urine analysis (severe proteinuria)
	High and/or rising terminal serum creatinine level (>2.3 mg/dl)
Generalized viral or bacterial infections	Creatinine clearance ≤60 ml/min
Human immunodeficiency virus carrier state	Preterminal urine output less than 0.5 ml/kg per hour
	Profound preterminal use of inotropic or vasoconstrictor drugs
	Disseminated intravascular coagulation
	Hepatitis B or C

Table 4.3. Contraindications for cadaver kidney procurement

Vascular/urological abnormalities
Arterial hypertension
Elevated last plasma creatinine
Long cold ischemia time
Older age/age under 5 years
HBV-HCV positivity
Poisoning
Mild renal diseases

Table 4.4. Marginal cadaveric donors

tumors that do not tend to metastasize. However, cases have been reported of cancer transmission from donors with primary brain tumors that have been palliated by means of ventricular shunts (Lefrançois et al 1987; Morse et al 1990) or extensive craniotomy (Ruiz et al 1993). Reports of donor-to-recipient transmission of chorioncarcinoma (Penn 1991; Doutrelepont et al 1995) have led to the recommendation that chorionic gonadotropin be measured in all women of childbearing age who have died from cerebral hemorrhage. Of particular concern is the transmission of unrecognized carcinoma in the donor kidney, a condition that can often lead to recipient fatalities (Penn 1995).

To minimize the risks of cancer transmission, a few guidelines should be followed. First, donor screening should include a careful history with special attention to any suspicion of neoplasia, a kidney ultrasonography, a chest radiograph, and measurement of human chorionic gonadotropins. Second, after nephrectomy, the kidneys should be carefully inspected, with removal and histological examination of any small suspected tumors. Third, in the case of an incidental malignant tumor found at autopsy, the clinician should consider the strong probability that the tumor could develop in the recipient (Penn 1988), although in some cases nephrectomy of the transplanted kidney may cure the transmitted cancer.

Presence of infections

The presence of the human immunodeficiency virus (HIV) should preclude the use of the organs of the potential donor, as the transmission of virus with development of fatal infection in the recipient is well documented (Erice et al 1991). In children with brain death, it is important to exclude underlying varicella virus infection, which may be transmitted to the recipient and thereby introduce a high risk of fatal encephalitis. Serologic assays for latent viruses such as cytomegalovirus and Epstein–Barr virus are useful not for deciding whether to accept or refuse the donor, but to allocate the organ to, or at least plan preventive strategies in, the recipient (Rubin 1994).

Many transplant centers exclude from donation carriers of hepatitis B or C virus (HCV), as the ability to transmit these viruses through the transplanted kidney also has been well documented (Pereira et al 1995; Wachs et al 1995). However, the presence of hepatitis B virus in kidney transplant recipients was found to have an adverse effect on patient survival only after 10 years or more (Kliem et al 1994; Morales 1998), and it is possible that preimmunization of recipients with Heptavax will attenuate disease transmission. Furthermore, transplantation of kidneys from HCV-positive donors to HCV-positive recipients was associated with 5-year patient and graft survival rates similar to those observed with HCV-negative donors to HCV-negative recipients (Morales et al 1995; Ali et al 1998). Nevertheless, superinfection with a new viral genotype poses a potential problem. Pereira and Levey (1997) analyzed the impact of policies directing the use of HCV-positive donors in the United States. If HCV-positive kidneys were restricted to anti-HCV positive recipients, organ loss would be zero, transmission 2.4%, and new infection 0.5%; if these kidneys were restricted to HCV-RNA-positive recipients, organ loss would be zero, transmission 2.4%, and infection zero. In view of the good results observed at 5 years, this latter option seems an acceptable strategy to help reduce the donor shortage without incurring risks for the recipient.

Many potential donors acquire bacterial or fungal infections in the intensive care unit. Transplanting an infected kidney or a kidney from a patient with bacteremia or fungemia may expose the vascular suture lines, leading to the development of mycotic aneurysms with the consequence of catastrophic rupture (Rubin 1994). However, grafts from donors with syphilis (Caballero et al 1998a), bacterial meningitis (López-Navidad et al 1997), or bacterial endocarditis (Caballero et al 1998b) have been successful in anecdotal reports. Recently, Rubin and Fishman (1998) proposed that donors with systemic infection might also be accepted if certain recommendations were followed. These recommendations included using only those donors displaying bacteremia with a relatively bland organism—for example, Enterobacteriaceae (with the exception of *Salmonella* and *Streptococcus viridans*), or with an organism that has a high success rate of being rapidly cleared with bactericidal therapy. Bacteremia due to *Staphylococcus aureus*, *Pseudomonas aeruginosa*, or penicillin-resistant streptococci should be treated for at least 2 weeks, with blood cultures negative over a period of 1 week off antibiotics to assure adequate coverage. In contrast, one should exclude donors with septicemia caused by difficult-to-eradicate organisms: vancomycin-resistant enterococci, *S. milleri*, *Salmonella*, or fungal, nocardial, or mycobacterial etiologies.

Poisoning

Poisoning as a cause of death does not necessarily represent an absolute contraindication to donation. Organs have been successfully transplanted from donors who died from carbon monoxide (Hebert et al 1992), cyanide (Barkoukis et al 1993), methanol (Freidlaender et al 1996), or anticoagulant rodenticide (Ornstein et al 1999) poisoning.

Renal diseases

A history of diabetes mellitus and the presence of more than minimal proteinuria are each usually considered contraindications to donation. However, favorable results have been obtained with kidney transplants harvested from donors with hepatorenal syndrome (Koppel et al 1969), early diabetic nephropathy (Alexander 1992), or IgA nephropathy (Cosyns et al 1998).

Renal anatomic abnormalities

Preretrieval vasoconstrictive pressor support represents a relative contraindication because of the adverse effects on renal vasculature. Most vascular and/or urological abnormalities do not represent a contraindication to donation. Kidneys with multiple vessels, benign cysts, and other urological abnormalities have been transplanted with success (Vegeto and Berardinelli 1982; Schulak et al 1997).

Arterial hypertension

Little information is available on the outcome of kidneys harvested from hypertensive donors. Although this condition usually represents a relative contraindication, particularly for donors on chronic medical therapy, good results using hypertensive cadaveric donors have been reported in a small series (Lee et al 1996). A recent retrospective analysis of the UNOS database (Cho 1999) showed that the duration of hypertension in the donor affected graft survival. Kidneys transplanted from donors with less than a 5-year history of hypertension were intermediate between the results with kidneys from normotensive donors and those with kidneys from donors with a longer history of hypertension.

Renal hemodynamic instability

Many transplant units reject donors that display renal dysfunction before operation. However, a retrospective analysis of French data showed no difference between patients whose last plasma creatinine concentration was higher, versus patients whose concentration was lower, than 2.3 mg/dl (Alexandre et al 1996). A review of 1157 renal transplant patients suggested that neither oliguria nor hypotensive episodes in the donor influenced the risk of delayed graft function (Groenewoud and De Boer 1995).

Cold ischemia time

Prolonged preservation or anastomosis times significantly increase the incidence of chronic cyclosporine (CsA) nephrotoxicity (Table 4.5). More importantly, cold ischemia times longer than 24 hours are usually considered a major risk factor for delayed graft function—a major complication that is associated with reduced graft, but not patient, survival (Figure 4.1). Indeed, Held et al (1994) identified prolonged cold storage of the kidney to be the major factor to reduce 5-year graft survival; extension of the cold storage time from 15.9 to 24.4 hours reduced the 5-year graft survival rate by 2.2% (Figure 4.2).

Factor	Outcome		P
	Good function	Chronic toxicity	
Preservation			
Mean time (min)	1072	1920	0.01
Incidence ≥24 hours	14%	72%	0.01
Anastomosis			
Mean time (min)	39	49	0.05
≥45	24%	60%	0.05
*Adapted from Keown et al 1985			

Table 4.5. Risk factors for chronic CsA toxicity*

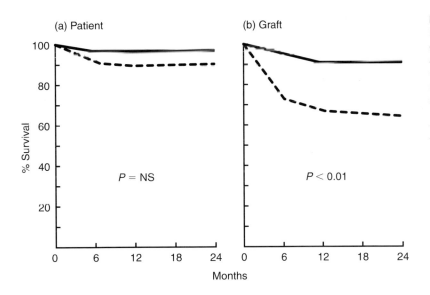

Figure 4.1. Impact of initial nonfunction on graft and patient survival (Stiller 1984). Graph (a) shows patient, and Graph (b) shows graft, survival rates for patients without (———) and with (– – – –) initial renal transplant nonfunction.

Older age

The effect of older age on the outcome of transplantation remains controversial. Although strict criteria demand that donors be previously healthy individuals between 18 months and 55 years of age, individuals outside this age range are increasingly being used (Lloveras et al 1993). It is well known that renal reserve is reduced after the sixth decade of life: the number of sclerotic glomeruli increases, the tubules may show signs of degeneration, interstitial fibrosis can develop, and the glomerular filtration rate may progressively decrease (Rodriguez-Puyol 1998). However, about one-third of older patients show no change in glomerular filtration rate (Lindeman et al 1985). It has been

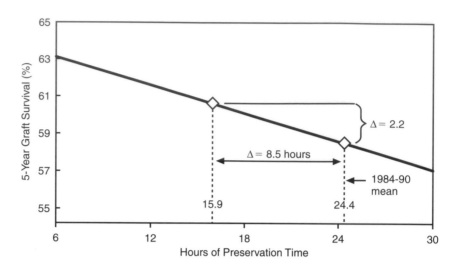

Figure 4.2. The 5-year graft survival rate as a function of mean hours of total preservation time for first cadaver renal transplants performed between 1984 and 1990 in recipients aged 10–60. Line is derived from Cox multivariate analysis. (Held PJ, Kahan BD, Hunsicker LG et al. *N Engl J Med* **331**(12):765–770. © 1994 Massachusetts Medical Society. All rights reserved.)

hypothesized that the renal dysfunction of the elderly owes to an accumulation of damage induced by minimal, clinically undetected renal disease rather than by aging itself (Rodriguez-Puyol 1998).

Several studies reported a negative impact of older donor age on graft survival (Cecka and Terasaki 1995; Hariharan et al 1997; Terasaki et al 1997; Miranda and González-Posada 1998). However, good results have been reported with the use of elderly donors in single-center experiences (Alexander et al 1994; Busson et al 1995; Kuo et al 1996; Solá et al 1998). These studies suggested that the values of creatinine clearance and the physiological age of the donor are more important than the chronological age. Thus, attention should be paid to the history and to the toxic habits of the older patient. A study of the retinal vessels may help to predict the severity of renal lesions caused by hypertension, atherosclerosis, or diabetes. Renal echography may provide useful information about kidney size, parenchymal echogenicity, and corticomedullary ratio, all of which are indirect indices of the degree of renal parenchymal sclerosis. The serum creatinine value on admission is an important index, but, in elderly subjects or in patients with small muscle mass, serum creatinine per se is not a reliable index of the glomerular filtration rate. A rapid and reliable estimation of the creatinine clearance is afforded by the formula of Cockroft–Gault (1976):

$$\frac{140 - \text{age} \times \text{body weight (kg)}}{72 \times \text{serum creatinine (mg/dl)}} = \text{creatinine clearance (ml/min)}.$$

The result must be multiplied by 0.85 in females. A more recent formula has been claimed to better correlate with glomerular filtration rate in elderly people (Baracsksy et al 1997):

$$\frac{1}{2}\left(\frac{100}{\text{serum creatinine}}\right) + (88 - \text{age}).$$

Even this formula, however, has a standard error of around 16 ml/min when the calculations are compared with measured iothalamate clearance.

It has been recommended that elderly donors with creatinine clearance lower than 50 ml/min not be utilized (Lloveras 1991; Kuo et al 1996), particularly if the patient is atherosclerotic, hypertensive, and/or diabetic. A final decision must be made in the operating room, particularly in cases of a disparity in renal size. Macroscopic inspection of the kidneys is a valuable tool for assessing the quality of the organs, particularly when there is evidence of scarring. Ex vivo renal allograft perfusion provides information about intrarenal vascular resistance. The presence of a benign macroscopic appearance and nonimpeded perfusion have been found to correlate with the presence of less than 20% of glomeruli that are sclerotic. In dubious cases, the quality of the kidney must be assessed by a renal biopsy.

Pediatric age

Some groups are reluctant to transplant the kidney of a pediatric donor to an adult recipient, fearing that a hyperperfusion injury might have a detrimental impact on renal outcome. A study comparing renal function in adults who received pediatric kidneys to that in recipients of adult kidneys showed no significant differences in either the creatinine clearance or the level of proteinuria at 3 years (Al-Bader et al 1996). On the other hand, transplantation in adults of single kidneys harvested from children younger than 5 years is often associated with poor graft survival. Vascular thrombosis (Sing et al 1997) and insufficient recovery of renal function often lead to progressive graft failure. To overcome these problems, en bloc transplant of both kidneys in an adult recipient has been recommended when the kidney has a length less than 6 cm (Satterthwaite et al 1997) or when the donor weighs less than 15 kg (Bretan et al 1997). Nevertheless, kidneys from donors younger than 2 years frequently (Satterthwaite et al 1997), but not necessarily (Amante and Kahan 1996), perform poorly when transplanted en bloc.

Gender

A detrimental influence of female donor gender on the outcome of cadaver kidney grafts has been observed in both primary and retransplant situations (Neugarten and Silbiger 1994). Nephron overload, induced by the smaller size of female donor kidneys, is hypothesized to be responsible for the poor outcome of female organs in male recipients. However, the possibilities of increased risks of acute rejection or technical failures may also contribute to the poor outcome of female-to-male transplants (Vereerstraeten et al 1999).

Limited nephron mass

Another risk factor associated with donor selection is limited nephron mass, due to elderly age, small donor size relative to the recipient, and/or female gender (Table 4.6). To minimize the potential risks of nephron underdosing with the use of older kidneys, several strategies have been proposed: transplantation of an elderly kidney to a recipient with a small body mass (Mizutani et al 1997) or to a female (Terasaki et al 1997), allocation of the kidney to an aged recipient (Cecka and Terasaki 1995), and/or routine biopsy to disqualify kidneys with severe histologic lesions (Delmonico 1997).

Recently, investigators have explored the option of grafting two kidneys from a marginal donor into a single recipient in an effort to increase the nephron mass (Johnson et al 1996; Alfrey et al 1997; Stratta and Bennett 1997). Save for the further attenuation of the disparity between numbers of cadaveric donors and recipients, the technique imposes some minor disadvantages to the recipient, including prolonged anesthesia time, a larger field of dissection, and a surgical complication rate that might, in theory, be twice that of conventional, single-kidney grafting. Alfrey et al (1997) studied the outcome of 52 recipients of cadaveric-donor kidneys that had been rejected by other centers. Of these, 15 received dual transplants while the remaining 37 received single kidneys. In the subgroup with donor creatinine clearance less than 90 ml/min, the risk of delayed graft function was 45% in single-kidney recipients, compared with 9% in dual-transplant recipients. In the subgroup of donors aged more than 59 years, the recipients of a single kidney had significantly higher serum creatinine values at 12 weeks than the recipients of dual kidneys. However, single- and dual-kidney recipients showed similar overall 1-year patient (96% versus 93%) and graft (81% versus 87%) survival rates. Presently, the partisans of the dual-graft program recommend use of this technique if the creatinine clearance of the donor is above 40 ml/min and below 90 ml/min (Dafoe and Alfrey 1998).

Donor	Gender/size disparity (nephron mass)
	Age (>60 years)
	Pre-existing disease
	Vasoconstrictor Rx
Storage	>24 hours
Recipient	Vascular disease
	Anastomotic time
	Hypertension
	Acidosis

Table 4.6.   Renal allograft risk factors

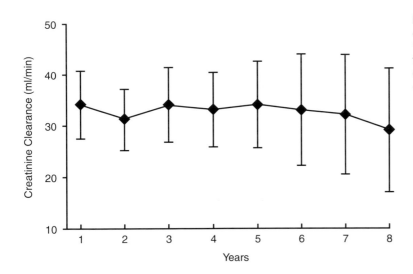

Figure 4.3. Mean values of creatinine clearance in 14 cadaveric renal transplant recipients with creatinine clearance <40 ml/min at 1 year.

The use of two kidneys is based on the assumption that the creatinine clearance of the donor is halved by using individual kidneys, and further decreased by the use of nephrotoxic drugs such as the calcineurin inhibitors CsA and tacrolimus. However, patients who receive kidneys with low preharvest levels of creatinine clearance and prolonged treatment with CsA posttransplant may maintain stable renal function for several years (Figure 4.3). We believe that the criteria for dual-kidney transplantation should be revisited to avoid halving, rather than increasing, the number of available kidneys. The use of two kidneys from a marginal donor presumes that the overload of a reduced nephron mass inexorably leads to progressive allograft dysfunction. However, if chronic graft nephropathy is primarily due to a problem with the kidney itself (Halloran et al 1999), the benefit of dual-renal transplantation would be less than expected. Clearly, further studies are needed to examine whether dual- versus single-renal transplantation has a superior impact on patient and graft survival, and thus to define the indications for dual-renal transplantation.

Cadaveric donor nephrectomy

Preretrieval procedures

After consent for organ donation has been obtained from the next of kin, the intravascular volume of the cadaveric donor is expanded to maintain a satisfactory mean blood pressure greater than 90 mmHg and a urinary output greater than 1.5 ml/kg per hour (Table 4.7). Vasopressors are withheld if possible, or reduced to the lowest level required to maintain a satisfactory blood pressure. To avoid renal vasoconstriction, dopamine

State of active diuresis (1.5 ml/kg per hour)
    Crystalloid fluids
    Colloid fluids
    Furosemide
    Mannitol
Correction of acidosis
Maintenance of perfusion (systolic blood pressure >90 mmHg)

Table 4.7. Cadaveric kidney donor: optimal conditions for procurement

infusions should not exceed 15 µg/kg per minute. Intravenous mannitol (1 g/kg) or intravenous furosemide (1 mg/kg) is often required to sustain an adequate urinary output. In contrast, diabetes insipidus frequently develops in brain-dead patients, requiring administration of 5–10 units of subcutaneous vasopressin, as well as aggressive replacement of excessive urinary fluid loss with intravenously administered fluids. Heparinization is withheld to facilitate the operative procedure, unless the donor displays severe hypotension and/or cardiac arrest, in which case 25 000 units is delivered intravenously to forestall coagulation of the renal bed. In the case of a nonheart-beating donor with delay in transport to the operating room, cut-down to the femoral artery is performed immediately, with retrograde infusion of preservation solution containing heparin. Although the incidence of delayed graft function is high in this situation, renal recovery is usually observed by 3 months.

Surgical technique for cadaveric organ retrieval

During a multiorgan harvest, the kidneys are usually recovered together. A midline incision is extended from the sternal notch to the symphysis pubis (Figure 4.4a). The Sarns saw or a Lebsche knife and mallet are used to split the sternum. Blood loss is limited by the application of bone wax and electrocautery. Self-retaining retractors are positioned in the sternal and abdominal components of the incision to maintain exposure. Occasionally, a combined midline and transverse abdominal incision (Figure 4.4b) is necessary for obese donors. For kidney retrieval, the posterior peritoneum on the right is incised lateral to the ascending colon, and then medially around the cecum and upward to the ligament of Treitz (Figure 4.5). Similarly, the surgeon incises the white line of Toldt lateral to the descending and sigmoid portions of colon. The right colon and small bowel, as well as the left colon, are reflected superiorly by developing a plane superficial to the gonadal vessels. The abdominal aorta and the inferior vena cava are exposed just proximal to the iliac bifurcation and individually encircled with umbilical tapes. The inferior mesenteric artery is divided at its aortic origin between ligatures. During the dissection, care is taken to avoid injury to polar renal arteries that may cross anterior to the surface of the inferior vena cava to supply the lower pole of the right

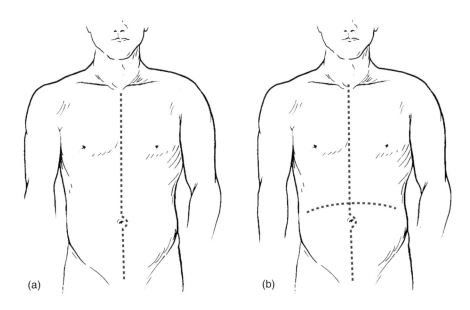

Figure 4.4 Incisions for multiorgan retrieval from a cadaver donor. (a) Midline incision; (b) combined midline and transverse abdominal incisions.

kidney or distally from the aorta to the left kidney. As the bowel and its mesentery are reflected cephalad, the left renal vein is identified as it crosses anterior to the aorta; it serves as a landmark for the origin of the superior mesenteric artery (SMA). The SMA, usually surrounded by a thick cover of lymphatic, neural, and connective tissue that requires sharp division, is ligated and divided. Isolation of the abdominal aorta above the SMA is facilitated by division of the crura of the diaphragm, following either direct entry via the lesser omental sac or by dissection extending medially above the spleen, for proximal control of the aorta at the point where it exits through its diaphragmatic hiatus. Division of the crural fibers above the aorta facilitates sharp and blunt, finger dissection to establish a plane between the adjacent esophagus and the aorta well above the SMA and the celiac axis. A large, right-angle clamp is used to encircle the aorta with an umbilical tape. Proximal control of the vena cava has usually been provided by the liver retrieval team, but, in instances in which hepatic recovery does not occur, an umbilical tape is placed just below the liver.

After administration of intravenous heparin (100 units/kg), a cannula is placed into the distal aorta and passed retrograde from above the iliac bifurcation to the origins of the renal arteries. The distal vena cava is ligated with an umbilical tape after a large bore cannula has been placed for drainage by gravity (Figure 4.6). The supradiaphragmatic portion of the inferior vena cava is then incised to allow venous blood to vent into the chest cavity (Figure 4.6a). After application of a clamp just below the diaphragm to occlude its proximal segment, the abdominal aorta is perfused in retrograde fashion with University of Wisconsin (UW) preservation solution (DuPont, Wilmington, DE, USA) to

161

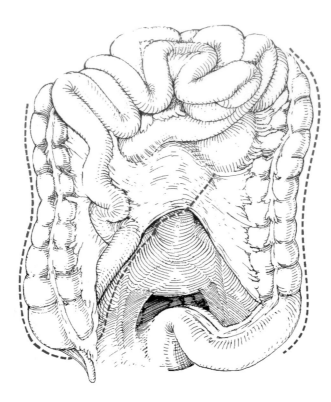

Figure 4.5. Incision of posterior peritoneum lateral to ascending colon, around cecum, and upward to the ligament of Treitz and on the other side lateral to the sigmoid and descending colon, as well as the spleen.

achieve in situ flushing of the kidneys. Iced slush of sterile saline solution is then applied to the kidneys to achieve surface cooling. During flushing with perfusion solution (Figure 4.6b), care must be taken to avoid either introducing air into the aorta, which may embolize into the kidneys, or obstructing the flow of perfusate into the kidneys by inadvertent placement of the cannula (Figure 4.6c) above the renal artery orifices.

The final stage of kidney retrieval begins by mobilizing and dividing the ureters deep in the pelvis. The distal ends of the ureters are tagged with mosquito clamps to facilitate identification. The kidneys are mobilized by sharply dissecting Gerota's fascia off the iliopsoas muscle and dividing peritoneal reflections. The left kidney is freed from the splenorenal ligament and brought through a mesenteric window created in the mesocolon. The lumbar arteries arising from the aorta may be controlled with hemoclips. The aorta and vena cava are transected above the level of the celiac axis, and the flushing procedure is terminated. As both kidneys with their ureters attached are gently lifted from the field, restraining bands of paravertebral muscles are divided to establish a plane above the bodies of the last thoracic vertebra and lumbar vertebrae to the sacral promontory. This en bloc technique avoids injury to the posterior wall of the aorta and vena cava during dissection; however, care must be exercised in the delivery of the organs during this final stage to avoid avulsion or intimal traction injuries of the renal vessels. The distal aorta and vena cava are divided above iliac ligatures to release the en bloc organs (Figure 4.6f).

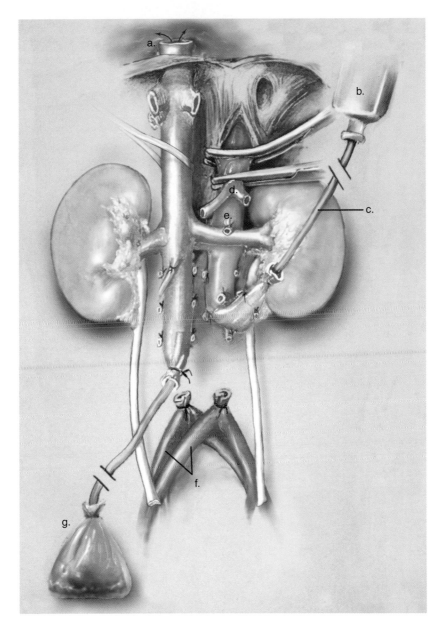

Figure 4.6. En bloc dissected specimen in cadaver donor. (a) Venous effluent from perfusion drains into the chest. (b) University of Wisconsin fluid delivered by (c) perfusion cannula solution in distal aorta, (d) celiac axis, and (e) superior mesenteric artery shown in sites after transection of distal portions. (f) Common iliac artery and vein ligated. (g) 'Bleeding bag' to catch venous effluent to insure a low-pressure efflux.

Ex vivo dissection and preparation of the kidney

The en bloc specimen is placed in a pan of cold saline. The left renal vein is first carefully dissected toward and divided flush with the vena cava to preserve adequate length (Figure 4.7a). The specimen is turned over (Figure 4.7, arrow) to expose the posterior wall of the aorta, which is then incised longitudinally to avoid injury to the renal arteries. After incision of the anterior wall of the aorta, the two kidneys are separated (Figure 4.7b), leaving the right renal vein attached to the inferior vena cava to permit extension of a short renal vein if necessary. Excess adherent fat is dissected from the kidney surface, and care is taken to preserve the triangular wedge of tissue between the lower pole and the ureter (Figure 4.7c). Each kidney is then placed in a sterile plastic jar holding iced-cold Collin's solution. The container is wrapped in three layers of sterile barriers and packed in ice for storage and shipping. In addition, 15–20 lymph nodes and 15 g of splenic tissue are removed for histocompatibility testing, and the incision is closed by approximating the skin with a continuous No. 1 nylon suture.

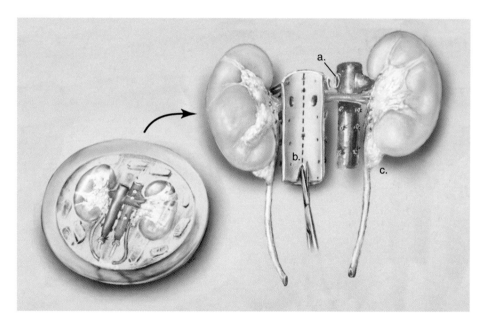

Figure 4.7. Dissection of the en bloc specimen. The left renal vein is transected at the vena cava (a). The anterior wall of the aorta is carefully incised (b). The kidneys are dissected free of adherent fat, preserving the fibroadipose triangle between the lower pole and the ureter (c).

LIVING-DONOR EVALUATION AND RENAL TRANSPLANT

Living donation is accepted by law, religion, and bioethics, provided that the donor is aware of the consequences of his/her act and makes the decision without outside pressure or commercialism (Spital 1998). A poll of the general population showed that most people would be willing to donate a kidney to a relative or to receive a kidney from a living donor (Sanner 1998). However, living-donor kidney transplant activity varies widely among countries (Table 4.8). In addition, the selection of living donors has created controversy among members of the transplant community. Some nephrologists do not encourage living-related donation, and some transplant centers rarely or never perform these procedures.

The main arguments against living donation are that cadaveric donation represents a valid alternative, that donation is not risk-free, and that living-donor transplantation may represent an excuse not to harvest every possible cadaveric donor (Michielsen 1992; Isoniemi 1997). On the other hand, the point remains that not a single country in the world can offer cadaveric kidneys to all potential recipients. In many countries, the shortage of organs is dramatic, and, in countries without facilities for full renal replacement therapy, the shortage of kidneys for transplantation simply means death for uremic

Country/Organization	Living-donor kidney transplants (per million population)
United States	14.1
Scandiatransplant	10.1
Canada	9.5
Greece	7.8
Switzerland	7.6
Australia	7.4
Eurotransplant	3.6
United Kingdom	2.8
Italy	2.1
Czech Republic	1.2
France	1.2
Spain	0.5
* Adapted from Transplantation Committee of the Council of Europe 1998	

Table 4.8. International data on living-donor kidney transplants per million population in 1997*

Shortage of cadaveric donors
Minimal risk to the living donor
Potential psychological benefits for the donor
Benefits for society and the recipient
Pre-emptive transplantation
Better results compared to cadaveric-donor transplantation

Table 4.9. Reasons for continuing and expanding living-donor kidney transplantation

Donors	Number of transplants	3-year graft survival rate (%)
HLA-identical siblings	1255	95
Parent	1974	86
Unrelated-living	1000	86
HLA-matched cadaveric	2023	80
* Adapted from Cecka 1999		

Table 4.10. Results of living-donor kidney transplants performed at 173 centers in the United States, 1994–1997*

patients. Moreover, several clinical considerations support the continuation or implementation of the use of living donors for renal transplant (Table 4.9). The results of living kidney transplantation are superior to those of cadaveric renal transplantation, both for related and nonrelated donors (Table 4.10).

Informed consent

A fully informed consent of the potential living donor and the exclusion of coercion and/or commercial practices are not only ethically necessary, but also mandated by most nations. Thus, even before considering clinical evaluation, it is important to verify that the potential donor is acting voluntarily and altruistically, and not under pressure or due to commercialism. It is the physician's responsibility to assess the motivation of the donor and to confirm the voluntary nature of the decision to donate an organ. Individuals who cannot be regarded as voluntary for reasons of age (children), mental retardation, or incarceration (prisoners) cannot serve as organ donors unless judicial consent is granted. The living donor must recognize the risks of the procedure, including the risks of mortality and postoperative morbidity, financial costs, and inconvenience. Donors should be made aware of the maximum level of risk they may incur, as well as the fact that they can change their mind at any point before the operation. A number of transplant centers also require a routine psychological evaluation of the potential donor, both to uncover psychiatric disorders that would preclude donation and to ensure that the donor has been informed of the potential risks and benefits of donating a kidney. (See further Chapter 20.)

Risks to donors

The use of living donors requires nephrectomy not to have severe consequences. The most dreaded complication is donor death. Two studies in the United States estimated perioperative mortality at about 0.03% (Najarian et al 1992; Bia et al 1995). However, these data included donations made in the early years of transplantation; it is likely that the perioperative mortality has since declined. For example, most of the few deaths were caused by pulmonary emboli, which can now be prevented with early ambulation and adequate anticoagulant prophylaxis. In the long term, donor survival is even better than that of the general population. In a Swedish experience, 85% of donors were alive after 20 years of follow-up, whereas the expected survival rate was 66%. This discrepancy owes probably to the fact that only healthy persons are accepted for living donation (Fehrman-Ekholm et al 1997), but it is also possible that regular follow-up visits after donation may contribute to a longer survival.

Apart from the risk of mortality, major complications of nephrectomy are very rare, around 0.2%, while minor complications occur in about 8% of cases. Wound infection, pneumothorax, and unexplained fever are the most frequent complications (Johnson et al 1997). One study found that donors returned to work after 5 ± 2 weeks, although their ability to cope fully with all aspects of daily life returned only after 9 ± 2 weeks (Binet et al 1997).

Concern has been raised that mononephrectomy could expose the remaining kidney to morphological and functional damage in the long term. Experimental studies showed that a five-sixths nephrectomy in rats with a high-protein intake may cause glomerular hyperfiltration by the remnant nephrons, resulting in proteinuria and glomerulosclerosis. It has been hypothesized that the reduced renal mass might lead to progressive kidney failure in humans as well (Brenner et al 1982). However, it has been demonstrated that glomerulosclerosis does not develop in all animal models of reduced renal mass. Even within the same species, the development of glomerular sclerosis does not occur in all animals, but is controlled by genetics (Striker 1998). Several studies in the 1980s in humans showed no evidence of renal abnormalities in subjects nephrectomized for living donation (Vincenti et al 1983; Anderson et al 1985; Williams et al 1986). One may argue that the 10- and 20-year follow-up periods of the studies may be too short to reveal detrimental effects of the reduced renal mass. However, more recent, well-designed studies confirmed that the long-term risk of kidney donation is low to nonexistent. At 20 years or more after donation, Najarian et al (1992) showed similar mean creatinine clearance, blood pressure, and proteinuria values between 57 donors (mean age 61 years) and 65 healthy siblings (mean age 58 years). Narkun-Burgess et al (1993) examined, in 62 men, the consequences 45 years after unilateral nephrectomy following traumatic injuries during World War II: mortality rates were similar to those of World War II servicemen of the same age, and the prevalence of hypertension was not increased. Five of 28 surviving subjects had levels of proteinuria between 377 and 535 mg/day, and three had increased serum creatinine values (1.7–1.9 mg/dl). The authors assert that conditions other than nephrectomy could have contributed to the impaired renal function in these patients. Glomerular sclerosis was not increased in 10 subjects who had autopsy examinations. Kasiske et al (1995) conducted a meta-analysis of 48 studies of 3124 patients that had been unilaterally nephrectomized for a variety of reasons, as well as 1703 normal persons. After nephrectomy, there was a mean decrement of glomerular filtration rate by 17.1 ml/min. However, this decline was not progressive, but tended to improve with each 10 years of follow-up (1.4 ml/min per decade). Although proteinuria progressively increased (76 mg/day per decade) among patients nephrectomized for other reasons, it was negligible after nephrectomy for kidney donation. The prevalence of hypertension did not change after nephrectomy, but systolic blood pressure increased slightly (1.1 mmHg/decade).

Thus, most nephrologists agree that unilateral nephrectomy in healthy subjects does not cause progressive renal dysfunction, but at most may be associated with microalbuminuria and a slight increase in blood pressure. Although these abnormalities are mild and not alarming, it may be prudent to perform a systematic follow-up of kidney donors to detect possible early renal complications (Bia et al 1995; Saran et al 1997).

Benefits to donors

In addition to benefiting recipients and society, living donation may also benefit donors. The immediate postoperative period is commonly marked by minor feelings of depression, especially if the donated kidney has failed. However, after the first days or weeks, most donors have feelings of increased self-esteem and lower scores of depression than normal controls. These feelings often persist for many years, especially when the recipient does well (Gouge et al 1990). Furthermore, the vast majority of donors would again donate their kidney if they could, even in cases in which the transplant has failed (Smith et al 1986; Westlie et al 1993; Spital 1997).

Benefits to recipients

Pre-emptive transplantation

Living donation can allow dialysis to be bypassed completely. The advantages are substantial for the patient, as transplantation improves the quality of life: no time is lost due to dialysis, and full employment can be maintained. Pre-emptive transplantation also represents an advantage for society, as it eliminates dialysis costs and disability allowance (Katz et al 1991; Thiel 1997). Moreover, two recent reports suggest that pre-emptive kidney transplantation is associated with better graft survival, particularly in living-donor recipients, compared with the outcomes among patients that received a kidney allograft after starting dialysis (Roake et al 1996; Asderakis et al 1998). Spousal donors further increase the possibility of pre-emptive transplantation. In Norway, about 66% of kidney transplants are now performed pre-emptively, of which 25% are related-donor transplants (Jakobsen 1997).

Results of living kidney donation

Even in the modern era of immunosuppressive therapy, living-donor kidney transplantation offers better results than cadaveric kidney transplantation in both the short and the long term. In the rare cases of transplantation between identical twins, no immunosuppressive therapy is needed. With the exception of potential surgical complications, the only risk to the recipient is that of recurrence of the original disease in the transplanted kidney (Tilney 1986). Apart from identical twins, the best combination for renal transplantation is HLA-identical siblings. A recent UNOS study revealed that the 3-year graft survival rate was 95% for HLA-identical sibling transplants performed between 1994 and 1997, compared to 86% for HLA-haploidentical parental-donor transplants performed during the same period (Cecka 1999).

Over the last few years, a number of studies have shown excellent results with transplantation from living-unrelated kidney donors, mostly spouses (Terasaki et al 1995; Lowell et al 1996; Alfani et al 1997; Binet et al 1997; Said and Curtis 1998). According to the most recent UNOS data, the results with 1000 living-unrelated donors were similar to those obtained in 1974 HLA-haploidentical living-parent donors, namely, a 3-year graft survival rate of 86% for both living-unrelated and parental-donor transplants. These results are superior to the 82% 3-year graft survival observed among 2023 cadaveric-donor renal transplant recipients (Cecka 1999) (Table 4.10). The superior survival rate of grafts from living-unrelated donors could not be attributed to better HLA matching, white race, younger donor age, or shorter cold-ischemia times (Terasaki et al 1995).

Since cadaveric and living-unrelated donors are equally genetically disparate from their recipients, the better survival rates of organs from living volunteers (Levy and Milford 1989; De Marco et al 1982; Terasaki et al 1995) compared to those from cadaver donors owe at least in part to the elective nature of living-donor transplantation. A thorough medical evaluation and preparation of the living donor increases the probability that the allograft will be healthy, functional, and anatomically normal. The circumstances of retrieval of organs from living donors can be controlled to avoid donor hypotension, bacteremia, warm ischemia, and/or prolonged cold preservation. In contrast, the emergent nature of cadaveric-organ transplantation poses several disadvantages. Not only may cadaveric kidneys suffer profound physiological derangement due to brain death, but it has also been hypothesized that irreversible central nervous system injury may upregulate the expression of proinflammatory mediators and cell surface molecules in cadaveric-donor organs, making them more vulnerable to host inflammatory and immunological responses (Takada et al 1998). Moreover, the damage produced by ischemic/reperfusion injuries may produce physiological changes (Ojo et al 1997), including the release of cytokines that upregulate HLA antigen expression on tubular and endothelial cells, thereby producing an increased risk of rejection (Goes et al 1995).

In addition to a better functioning graft, the living-donor transplantation procedure offers several advantages. Particularly in cases of familial donation, living donors may provide a higher degree of histocompatibility than is obtained with a cadaver donor. Recipients of living-donor kidneys also may receive preoperative immunosuppression, whereas cadaveric allograft recipients can only begin their treatment perioperatively. Moreover, living donation can facilitate pre-emptive transplantation, thereby eliminating the need for dialysis. In addition to all of these factors that may improve outcome, living-donor transplantation is associated with lower healthcare costs than those for cadaveric-donor transplants. Finally, living kidney donation poses minimal risk to the donor, in both the short and the long term, and seems to offer potential psychological benefits to the donor (Kasiske and Bia 1995).

Thus, there are many reasons to believe that related- and unrelated-living donors are ethically and clinically acceptable. In the United States, 90% of transplant centers accept emotionally related donors, while 60% actually encourage this practice (Spital 1996b). The increased use of emotionally related living donors could substantially mitigate the severe organ shortage worldwide. However, just as every effort should be made to fight any form of coercion or commercialism (Morris 1985; Chugh 1996; Broumand 1997), an excessive medical paternalism should also be avoided. The transplant center must evaluate and advise transplant candidates, but, in general, the donor should make the final decision (Spital 1997). As stated by the Ethics Committee of UNOS, 'The donor has a right to take a reasonable risk in order to achieve substantial benefit for the recipient' (Ethics Committee, UNOS 1992).

Living donor evaluation

Medical evaluation

Several considerations affect the identification of a living donor and/or the selection of an operative approach (Table 4.11). Living-donor evaluation, including a medical history and physical examination, laboratory tests, serologic screening for infectious diseases, excretory urograms, and renal arteriography, seeks to exclude donors with evidence of ongoing illness, as well as individuals at significant risk for subsequent development of hypertension or renal disease (Table 4.12). In the medical history, attention should be paid to diseases that can preclude transplantation, such as cancer, hypertension, renal disease, diabetes, or systemic diseases with potential renal involvement. Physical examination should uncover any condition that may contraindicate donation,

Healthy volunteer family member, spouse, or friend

Normal renal function

ABO compatibility and negative crossmatch

Normal or acceptable renal anatomy

Additional considerations

    Older age

    Obesity

    Vascular anomalies

    Atherosclerosis

    Skeletal deformities

Table 4.11. Criteria for living kidney donors

Laboratory tests

    Viral tests (CMV, EBV, HBV, HCV, HIV)

    Hematology

    Cardiovascular evaluation (ECG, chest radiograph, others)

    Abdominal ultrasound

    Mammography, occult blood in stool, PSA (in older donors)

    Serum glucose, cholesterol, transaminases, bilirubin

Renal evaluation

    Creatinine clearance (double-check)

    BUN, serum electrolytes

    Urinalysis

    Urine culture

    Kidney, bladder, and prostate echography

    Sequential renal scintigraphy

    Intravenous pyelography (optional)

    Renal angiography

Table 4.12. Evaluation of potential living kidney donors

such as hypertension, chronic cardiovascular disease, chronic pulmonary disease, chronic infection, or malignancy.

In addition to taking a careful history and performing a meticulous physical examination, a number of virological and laboratory tests should be performed routinely (Table 4.12). In younger donors without apparent risk factors, an electrocardiogram and a chest roentgenogram may be sufficient to evaluate the cardiac status. For older donors with cardiovascular risk factors, and/or for those with cardiac symptoms or an abnormal electrocardiogram, noninvasive cardiac stress testing and echocardiogram should be obtained. Glucose tolerance tests are usually limited to donors with elevated fasting glucose or with a strong family history of diabetes; glycosylated hemoglobin A_1C values may also be useful. To exclude the presence of neoplasia in donors above 50 years, we also recommend ultrasonography of the abdomen and a search for occult blood in the stool, as well as a mammogram and a pap cervical smear test in women or a prostatic-specific antigen determination in men.

Medical contraindications

Patients with HIV infections should be excluded from donation, since the virus is transmittable with the transplanted kidney. For the same reason, carriers of hepatitis viruses should also be excluded, with the possible exception of desperate cases in which both donor and recipient give informed consent. Evidence of an active infection should delay the transplantation until the infection is completely cured.

Generally, patients being considered for donation should be healthy or have only mild diseases that do not cause functional limitations. Patients with jugular venous distension, recent infarction, premature atrial or ventricular contractions, important aortic valvular stenosis, or poor general condition should be excluded due to the increased risk for cardiac complications (Goldman et al 1977). Diabetics are generally excluded because of the increased risk of postoperative complications in the short term and because of the potential risk of developing diabetic nephropathy in the long term (Kasiske et al 1996). The presence of skeletal deformities, particularly of the thoracolumbar spine, may also be an exclusionary factor, as this condition may contraindicate a flank approach for nephrectomy.

There are no precise guidelines for donation from patients with arterial hypertension. Although more than half of the transplant centers in the United States exclude as donors patients who display persistent borderline hypertension or take antihypertensive agents (Bia et al 1995), there is little evidence that well-controlled hypertension may lead to kidney damage in an otherwise healthy subject. Thus, it may not be unreasonable to accept as a donor a patient more than 40 years of age who has a normal blood pressure on therapy with one antihypertensive agent and displays no evidence of cardiac, retinal, or renal disease.

Other conditions of concern include obesity, due both to technical considerations to retrieve a well-functioning kidney and to the increased likelihood of postoperative complications such as atelectasis, wound infection, and deep venous thrombosis. Potential donors who are smokers are also at greater risk for postoperative complications. To minimize these risks, obese donors are encouraged to lose weight, and smokers to stop smoking. Most centers accept potential donors with a drug or alcohol abuse history, if abstinent for a suitable period (Bia et al 1995).

Renal evaluation

Creatinine clearance, blood urea and electrolytes, urinalysis, and urine culture must be obtained prior to acceptance of a living donor for kidney transplantation. Renal echography and sequential scintigraphy are useful but not essential tests for assessing the morphological and functional characteristics of the two kidneys. The greatest hurdle for the potential donor to accept in the evaluation process has been the aortogram, which seeks to define the renal artery anatomy and carries a 1.4% complication rate from puncture site bleeding, groin hematoma, arterial dissection, thrombosis, contrast reactions, contrast-induced renal failure, and, rarely, angina and neurotropic injuries (Egglin et al 1995). Advances in computerized tomography, using magnetic resonance angiography (MRA) or spiral computerized tomography methods, have simplified the procedure of defining donor vascular anatomy. Indeed, computer software programs incorporate these data into three-dimensional images (Lerner et al 1999). These techniques permit intravenous rather than intra-arterial delivery of modest amounts of contrast and overcome all the complications of angiography except for allergic reactions. In addition, these methods identify with a greater degree of accuracy the presence of multiple renal arteries, ureteral duplication, vascular plaques and calcifications, and/or aberrant or anomalous retro- or circumaortic renal veins. Some transplant centers also require that an intravenous pyelogram be performed to study the excretory apparatus; this measure may not be necessary with delayed MRA films. Only in patients with screening studies suggesting vascular abnormalities is it useful to perform an angiogram with selective renal artery injections (Table 4.12).

Renal diseases

Adult relatives of patients with polycystic kidney disease can be accepted for donation if they have a normal computerized tomography scan or renal ultrasound. Opinions differ about the acceptance of potential donors with nephrolithiasis. After nephrectomy, the donor could develop recurrent stones, obstruction, and/or infection, which might injure the remaining kidney. It seems reasonable to accept as donors only those subjects without stones at the time of evaluation and with normal values within a 24-hour urine collection of calcium, urate, and oxalate.

In families with inherited Alport's syndrome, inheritance may be X-linked; however, in up to 15% of cases, the syndrome develops due to a new mutation. Male relatives without hematuria do not carry the abnormality and can be considered to be suitable donors. Female relatives with isolated hematuria rarely progress to renal failure. The decision whether to accept a mother for kidney donation depends on the age of the woman and on the presence of other mild renal abnormalities. Female relatives without hematuria may donate, although the absence of hematuria does not completely exclude the possibility that the woman is a carrier of Alport's syndrome (Kasiske et al 1996).

Renal anatomic abnormalities

The vascular anatomy constitutes another important consideration. Because renal veins collateralize, only the largest vein must usually be anastomosed to drain the kidney. However, a particularly short right renal vein or a retroaortic left renal vein may present an operative challenge. In contrast, renal arteries are end-arteries and must all be anastomosed. Atherosclerosis of the renal artery, a not-infrequently encountered finding, generally tends only to involve the aortic origin and not to present a problem for organ retrieval. In contrast, a tortuous, bead-like appearance of the artery suggests the presence of fibromuscular hyperplasia, an absolute contraindication to donation.

Isolated microhematuria

The detection of microscopic hematuria in an adult donor necessitates careful evaluation (Fogazzi and Ponticelli 1996; Figure 4.8). In young adults, particularly women, the risk of an underlying cancer is small if the ultrasound is normal. There is a much higher risk of hematuria reflecting an underlying cancer among men aged more than 45–50 years; such donors require careful investigation.

An accurate study of the urine sediment using a phase contrast microscope may also be helpful. The presence of more than 75–80% of the red blood cells in distorted shapes is a finding strongly suggestive of glomerular disease, particularly when more than 4–5% of cells are acanthocytes (Figure 4.9). The finding of monomorphic erythrocytes sug-

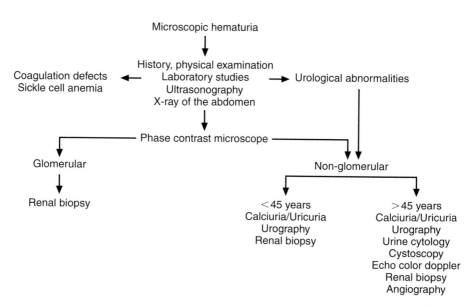

Figure 4.8. Algorithm for screening potential kidney donors having microscopic hematuria.

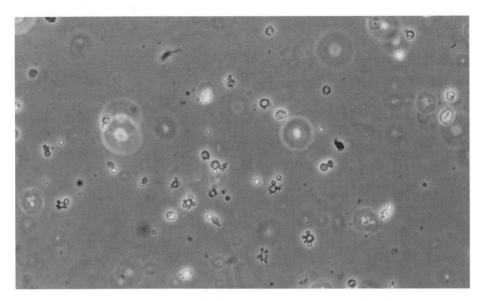

Figure 4.9. Dysmorphic erythrocyturia. Most erythrocytes appear to be distorted; many show characteristic protrusions of different size and shape (acanthocytes). This image is typical of glomerular diseases.

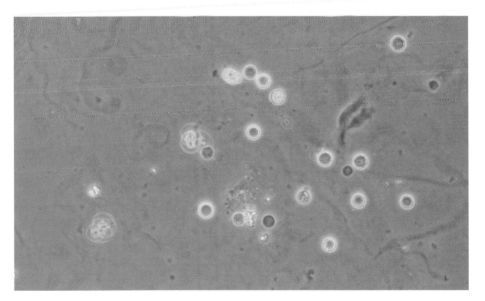

Figure 4.10. Monomorphic erythrocyturia. The erythrocytes are isomorphic and round, with differing hemoglobin content.

gests a possible lower urinary tract abnormality as the cause of the hematuria (Figure 4.10), although exceptions may occur, particularly in patients afflicted with IgA nephropathy.

Proteinuria

If a patient is polyuric, evaluation of spot urine tests for protein can produce a negative result despite the presence of proteinuria. Thus, assessment of proteinuria should be performed on a 24-hour urine collection. Urinary protein excretion in healthy subjects is less than 150 mg/day. An amount of proteinuria below this value is not considered a contraindication to donation in the absence of microhematuria, hypertension, or pyuria. Postural proteinuria is now recognized as a benign condition and does not represent a contraindication to donating a kidney.

Leukocyturia

Pyuria may be caused by a trivial urinary tract infection, but may also be associated with chronic pyelonephritis, tubulointerstitial disorders, or renal parenchymal diseases. The persistence of a significant leukocyturia in a potential donor necessitates a thorough investigation to determine possible nephrological or urological abnormalities.

Renal function

Most centers use serum creatinine and creatinine clearance to estimate the glomerular filtration rate. In the United States, 58.8% of transplant centers exclude living donors with a creatinine clearance below 80 ml/min, 21.2% accept donors with a creatinine clearance below 60 ml/min, and 10% do not exclude donors on the basis of creatinine clearance alone (Bia et al 1995). In evaluating whether the values of glomerular filtration rate are normal, one should consider the impact of multiple factors, including diet, muscle mass, and ability to accurately perform a urine collection. In particular, the values of glomerular filtration are strongly influenced by age, with a progressive decline after age 30–40 years.

Histocompatibility

Donors should be tested for blood and tissue compatibility with the recipient. ABO compatibility should be assured, although good results have been obtained with plasma-pheresis and splenectomy even when ABO-incompatible kidneys were transplanted. HLA-A, B, and DR testing of donor and recipient should be performed. Generally, one-quarter of siblings will be HLA-identical to the potential recipient, half of siblings will share one haplotype, and the remaining one-quarter will not share any HLA antigen. All parents will share one haplotype with their children. A T cell crossmatch between the serum of the recipient and the lymphocytes of the donor should be performed in an attempt to discover preformed antibodies against donor HLA antigens. More debatable is the significance of the B cell crossmatch, which some investigators alleged to have some deleterious effect (Feucht and Opelz 1996).

Older age

While there is no universally accepted maximum age for exclusion of donors, the upper limit for living donors was frequently proposed to be 55 years (Bay and Hebert 1987). More recently, however, several studies reported excellent graft survival and function, as well as little morbidity, using kidneys from older living donors (Berardinelli et al 1997; Kostakis et al 1997; Nyberg et al 1997). However, aged individuals, even those who fulfill all criteria for donation, may have the disadvantages of subclinical glomerulosclerosis and/or a reduced likelihood to display compensatory hypertrophy of the remaining native kidney necessary to regain renal reserve. Although we have had good results with kidneys from donors older than 70 years of age, a review of 960 living-donor transplants suggests reduced graft survival rates and higher baseline creatinine values among recipients of kidneys from donors over the age of 60 years (Kasiske and Bia 1995). Thus, while the use of carefully selected older living donors is currently considered an acceptable practice (Kasiske et al 1996; Spital 1998; Kerr et al 1999), such donors and their recipients should be informed of the possibility that allograft function may be compromised due to donor age.

Pediatric age

Most laws do not allow minors to donate organs. In some countries, the law permits a minor to donate if he or she possesses the mental capacity to make such a decision, or if he or she does not object. However, a questionnaire among centers in the United States showed that only 11% of these centers would exclude a younger donor due to age alone (Bia et al 1995).

Size

It has been hypothesized that the kidneys of small donors may have too few nephrons for a large recipient, and that this size mismatch could eventually lead to graft failure (Brenner et al 1992). However, a review of the results with transplants between spouses showed a tendency to better graft survival when the donor was the wife rather than the husband (Terasaki et al 1995). Other investigators did not find any significant impact of donor/recipient size matching on outcomes of living-donor kidney recipients (Gaston et al 1996; Miles et al 1996). Only 5% of centers in the United States reject a living donor if she or he is considerably smaller than the potential recipient (Bia et al 1995).

Living donor nephrectomy

Anesthetic principles and intraoperative preparation

Prior to the procedure and following hospital admission, the living donor undergoes hydration. At most renal transplant centers, the donor receives overnight preoperative hydration with intravenous infusions of dextrose (5%) in 0.45% saline at a rate of

150 ml/hour; however, some centers have been forced by insurance entities to perform a rapid hydration immediately preoperatively during a same-day admission (Friedman et al 1996). After inhalation anesthesia is administered, the legs are wrapped with compressive bandaging to reduce venous pooling in the lower extremities, and a Foley catheter is introduced aseptically into the bladder. The patient is placed in the lateral decubitus position. The kidney rest is raised and the table is flexed so that the flank is taut. Pillows and foam are used liberally to prevent undue pressure points. The upper arm may be supported on pillows, a padded Mayo stand, or a hammock support. The dependent arm and axilla are protected by placing an axillary roll to avoid injury to the brachial plexus. Through proper padding and support of the head, the cervical spine remains aligned with the thoracic spine, thus preventing impaired venous drainage of the head and the development of a transient Horner's syndrome due to overstretching or neurapraxia of the cervical sympathetic chain. The patient is then secured to the table with wide strips of adhesive tape over the shoulders and buttocks.

Following induction of anesthesia and stabilization of the vital signs, mannitol (12.5 g) is delivered intravenously as a cytoprotectant before manipulation of the kidney. For colloid support, administration of boluses of 5% albumin coupled with small 20 mg doses of intravenous furosemide may be necessary to maintain a brisk diuresis during the organ retrieval procedure. The anesthesiologist must remember that only the surgeon can monitor the state of the donor kidney, because its ureter has been transected and brought into the field; the urinary output via the Foley catheter observed by the anesthesiologist only reflects the activity of the remaining native kidney.

Systemic heparinization (1 mg/kg intravenously) is delivered 10 minutes before the vascular clamps are placed. Following organ recovery, the heparinization is reversed with slow infusion of an equal dose of protamine. The estimated blood loss during an uncomplicated donor nephrectomy ranges from 100 to 150 ml. Perioperative complications include pleural tears with pneumothorax, which, if greater than 15%, requires tube thoracostomy, or bleeding from the stumps of the renal artery or vein (De Marco et al 1982).

Flank approach

The left kidney is preferred for recovery because of its longer renal vein and the easier access to the origin of the renal artery. If the patient has multiple arteries to the left kidney, the right kidney may be harvested instead. The kidney is usually approached via an oblique 12 cm incision through the bed of the eleventh or twelfth rib, extending from the lateral edge of the rectus muscle ventrally to the midaxillary line dorsally (Figure 4.11a). After the muscles have been divided by electrocautery, a 4–6 cm length of rib is resected. Because attempts to approach the kidney via an intercostal space frequently result in incidental rib fractures, deliberate and limited rib resection generally seems, in our experience, to cause less morbidity than an intercostal approach. In some cases, a subcostal approach without rib resection offers less morbidity.

The retroperitoneal space is carefully developed without injuring the pleura, for this

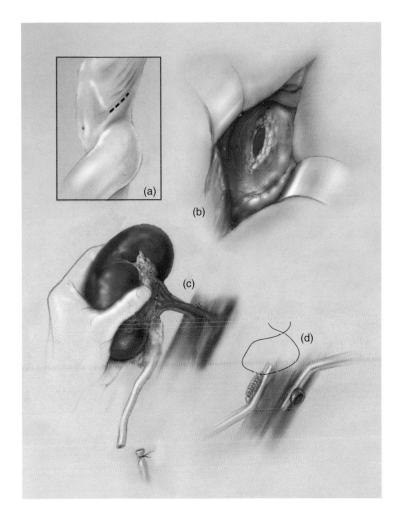

Figure 4.11. Flank approach for living-donor nephrectomy. (a) Line of incision indicated by dotted line. (b) Opening in Gerota's fascia revealing surface of the kidney. (c) Dissection of the origins of the renal artery and renal vein. Note that the ureter has been ligated and transected. (d) Oversewing of the proximal end of the renal vein showing the clamp on the vena cava.

complication produces a pneumothorax. Gerota's fascia is first incised to examine the surface of the kidney to exclude occult polycystic disease, scarring, or other malformations (Figure 4.11b). If the organ is not deemed appropriate, the procedure is aborted with minimal risk to the donor. Once reassured of the health of the kidney, the surgeon sweeps the peritoneum medially to identify the ureter in the vicinity of the gonadal vein. The ureter is divided at a level distal to its crossing over the iliac vessels. The distal, retained segment is suture-ligated with 2-0 resorbable material (Figure 4.11c). The proximal segment of ureter is mobilized—encased in a generous sleeve of periureteral tissue to preserve its blood supply, which emanates from the donor's renal artery. The kidney is then gently retracted upward to identify the renal vein (see Figure 4.11c). On the left side, communicating gonadal, adrenal, and lumbar veins are divided between ligatures

(Yang et al 1992). On the right side, the junction of the short renal vein and the inferior vena cava is gently exposed by sharp dissection of the connective tissues and by medial reflection of the duodenum and peritoneum. Generally, the right renal vein is procured with a 3 mm cuff of vena cava.

The left renal artery usually lies posterosuperior to the renal vein, whereas the right renal artery usually runs immediately posterior to the vein. During the left nephrectomy, the renal artery is mobilized to its aortic origin. Lymphatic, nervous, and connective tissues that course between the renal hilus and aorta are divided and ligated with 3-0 silk ties. If the renal artery displays spasm, producing a loss of normal kidney tone, a sponge soaked in 1% xylocaine (without epinephrine) may be applied to the artery, and manipulation of the kidney is avoided until the condition resolves. Topical application of warm saline may facilitate the process. At 10 minutes before donor nephrectomy, 50 mg (5000 units) of heparin is administered intravenously under anesthesia. After application of occlusion clamps and ligation of the vascular stumps (Figure 4.11d), the heparinization is reversed with protamine. The wound is closed in layers. Recent reports document improved outcomes with the flank procedure (Johnson et al 1997; Shaffer et al 1998).

The excised kidney is transferred to a back table, where it is flushed first with warm and then with chilled Collins solution. Initial intrarenal flushing with warm solution minimizes vasospasm and helps to prevent intraluminal thrombosis. Flushing with chilled solution thereafter achieves rapid core cooling and is complemented by direct surface cooling with 500 ml chilled saline. Because live-donor organs are stored for only short periods, the content of preservation solution is less important than in situations of cadaveric-donor kidney transplantation; indeed, Ringer's lactate has been used as the flushing solution without jeopardizing renal functional recovery.

Anterior extraperitoneal approach

An alternative to the flank approach is the anterior extraperitoneal exposure of the kidney, as originally described by Lyon (1958) and reintroduced in the early 1980s (Connor et al 1981). This approach affords better visualization of multiple arteries and the opportunity to use the supine position—a necessity for patients with skeletal deformities—rather than the flexed lateral decubitus position required for flank nephrectomy. A curvilinear subcostal incision is made from the level of the eighth costochondral junction anteriorly, to the eleventh rib laterally at least 3 cm inferior to the costal margin, to ensure adequate fascia for closure. The fascia and muscle are divided either by muscle splitting or by transection. The retroperitoneal space is developed by separating the parietal peritoneum from the anterior and lateral abdominal walls over the area from the diaphragm to below the pelvic brim. This maneuver exposes the entire abdominal aorta inferior to the celiac axis (Figure 4.12). Dissecting the colon from the anterior surface of the perinephric structures exposes the contents of the Gerota's fascia. After its upper pole has been released, the kidney shifts inferior and the renal vessels enter the center of the field. On the left side, the adrenal and gonadal veins are ligated and separated from

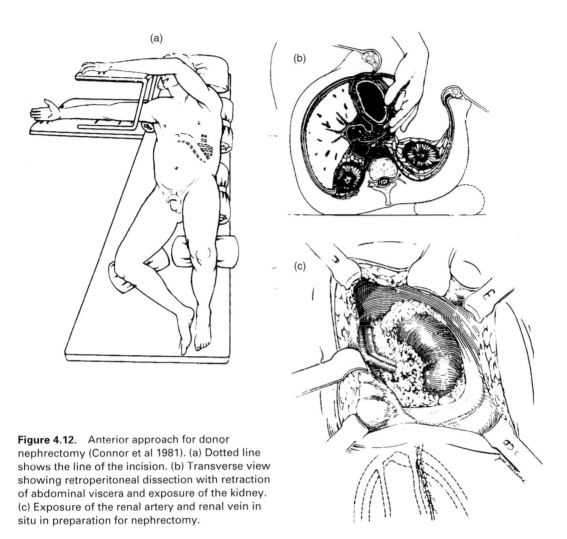

Figure 4.12. Anterior approach for donor nephrectomy (Connor et al 1981). (a) Dotted line shows the line of the incision. (b) Transverse view showing retroperitoneal dissection with retraction of abdominal viscera and exposure of the kidney. (c) Exposure of the renal artery and renal vein in situ in preparation for nephrectomy.

the renal vein. Approximately one-third of the patient population has a large lumbar tributary to the left renal vein that requires ligation to avoid injury to the posterior wall of the renal vein and to adequately expose the renal artery. The adrenal gland is separated from the perinephric structures to complete the mobilization of the upper pole of the kidney. The left renal artery is exposed at its origin by cautiously retracting the renal vein. A right nephrectomy requires mobilization of the renal vein and vena cava to obtain an adequate length of vein. Thereafter, the ureter is dissected to a level below the iliac vessels with a wide cuff of fatty areolar tissue and then divided. From this point onward, the procedure is performed as described above for a flank nephrectomy.

Unfortunately, patients who undergo the anterior extraperitoneal as opposed to the flank approach for nephrectomy experience an increased rate of pulmonary atelectasis,

181

namely, 43.7% compared to 15%, respectively (Connor et al 1981). In addition, the anterior approach is associated with greater blood loss: seven patients in the extraperitoneal nephrectomy group received 1–3 units packed red blood cells intraoperatively, whereas only one patient in the flank nephrectomy group received red blood cells. Thus, preoperative banking of autologous blood is recommended for donors who appear to be better suited to anterior extraperitoneal nephrectomy.

Laparoscopic approach

To reduce the magnitude of the donor operation—and thus the period of convalescence and hospitalization as well as the perioperative pain—and to improve the cosmetic result, laparoscopic living-donor nephrectomy was introduced by Gill et al (1994) and Ratner et al (1995). Relative contraindications to the procedure include obesity, previous operations in the area, and pediatric age group. Many surgeons restrict the procedure to left nephrectomies. The procedure is performed under general anesthesia with the patient in the right decubitus (45° oblique) position. After creation of a 15 mmHg carbon dioxide pneumoperitoneum to allow adequate visualization, the left kidney is mobilized and dissected via four incisions using special abdominal wall retractors/lifters. The ureter is dissected with a harmonic scalpel to minimize collateral tissue damage. Following anticoagulation, a laparoscopic stapler is used to divide the ureter, renal artery, and renal vein. The kidney is extracted via a 6 cm umbilical median, pararectus, or Pfannenstiel incision using an extraction sac deployed over the spleen (Flowers et al 1997). A valuable modification was recently introduced by Wolf et al (1998): an occlusive Pneumo Sleeve™ (Dexterity Surgery, Inc., San Antonio, TX, USA) is used over the left arm to encase the surgeon's hand, which is introduced via an 8 cm midline incision above or below the umbilicus to assist in the dissection and mobilization of the kidney and to facilitate more rapid extraction than can be obtained with a bag.

The major concerns about the laparoscopic procedure, other than the possibilities of injury to vital structures due to the indirect nature of the manipulations, are the long operating time, the increased incidence of ureteral complications, the requirement for extensive laparoscopic experience, and the prolonged warm ischemia time during the renal extraction phase. At least as presently practiced, laparoscopically recovered organs show delayed recovery of kidney function (Nogueira et al 1999), possibly due to the longer warm ischemia time; the operative trauma due to the indirect, distant manipulation of the renal artery; and/or the use of pneumoperitoneum, which has been shown to attenuate renal blood flow.

Postoperative care

Three major management problems arise during the early postoperative period. First, pain control is critical and may be treated by the use of an epidural catheter for instillation of and/or preferably by patient-controlled intravenous delivery of a narcotic infusion. Second, due to the sedation for pain control, the medical team must provide aggressive pulmonary toilet to prevent significant atelectasis and consequent development of pneumonia, as well as perform active and passive motion of the patient's extremities to avert deep venous thrombosis due to extended periods of bed rest. Third, urine output during the early postoperative period should be maintained, with fluid and diuretics, at levels greater than 1 ml/kg per hour. The Foley catheter is removed the morning after surgery, and virtually all patients void without difficulty within 6 hours. Alimentation is begun slowly at about 48 hours and progressively advanced. The patient is discharged from the hospital when intestinal function returns, usually on the fourth or fifth postoperative day. The major postoperative complications, which in aggregate occur in 0.23% of donors, include pneumonia, atelectasis, urinary tract infection, wound infection, and pneumothorax.

CONCLUSION

Alternative sources of kidney allografts will continue to be explored to bridge the ever-widening gap between supply and demand of heart-beating cadaveric renal allografts. Such sources include nonheart-beating donors, 'marginal' cadaveric donors that exhibit conditions that in the past might have caused reservations, and, most importantly, highly mismatched living-related and -unrelated donors. Living-donor transplantation offers several benefits over cadaveric organ transplantation: for the recipient, better graft survival rates and immediate renal replacement pre-empting the need for dialysis, and, for the donor, potential long-term psychological benefits. In view of the continuing worldwide shortage of cadaveric-donor organs and the success with living-donor transplantation, potential kidney donors must be sought both among living-related and among living-unrelated, such as spousal, individuals, before a patient accepted for transplantation is placed on a cadaver-donor waiting list. Although highly effective surgical procedures for both cadaveric- and living-donor sources for renal transplantation are now well established, procedural innovations continue to be developed to enhance the success of the endeavor.

REFERENCES

Ad Hoc Committee of the Harvard Medical School (1968) A definition of irreversible coma. *JAMA* 6:85–88.

Al-Bader W el-R, Landsberg D, Manson AD, Levin A (1996) Renal function changes over time in adult recipients of small pediatric kidneys. *Transplantation* 62:611–615.

Alexander JW (1992) High-risk donors: diabetics, the elderly and others. *Transplant Proc* 24:2221–2222.

Alexander JW, Vaughn WK (1991) The use of 'marginal' donors for organ transplantation. The influence of donor age on outcome. *Transplantation* 51:135–141.

Alexander JW, Bennett LE, Breen TJ (1994) Effect of donor age on outcome of kidney transplantation: a two-year analysis of transplants reported to the United Network for Organ Sharing Registry. *Transplantation* 57:871–876.

Alexandre GPJ, Squifflet JP, De Bruyere M (1985) Splenectomy as a prerequisite for successful human ABO-incompatible renal transplantation. *Transplant Proc* 17(Suppl 2):138–140.

Alexandre L, Eschwege P, Blanchet P et al (1996) Effect of last donor creatininemia >200 μmol/L on kidney graft function. *Transplant Proc* 28:188.

Alfani D, Pretagostoni R, Rossi M et al (1997) Living unrelated kidney transplantation: a 12-year single center experience. *Transplant Proc* 29:191–194.

Alfrey EJ, Lee CM, Scandling JD et al (1997) When should expanded criteria donor kidneys be used for single versus dual kidney transplants? *Transplantation* 64:1142–1146.

Ali MK, Light JA, Barhyte DY et al (1998) Donor hepatitis C virus status does not adversely affect short-term outcomes in HCV$^+$ recipients in renal transplantation. *Transplantation* 66:1694–1697.

Amante AJ, Kahan BD (1996) En bloc transplantation of kidneys from pediatric donors, *J Urol* 155:852–857.

Anderson CF, Velosa JA, Frohnert PP et al (1985) The risks of unilateral nephrectomy: status of kidney donors 10 to 20 years postoperatively. *Mayo Clin Proc* 60:367–374.

Asderakis A, Augustine T, Dyer P et al (1998) Pre-emptive kidney transplantation: the attractive alternative. *Nephrol Dial Transplant* 13:1799–1803.

Baracsksy D, Jarioura D, Cugino A et al (1997) Geriatric renal function: estimating glomerular filtration in an ambulatory elderly population. *Clin Nephrol* 47:222–228.

Barkoukis TJ, Sarbak CA, Lewis D, Whitter FC (1993) Multiorgan procurement from a victim of cyanide poisoning: a case report and review of the literature. *Transplantation* 55:1434–1436.

Bay WH, Hebert LA (1987) The living donor in kidney transplantation. *Ann Intern Med* 106:719–727.

Berardinelli L, Raiteri M, Vegeto A (1997) Aging living donor: the best source for kidney transplantation? *Transplant Proc* 29:195–197.

Bia MJ, Ramos EL, Danovitch GM et al (1995) Evaluation of living donors. The current practice of US transplant centers. *Transplantation* 60:322–327.

Binet I, Bock AH, Vogelbach P et al (1997) Outcome in emotionally related living kidney donor transplantation. *Nephrol Dial Transplant* 12:1940–1948.

Booster MH, Wijnen RMH, Vroemen JP et al (1993) In situ preservation of kidneys from non-heart-beating donors: proposal for a standardized protocol. *Transplantation* 56:613–617.

Brenner BM, Meyer TW, Hostetter TH (1982) Dietary protein intake and the progressive nature of renal disease. The role of hemodynamically mediated glomerular injury in the pathogenesis of progressive glomerular sclerosis in aging, renal ablation, and intrinsic renal disease. *N Engl J Med* 307:652–659.

Brenner BM, Cohen RA, Milford EL (1992) In renal transplantation one size may not fit all. *J Am Soc Nephrol* 3:162–169.

Bretan PN, Friese C, Goldstein RB et al (1997) Immunologic and patient selection strategies for successful utilization of less than 15 kg pediatric donor kidneys—long-term experience with 40 transplants. *Transplantation* 63:233–237.

Broumand B (1997) Living donors: the Iran experience. *Nephrol Dial Transplant* 12:1830–1831.

Busson M, N'Doye P, Benoit G et al (1995) Donor factors influencing organ transplant prognosis. *Transplant Proc* 27:1662–1664.

Caballero F, Domingo P, Rabella N, López-Navidad A (1988a) Successful transplantation of organs retrieved from a donor with syphilis. *Transplantation* 65:598–599.

Caballero F, López-Navidad A, Domingo P et al (1988b) Successful transplantation of organs retrieved from a donor with enterococcal endocarditis. *Transplant Int* 11:387–389.

Cecka JM (1999) Results of more than 1000 recent living-unrelated donor transplants in the United States. *Transplant Proc* 31:234.

Cecka JM, Terasaki PI (1995) Optimal use for older donor kidneys: older recipients. *Transplant Proc* 27:801–802.

Cho YW (1999) Expanded criteria for donors. In: Cecka JM, Terasaki PI (eds). *Clinical Transplants 1998*, Los Angeles: UCLA Tissue Typing Laboratory, pp. 421–436.

Chugh K (1996) Commerce in transplantation in third world countries. *Kidney Int* 49:1180–1181.

Cockroft D, Gault MH (1976) Prediction of creatinine clearance from serum creatinine. *Nephron* 16:31–41.

Cohen B, McGrath SMC, De Meester J et al (1998) Trends in organ donation. *Clin Transplant* 12:525–529.

Connor WT, Van Buren CT, Floyd M, Kahan BD (1981) Anterior extra peritoneal donor nephrectomy. *J Urol* 126:443–447.

Cosyns JP, Malaise J, Hanique G et al (1998) Lesions in donor kidneys: nature, incidence, and influence on graft function. *Transplant Int* 11:22–27.

Daemen JW, Oomen APA, Kelders WPA, Kootstra G (1997) The potential pool of non-heart-beating kidney donors. *Clin Transplant* 11:149–154.

Dafoe DC, Alfrey EJ (1998) Dual renal grafts: expansion of the donor pool from an overlooked source. *Transplant Int* 11:164–168.

De Marco T, Amin H, Harty JI (1982) Living donor nephrectomy: factors influencing morbidity. *J Urol* 127:1082–1083.

Delmonico FL (1997) Discarding the older age kidney: establishing the need for innovative utilization. *Transplant Proc* 29:130–131.

Dew MA, Switzer GE, Goycoolea JM et al (1997) Does transplantation produce quality of life benefits? A quantitative analysis of the literature. *Transplantation* 64:1261–1273.

Donnelly PK, Price D, Henderson R, Garwood-Gowers A (1997) Questioning attitudes to living donor transplantation. In: Donnelly PK, Price D (eds). *Commission of the European Community Project Management Group: The Eurotold Project*, Leicester: Leicester University, pp. 18–33.

Doutrelepont JM, Mat O, Abramowicz D et al (1995) Inadvertent transfer of choriocarcinoma with renal transplantation: characteristics of the donor-recipient pairs. *Transplant Proc* 27:1789–1790.

Edwards EB, Bennett LE, Cecka JM (1997) Effect of HLA matching on the relative risk of mortality for kidney recipients. A comparison of the mortality risk after transplant to the mortality risk of remaining on the waiting list. *Transplantation* 64:1274–1277.

Egglin TK, O'Moore PV, Feinstein AR, Waltman AC (1995) Complications of peripheral arteriography: a new system to identify patients at increased risk. *J Vasc Surg* 22:787–794.

Erice A, Rhame FS, Heussner RC et al (1991) Human immunodeficiency virus infection in patients with solid organ transplants: report of five cases and review. *Rev Infect Dis* 13:537–542.

Ethics Committee United Network for Organ Sharing (1992) Ethics of organ transplantation from living donors. *Transplant Proc* 24:2236–2237.

Evans RW, Orians CE, Ascher NL (1992) The potential supply of organ donation: an assessment of the efficacy of organ procurement efforts in the United States. *JAMA* 267:239–246.

Fehrman-Ekholm I, Elinder CG, Stenbeck M et al (1997) Kidney donors live longer. *Transplantation* 64:976–978.

Feucht E, Opelz G (1996) The humoral immune response towards HLA class II determinants in renal transplantation. *Kidney Int* 50:1464–1475.

Flowers JF, Jacobs S, Cho E et al (1997) Comparison of open and laparoscopic live donor nephrectomy. *Ann Surg* 226:483–489.

Fogazzi GB, Ponticelli C (1996) Microscopic hematuria. Diagnosis and management. *Nephron* 72:125–134.

Friedlaender MM, Rosenmann E, Rubinger D et al (1996) Successful renal transplantation from two donors with methanol intoxication. *Transplantation* 61:1549–1552.

Friedman AL, Goker O, Dennis MJ et al (1996) Must living renal donors be hospitalized overnight prior to surgery? *Clin Transplant* 10:444–446.

Garvin PJ, Buttorf JD, Morgan R, Codd JE (1980) In situ cold perfusion of kidneys for transplantation. *Arch Surg* 115:180–182.

Gaston RS, Hudson SL, Julian BA et al (1996) Impact of donor/recipient size matching on outcomes in renal transplantation. *Transplantation* 61:383–388.

Gill IS, Carbone JM, Clayman RV et al (1994) Laparoscopic live-donor nephrectomy. *J Endourol* 8:143–148.

Goes N, Umson J, Kamassar V, Halloran PF (1995) Ischemic acute tubular necrosis induces an extensive local cytokine response: evidence for induction of interferon-gamma, transforming growth factor-beta 1, granulocyte–macrophage colony stimulating factor, interleukin-2, and interleukin-10. *Transplantation* 59:565–572.

Goldman L, Caldera DL, Nussbaum SR et al (1977) Multifactorial index of cadaveric risk in noncardiac surgery. *N Engl J Med* 297:845–850.

Gouge F, Moore J, Bremer BA et al (1990) The quality of life of donors, potential donors, and recipients of living-related donor renal transplantation. *Transplant Proc* 22:2409–2413.

Groenewoud A, De Boer J (1995) Potential risk factors affecting delayed graft function after kidney transplantation. *Transplant Proc* 27:3527.

Halloran PF, Melk A, Barth C (1999) Rethinking chronic allograft nephropathy: the concept of accelerated senescence. *J Am Soc Nephrol* 10:167–181.

Hariharan S, McBride MA, Bennett LE, Cohen EP (1997) Risk factors for renal allograft survival from older cadaver donors. *Transplantation* 64:1748–1754.

Hauptman PJ, O'Connor KJ (1997) Procurement and allocation of solid organs for transplantation. *N Engl J Med* 336:422–431.

Hebert MJ, Boucher A, Beaucage G (1992) Transplantation of kidneys from a donor with carbon monoxide poisoning. *N Engl J Med* 326:1571.

Held PJ, Kahan BD, Hunsicker LG et al (1994) The impact of HLA mismatches on the survival of first cadaveric kidney transplants. *N Engl J Med* 331:765–770.

Hilbrands LB, Hoitsma AJ, Koene RAP (1995) The effect of immunosuppressive drugs on quality of life after renal transplantation. *Transplantation* 59:1263–1270.

Isoniemi H (1997) Living kidney donation. A surgeon's opinion. *Nephrol Dial Transplant* 12:1828–1829.

Jacobbi LM, McBride VA, Etheredge EE et al (1995) The risks, benefits, and costs of expanding donor criteria: a collaborative prospective three-year study. *Transplantation* 60:1491–1496.

Jakobsen A (1997) Living renal transplantation—the Oslo experience. *Nephrol Dial Transplant* 12:1825–1827.

Johnson EM, Remucal MJ, Gillingham KJ et al (1997) Complications and risks of living donor nephrectomy. *Transplantation* 64:1124–1128.

Johnson LB, Kuo PC, Dafoe DC et al (1996) Double adult renal allografts: a technique for expansion of the cadaveric kidney donor pool. *Surgery* 230:580–584.

Kasiske BL, Bia MJ (1995) The evaluation and selection of living kidney donors. *Am J Kidney Dis* 26:387–398.

Kasiske BL, Ma JZ, Louis TA, Swan K (1995) Long-term effects of reduced renal mass in humans. *Kidney Int* 48:814–819.

Kasiske BL, Ravenscraft M, Ramos EL et al (1996) The evaluation of living renal transplant donors: clinical practice guidelines. Ad Hoc Clinical Subcommittee of the Patient Care and Education Committee of the American Society of Transplant Physicians. *J Am Soc Nephrol* 17:2288–2313.

Katz SM, Kerman RH, Golden D et al (1991) Preemptive transplantation—an analysis of benefits and hazards in 85 cases. *Transplantation* **51**:351–355.

Keown PA, Stiller CR, Wallace AC et al (1985) Cyclosporine nephrotoxicity: exploration of the risk factors and prognosis of the renal injury. *Transplant Proc* **17**(Suppl 1):247–253.

Kerr SR, Gillingham KJ, Johnson EM, Matas AJ (1999) Living donors >55 years: to use or not to use? *Transplantation* **67**:999–1004.

Kliem V, Ringe B, Holhorst K, Frei U (1994) Kidney transplantation in hepatitis B surface antigen carriers. *Clin Invest Med* **72**:1000–1006.

Koppel MH, Coburn JW, Mims MM et al (1969) Transplantation of cadaveric kidneys from patients with hepatorenal syndrome. Evidence for the functional nature of renal failure in advanced liver disease. *N Engl J Med* **280**:1367–1371.

Kostakis A, Bokos J, Stamatiades D et al (1997) The 10 years single center experience of using elderly donors for living related kidney transplantation. *Geriatric Nephrol Urol* **7**:127–130.

Kuo PC, Johnson LB, Schweitzer EJ et al (1996) Utilization of the older donor for renal transplantation. *Am J Surg* **172**:551–557.

Laupacis A, Keown P, Pus N et al (1996) A study of the quality of life and cost-utility of renal transplantation. *Kidney Int* **50**:235–242.

Lee CM, Scandling JD, Shen GK et al (1996) The kidney that nobody wanted. *Transplantation* **62**:1832–1841.

Lefrançois N, Touraine JL, Cantarovich D et al (1987) Transmission of medulloblastoma from cadaveric donors to three organ transplant recipients. *Transplant Proc* **19**:2242–2243.

Lerner LB, Henriques HF, Harris RD (1999) Interactive 3-dimensional computerized tomography reconstruction in evaluation of the living renal donor. *J Urol* **161**:403–407.

Levy AS, Milford EL (1989) Donor and recipient selection. In: Milford EL (ed.). *Renal Transplantation*. New York: Churchill Livingstone, pp. 247–294.

Light JA, Kowalski AE, Ritchie WO et al (1996) New profile of cadaveric donors: what are the kidney donor limits? *Transplant Proc* **28**:17–20.

Lindeman RD, Tobin J, Shock NW (1985) Longitudinal studies on the rate of decline in renal function with age. *J Am Geriatr Soc* **33**:278–285.

Lloveras J (1991) The elderly donor. *Transplant Proc* **23**:2592–2595.

Lloveras J, Arias M, Puig JM et al (1993) Long-term follow-up of recipients of cadaver kidney allografts from elderly donors. *Transplant Proc* **6**:3175–3176.

López-Navidad A, Domingo P, Caballero F et al (1997) Successful transplantation of organs retrieved from donors with bacterial meningitis. *Transplantation* **64**:365–368.

Lowell JA, Brennan DC, Shenoy S et al (1996) Living-unrelated renal transplantation provides comparable results to living-related renal transplantation: a 12-year single-center experience. *Surgery* **119**:538–543.

Lyon R (1958) An anterior extraperitoneal incision for kidney surgery. *J Urol* **79**:383–392.

Matas AJ, Lawson W, McHugh L et al (1996) Employment patterns after successful kidney transplantation. *Transplantation* **61**:729–733.

Merrill JP, Murray JE, Harrison JH, Guild WR (1956) Successful homotransplantation of the human kidney between identical twins. *JAMA* **160**:277–282.

Michielsen P (1992) Organ shortage—what to do? *Transplant Proc* **24**:2391–2392.

Miles AM, Sumrani N, John S et al (1996) The effect of kidney size on cadaveric renal allograft outcome. *Transplantation* **61**:894–897.

Miranda B, González-Posada JM (1998) Cadaver kidney procurement. *Curr Opin Organ Transplant* **3**:197–204.

Mizutani K, Yamada S, Katoh N et al (1997) Cadaveric kidneys from older donors and their effective use in transplantation: a risk factor for long-term graft survival. *Transplant Proc* **29**:113–115.

Mollaret P, Goulon M (1959) Le coma dépassé [in French]. *Rev Neurol* 101:3–15.

Morales JM (1998) Renal transplantation in patients positive for hepatitis B or C (pro). *Transplant Proc* 30:2064–2069.

Morales JM, Campistol JM, Bruguera M et al (1995) Hepatitis C virus and organ transplantation. *Lancet* 345:1174–1175.

Morris PJ (1985) Presidential address: transplantation study 1984. *Transplant Proc* 17:1615–1616.

Morse JH, Turcotte JG, Merion RM et al (1990) Development of malignancy from a donor with a cerebral neoplasm. *Transplantation* 50:875–877.

Najarian JS, Chavers BM, McHugh LE, Matas AJ (1992) 20 years or more of follow-up of living kidney donors. *Lancet* 340:807–810.

Narkun-Burgess DM, Nolan CR, Norman JE et al (1993) Forty-five year follow-up after uninephrectomy. *Kidney Int* 43:1110-1115.

Nathan HM, Jarrell BE, Broznik B et al (1991) Estimation and characterization of the potential renal organ pool in Pennsylvania: Report of the Pennsylvania Statewide Donor Study. *Transplantation* 51:142–149.

Neugarten J, Silbiger S (1994) The impact of gender on renal transplantation. *Transplantation* 58:1145–1152.

Nogueira JM, Cangro CB, Fink JC et al (1999) A comparison of recipient renal outcomes with laparoscopic versus open live donor nephrectomy. *Transplantation* 67:722–728.

Nyberg SL, Manivel JC, Cook ME et al (1997) Grandparent donors in a living related renal transplant program. *Clin Transplant* 11:349–353.

Ojo AO, Wolfe RA, Held PJ et al (1997) Delayed graft function: risk factors and implications for renal allograft survival. *Transplantation* 63:968–972.

Ornstein DL, Lord KE, Yanofsky NN et al (1999) Successful donation and transplantation of multiple organs after fatal poisoning with brodifacoum, a long-acting anticoagulant rodenticide: case report. *Transplantation* 67:475–478.

Penn I (1988) Transmission of cancer with donor organs. *Transplant Proc* 20:739–741.

Penn I (1991) Donor transmitted disease: cancer. *Transplant Proc* 23:2629–2631.

Penn I (1995) Primary kidney tumors before and after renal transplantation. *Transplantation* 59:480–485.

Pereira BJ, Levey AS (1997) Hepatitis C virus infection in dialysis and renal transplantation. *Kidney Int* 51:981–999.

Pereira B, Wright T, Schmid C, Levy AS (1995) A controlled study of hepatitis C transmission by organ transplantation. The New England Organ Bank Hepatitis C Study Group. *Lancet* 345:484–487.

Randall T (1991) Too few human organs for transplantation, too many in need . . . and the gap widens. *JAMA* 265:1223–1227.

Ratner LE, Ciseck LJ, Moore RG et al (1995) Laparoscopic live donor nephrectomy. *Transplantation* 60:1047–1049.

Roake JA, Cahill AP, Gray CM et al (1996) Preemptive cadaveric renal transplantation. Clinical outcome. *Transplantation* 62:1411–1416.

Rodriguez-Puyol D (1998) The aging kidney. *Kidney Int* 54:2247–2265.

Rubin RH (1994) Infection in the organ transplant recipient. In: Rubin RH, Young LS (eds). *Clinical Approach to Infection in the Immunocompromised Host*, 3rd edn. New York: Plenum Press, pp. 629–705.

Rubin RH, Fishman JA (1998) A consideration of potential donors with active infection—is this a way to expand the donor pool? *Transplant Int* 11:333–335.

Ruiz JC, Cotorruello JG, Tudela V et al (1993) Transmission of glioblastoma multiforme to two kidney transplant recipients from the same donor in the absence of ventricular shunt. *Transplantation* 55:682–683.

Said MR, Curtis JJ (1998) Living unrelated renal transplantation: progress and potential. *J Am Soc Nephrol* **9**:2148–2152.

Sanner M (1998) Giving and taking—to whom and from whom? People's attitudes toward transplantation of organs and tissues from different sources. *Clin Transplant* **12**:530–537.

Saran R, Marshall SM, Madsen R et al (1997) Long-term follow-up of kidney donors: a longitudinal study. *Nephrol Dial Transplant* **12**:1615–1621.

Satterthwaite R, Aswad S, Sunga V et al (1997) Outcome of en bloc and single kidney transplantation from very young cadaveric donors. *Transplantation* **63**:1405–1410.

Schnuelle P, Lorenz D, Trede M, Van der Woude F (1998) Impact of cadaveric renal transplantation in end-stage renal failure: evidence for reduced mortality risk compared with hemodialysis during long-term follow-up. *J Am Soc Nephrol* **9**:2135–2141.

Schulak JA, Matthews LA, Hricik DE (1997) Renal transplantation using a kidney with a large cyst. *Transplantation* **63**:783–785.

Shaffer D, Sahyoun AI, Madras PN, Monaco AP (1998) Two hundred and one consecutive living-donor nephrectomies. *Arch Surg* **133**:426–431.

Siminoff LA, Arnold RM, Caplan AL et al (1995) Public policy governing organ and tissue procurement in the United States. Results from the National Organ and Tissue Procurement Study. *Ann Intern Med* **123**:10–17.

Sing A, Stablein D, Tejani A (1997) Risk factors for vascular thrombosis in pediatric renal transplantation. A special report of the North American Pediatric Renal Transplant Cooperative Study. *Transplantation* **63**:1263–1267.

Slakey DP, Patel S, Joseph V et al (1997) Patient acceptance of cadaveric kidneys from expanded criteria donors. *Transplant Proc* **29**:116–117.

Smith MD, Kappel DF, Province MA et al (1986) Living-related kidney donors: a multicenter study of donor education, socioeconomic adjustment, and rehabilitation. *Am J Kidney Dis* **8**:223–233.

Solá R, Guirado L, López-Navidad A et al (1998) Renal transplantation with limit donors: to what should the good results obtained be attributed? *Transplantation* **66**:1159–1163.

Spital A (1996a) Mandated choice for organ donation: time to give it a try. *Ann Intern Med* **125**:66–69.

Spital A (1996b) Do US transplant centers encourage emotionally related kidney donation? *Transplantation* **61**:374–377.

Spital A (1997) Ethical and policy issues in altruistic living and cadaveric organ donation. *Clin Transplant* **11**:77–87.

Spital A (1998) Living kidney donors: still a valuable resource. *Curr Opin Organ Transplant* **3**:205–211.

Stiller CR (1984) Update for the Canadian multicenter trial of cyclosporine in renal allografts. *N Engl J Med* **310**:1464–1465.

Stratta RJ, Bennett L (1997) Preliminary experience with double kidney transplants from adult cadaveric donors. Analysis of United Network for Organ Sharing data. *Transplant Proc* **29**:3375–3376.

Striker L (1998) Nephron reduction in man—lessons from the Os mouse. *Nephrol Dial Transplant* **13**:543–545.

Takada M, Nadeau KC, Hancock WW et al (1998) Effects of explosive brain death on cytokine activation of peripheral organs in the rat. *Transplantation* **65**:1533–1542.

Terasaki PI, Cecka JM, Gjertson DW, Takemoto S (1995) High survival rates of kidney transplants from spousal and living unrelated donors. *N Engl J Med* **333**:333–336.

Terasaki PI, Gjertson DW, Cecka JM et al (1997) Significance of the donor age effect on kidney transplant. *Clin Transplant* **11**:366–372.

Thiel G (1997) Emotionally related living kidney donation: pro and contra. *Nephrol Dial Transplant* **12**:1820–1824.

Tilney NL (1986) Transplantation between identical twins: a review. *World J Surg* 10:381–385.

Transplantation Committee of the Council of Europe (1998) *Organs and Tissues*, Strasbourg: Council of Europe.

Vegeto A, Berardinelli L (1982) Outcome of renal graft with multiple damage vessels. *Proc EDTA* 19:477–481.

Vereerstraeten P, Wissing M, De Pauw L et al (1999) Male recipients from female donors are at increased risk of graft loss—from both rejection and technical failure. *Clin Transplant* 13:181–186.

Vincenti F, Amend WJC, Kaysen G et al (1983) Long-term renal function in kidney donors. Sustained compensatory hyperfiltration with no adverse effects. *Transplantation* 36:626–629.

Wachs ME, Amend WJ, Ascher NL et al (1995) The risk of transmission of hepatitis B from HbsAg(−), HbcAb(+), HBIgM(−) organ donors. *Transplantation* 59:230–234.

Westlie L, Fauchald P, Talseth T et al (1993) Quality of life in Norwegian kidney donors. *Nephrol Dial Transplant* 8:1146–1150.

Whiting JF, Golconda M, Smith R et al (1998) Economic cost of expanded criteria donors in renal transplantation. *Transplantation* 65:204–207.

Wight C, Cohen B, Beasley C et al (1998) Donor action: a systemic approach to organ donation. *Transplant Proc* 30:2253–2254.

Wijnen RM, Booster MH, Stubenitsky BM et al (1995) Outcome of transplantation of non-heart-beating donor kidneys. *Lancet* 345:1067–1070.

Williams SL, Oler J, Jorkasky DK (1986) Long-term renal function in kidney donors. A comparison of donors and their siblings. *Ann Intern Med* 105:1–8.

Wolf JS Jr, Moon TD, Nakada SY (1998) Hand-assisted laparoscopic nephrectomy: comparison to standard laparoscopic nephrectomy. *J Urol* 160:22–27.

Yang SC, Suh DH, Suh JS et al (1992) Anatomical study of the left renal vein and its draining veins as encountered during living donor nephrectomy. *Transplant Proc* 24:1333–1334.

Youngner SJ, Arnold RM (1993) Ethical, psychosocial, and public policy implications of procuring organs from non-heart-beating cadaver donors. *JAMA* 269:2769–2774.

5 SURGICAL PRINCIPLES OF THE OPERATION

Carrel (1902) and Guthrie (1912) described the vascular anastomotic techniques for transplantation in 1904. In 1905, Floresco (1905) described implantation of a renal graft in the recipient iliac fossa. The first transplant procedure was performed in humans in 1906 by Jaboulay (1906), who anastomosed the brachial vessels of a human recipient who suffered from acute nephritis to pig kidneys, each of which functioned for approximately 1 hour. For several decades, clinical transplantation was attempted with minimal success until 1955 when Hufnagel, Landsteiner, and Hume (Hume et al 1955) connected a human pediatric cadaver donor kidney to the brachial vessels of a young woman dying of acute renal failure. The graft initially functioned, but had to be removed after 2 days. However, fear of anastomotic disruption of a ureteroureterostomy or a ureteroneocystostomy led to a prolonged period during which surgeons preferred to implant the ureter cutaneously. Hume et al (1952) used anastomoses to the femoral vessels and cutaneous ureterostomies in a series of cadaver donor kidney transplants. Although none of the kidneys exhibited long-term function, a few grafts displayed significant diuresis for more than a month. The procedure described by Lawler et al (1950), in which a renal transplant was placed orthotopically, was probably a technical failure; when the graft was removed at 7 months, it was the size of a walnut. The retroperitoneal technique was rediscovered by Kuss (1951), and then used by Murray et al (1955) to perform transplants between monozygotic twins that resulted in excellent long-term graft survival rates. The surgical techniques in transplantation have undergone only a modest evolution during the past 40 years despite the tremendous advances in immunosuppression.

Although technical pitfalls becloud all major surgical procedures, additional risks, such as impaired wound healing and diminished host resistance, are engendered by the immunosuppressive therapy required after transplantation. Wound healing also may be adversely affected by protein-calorie malnutrition or hypercatabolism, which may be observed in patients with end-stage renal disease (ESRD) resulting from a number of causes. (1) Anorexia or inadequate intake of nutrients (Schoenfel et al 1983) may engender an immunodeficient state (Mattern et al 1982). (2) Dialysis may exacerbate protein degradation, inhibit protein synthesis (Delaporte et al 1980), and trigger abnormal amino acid metabolism (Kopple 1978; Ward et al 1979; Garber 1983), particularly in the presence of underlying metabolic illnesses such as diabetes mellitus. (3) End-stage renal disease patients display decreased biological activity of anabolic hormones, such as insulin (Defronzo et al 1981a, b) and somatomedins, and contrariwise increased activity of catabolic hormones, such as glucagon (Corry and Kelley 1978) and parathyroid hormone (Hutchinson et al 1993). Furthermore, patients afflicted with renal failure experience enhanced susceptibility to infection, possibly resulting from inhibited humoral and cellular immunity, including adverse effects of (1) azotemia on phagocytes (Vanholder et al 1991); (2) guanidine on natural killer and T cell responses to interleukin-2 (IL-2; Dubrow and Levin 1995); or (3) bioincompatible dialyzer membranes on neutrophils and monocytes (Burt et al 1989). These immunodeficiencies, combined with the intensive medical immunosuppressive regimen, substantially increase susceptibility to infection, which continues to be a major cause of morbidity and mortality.

To minimize the risk of infection, particularly from commensal respiratory-, skin-, or gut-derived organisms, strict asepsis and meticulous hemostasis are essential. Careful skin preparation, aseptic insertion of indwelling catheters, avoidance of the use of drains with their proclivity to retrograde contamination, and rigorous postoperative surveillance are critical factors to minimize infection risk. Hematoma formation occurs not uncommonly, owing to the frequent use of anticoagulants to maintain the patency of vascular access, as well as intrinsic hemostatic abnormalities of uremic patients, including thrombocytopathy, which results from the direct effects of urea, guanidinosuccinic acid and hydroxy phenols, and plasma factor deficiency (factor VIII: von Willebrand factor).

RENAL TRANSPLANT OPERATION

Preoperative preparation of recipient

Potential recipients of cadaver-donor kidneys are admitted to the hospital on an urgent basis to receive a transplant within 6–24 hours. Although current preservation techniques allow storage of allografts with reasonable viability for up to 72 hours, grafts implanted with cold ischemia times of less than 24 hours function better in the immediate posttransplant period (Held et al 1994; UNOS 1994). Upon admission, the potential transplant candidate undergoes a chest radiograph, electrocardiogram, complete blood count, electrolyte panel, prothrombin and partial thromboplastin times, and crossmatch tests for ABO blood type compatibility and for transfusion of cytomegalovirus (CMV)-negative donor blood. The crossmatch tests include microcytotoxicity assays in which the most reactive historical and current (within 1 month) sera are used. Save for donor–recipient pairs that display no HLA-mismatch, the recipient is chosen from among the final pretransplant crossmatch-negative candidates based on whether the patient is presensitized. If no crossmatch-negative sensitized patient is available, the decision is based strictly on length of waiting time.

Patients who have received dialysis within 24 hours before transplantation are ideal candidates because they rarely show hyperkalemia ($K^+ > 5.5$ mEq/l) and/or acidosis, namely, a bicarbonate level less than 15 mEq/l. Although patients with hemoglobin concentrations greater than 6 g/100 ml may be anesthetized (Sears 1988), candidates with concentrations less than 8 g/100 ml may require transfusion during the procedure. Since intraoperative blood loss is generally estimated at 100–300 ml during an uncomplicated transplant, the liberal use of recombinant erythropoietin during dialytic therapy (Paganini 1995) usually precludes the need for routine preoperative blood transfusions.

The hypertensive status of the recipient must also be assessed. Poor pretransplant control of blood pressure by dialysis and oral antihypertensive medications may forebode hypertensive crises upon initiation of cyclosporine (CsA) therapy, which can exacerbate the ischemic injury to the organ. Furthermore, some patients experience either hypotension upon induction of anesthesia due to depressed myocardial contractility from beta-blocker therapy, or decreased total peripheral resistance due to chronic vasodilator therapy with alpha sympathetic and/or calcium channel blockade. The former situation generally responds to infusions of low doses of dopamine (1–5 µg/kg per min) and the latter condition to volume expansion. Finally, owing to concern about infection, patients are prophylactically treated preoperatively with intravenous broad-spectrum antibiotics (nafcillin and gentamycin) on call to the operating room and for 48 hours postoperatively.

Before the patient is anesthetized, the kidney allograft, which has been stored in iced electrolyte solution, is dissected at a back table to define the graft anatomy. The renal artery and vein are inspected for injury or anatomic variations. The perinephric fat is excised by sharp dissection, particularly seeking to preserve the tissue in the region of the lower pole of the kidney that envelops and provides the blood supply to the proximal third of the ureter. Lower renal polar arteries must be reconstructed to avoid ureteral ischemia or necrosis; multiple arteries joined as necessary; and the right renal vein lengthened using the vena caval segment. There are two approaches to address a short right renal vein. Division of the recipient internal iliac vein releases the venous axis and facilitates the venous anastomosis. Alternatively, Corry's (Corry and Kelley 1978) venous extension technique uses the attached segment of inferior vena cava to augment the length of the renal vein. Barry et al (Barry and Fuchs 1978; Barry and Lemmers 1995) reported two modifications to this technique: (1) use of a caval patch graft to repair the cephalic portion of the renal vein that may be inadvertently amputated during multiple organ retrieval; or (2) a transverse closure of the inferior vena caval orifices on the sides of the renal vein. When a double renal vein is present, one vein may be anastomosed and the other ligated due to Halstead's law that the venous circulation interanastomoses to provide drainage. During living-donor nephrectomy, it is possible to assess the dominance of venous drainage using a control loop to evaluate whether both veins need to be drained as a common ostium or whether one vein can be selected as a single anastomosis. Clearly, veins less than 5 mm in caliber can simply be ligated.

Anesthetic principles

Because optimal intravascular volume is critical for good renal transplant function, a central venous pressure (CVP) monitor inserted through either the internal jugular or the subclavian vein after induction of general anesthesia is extremely useful. The CVP monitors right heart filling pressures, as well as providing venous access for blood sampling and administration of intravenous fluids or vasoactive drugs. In patients suspected of cardiac compromise, a Swan–Ganz catheter is useful.

During the procedure, one liberally administers fluids to restore an adequate intravascular volume since many patients have been ultrafiltered preoperatively (Carlier et al 1982). Delayed graft function is a serious adverse factor for graft survival, both obfuscating the diagnosis of acute rejection episodes and reducing the extent of eventual renal recovery. One critical factor that minimizes the risk of delayed graft function is an adequate filling pressure. Unlike nontransplant procedures performed on chronic renal failure patients, in which the patient is required to be dry to prevent fluid overload and avoid postoperative dialysis, renal transplantation requires extreme hydration and luxuriant blood flow to the new renal transplant. We hydrate recipients to a minimum central venous pressure of 10–12 mmHg using 0.9% normal saline with or without 5% albumin (Davidson et al 1992) for initial volume expansion. Packed red blood cells are only transfused when the pretransplant hemoglobin is no more than 8 g% or the intraoperative blood loss is excessive. The mean arterial blood pressure is kept above 100 mmHg to optimize perfusion of the denervated, cold-preserved kidney. In addition, during the vascular anastomoses, recipients are administered a cocktail solution containing mannitol (adults, 25 g; children, 0.25 g/kg), albumin (50 g), and furosemide (adults, 100 mg; children, 1 mg/kg) to promote diuresis upon reperfusion. This regimen decreases the incidence of acute tumor necrosis (ATN) and early anuria (Luiani et al 1979; Weimar et al 1983; Lauzurica et al 1992). Occasionally, a low-dose dopamine infusion (2–4 µg/kg per min) is administered to improve renal perfusion (Hoffmann and Lefkowitz 1990; Sutherland et al 1993) or to maintain the mean blood pressure above 100 mmHg (Grundmann et al 1981). In addition, 100 mEq (2 ampules) of sodium bicarbonate may be slowly administered to reduce the acidosis caused by release of K^+-rich perfusion solution from the stored organ upon reperfusion.

The operative procedure

Preparation of the transplant bed

After induction of anesthesia, a 22-French urethral catheter is inserted into the bladder aseptically; any urine obtained is sent for analysis and culture. A large catheter is necessary, owing to the possibility of obstruction from blood clots from the cystotomy. The bladder is then distended with antibiotic solution (50 000 units of bacitracin:1 g kanamycin per litre normal saline) to facilitate intraoperative identification. It is critical to fill the bladder under gravity, since application of pressure may lacerate the fragile mucosa of the previously obsolescent viscus. The catheter is clamped and connected to a closed drainage system. The operative site is then prepared with iodine solution.

Three incisions have been used to perform renal transplantation: (1) the orthotopic lumbar approach; (2) the lower abdominal (hockey-stick) approach; and (3) the pelvic Gibson approach (Figure 5.1a). Orthotopic placement of the kidney in its normal posi-

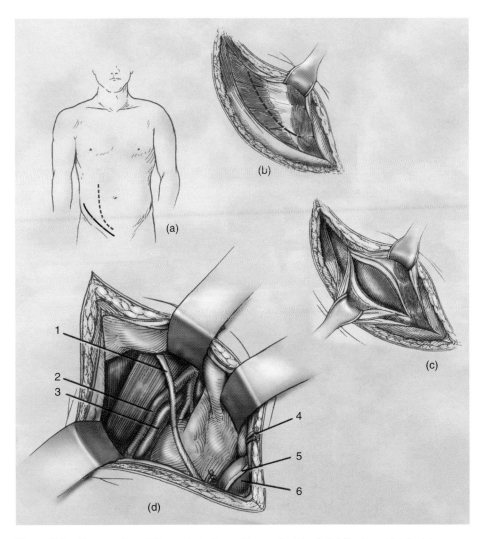

Figure 5.1. Preparation of the recipient renal transplant bed. (a) Hockey-stick incision (dotted) and the usual Gibson incision (solid). (b) Incision in the abdominus internus muscle; (c) splitting across the transversalis fibers to expose the peritoneal reflection. (d) The allograft bed showing host ureter (1), iliac artery (2)/vein (3), epigastric vessels (4) controlled by ligatures, and bladder (6). Note that the spermatic cord (5) is reflected medially.

tion in the left flank with restoration of continuity of the urinary tract, as attempted by Lawler et al (1950) and by Kuss et al (1951), is mentioned primarily for historical reasons, although it may represent the only option if there is occlusion of the infrarenal vena cava or if the kidney transplant is being performed en bloc as part of a cluster transplant operation. A single incision is used to remove the native kidney, with transplantation of the donor organ into the same bed. The allograft artery is anastomosed end-to-end, either to the stump of the recipient renal artery (if it is sufficiently large), or to the splenic artery after concomitant splenectomy. The donor vein is anastomosed to the stump of the recipient renal vein. The donor ureter is anastomosed end-to-end to the recipient ureter. Transplant surgeons rarely use this technique, since the renal pedicle provides only a tenuous support for the graft, because the graft is impalpable and relatively inaccessible to percutaneous biopsy or other manipulations. The primary indiction for orthotopic transplantation in the present era is an occluded infrarenal vena cava.

The usual strategy is to transplant the graft into the iliac fossa. The side for renal transplantation is selected to avoid areas of peripheral vascular disease, as assessed by preoperative angiogram or dampened femoral pulse, and/or the presence of a previously failed transplant. If there is no contraindication, the right iliac fossa is generally preferred, since the right iliac vein runs a more superficial and horizontal course.

One lower-abdominal technique uses a modified hockey-stick (J-type; Figure 5.1a) incision that can be extended cephalad toward the subcostal margin as originally advocated by Starzl et al (1964). This approach has the advantages of minimal muscle splitting, and of excellent access to the common iliac vessels, aortic bifurcation, and inferior vena cava. This strategy is particularly suitable for intraperitoneal transplantation in small pediatric recipients; for patients with previous iliac artery disease, arterial dissection, or transplantation; or for patients who require a venous anastomosis to the proximal common iliac vein or the lower inferior vena cava.

The most widely used technique is the Gibson incision (Figure 5.1a), which extends from the midline, namely, one and one-half finger-breadths above the symphysis pubis in curvilinear fashion to a point three finger-breadths medial to the anterior superior iliac spine. The external oblique muscle is divided in the direction of its fibers (Figure 5.1b). At the lateral corner of the incision, the muscle is split; medially, the incision is carried into the rectus sheath to facilitate exposure of the bladder. The internal oblique and transversus abdominis muscles (Figure 5.1c) are divided as a unit, a procedure that is facilitated by insinuating a Kelly clamp through the two muscle layers at the lateral corner of the incision. The properitoneal space is developed by sweeping the peritoneum cephalad from the undersurface of the transversus abdominis muscle. The internal oblique and transversus abdominis muscles are then divided simultaneously with an electrocautery, stopping at the medial corner just lateral to the rectus muscle. Division of the rectus muscle up to the midline is restricted for cases in which it is difficult to obtain adequate exposure of the bladder. The inferior epigastric vessels are ligated and divided. Exposure of the iliac fossa is obtained by reflecting the peritoneum superiorly to the level of the common iliac artery. The spermatic cord in males is preserved by reflecting it medially; the round ligament of females is ligated and divided. A self-retaining Bookwalter retractor affords exposure of the iliac vessels (Figure 5.1d). The lateral blades are padded to prevent injury to the lateral femoral cutaneous nerve, and the inferior blade is padded to avoid compression of the femoral nerve. Traction injuries to these structures can cause sensorimotor deficits on the ipsilateral anterior thigh. The superficial femoral nerve may be injured as it emerges proximal to the inguinal ligament and lateral to the femoral vessels. The symptoms of quadriceps weakness or painless cutaneous numbness of the lateral thigh typically present within the first 2–5 postoperative days and resolve within 2–12 months.

Revascularization of the kidney: usual approaches

The transplant procedure starts when the flushed, cooled kidney is brought to the operative field. During the vascular anastomoses, the kidney must be kept cold by continuous surface irrigation with iced-cold saline. The kidney is placed where it lies most naturally within the renal pelvis, with the ureter oriented distally. Unless the artery is particularly short or the anastomosis is deemed difficult, the deeper venous anastomosis is usually performed first. After application of proximal and distal vascular occlusion clamps and incision of a 10–15 mm venotomy, the host venous lumen is flushed with 20 ml 10% heparin solution, which is delivered through a blunt metal cannula. The venous anastomosis is constructed with either 6-0 or 5-0 monofilament sutures, beginning with a horizontal mattress technique between the corner of the renal vein and the venotomy end of the external iliac vein. After the distal suture is tied, a Linton mattress stitch is placed, namely, from host vein to donor and then donor to host. Thereafter, the sides are apposed using a continuous everting suture, which starts first at the lower and then at the upper end, and is tied at the midpoint. The kidney is then reflected to the other side for another running suture in the same fashion from both angles. It is important to avoid traction on the kidney to prevent tearing of the vein, particularly the short, friable right renal vein, during the anastomosis.

The arterial site for anastomosis is selected based on the vascular anatomy of the graft and the host. We prefer to use the internal iliac artery, provided that the hypogastric artery is free of atherosclerotic plaque at its origin (Figure 5.2a). If the internal iliac artery is used, dissection is limited to mobilize this artery, as well as the distal common and proximal external iliac arteries, in order to facilitate delivery of the anastomosis anteriorly. If the hypogastric artery cannot be used, an end-to-side anastomosis to the external iliac follows dissection of a small segment of the external iliac artery (Figure 5.2b). Meticulous ligation and division of the lymphatic tissues that encompass the vascular structures is mandatory to reduce the incidence of postoperative lymphocele formation.

When an end-to-end anastomosis to the hypogastric artery is used, the distal vessel is double-ligated with 2-0 silk suture just above its trifurcation into the superior vesicle, pudendal, and deep gluteal arteries. The vascular stump is secured with a figure-of-eight suture ligature. The origin of the hypogastric artery is controlled with a vascular clamp,

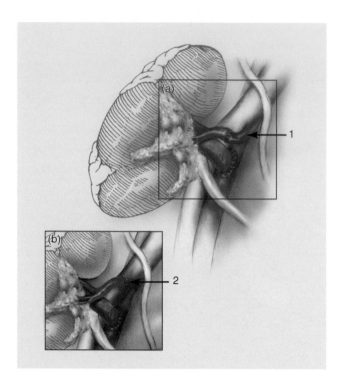

Figure 5.2. Vascular anastomoses of renal transplant artery. (a) End-to-end renal to internal iliac artery (1) to renal artery anastomosis. (b) End-to-side renal artery to external iliac artery (2) anastomosis.

and the artery is divided. After the lumen has been irrigated with heparinized saline, and the common iliac artery flushed in retrograde fashion, the internal iliac artery is aligned and tailored to the donor renal artery using a longer medial donor segment to prevent angulation. The anastomosis is performed using simple interrupted sutures of 6-0 monofilament, a continuous everting suture, or a combination of a continuous posterior and a series of interrupted anterior sutures. Endarterectomy of the hypogastric artery may be necessary when there is atherosclerotic narrowing of the lumen (Figure 5.3a); indeed, extensive distal atherosclerotic disease may be best addressed with a 'butt' anastomosis of the renal artery to the origin of the internal iliac vessel. If the origin of the internal iliac is extensively diseased, it is preferable to perform an end-to-side anastomosis to the common or the external iliac artery, provided that endarterectomy successfully removes vascular plaque (Figure 5.3b).

An end-to-side arterial anastomosis (Figure 5.2b) is performed to the common iliac or external iliac artery, particularly in situations of extensive atherosclerosis of the hypogastric artery as in diabetics. It is also performed in cases of significant disparity between the calibers of the renal and hypogastric arteries; of multiple donor renal arteries readily encompassed by a Carrel aortic patch; or, in male patients, of previous transplants using the contralateral hypogastric artery, thus rendering the patient at risk of postoperative impotence if both internal iliac arteries are ligated. The end-to-side arterial

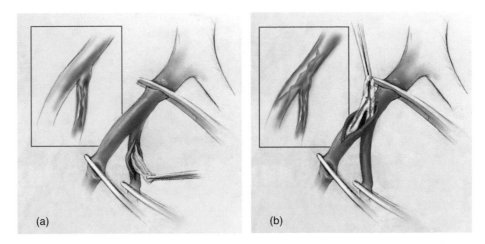

Figure 5.3. Endarterectomy to facilitate vascular anastomosis. (a) Recovery of an arterial plaque from the internal iliac artery. (b) Removal of a plaque at the bifurcation of the common iliac artery.

anastomosis is performed with either an interrupted suture or a continuous 6-0 vascular monofilament sutures. It is particularly important to preserve growth of the vascular anastomosis by using interrupted sutures over at least one-half of the circumference, especially for recipients either of pediatric donor kidneys or of grafts supplied by a renal artery not attached to an aortic patch.

Upon completion of the arterial anastomosis, and after confirming the absence of leakage by testing under distal renal arterial occlusion, the vascular clamps are removed in quick succession. First, the low-pressure clamps—the superior venous clamp and inferior arterial clamp—are removed. Then the high-pressure clamps—the inferior venous clamp, and the upper arterial clamp on the external iliac artery—are removed. The vascular anastomoses are inspected and packed with oxidized cellulose (Oxycel™; Becton Dickenson, Menlo Park, CA, USA) if hemostatic control is necessary at the suture line. Ligature of bleeding points is preferred over metal clips, which may interfere with future radiologic evaluation. The kidney should regain its normal pink color and turgor. It is important at this time to ensure that the patient has an adequate circulating blood volume. Mottling of the graft surface owing to arterial spasm is not uncommon, but generally resolves within 30 min. Occasionally, dramatic improvement in the mottled look is attained by topical application of 1% xylocaine solution (without epinephrine) on the renal artery. Intravascular delivery of a dopamine drip (1–5 mg/kg per min) may also improve perfusion. Direct injection of calcium channel blockers into the renal artery is generally avoided, owing to the possibility of elevating an intimal flap.

Sometimes the allograft fails to reperfuse well intraoperatively, owing to the problems with arterial inflow, including dissection under an intimal flap, technical misadventures, or twisting of the vessels. Detection of these problems is facilitated by evaluation with a pencil doppler. In these cases, the arterial anastomosis must be immediately revised. After systemic heparinization (1 mg/kg) and establishment of proximal and distal vascular control over both the iliac artery and vein, the allograft is reflushed through the renal or external iliac artery using room temperature and then chilled solution with a venous venting via a tributary of the renal vein, such as the gonadal or adrenal branches, to avoid disrupting the venous anastomotic suture line. If no tributary is available, a small venotomy may be placed in the external iliac vein. After the arterial anastomosis has been revised, the organ is reperfused with blood, following closure of the venous vent with a Prolene (Anison Inc., Somerville, NJ, USA) 6-0 mattress suture. In other situations, revision of the venous anastomosis may be necessary; the need for this maneuver is usually evidenced by the presence of venous hypertension characterized by a dark blue color of the graft and excessive bleeding from hilar and renal capsular vessels.

Revascularization of the kidney: anatomic variations

Special techniques are necessary to address anatomic variations in donor kidneys, especially the presence of multiple renal arteries or disparities in length or caliber of the donor artery in relation to the recipient vessels. Approximately 10–20% of kidneys have multiple renal arteries (Pollak and Mozes 1986). Benedetti et al (1995) recently reported a significantly higher incidence of late renal artery stenosis in kidneys with multiple renal arteries, regardless of whether one or more arterial anastomoses were performed.

The most common technique to anastomose multiple arteries in cadaver donor kidneys uses an aortic Carrel patch that is anastomosed end-to-side to the external iliac artery (Figure 5.4a). Alternative techniques to anastomose multiple arteries include splicing of two, almost equal-sized renal arteries side-to-side to form a common ostium (Figure 5.4b), or excising a segment of aorta to reshape a Carrel patch for anastomosis (Figure 5.4c). An anastomotic technique that attaches one renal artery end-to-end to the internal iliac artery, and the other artery end-to-side to the common or external iliac artery (Figure 5.5a), is preferred over the use of two end-to-end anastomoses to distal branches of the internal iliac, owing to the frequent occurrence of distal disease (Figure 5.5b). End-to-side reimplantation of a smaller polar artery into the main renal artery using 7-0 polypropylene represents a less satisfactory option, owing to the increased incidence of thrombosis (Figure 5.5c), but may be preferable in cases of extensive recipient atherosclerotic disease. An alternate approach—that is, end-to-end anastomosis of the inferior epigastric artery to the lower polar artery—generally fails to provide adequate inflow. Therefore, a venous bypass to the external iliac artery is usually necessary when there is insufficient length of the smaller, particularly lower polar, renal artery to reach either the main renal artery or the external iliac artery (Figure 5.6). In contrast, upper polar renal arteries may be safely ligated if they feed less than 10% of the renal parenchyma, as verified by injection of dilute (1:1000) methylene blue.

Failure to revascularize accessory renal arteries, particularly those feeding the lower pole of the kidney, may lead to chronic obstruction resulting from segmental infarction,

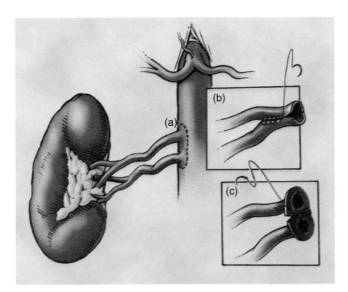

Figure 5.4. Alternate methods to anastomose multiple renal arteries, including (a) Carrel patch; (b) side-to-side anastomosis of equal-sized renal arteries; and (c) excision of an aortic segment and reanastomosis as a neoCarrel patch.

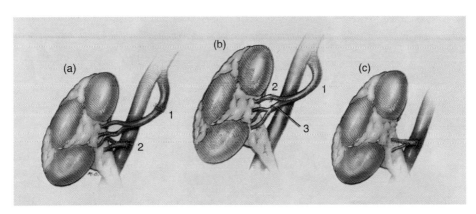

Figure 5.5. Alternate techniques for anastomosis of two renal arteries of disparate size. (a) Larger artery anastomosed end-to-end to internal (1) and smaller artery, end-to-side to external (2) iliac artery. (b) Anastomosis of each renal artery to a separate branch of the internal iliac artery (1), namely, superior vesicle (2) and pudendal (3) arteries. (c) End-to-side reimplantation of smaller polar artery into main renal artery.

calyceocutaneous fistula, ureteral necrosis, or chronic ischemic fibrosis of the transplant ureter. The donor renal artery may also present technical problems if it is slender, of small caliber, or friable in contrast to the recipient vessels, in which cases dilatation and spatulation are likely to injure the vessel. Small shallow bites provide an adequate anastomosis. Insufficient renal artery length may be addressed by the use of an autogenous vein bypass graft or, less preferably, by a synthetic segment of polytetrafluoroethylene (PTFE; IMPRA, Tempe, AZ, USA; Figure 5.7).

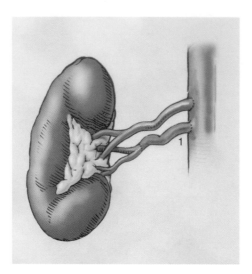

Figure 5.6. Use of interposition reversed saphenous vein (1) to reconstruct a lower polar renal artery inadvertently transected at the level of the renal hilum.

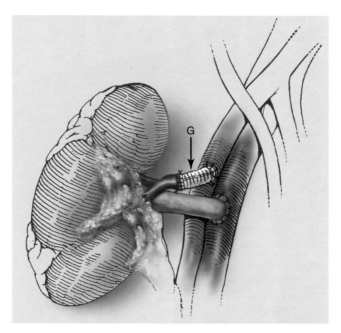

Figure 5.7. Arterial anastomosis of the kidney to the external iliac artery using a synthetic vascular graft (G).

Re-establishment of urinary tract continuity: ureteroneocystomy techniques

Continuity of the urinary tract is usually established with a ureteroneocystostomy technique. In the Leadbetter–Politano method (Leadbetter et al 1966; intravesical; Figure 5.8), an anterior cystostomy is performed to visualize the interior of the bladder. A 2–3-cm submucosal tunnel is constructed to implant transplant ureter into the bladder mucosa superior and medial to the native ureteral orifice in the trigone (Figure 5.8a, b).

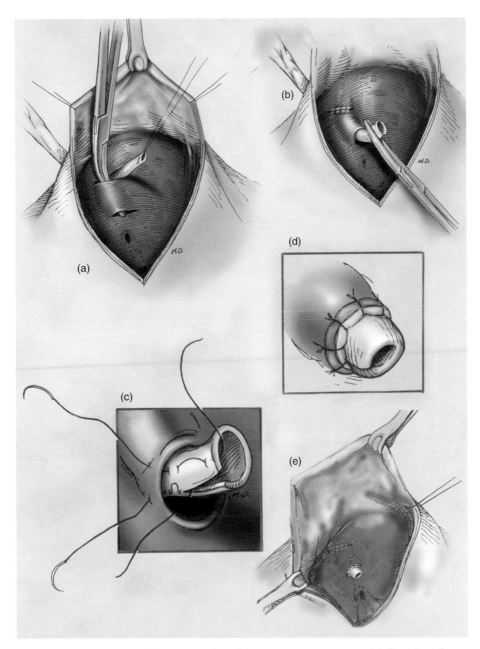

Figure 5.8. Leadbetter–Politano procedure for ureteroneocystostomy. (a) Creation of submucosal tunnel shown by position of tonsil clamp. (b) Ureter tunneled and ready for implantation in the supra-trigonal area after bladder counter-incision is closed. (c) Ureter spatulated and anchored with quadrant sutures. (d) Ureteral nipple. (e) Overview of completed implant.

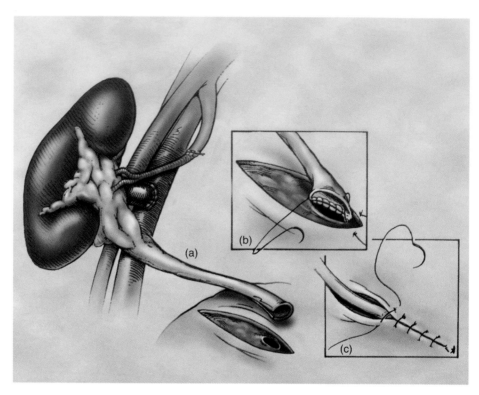

Figure 5.9. Lich–Gregoir procedure for ureteroneocystostomy. (a) Extravesical ureteroneocystostomy with spatulated distal ureter and a small bladder mucosal nick made after myotomy incision. (b) Ureterovesical anastomosis using continuous suture of Maxxon 5-0. (c) Creation of submucosal tunnel by approximation of seromuscular layers.

After the distal ureter is spatulated anteriorly (Figure 5.8c), it is anchored to the bladder mucosa using three monofilament absorbable 4-0 Maxxon sutures after the fashion of a Brook ileostomy. Between these stitches 5-0 Maxxon sutures are placed to create a nipple (Figure 5.8d). Figure 5.8e shows the completed ureteroneocystostomy. In the absence of brisk urine flow, ureteral patency is checked by inserting a French 5-0 pediatric feeding tube past the vesical wall up to the midureter. The tube may be left as a stent if the ureteral caliber is particularly small, or if the bladder is contracted owing to disuse or disease. A watertight cystorrhaphy is achieved with a three-layer closure. Foley catheter drainage is used for 3–5 days, depending on the strength of the bladder tissue. Prevesical drains are not routinely used.

The extravesical approach (Figure 5.9a–c) was described by Lich et al (1961) and Gregoir et al (1964) for the correction of vesicoureteral reflux, and by MacKinnon et al (1968) for clinical transplantation. A 4-cm myotomy incision is made on the anterolateral surface of the bladder using electrocautery (Figure 5.9). The incision is continued through the seromuscular layer until the bladder mucosa bulges. The edges of the muscularis are undermined to facilitate closure. A small nick is made in the mucosa in the distal aspect of the muscular incision. An anastomosis of the donor ureter, which is spatulated posteriorly, is made with a transfixing horizontal mattress stitch anastomosing the 'toe' end of the spatulated ureter to the entire thickness of the bladder wall (Figure 5.9b). The full thickness of the remaining free edge of the ureter is sewn to the bladder mucosa using 5-0 polygyconate suture in running fashion, thereby creating a watertight closure. The seromuscular layer is closed over the ureter with interrupted 3-0 polydiaxonone sutures, thereby attempting to create a 2–3-cm submucosal tunnel (Figure 5.9c). Care must be taken to avoid ureteral strangulation at the proximal end of the tunnel. The extravesical technique is advantageous because of the smaller cystotomy, which reduces the risk of contamination and urinary leakage, and because the shorter length of ureter is less likely to suffer distal ureteral ischemia. However, this technique is not suitable for a bladder with a thin or scarred wall. Drains are not routinely used. A Foley catheter drains the bladder for 48–72 hours. There is no uniformity in opinion on the use of ureteral stents, which can ensure free drainage despite anastomotic edema and avoid ureteral distension that can lead to ischemia.

Re-establishment of urinary tract continuity: ureteropyelostomy techniques

Although most surgeons prefer to establish urinary tract continuity with a ureteroneocystostomy, Cosimi et al (Whelchel et al 1975; Hughes et al 1987) have advocated the use of ureteropyelostomy connecting the ipsilateral recipient native ureter to the donor renal pelvis (Figure 5.10). This anastomosis affords a large stoma, which reduces the chance of ureteral obstruction or stenosis, ensures a better blood supply to the anastomosis coming via the native vessels, and increases the possibility for early removal of the Foley catheter. The donor pelvis and recipient ureter, which have been spatulated to create a 1.5-cm ostium, are anastomosed in running fashion using 7-0 polydioxanone sutures under ×3 loupe magnification. An internal stent helps to provide alignment of the structures and facilitates emptying of the donor pelvis. Ipsilateral native nephrectomy is not necessarily required at the time of transplantation, especially if the recipient has neither appreciable urine output nor history of pyelonephritis. A Jackson–Pratt closed suction drain is left in the perinephric space for 5–7 days following transplant or until drainage is less than 30–50 ml for a 24-hour period. However, the major complication of ureteropyelostomy, namely, an infected urinoma, is sufficiently grave that this technique is rarely used. Additional complications include the frequent occurrence of urinary fistula, the not infrequent stricture formation, the greater risk of vascular disruption owing to extension of infection from the urinary connection to the hilar vessels, the not infrequent need to perform an ipsilateral native nephrectomy, and the need to sacrifice the host's other native ureter to rectify urological complications.

An alternate ureteroureterostomy technique, described by Hamburger et al (1962), may be useful, particularly when ureteroneocystostomy is not feasible owing to a

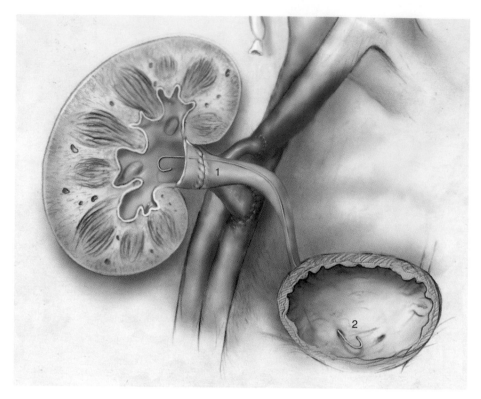

Figure 5.10. Ureteropyelostomy technique for urinary reconstruction. Anastomosis of host ureter to donor renal pelvis (1) stabilized by double J-stent (2).

foreshortened donor ureter from a surgical misadventure during organ harvesting or during ureteral re-exploration. The donor ureter is divided 2–3 cm from the uretero-pelvic junction. The proximal native ureter is ligated. The spatulated ureteral ends are anastomosed end-to-end with either an interrupted or a continuous technique using 6-0 monofilament suture. A double-J stent is placed to protect the anastomosis. Unfortunately, this technique is not uncommonly associated with urinary leaks—which require prolonged drainage with eventual ureteral strictures—and with stone formation at the suture line.

Re-establishment of urinary tract continuity: implantation into an augmented bladder or into an ileal conduit

The surgical approach to urinary drainage must be modified in patients afflicted with the abnormalities of a pathologically scarred bladder resulting from chronic infection (e.g. tuberculous cystitis); multiple previous surgical procedures; long-standing neurogenic detrusor dysfunction secondary to meningomyelocele, spinal cord trauma, and

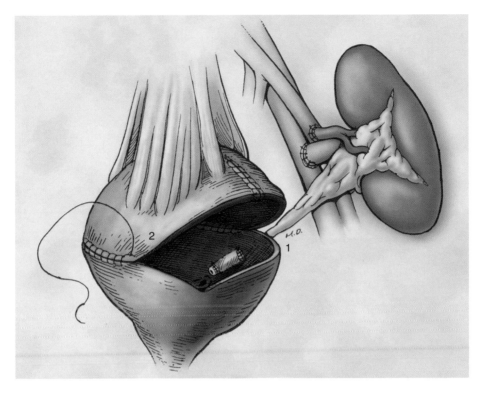

Figure 5.11. Implantation of transplant ureter (1) into a bladder augmented with a cecal cap (2).

other neurological diseases; and/or bladder neck contractures or urethral strictures secondary to prostatic disease, vesicoureteral reflux, bladder exstrophy, or posterior urethral valves. Although it is preferable to correct these bladder abnormalities before transplantation, they may have to be addressed postoperatively with treatments ranging from intermittent clean self-catheterization (ICSC) to supravesical urinary diversion (Barnett et al 1987).

The transplant ureter can be implanted either into the remaining segment of native bladder or into the augmented bowel segment using a tunneled Leadbetter–Politano ureteroneocystostomy (Figure 5.11) or a nontunneled direct anastomosis, respectively. The neobladder is drained via a suprapubic or a urethral catheter for at least 10–14 days. The almost inevitable bacteruria from long-term ICSC produces chronic urinary tract infections, requiring antibiotic prophylaxis.

The transplant procedure using an ileal conduit must place the kidney more cephalad than its usual position, usually on the side ipsilateral to the stoma (Figure 5.12). The conduit is established pretransplant by mobilizing an ileal segment (Figure 5.12a) with a closed distal end and a proximal end in a lower abdominal quadrant (Figure 5.12b) with

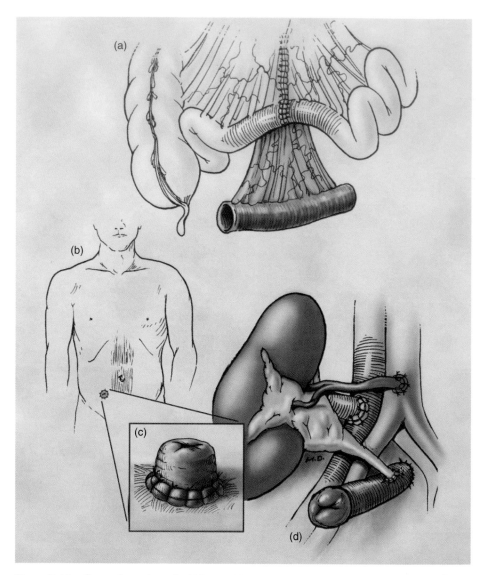

Figure 5.12. Transplantation of a kidney with urinary drainage into an ileal conduit. The conduit has been prepared prior to transplant by isolation of an ileal segment (a) with the proximal end anastomosis in a lower quadrant (b) using maturation with the Brooke technique (c). Anatomy of ureteral anastomosis into distal ileal loop (d). Note arterial and venous anastomoses to the aorta and vena cava, respectively.

a matured orifice using the Brooke ileostomy technique (Figure 5.12c). The blind end of the conduit is identified through a peritoneal window and placed in a dependent position in the pelvis, preferably just below the sacral promontory. After a full thickness ellipse of the conduit is excised 2–3 cm above its closed end, a 1-cm spatulated anastomosis is performed with interrupted 4-0 chromic catgut or polyglycolic-acid sutures (Figure 5.12d). The sutures encompass the full thickness of the ureter and a generous portion of the serosa and muscularis of the conduit, but only the edge of the ileal mucosa, thereby telescoping the anastomosis into the ileal lumen and reducing ureteral tension. A single-layer anastomosis is used to reduce the risk of stenosis at the ureteroileal level, and is stented using an indwelling 5-French feeding tube, which courses to the exterior through the stoma. The peritoneum is closed around the conduit to reduce the possibility of herniation. Two weeks later, just prior to stent removal, radiological contrast is gravity-dripped through the splint to detect anastomotic stenosis or urinary leak.

A recent modification by Lucas et al (1992) utilizes an ileal segment just long enough to reach below the posterior rectus fascia for urinary diversion. The full length of ureter, which has traversed the properitoneal space to the ileal conduit, is advanced through a small opening created in the antimesenteric ileal wall, without any anchoring sutures. Its end is sutured to a pig-tail catheter that hangs out through the stoma. Several weeks after transplantation, the stent is removed, and the ureter is trimmed to a point just inside the stoma.

Although urinary tract infection is the most common complication following conduit drainage of kidney transplants (Hatch et al 1994), upper tract deterioration, stenosis of the stoma, peristomal hernia, calculus formation, ureterointestinal stenosis, pyocystis of the isolated bladder, small bowel fistula, bowel obstruction, and electrolyte abnormalities occur not infrequently (Hatch et al 1993), particularly among pediatric recipients.

Modifications for pediatric transplantation

Recipient operation

A transperitoneal incision or an extraperitoneal incision that extends from the tip of the twelfth rib to the symphysis pubis can be used to perform transplantation procedures in children who weigh less than 20 kg. The cecum and ascending colon are reflected medially to expose the aorta, vena cava, and common iliac vessels. A limited portion of these vessels is then isolated, taking care to ligate all lymphatics and small lumbar vessels in the area of dissection. The graft is placed in a more cephalad position, retroperitoneal to the cecum. The vascular anastomoses are performed in an end-to-side manner, with the renal vein anastomosed to either the vena cava or the right common iliac vein using 5-0 continuous polypropylene sutures. An end-to-side arterial anastomosis is made with either the aorta or the right common iliac artery using running 6-0 polypropylene sutures (Figure 5.13). Before completion of the vascular anastomosis, the recipient receives a renal cocktail containing 250 ml/kg 5% albumin, 12.5 g/kg mannitol, and 20 mg/kg furosemide. An additional 300 ml of blood products or albumin solution should be administered to compensate for a reduction of the intravascular volume as the adult allograft kidney fills with blood. The ureter is positioned in the retroperitoneal space and an extravesical or intravesical ureteroneocystostomy is performed in the same fashion as in adult recipients.

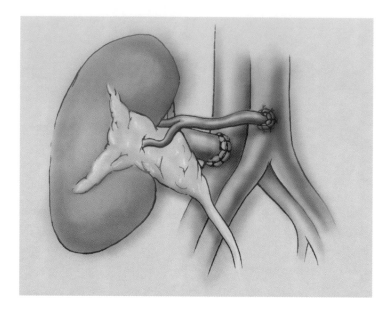

Figure 5.13. Renal transplant operation in a pediatric recipient with anastomosis to distal aorta and vena cava.

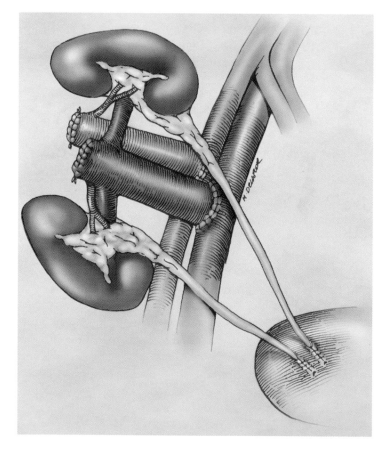

Figure 5.14. Method for en bloc transplantation of small pediatric kidneys: end-to-side aortic and venal caval anastomoses to external iliac artery and vein, respectively.

En bloc transplantation of pediatric kidneys from young donors

Organs from donors under 2 years of age are generally transplanted in pairs to provide sufficient renal reserve in the nephron mass. End-to-side anastomoses of the distal aorta and the vena cava to the recipient's external iliac artery and vein, respectively, represent the most widely used technique. Urinary continuity is established by creating two ureteroneocystostomy sites to drain each kidney separately (Figure 5.14). Stenting of the ureteral anastomoses minimizes the risk of complications attributed to the relatively small caliber of the pediatric ureters, as well as to their tenuous blood supply. Owing to turbulent blood flow in the cul-de-sacs at the distal ends of the vessels, this approach predisposes to thrombosis, particularly when blood flow is reduced during rejection episodes, or to a hypercoagulable state during CsA therapy. Furthermore, end-to-side anastomoses also pose the difficulty of properly positioning the en bloc grafts to prevent rotation of the small, paired kidneys.

An alternative approach places the allografts 'in continuity' using end-to-end vascular anastomoses, interposing the donor aorta and vena cava between the divided ends of the recipient external iliac artery and vein (Figure 5.15). The ureters are anastomosed to the

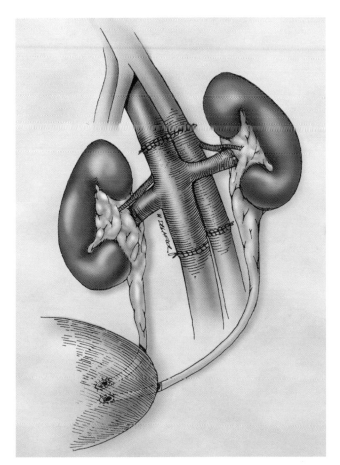

Figure 5.15. In continuity interposition technique anastomosing the aortic segment into the transected external iliac artery and the vena cava into the transected external iliac vein.

211

bladder via separate ureteroneocystostomy sites using either the Leadbetter–Politano or the extravesical Lich method. None of the patients in our series developed venous or arterial thrombosis following transplantation. Among the seven patients reported in our series, ureteral leaks occurred only twice, possibly associated with neither patient having been treated by placement of ureteral stents (Amante and Kahan 1996).

TRANSPLANT NEPHRECTOMY

Although most transplant units remove all grafts that fail within 90 days, after this time, nephrectomy is reserved for only those grafts that display an indication for the operation. Persistent rejection or pyelonephritis, as evidenced by fever, pain, or hematuria, occurs in about 10% of transplants (Jeevanandam et al 1992). Particularly after 6 months posttransplant, these events are rare unless the physician withdraws immunosuppression rapidly. A small number of grafts continue to lose large amounts of protein, due to recurrence of original disease or progressive transplant glomerulopathy. Other transplants cause refractory hypertension, particularly due to severe renal artery stenosis (Table 5.1). Although transplant nephrectomy was once considered a hazardous procedure with high morbidity and mortality rates, it is now generally accomplished with minimal problems (Sharma et al 1989; Southard and Belzer 1993).

An extracapsular approach (Figure 5.16a–d) to nephrectomy is readily performed within the first 3 posttransplant weeks. After 4–8 weeks, the dense inflammatory reaction between the renal capsule and the surrounding structures necessitates a subcapsular approach (Toledo-Pereyra et al 1987) to avoid injuring the host vasculature. The previous transplant incision is opened with special care to avoid the peritoneum, especially in patients on peritoneal dialysis so that they may continue their treatments immediately

Hyperacute rejection
Allograft thrombosis and infarction
Renal artery stenosis induced hypertension not amenable to open repair or angioplasty
Recurrent renal disease producing severe proteinuria
Chronic and recurrent pyelonephritis in a failed graft
Recurrent troublesome hematuria from a failed graft

Table 5.1. Indications for transplant nephrectomy

after the operation. When the kidney is removed in an extracapsular fashion, the renal artery and vein are exposed, individually ligated, and sutured. With the subcapsular nephrectomy (Figure 5.16a), the renal capsule is incised along the entire length of the kidney, and a plane is developed between the parenchyma and the overlying capsule. Although this procedure often results in bleeding from the renal surface as the kidney is separated from the capsule by gentle finger dissection toward the renal hilus (Figure 5.16b), it can be minimized by not lacerating or fracturing the renal parenchyma. Exposure of the renal vasculature and ureter is facilitated by incising the anteromedial or posteromedial renal capsule that is draped over the hilus (Figure 5.16c). The ureter is identified, ligated, and divided. Although it is necessary to isolate and individually divide and ligate the renal artery and vein, the pedicle may need to be initially controlled with a large Satinsky clamp close to the hilus, encompassing both renal vessels (Figure 5.16d), to deliver the allograft out of the operative field. The arterial stump or its branches are double ligated with silk-0 ligatures, while the vein is closed with continuous polypropylene 5-0 vascular suture. The distal ureter is dissected from the adherent fibrous connective tissue and traced toward the bladder, where it is subsequently ligated and divided. Residual parenchymal tissues adherent to the renal capsule must be debrided to reduce the risks of persistent drainage or recurrent abscess formation. Hemovac drains are placed in the operative field to drain the renal fossa for 24–48 hours. The fascia is closed with interrupted Ticron-0 (Davis and Geck, American Home Products, Mathison, NJ, USA) sutures.

The major intraoperative complications include bleeding from anastomotic disruption, parenchymal fractures or uremic coagulopathy, and inadvertent ligation of the external iliac artery (Kohlberg et al 1980). The blood loss may vary from 250 ml to almost 2 liters in complicated cases (Sutherland et al 1978). Postoperative complications include wound infections, hematoma formation, abscess formation, and acute exsanguinating hemorrhage from vascular breakdown owing to an infected arterial or venous suture line (Sinha and Castro 1976; Chiverton et al 1987). Due to the ongoing or previous immunosuppressive therapy, administration of prophylactic antibiotics is advised after nephrectomy to decrease the incidence of infection (Rosenthal et al 1993).

OPEN BIOPSY OF TRANSPLANT KIDNEY

Renal biopsies are performed to determine the cause of allograft dysfunction. Percutaneous needle biopsy, particularly with the fine needle Biopty Gun® (CR Bard, Inc., Murray Hill, NJ, USA), guided by ultrasonography, is frequently the procedure of choice. However, in 5–20% of cases, the kidney is not accessible due to its small size, to recipient obesity, or to the percutaneously obtained renal tissue sample being insufficient for histologic interpretation (Starnes et al 1984; Table 5.2). Intraperitoneal grafts are not amenable to the percutaneous approach, due to the possibility of bowel injury. Furthermore, the open biopsy is performed under direct vision, and this can be safely

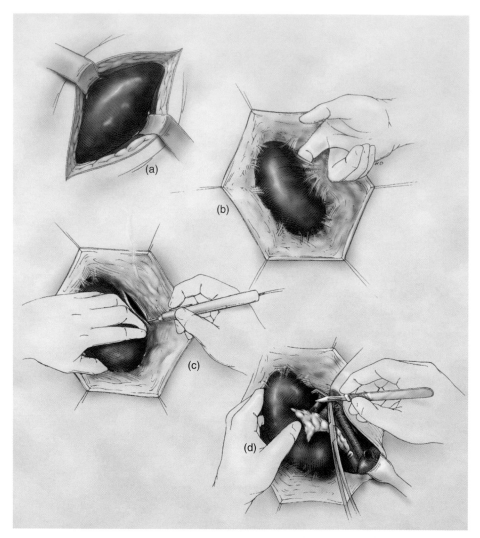

Figure 5.16. Subcapsular transplant nephrectomy. (a) Exposure of the transplant. (b) Finger dissection of subcapsular plane. (c) Incision of anteromedial renal capsule to expose hilar structures. (d) Isolation and transection of renal transplant vessels.

performed on patients under treatment with anticoagulants. Finally, we prefer the open technique to the percutaneous approach in long-term patients because of the high incidence of arteriovenous fistulas in the latter setting (Dunn et al 1990; Lawen et al 1990).

For open renal biopsies, the most superficial portion of the graft is exposed through a 2–4-cm opening in the old incision. Electrocautery is used to incise through the fibrotic fascia and muscle layers to reach the underlying kidney. The subcapsular plane is identified and developed, and exposure is achieved using self-retaining retractors. It is generally advisable to use an elliptical incision in a radial orientation to sample the renal

Failure to obtain adequate specimen by needle biopsy

Bleeding diathesis precluding needle biopsy

Massive obesity

Intra-abdominal location of the allograft

Presence of a transplant kidney that is more than 2 years old (because these grafts show an increased risk of arteriovenous fistula)

Table 5.2. Indications for open renal biopsy

cortex (Figure 5.17). The incision should be 5–10 mm in length and 5–7 mm deep. A core biopsy of the corticomedullary tissue is then obtained using an 18-gauge automated biopsy needle (Biopty Gun®). The kidney is punctured with the needle oriented tangentially to the exposed surface of the graft. The graft is manually compressed for 5–10 minutes to achieve hemostasis. The open biopsy site is closed with interrupted simple 4-0 polyglycolic acid sutures that are buttressed with a small piece of surgicel (oxidized, regenerated cellulose; Johnson & Johnson, Arlington, TX, USA; Figure 5.17). After adequate hemostasis is achieved, the wound is closed in separate layers with interrupted heavy Ticron-0 sutures. Drains are rarely required. The following complications develop in approximately 5% of cases (Walsh et al 1977; Sullivan et al 1994): hemorrhage requiring transfusion or re-exploration; hematoma formation; wound infection or

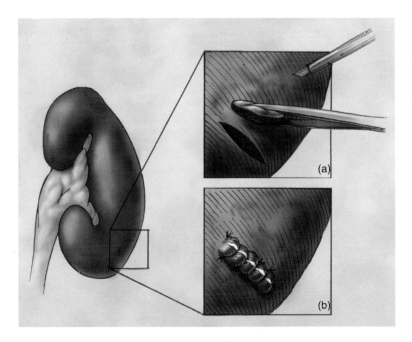

Figure 5.17. Wedge biopsy of the transplant kidney: (a) excision of wedge; (b) closure with mattress stitches with buttress of gel foam in the tissue gap.

abscess formation; arteriovenous fistula formation; or postoperative hematuria without or with clot obstruction in the ureter and/or renal pelvis.

CONCLUSION

Forty years of experience has led to secure surgical techniques for renal transplantation. Anastomosis of all renal arteries is mandatory, but may require host vessel endarterectomy, donor artery reconstruction, and/or the use of vascular bypass grafts. Urinary reconstructions via extra- or intravesicle techniques are now associated with low rates of complications; however, implantations into an augmented bladder or into an ileal conduit may pose technical challenges. Special considerations must be addressed for pediatric patients, both as donors and as recipients. Using a variety of techniques, surgeons can now anticipate a successful procedure in virtually every transplant case.

REFERENCES

Amante AJ, Kahan BD (1996) En bloc transplantation of kidneys from pediatric donors. *J Urol* 155:852–857.

Barnett MG, Bruskewitz RC, Belzer FO et al (1987) Ileocecocystoplasty bladder augmentation and renal transplantation. *J Urol* 138:855–858.

Barry JM, Fuchs EF (1978) Right renal vein extension in cadaver kidney transplant. *Arch Surg* 113:300.

Barry JM, Lemmers MJ (1995) Patch and flap techniques to repair right renal vein defects caused by cadaver liver retrieval for transplantation. *J Urol* 153:1803–1804.

Benedetti E, Troppmann C, Gillingham K et al (1995) Short- and long-term outcomes of kidney transplants with multiple renal arteries. *Ann Surg* 221:405–414.

Burt RK, Gupta-Burt S, Suki WN et al (1989) Reversal of left ventricular dysfunction after renal transplantation. *Ann Intern Med* 111:635–640.

Carlier M, Squifflet J, Pirson Y et al (1982) Maximal hydration during anesthesia increases pulmonary arterial pressures and improves early function of human renal transplants. *Transplantation* 34:201–204.

Carrel A (1902) La technique operatoire des anastomoses vascularis, et la transplantation des visceres. *Lyon Med* 98:859–880.

Chiverton S, Murie JA, Allen RD et al (1987) Renal transplant nephrectomy. *Surg Gynecol Obstet* 164:324–328.

Corry RJ, Kelley SE (1978) Technique of lengthening the right renal vein of cadaver donor kidneys. *Am J Surg* 135:867.

Davidson IJ, Sandoz ZF, Carpenter L et al (1992) Intraoperative albumin administration affects the outcome of a cadaver renal transplantation. *Transplantation* 53:774–782.

Defronzo RA, Tobin JD, Rowe JW et al (1981a) Glucose intolerance in uremia: quantification of pancreatic beta cell sensitivity to glucose and tissue sensitivity to insulin. *J Clin Invest* 62:425–435.

Defronzo RA, Alerstand A, Smith D et al (1981b) Insulin resistance in uremia. *J Clin Invest* 67:563–568.

Delaporte C, Gros F, Anagnostopolos T (1980) Inhibitory effects of plasma dialysate on protein synthesis in vitro: Influence of dialysis and transplantation. *Am J Clin Nutr* 33:1407–1410.

Dubrow A, Levin NW (1995) Biochemical and hormonal alterations in chronic renal failure. In: Jacobson HR, Striker GE, Klahr S (eds). *The Principles and Practice of Nephrology*, 2nd edn. St Louis: Mosby-Year Book, pp. 596–663.

Dunn J, Golden D, Van Buren CT et al (1990) Causes of graft loss beyond two years in the cyclosporine era. *Transplantation* **49**:349–353.

Floresco M (1905) Transplantation des organs; conditions anatomiques et techniques de la transplantation du rein. *J Physiol Path Gen* 7:27–31.

Garber AJ (1983) Effects of parathyroid hormone on skeletal muscle protein and amino acid metabolism. *J Clin Invest* 71:1806–1821.

Gregoir W, Van Regemorter G (1964) Le reflu vesico-ureteral congenital. *Rol Int* **18**:122–126.

Grundmann R, Kammerer B, Franke E et al (1981) Effect of hypotension on the results of kidney storage and the use of dopamine under these conditions. *Transplantation* **32**:184–187.

Guthrie CC (1912) *Blood Vessel Surgery and Its Application.* New York: Longmans Green.

Hamburger J, Vaysse J, Crosnier J et al (1962) Renal homotransplantation in man after radiation of the recipient: experience with six patients since 1959. *Am J Med* **32**:854–871.

Hatch DA, Belitsky P, Barry JM et al (1993) Fate of renal allografts transplanted in patients with urinary diversion. *Transplantation* **56**:838–842.

Hatch DA, Belitsky P, Barry JM et al (1994) Kidney transplantation in patients with an abnormal lower urinary tract. *Urol Clin North Am* **21**:311–320.

Held PJ, Kahan BD, Hunsicker LG et al (1994) The impact of HLA mismatches on the survival of first cadaveric kidney transplants. *N Engl J Med* **331**:765–770.

Hoffmann BB, Lefkowitz RJ (1990) Catecholamines and sympathomimetic drugs. In: Gilman AG, Rall TW, Nies AS et al (eds). *The Pharmacological Basis of Therapeutics*, 8th edn. New York: Pergamon Press, pp. 200–210.

Hughes JD, Delmonico FL, Auchincloss H Jr et al (1987) Ureteropyelostomy reconstruction in renal transplantation [brief communication]. *J Urol* **138**:459–461.

Hume DM, Merrill JP, Harrison JH (1952) Homologous transplantation of human kidneys. *J Clin Invest* **31**:640–654.

Hume DM, Merrill JP, Miller BF et al (1955) Experiences with renal homotransplantation in the human: report of nine cases. *J Clin Invest* **34**:327–382.

Hutchinson AJ, Whitehouse RW, Boulton HF et al (1993) Correlation of bone histology with parathyroid hormone, vitamin D3 and radiology in end-stage renal disease. *Kidney Int* **44**:1071–1077.

Jaboulay M (1906) Greffe de reins sau pli du conde sor dures arterielles et veinuses. *Lyon Med* **107**:575–576.

Jeevanandam V, Auteri JS, Sanchez JA et al (1992) Cardiac transplantation after prolonged preservation with the University of Wisconsin solution. *J Thorac Cardiovasc Surg* **104**:224–228.

Kohlberg WI, Tellis VA, Bhat DJ et al (1980) Wound infections after transplant nephrectomy. *Arch Surg* **115**:645–646.

Kopple JD (1978) Abnormal amino acid and protein metabolism in uremia. *Kidney Int* **14**:340–348.

Kuss R, Teinturier J, Milliez P (1951) Quelques essais de greffe de rein chez l'homme. *Mem Acad Chir* (Paris) 77: 755–759.

Lauzurica R, Teixido J, Serra A et al (1992) Hydration and mannitol reduce the need for dialyses in cadaveric kidney transplant recipients treated with CyA. *Transplant Proc* **24**:46–47.

Lawen JG, Van Buren CT, Lewis RM, Kahan BD (1990) Arteriovenous fistulas after renal allograft biopsy: a serious complication in patients beyond one year. *Clin Transplant* **4**:357–369.

Lawler RH, West JM, McNulty PH et al (1950) Homotransplantation of the kidney in humans. *JAMA* **144**:844–845.

Leadbetter GW, Monaco AP, Russell PS (1966) A technique for reconstruction of the urinary tract in renal transplantation. *Surg Gynecol Obstet* **123**:839–841.

Lich R, Howerton LW, David LA (1961) Recurrent urosepsis in children. *J Urol* **86**:554–558.

Lucas BA, Munch LC, Waid TH et al (1992) Pull-through skin-level allograft ureterostomy to isolated ileal stoma: report of 10 cases. *J Urol* **147**:3264–3268.

Luiani J, Frantz P, Thibault P et al (1979) Early anuria prevention in human kidney transplantation. *Transplantation* **28**:308–312.

MacKinnon KJ, Oliver JA, Morehouse DD et al (1968) Cadaver renal transplantation: emphasis on urological aspects. *J Urol* **99**:486–490.

Mattern WD, Hak LJ, Lamanna RW et al (1982) Malnutrition, altered immune function, and the risk of infection in maintenance hemodialysis patients. *Am J Kidney Dis* **1**:206–218.

Murray JE, Marrill JP, Harrison JH (1955) Renal homotransplantation in identical twins. *Surg Forum* **6**:432–436.

Paganini EP (1995) Adapting the dialysis unit to increased hematocrit levels. *Am J Kidney Dis* **25**(Suppl 1):S12–S17.

Pollak R, Mozes M (1986) Anatomic abnormalities of cadaver kidneys procured for purpose of transplantation. *Ann Surg* **52**:233–235.

Rosenthal JT, Peaster ML, Laub D (1993) The challenge of kidney transplant nephrectomy. *J Urol* **149**:1395–1397.

Schoenfel PY, Henry RR, Laird NM et al (1983) Assessment of nutritional status of the National Cooperative Dialysis Study population. *Kidney Int* **23**(Suppl 13):80–88.

Sears JW (1988) Anesthesia in renal transplantation. In: Morris PJ (ed.). *Kidney Transplantation: Principles and Practice*. Philadelphia: W B Saunders, pp. 235–261.

Sharma DK, Pandez AP, Nath V et al (1989) Allograft nephrectomy: a 16-year experience. *Br J Urol* **64**:122–124.

Sinha SN, Castro JE (1976) Allograft nephrectomy. *Br J Urol* **48**:413–417.

Southard JH, Belzer FO (1993) The University of Wisconsin organ preservation solution: components, comparison, and modifications. *Transplant Rev* **7**:176–182.

Starnes HF, McWhinnie DL, Bradley JA et al (1984) Delayed major arterial hemorrhage after transplant nephrectomy. *Transplant Proc* **16**:1320–1323.

Starzl TE, Marchioro TL, Morgan WW et al (1964) A technique for use of adult renal homografts in children. *Surg Gynecol Obstet* **119**:106–108.

Sullivan D, Murphy DM, McLean P et al (1994) Transplant nephrectomy over 20 years: factors involved in associated morbidity and mortality. *J Urol* **151**:855–858.

Sutherland DER, Simmons RL, Howard RJ et al (1978) Intracapsular technique of transplant nephrectomy. *Surg Gynecol Obstet* **146**:950–952.

Sutherland F, Bloembergen W, Mohamed M et al (1993) Initial nonfunction in cadaveric renal transplantation. *Clin J Surg* **36**:141–145.

Toledo-Pereyra LH, Gordon C, Kaufmann R et al (1987) Role of immediate versus delayed nephrectomy for failed renal transplants. *Am Surg* **53**:534–536.

United Network for Organ Sharing (1994) *By-Laws and Policies*. Richmond: UNOS.

Vanholder R, Dell'Aquila R, Ringoir S (1991) Phagocyte function in uremia. *Adv Exp Med Biol* **297**:193–205.

Walsh TJ, Zachary JB, Hutchins GM et al (1977) Mycotic aneurysm with recurrent sepsis complicating post-transplant nephrectomy. *Johns Hopkins Med J* **141**:85–90.

Ward RA, Shirlow MJ, Hayes JM et al (1979) Protein catabolism during hemodialysis. *Am J Clin Nutr* **32**:2443–2449.

Weimar W, Geerlings W, Bijnen AB et al (1983) A controlled study on the effect of mannitol on immediate renal function after cadaver donor kidney transplantation. *Transplantation* **35**:99–101.

Whelchel JD, Cosimi AB, Young HH et al (1975) Pyeloureterostomy reconstruction in human renal transplantation. *Ann Surg* **181**:61–66.

6 SURGICAL COMPLICATIONS

The incidence and severity of technical complications following kidney transplantation have decreased over the past 30 years. However, complications resulting from technical misadventures, albeit infrequent, may cause renal dysfunction, graft loss, or even death. Although most problems occur in the early postoperative period, some may not be detected until several years after transplant. Today, transplant complications are being effectively avoided or managed through the use of more selective immunosuppressants such as cyclosporine, which preserves nonspecific host resistance; the development of minimally invasive percutaneous radiological approaches; and the emergence of secure surgical techniques.

COMPLICATIONS OF THE VASCULAR SYSTEM

The percentage of patients who experience vascular complications varies from 10% to 30% (Vidne et al 1976). Vascular complications may occur at any time during the immediate to the long-term posttransplant period. Renal artery thrombosis, stenosis, and hemorrhage occur more frequently than venous complications.

Renal artery complications

Thrombosis

Postoperative renal artery thrombosis occurs in slightly more than 1% of renal transplant recipients, usually due to a small caliber of the vessels. This complication frequently presents as sudden cessation of urine output from a previously functioning allograft. After the possibilities of a clogged Foley catheter or a prerenal cause have been excluded, the diagnosis is established using a ^{99m}Tc-diethylenetriamine pentaacetic acid (^{99m}Tc-DTPA) renal scan, a color-flow Doppler examination, and/or an angiogram to assess the patency of the renal artery. The presence of a clear area, denoting an absence

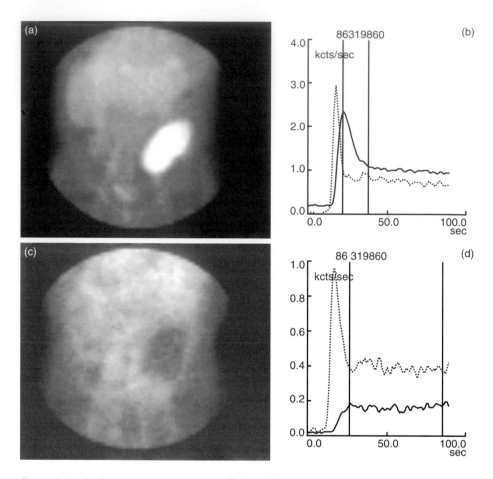

Figure 6.1. Radionucleotide scans using 99mTc-DTPA to assess renal allograft perfusion. (a) Immediate postoperative scan showing renal image. (b) Computer processed study showing aortic-iliac bolus (– – – –) and renal blood flow (——). (c) Absence of perfusion indicated by the clear (photopenic) image at the previously observed allograft site. (d) Computer-processed image showing good aortic-iliac flow (– – –) but little renal blood flow (——).

of perfusion on the 99mTc-DTPA scan, is diagnostic of graft thrombosis (Figure 6.1). Poor arterial flow demands immediate transplant exploration, because allograft damage progresses rapidly during warm ischemia; a delay in the time from diagnosis to surgical intervention frequently eventuates in primary nonfunction and graft nephrectomy (Vidne et al 1976; Louridas et al 1987). Allografts that suffer arterial thromboses within the first 16 posttransplant days virtually all require nephrectomy (Palleschi et al 1990). When thrombosis is accompanied by sepsis as an occult major complication, the mortality rate approaches 60% (Louridas et al 1987).

Technical misadventures represent the predominant cause of renal artery thrombosis. For example, dissection of the arterial wall, creating a distal intimal flap and a false lumen, may occur at donor nephrectomy and be occult at the time of transplantation; embolization of a plaque or a clot may occur prior to or at the time of transplant revascularization; extensive atherosclerotic plaque in the host external iliac artery at the anastomotic site may protrude into the vessel lumen; markedly size-disparate donor/recipient vascular segments may lead to improper suture techniques that further reduce luminal size; and kinking, malrotation, or torsion of the vessels may create turbulence or stasis of blood flow. A technical problem as a cause of renal dysfunction is strongly suggested when the renal transplant biopsy is 'bland'—that is, the kidney tissue shows no features of an alloimmune response. The second most frequent cause of arterial thrombosis is an immunologic etiology of allograft rejection, either of the hyperacute type of allorejection, as diagnosed histopathologically upon transplant biopsy by the presence of numerous polymorphonuclear leukocytes infiltrating glomerular and/or vascular structures, or of the irreversible accelerated acute type, presenting as interstitial hemorrhage, arteritis, edema, and venous congestion upon histopathologic examination. A third cause of arterial thrombosis is a generalized hypercoagulable state that may result from humoral factors associated with autoimmune diseases such as lupus erythematosus and/or antiphospholipid syndrome. Alternatively, large doses of cyclosporine have been associated with a 7% incidence of renal artery thrombosis, owing to the tendency of the drug to potentiate the action of intrinsic coagulation factors and/or to induce platelet aggregation (Kahan 1989). An increased incidence of thrombosis also has been reported upon administration of antilymphocyte sera.

Stenosis

Transplant renal artery stenosis occurs in 2–10% of cases (Benoit et al 1990), beginning as early as 2 days and as late as 22 months posttransplant. The sentinel findings that suggest an arterial stenosis include an abrupt onset of refractory hypertension, an unexplained impairment of renal function, and/or a change in the intensity of the bruit over an allograft (Table 6.1). While renal artery stenosis may be caused by a technical error of the types described above (but in lesser degree than that which produces thrombosis), other possible causes include an hyperplastic response of endothelial or smooth muscle cells to occult intraoperative trauma, or proliferative responses to immunological stimuli. Some authors report that technical errors occur more frequently with an end-to-end anastomosis than with an end-to-side anastomosis fashioned with a Carrel aortic patch (Miller et al 1989). Moreover, an excessively long donor artery may angulate or kink, producing turbulent blood flow with consequent anastomotic narrowing.

The arteriogram remains the gold standard for the diagnosis of arterial stenosis. The degree of narrowing is considered significant if the arterial luminal diameter is decreased by more than 50% (Figure 6.2). The diagnosis of renal artery stenosis may be suspected by noninvasive techniques, such as the Doppler duplex scan, the intra-arterial digital subtraction angiography (DSA), and, albeit rarely, the captopril radionuclide scan.

Symptoms/signs
- Progressive deterioration of renal function
- Bruit
- Refractory hypertension

Diagnostic tests
- Power Doppler
- Angiogram
- (Captopril renal scan)

Treatment
- Operative
- Percutaneous angioplasty

Table 6.1. Renal artery stenosis

Doppler duplex scanning displays a 58% sensitivity (Glicklich et al 1990) based upon the presence of an increased velocity of blood flow through the stenotic segment (>6 kHz) and marked turbulence downstream from the stenosis.

The captopril radionuclide scan procedure is said to display an 80% sensitivity (Glicklich et al 1990). An initial radionuclide scan examines renal function after intravenous administration of either 5 mCi of ^{99m}Tc-DTPA or 100 μCi ^{131}I-orthoiodohippurate. After oral administration of 25 mg of captopril, an angiotensin-converting enzyme inhibitor, the blood pressure is monitored at 10-min intervals for 1 hour, followed by a second radionuclide scan. If captopril produces a significant reduction in isotope uptake or excretion, the diagnosis of stenosis is confirmed, because captopril inhibition of angiotensin II-mediated efferent arteriolar vasoconstriction leads to an acute fall in the glomerular filtration rate, as evidenced by deterioration of the uptake of radionuclide. In our experience, this study is rarely useful, particularly in patients with serum creatinine values of at least 4 mg/dl.

Three strategies are currently available to manage renal artery stenosis, depending upon its location and degree. First, medical management with escalating doses of pharmacologic agents seeks to control the hypertension. Second, direct surgical repair may be performed by resection of the stenotic segment of an end-to-end connection either employing a primary reanastomosis (Figure 6.2b), or using a bypass graft to relieve a narrowing either at or just distal to an end-to-side connection (Figure 6.3). The alternative methods of surgical repair, namely, lysis of adhesions at the site of occlusion, or patch angioplasty wherein a detubularized segment of saphenous vein is used to widen the arterial lumen, rarely yield satisfactory long-term results. Use of a transperitoneal

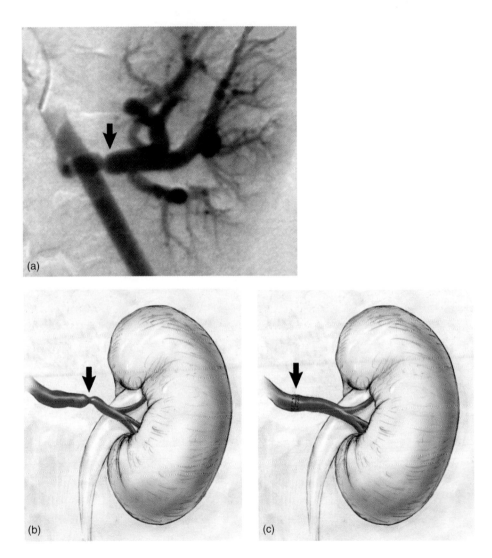

Figure 6.2. Renal artery stenosis of an end-to-end anastomosis. (a) Digital subtraction angiogram of a transplanted kidney showing an 80% stenosis at the anastomotic site of the recipient internal iliac artery to the donor renal artery (indicated by the arrow). (b) Diagrammatic representation of the stenosis (shown by the arrow). (c) Diagrammatic representation of the result after resection and reconstruction with an end-to-end anastomosis using interrupted sutures.

approach is critical for successful surgical repair of end-to-end anastomoses, whereas correction of end-to-side anastomoses may be more conveniently performed in some patients through the Gibson incision used for the transplant. Third, recalcitrant cases of localized lesions in the distal arterial tree may be managed by percutaneous transluminal angioplasty (PTA) without (Figure 6.4) or with an endovascular stent.

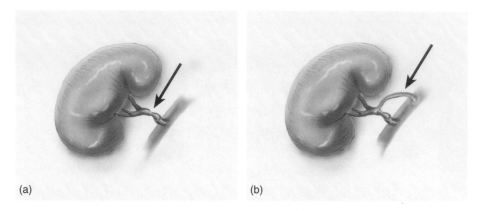

(a)   (b)

Figure 6.3. Renal artery stenosis after an end-to-side anastomosis. (a) Diagrammatic representation of a postanastomotic stenosis of the renal artery (indicated by arrow). (b) Diagrammatic representation of a saphenous vein bypass graft (indicated by arrow) from the external iliac artery to the poststenotic dilated arterial segment.

Increased success rates were recently reported when PTA was combined with placement of expandable metallic vascular stents (Figure 6.5), which are either balloon-expandable (Palmaz stent; Johnson and Johnson, Brunswick, NJ) or spring-loaded (Wallstent endoprosthesis; Medinvent, Lausanne, Switzerland). Stents appear to provide both mechanical support of the disrupted intima, thus preventing elastic recoil, and a scaffolding for controlled thrombosis and endothelial proliferation, which begin to form immediately following PTA. In four patients, Newman-Sanders et al (1994) reported apparent slowing of a previously aggressive, recurrent stenosis of the transplant renal artery, as well as maintenance of a satisfactory blood pressure and of stable allograft function. Wilms et al (1991) successfully used a Wallstent endoprosthesis in five of 15 patients; however, the serious complications of the procedure included acute stenosis leading to thrombosis that was successfully reversed by thrombolysis in one patient; massive cholesterol embolization necessitating dialysis in one patient; and recurrent stenosis in a few patients.

One recent review of 49 PTA and 39 surgical procedures to correct arterial stenoses reported 69% and 92.1% success rates, respectively (Roberts et al 1989). The superior results of the surgical repairs were achieved with low rates of morbidity or mortality, whereas serious complications were occasionally reported after PTA, including renal artery thrombosis or hemorrhage, both of which required surgical exploration (Majeski and Munda 1981; Lohr et al 1986). Percutaneous transluminal angioplasty seems to yield the best results for treatment of postanastomotic stenoses, while surgery gives better results for anastomotic stenoses. Surgical intervention is also favored when the transplant renal artery stenosis is due to a twisted, narrowed, or kinked renal artery anastomosis, or when the anastomotic narrowing appears to be due to a technical misadventure; such conditions render a percutaneous angioplasty procedure either difficult or dangerous.

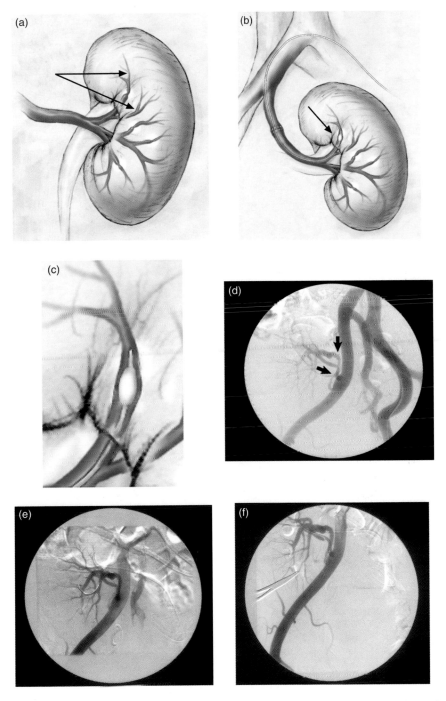

Figure 6.4. Percutaneous approach to relief of stenosis in the distal renal arterial tree. (a) Diagrammatic representation of distal stenoses (arrows). (b) Diagrammatic representation of percutaneous transvascular balloon dilatation (arrow). (c) A magnified field. (d) Digital subtraction angiogram showing stenoses of two renal arteries at sites indicated by arrows. (e) Results of percutaneous balloon angioplasty. (f) Oblique view of postangioplasty result.

225

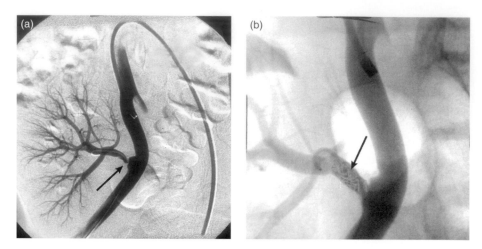

Figure 6.5. Endovascular stent. (a) Digital subtraction angiogram with area of stenosis distal to an end-to-side anastomosis. (b) Presence of endovascular stent dilating the region.

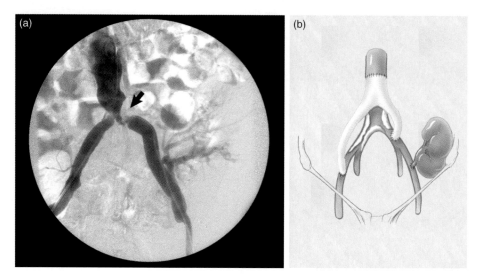

Figure 6.6. Proximal iliac occlusion producing renal ischemia. (a) Digital subtraction angiogram showing proximal left iliac artery occlusion just distal to the aortic bifurcation, with more extensive disease on the right. (b) Operative correction by right aortofemoral and left aortoiliac Dacron interposition graft.

The two criteria for successful relief of an arterial anastomotic stricture are a reduction in diastolic blood pressure below 90 mmHg without the need for antihypertensive medications, and a normalization of the serum creatinine value. A partial response may be defined as either a 15% decrease in the diastolic blood pressure or a reduction in the number of antihypertensive medications (Roberts et al 1989).

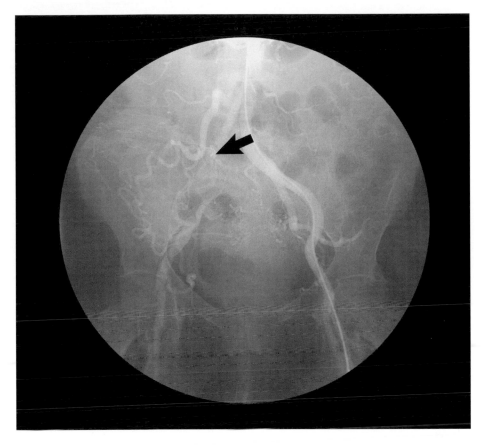

Figure 6.7. Aortoiliac study of a renal transplant recipient demonstrating a right common iliac artery occlusion (indicated by arrow) proximal to the renal transplant with abundant collateral blood flow and modest retrograde perfusion of the allograft.

In some patients, the renal ischemia is not due to an arterial stenosis, but rather to an arterial lesion proximal to the graft. The lesion may be occult and undetected prior to transplant. For example, one of our recent nondiabetic patients failed to gain normal renal function after living-related donor renal transplantation until an aortoiliac bypass was performed at about 3 months posttransplant to correct an isolated proximal stenosis (Figure 6.6). The angiogram shown in Figure 6.7 was performed on a patient who, at 12 years posttransplant, presented with compromised renal function and a relatively bland kidney biopsy. The angiogram shows an occluded common iliac artery above the renal allograft, which receives its blood supply in a retrograde direction from the distal external iliac artery via an abundant collateral blood flow. Interestingly, the contralateral iliac system shows no evidence of disease in the major vessels. These cases illustrate the need for detailed angiographic evaluation in cases of unexplained functional deterioration of a renal transplant.

Complications of the venous system

Renal allograft venous thrombosis is a relatively uncommon complication, ranging from a 0.3 to a 4.2% incidence (Merion and Calne 1985; Debleke et al 1989; Duckett et al 1991). Although this complication tends to occur in the early postoperative period, it is usually discovered after the graft has undergone infarction. Thrombosis of the main renal vein generally produces permanent graft damage, primarily because transplanted kidneys have only a single venous drainage system without any collateral anastomoses via capsular veins. The increased outflow impedance compromises arterial inflow. The causes of renal vein thrombosis include angulation, kinking, or stenosis of the anastomosis; compression by hematoma or lymphocele; or ascending thrombophlebitis from the ipsilateral femoral and/or iliac veins.

Renal vein thrombosis produces the nonspecific symptoms of acute allograft swelling accompanied by pain and tenderness, as well as oliguria or gross hematuria (Table 6.2). Prompt clinical diagnosis demands a high index of suspicion. The early diagnosis of renal vein thrombosis may be made by duplex Doppler sonography and renal scintigraphy. Doppler sonography showing a highly abnormal arterial signal with a sharp systolic peak and a plateau-like reversed diastolic flow with complete absence of venous flow is suggestive of, but not diagnostic for, renal vein thrombosis (Baxter et al 1972). Although renal scintigraphy using ^{99m}Tc-DTPA may fail to demonstrate perfusion, the transplant itself is not photopenic (as is seen in arterial infarction). A recent publication found that both Doppler sonography and scintigraphy examination were useful tools to diagnose renal vein thrombosis in two of three patients (Debleke 1989). Because renal vein thrombosis shows similar findings as acute rejection on both sonography and

Symptoms/signs
- Swelling ipsilateral extremity
- Proteinuria
- Distal thrombophlebitis

Diagnostic tests
- Venogram
- Arterial/venous Doppler
- Contrast angiogram

Treatment
- Thrombectomy (frequent recurrence)
- Heparinization

Table 6.2. Renal vein thrombosis

scintigraphy, most cases are diagnosed at the time of surgical exploration performed because a percutaneous transplant biopsy is not diagnostic of rejection (bland appearance).

Early exploration and thrombectomy have been reported to allow salvage of allografts afflicted with renal vein thrombosis. However, usually the transplant is no longer viable at the time of exploration, owing to the prolonged venous hypertension or to the propagation of the clot into the smallest venous tributaries (Clarke et al 1972). Thus, most patients require nephrectomy. Even when the allograft is salvageable, there tends to be persistent renal compromise.

The usual operative strategy is to remove the clot through a renal venotomy and then perfuse the kidney with cold Collins' solution to rinse out static blood within the graft. Chiu and Landsberg (1991) reported one case of successful, nonoperative relief of acute renal vein thrombosis using a 4-day intra-arterial infusion of streptokinase selectively into the transplant. However, streptokinase infusions may induce life-threatening hemorrhage or cause clot migration, thereby necessitating prophylactic placement of a vena caval filter prior to the initiation of lytic therapy. In addition, even if the patient experiences immediate relief following streptokinase infusion, the anastomotic error that led to the thrombosis must be corrected to achieve a durable result.

Arteriovenous fistula

Arteriovenous (AV) fistulas almost invariably represent an iatrogenic complication of percutaneous needle biopsies of the kidney. Because these complications occur so rarely after wedge biopsies, it has been assumed that they are due to penetration by the biopsy needle of a renal arteriole and then a vein, producing an injury that undergoes healing as an 'AV fistula'. Figure 6.8 shows a fistula that lies proximally in the renal hilum, as evidenced on this renal arteriogram by rapid visualization of the renal and external iliac veins. Although AV fistulas that occur after biopsy of native kidneys tend to display a benign course (Bennett and Wiener 1965; DeBeukelaer et al 1971; O'Brien et al 1974; Grau et al 1979; Gault and Meuhrcke 1983), the evolution of the lesion may be quite pernicious in the transplant setting (Lawen et al 1990).

The diagnosis of an AV fistula demands a high degree of suspicion, particularly when the patient is known to have experienced hematuria after a percutaneous biopsy. Other signs of AV fistula formation include the onset of a bruit and, rarely, a thrill over the graft; deterioration of renal function, marked particularly by an increased blood urea nitrogen to serum creatinine ratio; a prior history of incompletely controlled hypertension; and the presence of fibrosis and arteriolopathy on the biopsy specimen. Confirmation of the diagnosis of an AV fistula is generally made by angiography: namely, the rapid appearance of contrast in the renal vein. The treatment algorithm for an AV fistula depends upon its size and hemodynamic significance, as determined by the degree of vascular steal, that is the relative amount of blood flow via the fistula versus the amount of flow into the arterioles leading to the renal cortex. Embolization using either an auto-

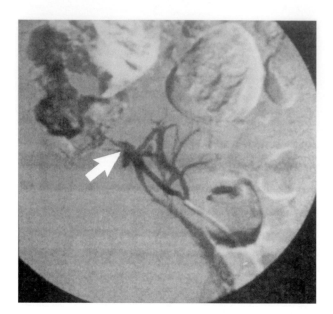

Figure 6.8. Digital subtraction angiogram demonstrating an arteriovenous (AV) fistula, presumably produced by a percutaneous biopsy. The arrow shows a pool of blood in the AV fistula, which lies in the hilum of the allograft.

genous blood clot or a spring is the only therapeutic maneuver to close the anomaly (Morse et al 1985; Baquero et al 1985), since these fistulas are generally too deep to approach surgically. Embolization produces infarction of the tissue receiving its arterial supply from that vessel, generally 20–33% of the distal renal mass. The two major complications of the procedure are propagation of the thrombus proximally, which further compromises renal function, and superinfection of the infarcted tissue. Overall, embolization does not seem to ameliorate the renal dysfunction, although it may slow progression of the disorder. Thus, an AV fistula represents a serious complication that is likely to shorten significantly the length of allograft survival.

Hemorrhage

Arterial or venous anastomotic hemorrhage represents a rare complication after transplantation. The usual causes of this complication are a mycotic aneurysm, a perianastomotic infection, a surgical misadventure, or an anastomotic disruption due to excessive tension. Hemorrhage distal to an anastomosis may be caused by an arterial laceration that was unrecognized at the time of procurement, an unligated small arterial branch, or a displaced ligature. Since the graft is cooled during storage, producing at least some degree of vasoconstriction, the bleeding may only be evident several hours later, upon complete rewarming and vasodilation. Hemorrhage also may result from capsular disruption due to a parenchymal tear, an event that is particularly associated with the accelerated form of acute rejection.

Allograft hemorrhage usually presents as intense graft site or back pain that may radiate to the flank or rectum, and that may be accompanied by a fall in hematocrit or even symptoms of vascular collapse. Prompt exploration is mandatory to preserve the patient's life. Attempts to repair anastomotic suture line disruptions are only rarely justified, due to the high rate of recurrence. Small parenchymal tears may be best treated with topical application of thrombostatic agents; attempts to place hemostatic sutures in the parenchyma should be avoided, due to the friability of the tissue. Nephrectomy represents the conservative approach in most cases of massive bleeding, a complication that has been associated with 33–50% mortality rates (Vidne et al 1976).

COMPLICATIONS OF THE URINARY TRACT

Urinary tract complications, which occur in 2–10% of cases (Kinnaert et al 1985), may result from pathologic processes at any level of the urinary system. The transplant ureter has a proclivity toward complications, because it receives its entire blood supply from vessels that emanate in the hilar and upper periureteral areolar tissues, sites that are vulnerable to injury during donor nephrectomy. The donor ureter is deprived of blood that is supplied in situ in the donor from either the bladder or the lumbar vessels, both of which are transected during organ retrieval. Ureteral devascularization readily occurs unless caution is exercised during dissection of the perihilar fat and periureteral adventitial tissues. In addition, the blood supply may be compromised if the ureteral segment is either too long and redundant, or too short and under tension. Proper handling of the donor ureter during organ retrieval and during the transplant procedure is thus mandatory to reduce the incidence of complications.

The rates of complications with the Leadbetter–Politano versus the Lich–Gregoir ureteroneocystostomy techniques are similar—9.4% and 3.7%, respectively (Thrasher et al 1990). The choice of a given technique usually reflects the previous experience of the surgeon rather than the relative benefits of that procedure. However, patients with a history of reflux are probably best managed with the Leadbetter–Politano procedure, and implants of short ureters may be possible only with the Lich–Gregoir technique. Ureterovesical obstruction is observed more often after Leadbetter–Politano implants because of kinking of the ureter at the new hiatus created in the muscularis of the bladder, because of trauma to the adventitial blood supply during placement into the submucosal tunnel, and/or because of the longer distal ureteral segment required to construct the tunnel. In contrast, the incidences of urine leakage and of vesicoureteral reflux are greater with the Lich–Gregoir technique. Ureteral necrosis occurs at about an equal frequency with both techniques, presumably reflecting the fact that most complications are related to an injury to the ureteral adventitia that occurs during donor nephrectomy.

Ureteral obstruction

Ureteral obstruction, which is the most common urinary complication following renal transplantation, may present early or late in the postoperative course. The onset of ureteral obstruction at years posttransplant generally results from fibrosis due to chronic ischemia or extrinsic compression by a lymphocele or other mass. The clinical presentation of ureteral obstruction is decreased urine output progressing to oligoanuria, urinary tract infection progressing to sepsis, local pain over the graft site, or a gradual rise in serum creatinine (Table 6.3). This complication is readily differentiated from transplant rejection using ultrasonography, nuclear scintography, and/or antegrade pyelography. Sonography demonstrates pyelocaliectasis in about 86% of cases (Smith et al 1988; Figure 6.9). Renography is less sensitive, detecting ureteral stenosis in only 18% of cases, probably because the obstructed kidney also displays impaired radionuclide uptake, a sign suggestive of allograft rejection (Frentz et al 1981). Antegrade pyelography is the most accurate method to define anatomically the location and degree of obstruction.

A 'combined' Whitaker test (Schiff et al 1979) to differentiate true obstruction from a dilated (but unobstructed) urinary system is generally unnecessary. The Whitaker test simultaneously measures the pressure in the renal pelvis using a manometer device attached to a nephrostomy tube placed into the collecting system, and the pressure in the urinary bladder via a similar device attached to a Foley catheter during and after infusion of sterile saline at a rate of 10 ml/min. If the net renal pelvic minus bladder pressure at the plateau level is greater than 22 cmH$_2$O, the findings are deemed consistent with obstruction, and net pressures less than 15 cmH$_2$O, with the absence of obstruction.

Symptoms/signs
- Decreased urine volume (oliguria)
- Urinary tract infection (sepsis)
- Pain over graft site

Diagnostic tests
- Ultrasound shows calyceal dilatation
- Antegrade pyelogram, defines site of stenosis

Treatment
- Distal: resection and reimplantation of ureter
- Proximal: native host ureter to donor renal pelvis (ureteropyelostomy). If no donor ureter available, transplant pelvis to bladder (pyelovesicostomy) or Boari flap

Table 6.3. Ureteral stenosis

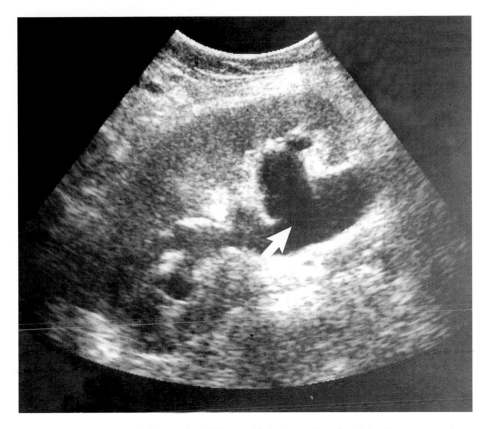

Figure 6.9. Ultrasound of transplant kidney with hydronephrosis arising from ureteral obstruction. The arrow shows the dilated transplant renal pelvis.

Before attempting percutaneous or surgical treatment, ureteric obstruction is initially managed by insertion of a nephrostomy catheter (Figure 6.10) to permit recovery of renal function and relief of the dilatation. At the time of insertion of the tube, an antegrade pyelogram is performed to define the level of obstruction. Obstruction may occur during the early posttransplant period due to blood clots (Figure 6.11); to edema and/or hematoma that exacerbate(s) the narrowing in a relatively tight submucosal tunnel; to malrotation (Figure 6.12) or to kinking (Figure 6.13) of the distal ureteral segment in the bladder. Although within 5 days the blood clot generally lyses or the tunnel edema decreases, malrotation, kinks, or profound degrees of obstruction require surgical intervention. A direct surgical approach, such as the revision of the ureteroneocystostomy with an indwelling stent, is the recommended approach, particularly for a distal obstruction in the presence of at least a modestly redundant ureter (Figure 6.14). The nephrostomy can be removed within 1 week, and the stent, at 4–6 weeks.

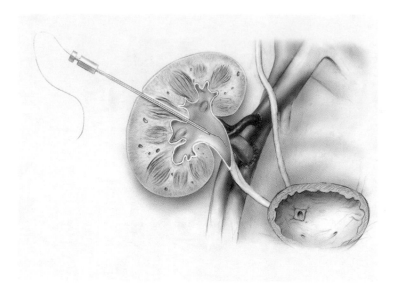

Figure 6.10. Insertion of a percutaneous nephrostomy for drainage of a dilated urinary drainage system.

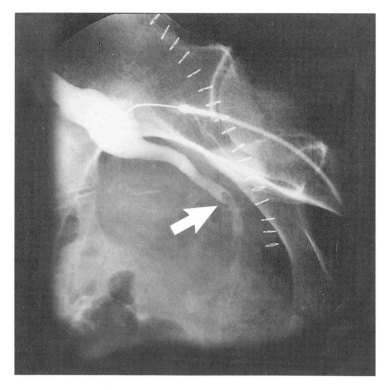

Figure 6.11. Antegrade pyelogram via a percutaneous nephrostomy, demonstrating that the ureteral occlusion was due to a blood clot (indicated by arrow).

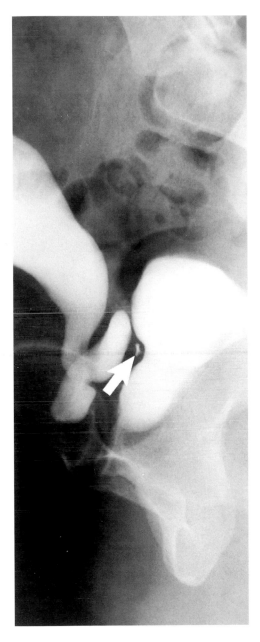

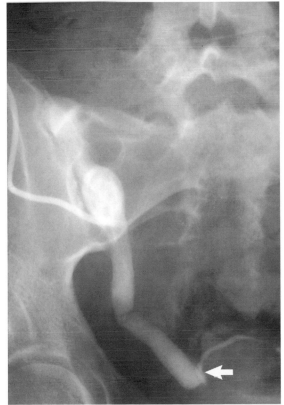

Figure 6.12. Antegrade pyelogram of a transplanted kidney via a percutaneous nephrostomy demonstrating obstruction of the distal transplant ureter. The arrowhead shows the obstructed segment resulting from malrotation of the ureter.

Figure 6.13. Antegrade pyelogram demonstrating that ureteral obstruction was due to kinking (at the site indicated by arrow) of the submucosal portion of a long tunnel within a Leadbetter–Politano ureteroneocystostomy.

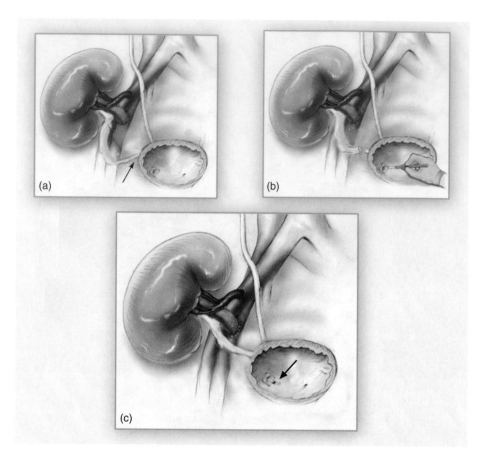

Figure 6.14. Reanastomosis of the transplant ureter in the presence of a distal stricture. (a) Anatomy of a stricture due to ischemia in the distal portion of the ureter (shown by an arrow). (b) Excision of the stenotic segment, which is pulled through the bladder after incision of the neo-orifice, as shown, using a scalpel. (c) Creation of a new ureteroneocystostomy with placement of a simple polyethylene tube (#5 pediatric feeding tube) as a stent (shown by arrow).

An alternative, conservative approach for first-line treatment is percutaneous transluminal antegrade or retrograde dilation with a 6–8-mm angioplasty balloon catheter and placement of a double J-stent for at least 35 days (Smith et al 1988). This procedure has been reported to have a success rate of 78% (Bennett et al 1986). However, technical difficulties in gaining access for the catheter to an upper polar calyx, or in negotiating a long, tight ureteral stricture, may render this approach impossible. Furthermore, percutaneous management of strictures may be complicated by persistent hematuria, perinephric hematoma, urinary leakage at the nephrostomy site, and/or sepsis.

In cases of a long stenotic segment or a limited length of donor ureter, the preferred

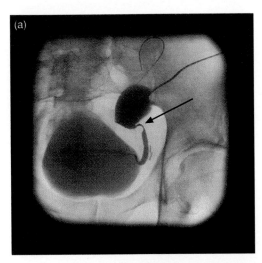

Figure 6.15. Diagnosis and ureteropyelostomy reconstruction for a ureteropelvic junction (UPJ) stricture. (a) Antegrade pyelogram showing a proximal dilated renal pelvis, a ureteropelvic junction narrowing (shown by arrow) with a normal-appearing ureter. (b) Schematic representation of operative correction by ureteropyelostomy performed by mobilizing the host ureter for an end-to-end anastomosis with the transplant pelvis and insertion of a double J-stent.

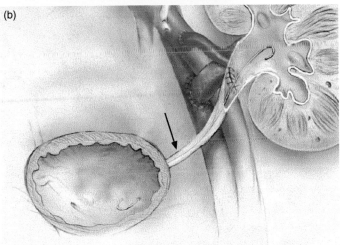

surgical approach is an anastomosis of the distal host ureter to the donor renal pelvis (Figure 6.15). The anastomosis is generally performed in running fashion with PDS (or Maxxon), a material that is resorbed by 6 weeks, thus reducing the likelihood of long-term concretions on the suture line. In cases in which the renal pelvis is friable, an interrupted suture technique is used, buttressing the anastomosis with adjacent tissues (or even an omental flap mobilized through a peritoneal window) with wide drainage of the potential area of urinary leakage. Despite persistence of the leakage for 3–6 months (or even longer), the area of the anastomosis usually heals without stricture. In most cases, the proximal host ureter may be ligated with impunity, save for situations of pre-existent chronic pyelonephritis and/or of subsequent host kidney infection. Although native

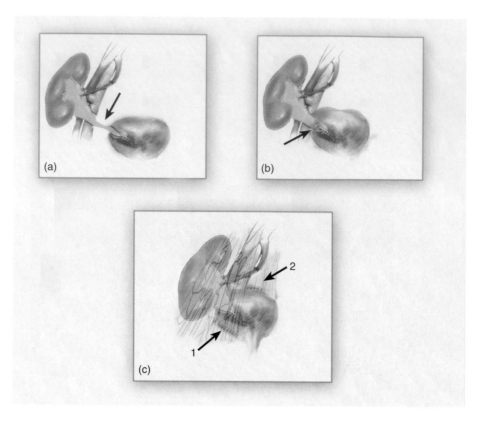

Figure 6.16. Diagrammatic representation of pyelovesicostomy procedure. (a) Long stenotic area in a short distal ureter anastomosed to the bladder by the Liche procedure. (b) Resection of distal ureter and anastomosis of renal pelvis to bladder. (c) Hitching of the bladder to the psoas (1) and/or to the rectus (2) muscles to stabilize the anastomosis.

nephrectomy can be performed at the time of ureteropyelostomy by extending the incision to the costal margin, it is usually preferable to defer the extirpation pending the presentation of symptoms. A semielective procedure can then be performed later via a transcostal approach to the native kidney. The alternative strategy of a ureteroureterostomy joining host ureter to donor ureter in either end-to-end or end-to-side fashion unfortunately has a high rate of stricture formation and is generally not recommended.

In patients whose host ureter has been previously extirpated, generally for treatment of reflux refractory to surgical intervention, primary restoration of urinary tract continuity may be established by mobilizing the contralateral distal ureter (although frequently it too has been extirpated) for a ureteropyelostomy. Two less satisfactory approaches are possible. Direct pyelovesicostomy, which is a direct anastomosis of donor urinary pelvis to the bladder, should be accompanied by a 'hitch' of the bladder to either the psoas or the posterior sheath of the rectus muscle (Figure 6.16c). Alternatively and

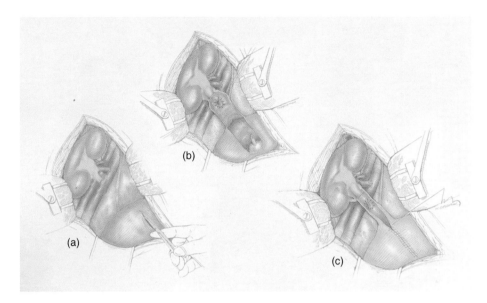

Figure 6.17. Schematic representation of Boari flap reconstruction of a devascularized fibrotic ureter by anastomosis of bladder to the renal pelvis. (a) Development of the bladder flap. (b) Onlay of bladder flap with neo-anastomosis of transplant pelvis to the posterior wall of the flap. (c) Closure of flap with construction of a 'neo-ureter'.

preferably, a Boari flap, a tubular segment of the host bladder, is created and anastomosed to viable margins of the transplant pelvis (Figure 6.17). The Boari flap offers several potential advantages over a pyelovesicostomy: (1) it allows as much as 15 cm of the ureter to be replaced if the bladder has a capacity of at least 400 ml; (2) it allows submucosal channeling of the transplant ureter (where possible) into the tubular flap and thus dampens the refluxing pressure; and (3) it reduces the degree of direct contamination of the collecting system during episodes of lower urinary tract infections (e.g. acute bacterial cystitis). Pyelovesicostomy is clearly the least acceptable of these options, since the free urinary reflux transmits both the high voiding pressure and any vesicle infection. However, pyelovesicostomy is preferable to permanent nephrostomy drainage of the urinary system, which almost always eventuates in chronic pyelonephritis and renal scarring.

Urinary leakage

Ureteral leakage may result from faulty handling of the donor ureter; undue tension created by a short ureter; ureteral or renal pelvis blowout due to severe obstruction; invasive wound infection; distortion by a pelvic hematoma; or, rarely, slow blood flow during a rejection episode. The clinical symptoms of leakage, which usually present

Symptoms/signs/laboratory findings
- Fever
- Decreased urine volume
- Pain and swelling at graft site, perineum, scrotum, or labia
- Wound drainage
- Sepsis
- Elevated serum creatinine

Diagnostic studies
- Ultrasound: fluid collection
- Renal scan: isotope extravasation
- Indigo carmine test
- Cystogram
- Antegrade pyelogram

Table 6.4. Urine leak: diagnosis

before the fifth posttransplant week, include decreased urine output; fever; pain and swelling over the graft site, perineum, scrotum, or labia; elevated serum creatinine values; oliguria; cutaneous urinary drainage; and/or sepsis (Table 6.4). Urinary leaks in patients with drainage are readily diagnosed by the higher creatinine content of fluid collected from the wound site than that of serum. The diagnosis of a ureterocutaneous fistula may be confirmed if intravenously administered indigo carmine produces a bluish color in the drainage fluid. Because most patients do not present with liquid issuing from the skin, radionuclide imaging studies are usually required for the diagnosis. While sonography may identify a peritransplant fluid collection in 67% of cases, nuclear renography, including delayed images obtained as long as 24 hours after isotope injection (Stratemeier et al 1987), represents a more specific, albeit less frequently positive (about 30% of patients) tool. However, among patients with good renal function and a large disruption, nucleide appearance in a nonphysiologic site indicates urine leakage (Figure 6.18). Because obstruction leading to caliectasis is also frequently present, percutaneous antegrade pyelography provides not only an 85% sensitivity to detect the complication, but also an anatomic definition of its site (Figure 6.19).

Urinary bladder leak

Management of the urine leak depends on the site and the degree of disruption (Table 6.5). Bladder complications usually manifest within the first 2 weeks of the posttransplant period as urine extravasation, elevation of the serum creatinine value, a palpable

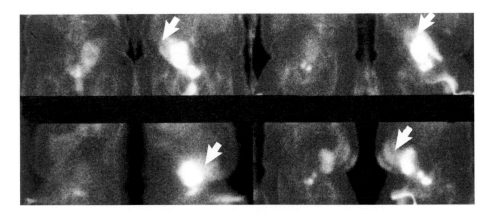

Figure 6.18. ^{99m}Tc-DTPA renal scan in a patient with urine leakage using images delayed 8 hours after isotope injection. The location of isotope outside the urinary system is indicated by arrows.

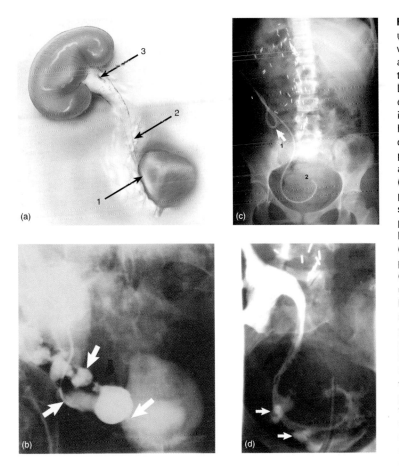

Figure 6.19. Multiple urinary leaks in a patient with severe ureteral stenosis and secondary blowout of the renal pelvis. (a) Diagrammatic representation of radiological findings including deviation of the bladder (1) to the contralateral side by the pressure of the urinoma (2), and concomitant renal pelvis (3) blow-out due to intense pressure in the collecting system. (b) Antegrade pyelogram showing multiple large urinary leaks (arrows). (c) Placement of a percutaneous nephrostomy (1) and via this tube a ureteral stent (2). Note the large number of clips in the native right renal fossa from previous nephroureterectomy performed at the patient's local hospital. (d) Antegrade nephrostogram performed 6 weeks later, showing less pronounced pelvic leakage with two residual, small ureteral leaks. Note that the nephrostomy has been removed, but that the ureteral stent and the Foley catheter remain in place.

241

Bladder: Foley catheter (14–42 days)
Distal ureter: reimplantation
Entire ureter: host ureter to donor pelvis (ureteropyelostomy)
Pelvis: indwelling stent/nephrostomy

Table 6.5. Urine leak: treatment as a function of site

suprapubic mass, pain over the graft site, or painful voiding. Bladder fistulas usually develop either at the site of the anterior cystotomy closure or at the ureteral hiatus. The diagnosis may be confirmed by ultrasonography or gravity cystography. Sonography may demonstrate a perivesical fluid collection, and gravity cystography identifies the site of urinary extravasation. Vesical fistulas of substantial size are generally managed by early exploration, primary repair, and 2–6 weeks of bladder decompression with a Foley catheter until a gravity contrast study fails to show extravasation. However, most bladder leaks can be controlled expectantly by bladder drainage alone; persistent leakage as detected by sonography represents an indication for surgical intervention.

Ureteral leak

In the absence of a frank abscess, distal ureteral leaks are best addressed by expedient surgical procedures that re-establish urinary tract continuity and provide effective drainage with less risk of sepsis or chronic fistula formation, two not-uncommon outcomes of prolonged periods of conservative management. Surgical options include revision of the ureteroneocystostomy with placement of an indwelling stent (Figure 6.15), donor-to-recipient pyeloureterostomy with an indwelling stent (Figure 6.15), or construction of a Boari flap that uses a bladder advancement in place of the necrotic ureter (Figure 6.17). The choice of the technique and timing of surgical repair depends on the length of viable ureter available for urinary reconstruction. Distal lesions at the ureterovesicle junction are usually managed aggressively, whereas lesions in the more proximal ureter tend to be managed conservatively.

In the presence of an abscess or of septicemia, the urinoma must be drained by either a percutaneous approach or a surgical procedure. In this setting, percutaneous approaches may be particularly useful, since they have been reported to achieve 63–87% success rates to heal transplant ureteral leaks (Bennett et al 1986; Warner et al 1987). A strategy combining a diverting nephrostomy with an antegrade ureteral stenting led to an 87% leak closure rate in one study (Matalon et al 1990). The double J-stent is particularly convenient for this complication, because it is unlikely to be accidentally passed per urethra. However, the procedure has been commonly associated with sepsis due to the requirement for prolonged catheter drainage to permit healing of the areas of ureteral slough. However, a good result is achieved in many cases, particularly if the prednisone dose has been reduced to modest levels (Figure 6.19).

Indwelling stents are generally removed after 14–45 days, depending upon the extent of the lesion. Failure to demonstrate extravasation by antegrade pyelogram upon gravity instillation of contrast is a sign of healing; however, it is generally wise to clamp the nephrostomy tube for a period of 5–7 days to ascertain a good functional result, as evidenced by little rise in the serum creatinine, before removing the tube.

Renal pelvis

Although it occurs infrequently, urine leakage resulting from necrosis of the transplant pelvis constitutes an emergent situation that requires immediate intensive investigation, beginning with ultrasound and nuclear scanning studies as well as an antegrade pyelogram when possible. However, definition of the lesion may require prompt surgical exploration. Pelvic wall necrosis may result from vascular insufficiency or incidental laceration at the time of excessive dissection of the renal transplant hilum, or from high intraluminal pressure due to ureteral obstruction.

Because the extent of necrosis may be deceptive at the time of initial exploration, the optimal treatment of this complication demands an individualized approach. The strategy is generally conservative: placement of percutaneous nephrostomy, and wide drainage of any surrounding infection. Once the inflammation process becomes quiescent, surgical re-exploration will afford a better opportunity to assess the blood supply to the renal pelvis. If the vascularization seems adequate, a primary repair may be performed, restoring the lower urinary tract continuity using a pyeloureterostomy with the ipsilateral native ureter, a Boari flap, a direct pyelovesicostomy, or an interposition of a segment of ileum between the renal transplant pelvis and bladder. If the blood supply seems inadequate, the renal pelvis is buttressed with a pedicle of omentum as a possible source of a parasitic blood supply, and nephrostomy drainage continued. It is exceedingly rare that surgical intervention cannot eventually correct the problem.

COMPLICATIONS OF THE TRANSPLANT BED

Lymphocele

Lymphoceles, which are lymph collections between the inferior pole of the kidney and the bladder, represent not-uncommon complications following transplantation, namely, a 0.6–18% incidence (Braun et al 1974; Thomalla et al 1985). The development of lymphoceles has been ascribed to inadequate ligation of the afferent lymphatics coursing over the recipient iliac vessels or lying within the allograft hilum, or to decapsulation of the kidney transplant (Kay et al 1980). Most lymphoceles are small and asymptomatic, and probably resorb. Some collections become clinically manifest between 18 and 180 days after surgery (Teruel et al 1983), owing to pressure on adjacent structures, including the

Symptoms/signs
- Leg swelling ipsilateral to graft
- ± Palpable mass

Diagnostic studies
- Ultrasound: fluid collection ± hydronephrosis

Treatment
- First line: percutaneous drainage
- Second line: operative peritoneocystostomy

Table 6.6. Lymphocele

urinary bladder, ureter, iliac vein, or lower extremity lymphatics. In severe cases, the patient displays hydronephrosis, azotemia, frequent urination, ipsilateral leg edema, a protuberant mass, or a cutaneous lymph fistula (Table 6.6).

The presence of a lymphocele is confirmed by ultrasonography (Figure 6.20) or by a renal scan. Cystograms or computed axial tomography (Figure 6.21) can also be useful to document bladder compression. Lymphangiograms do not tend to be diagnostic of either the presence or the site of the lymph leakage. The management strategy depends on the size and symptomatology. In most cases, the initial approach is a radiologically monitored, percutaneous aspiration with insertion of an 8 or 12 French drainage tube

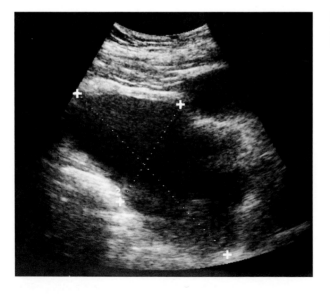

Figure 6.20. Large lymphocele cavity on ultrasonography. The greatest dimension is shown by the transecting dotted lines.

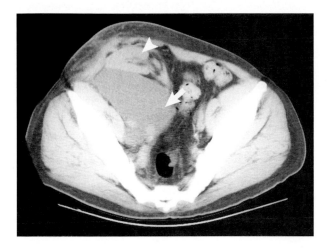

Figure 6.21. Computerized axial tomogram showing a large lymphocele cavity. The transplant kidney is compressed superolaterally (indicated by the arrowhead) by the fluid collection (shown by the full arrow).

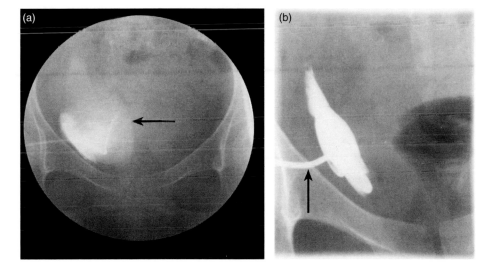

Figure 6.22. Percutaneous drainage of lymphocele. (a) Visualization of a lymphocele (shown by the arrow) that was subsequently drained. (b) Recurrence of lymphocele as a smaller collection producing venous compression. The panel depicts an inserted drainage tube (shown by the arrow).

until follow-up ultrasonography confirms the disappearance of the collection (Figure 6.22). If the condition recurs, sclerotherapy using a 10% povidone–iodine solution may be useful, provided that the lymphocele is relatively small and not loculated (Teruel et al 1983). However, this technique is associated with an 80–90% recurrence rate and has the potential to introduce exogenous infection (Zincke et al 1973).

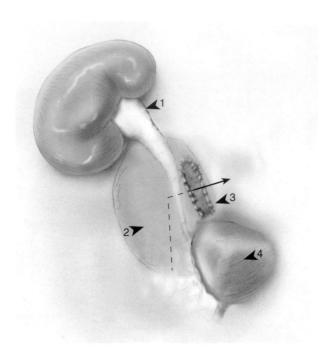

Figure 6.23. Schematic representation of peritoneocystostomy procedure for internal drainage of lymphocele. The figure shows the renal pelvis and ureter dilated secondary to compression (1) by the lymphocele (2); an incision in the peritoneal covering of the lymphocele is made to form a window (3). Note that the bladder (4) is deviated to the contralateral side. The arrow shows the drainage from the lymphocele into the peritoneal cavity.

In contrast to cutaneous marsupialization, which is associated with a high incidence of infection, the procedure of choice for noninfected fluid collections is intraperitoneal marsupialization, as described by Byron and coworkers (1966). A peritoneal window is constructed to connect the lymphocele with the peritoneal cavity, thereby allowing lymphatic fluid to drain freely into the abdominal cavity, where it is absorbed by the peritoneum (Figure 6.23). It is important to create a window sufficiently large to ensure patency and to use a running stitch of absorbable suture to maintain an oval window having dimensions not less than 2.5 × 5.0 cm. Extreme care must be exercised in opening and exploring the lymphocele cavity to avoid the ureter and the transplant vascular structures lying either within or in proximity to the lymphocele, which is not uncommonly involved in an inflammatory reaction, particularly in cases initially managed by aspiration. Omentum is placed adjacent to the peritoneocystostomy opening to facilitate fluid absorption and to avoid internal herniations of the small intestine. Although this procedure has a 90% success rate to decompress the lymphocele (Langle et al 1990), celiotomy has been associated with a variety of complications, including small bowel obstruction, or injury to the adjacent donor ureter or host vas deferens. Endoscopic laparoscopy has been used to avoid the lower midline abdominal incision and to shorten the length of hospitalization (Khauli et al 1992).

Perinephric hemorrhage and hematoma

Nonanastomotic postoperative bleeding is a not-uncommon complication caused by uremic coagulopathies, unappreciated injuries to small host or torn hilar donor vessels, as well as anticoagulant therapy to maintain the potency of vascular access grafts or to treat coagulation disorders. Because of innovations in technique and equipment, anticoagulation is no longer required during preoperative hemodialysis; thus this cause of bleeding is avoidable. Symptoms may include graft site or back pain radiating to the flank and rectum, decreased hematocrit, and a palpable mass in the graft site. The diagnosis can be confirmed by ultrasonography, by a radiolucent halo on renal scan, or, particularly when infection is suspected, by computed tomography (Figure 6.24). Early exploration is indicated to evacuate large or expanding hematomas before they occlude the arterial or venous supply. Although smaller hematomas usually resolve, some remain a potential site for bacterial colonization, and for extension to vascular structures with formation of a mycotic aneurysm. Whereas noninfected hematomas can be drained with primary closure of the wound, infected collections require wide drainage and healing by secondary intention.

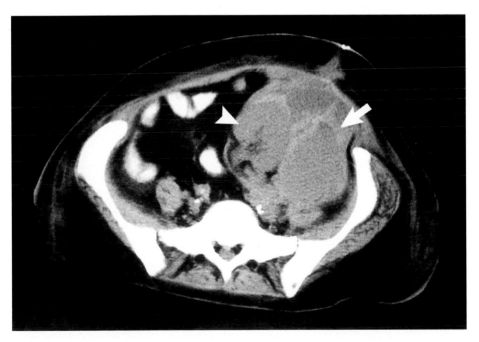

Figure 6.24. Computerized axial tomogram shows a large perinephric hematoma. The arrowhead shows the transplant kidney displaced medially by a huge perinephric hematoma (full arrow).

Posttransplant scrotal complications

The spermatic cord and accompanying vessels are usually mobilized and retracted medially during exposure of the iliac fossa to avoid tethering the allograft ureter with consequent compromise of the ureterovesical anastomosis. In the rare cases in which mobilization of the spermatic cord and vessels is restricted by scarring or is inadvertently neglected, these structures must be divided and ligated. The consequent hydrocele formation in the ipsilateral scrotal sac usually appears within 2–6 weeks after surgery. The cystic nature of the scrotal mass is confirmed by transillumination or ultrasonography. Generally, these relatively small and asymptomatic hydroceles are best managed without intervention; large collections may require hydrocelectomy or aspiration/sclerotherapy. More serious complications include testicular atrophy or necrosis, acute bacterial epididymitis, and recurrent scrotal pain. Acute epididymitis, which is usually a result of prolonged postoperative Foley catheterization, generally responds to broad-spectrum antibiotic therapy, preferably with ciprofloxacin for at least 4 weeks. In severe cases, orchidectomy may be necessary to prevent sepsis. Acute bacterial prostatitis, most likely related to an ascending urethral infection caused by an indwelling Foley catheter, is not uncommon. The patient may complain of a febrile illness associated with perineal discomfort or bladder outlet obstruction after catheter removal. Common organisms isolated from urine specimens are *Escherichia coli*, *Proteus mirabilis*, *Klebsiella pneumoniae*, *Pseudomonas aeruginosa*, Enterobacter and Serratia species. Treatment with parenteral antibiotics, usually ampicillin and aminoglycosides, is empirically initiated until sensitivity results are available. Oral antibiotic therapy should continue thereafter for 30 days.

CONCLUSION

After 40 years of clinical practice, the technical aspects of the renal transplant procedure are well understood. However, each procedure presents unique challenges for the surgeon because of the variable combinations of donor kidney and recipient anatomy and/or disease. Complications may occur due to technical misadventures or to an unanticipated evolution of minor problems. While the overall incidence of technical complications is approximately 5%, most problems are neither life-threatening nor hazardous to the outcome of the graft. Meticulous attention to surgical technique, combined with knowledge of the pathophysiology of the disorder, can reliably guide the surgeon to address these technical challenges effectively. Satisfactory long-term results demand early recognition and appropriate management of surgical complications involving the vascular anastomoses or urinary drainage system. These strategies demand that the surgeon recognize and compensate for the impaired wound healing and proclivity to infection characteristic of renal transplant recipients.

REFERENCES

Baquero A, Morris MC, Cope C et al (1985) Selective embolization of vascular complications following renal biopsy of the transplant kidney. *Transplant Proc* **17**:1751–1754.

Baxter GM, Morley P, Dall B (1972) Acute renal vein thrombosis in renal allografts: new Doppler ultrasonic findings. *Clin Radiol* **43**:125–127.

Bennett AR, Wiener SN (1965) Intrarenal arteriovenous fistula and aneurysm: a complication of percutaneous renal biopsy. *Am J Roentgenol* **95**:372–382.

Bennett LN, Voegli DR, Crummy AB et al (1986) Urologic complications following renal transplantation: role of interventional radiologic procedures. *Radiology* **160**:531–536.

Benoit G, Moukarzel M, Hiesse C et al (1990) Transplant renal artery stenosis: experience and comparative results between surgery and angioplasty. *Transplant Int* **3**:137–140.

Braun WE, Banowsky LH, Straffon RA et al (1974) Lymphocele associated with renal transplantation: report of 15 cases and review of literature. *Am J Med* **57**:714–729.

Byron RL, Yonemoto RH, Davajan V et al (1966) Lymphocysts: surgical correction and prevention. *Am J Obstet Gynecol* **94**:203–207.

Chiu AS, Landsberg DN (1991) Successful treatment of acute transplant renal vein thrombosis with selective streptokinase infusion. *Transplant Proc* **23**:2297–3000.

Clarke SD, Kennedy DA, Hewitt JC (1972) Successful removal of thrombus from renal vein after transplantation. *BMJ* **102**:29–31.

DeBeukelaer MM, Schreiber MH, Dodge WF, Travis LB (1971) Intrarenal arteriovenous fistulas following needle biopsy of the kidney. *J Pediatr* **78**:266–272.

Debleke D, Sacks GA, Sandler M (1989) Diagnosis of allograft renal vein thrombosis. *Clin Nucl Med* **14**:415–419.

Duckett T, Bretan P Jr, Cochran ST et al (1991) Noninvasive radiological diagnosis of renal vein thrombosis in renal transplantation. *J Urol* **146**:403–406.

Frentz GD, Schlegel JV, Hussey JL, Prima R (1981) Quantitative renal scintillation camera studies in renal transplantation. *Urology* **18**:546–555.

Gault MH, Meuhrcke RC (1983) Renal biopsy: current views and controversies. *Nephron* **34**:1–34.

Glicklich D, Tellis VA, Quinn T et al (1990) Comparison of captopril scan and Doppler ultrasonography as screening tests for transplant renal artery stenosis (Brief Communication). *Transplantation* **49**:217–218.

Grau JH, Gonick P, Wilson A (1979) Post-biopsy intrarenal arteriovenous fistula. *J Urol* **122**:233–236.

Kahan BD (1989) Cyclosporine. *N Engl J Med* **32**:1725–1738.

Kay R, Fuchs E, Barry JM (1980) Management of postoperative pelvic lymphocele. *Urology* **15**:345–349.

Khauli RB, Mosenthal AC, Caushaj PF (1992) Treatment of lymphocele and lymphatic fistula following renal transplantation by laparoscopic peritoneal window. *J Urol* **147**:1353–1355.

Kinnaert P, Hall M, Janssen F et al (1985) Ureteral stenosis after kidney transplantation. True incidence and long-term followup after surgical correction. *J Urol* **133**:17–20.

Langle F, Schurawitzki F, Muhlbacher R et al (1990) Treatment of lymphoceles following renal transplantation. *Transplant Proc* **22**:1420–1422.

Lawen JG, Van Buren CT, Lewis RM, Kahan BD (1990) Arteriovenous fistulas after renal allograft biopsy: a serious complication in patients beyond one year. *Clin Transpl* **4**:357–369.

Lohr JW, MacDougall ML, Chonko AM et al (1986) Percutaneous transluminal angioplasty in transplant renal artery stenosis: experience and review of literature. *Am J Kidney Dis* **7**:363–367.

Louridas G, Botha JR, Meyers AM, Myburgh JA (1987) Vascular complications of renal transplantation: the Johannesburg experience. *Clin Transplant* **1**: 240–245.

Majeski JA, Munda R (1981) Hazard of percutaneous transluminal dilation in renal transplant arterial stenosis. *Arch Surg* 116:1225–1226.

Matalon TAS, Thompson MJ, Patel SK et al (1990) Percutaneous treatment of urine leaks in renal transplant patients. *Radiology* 174:1049–1051.

Merion RM, Calne RY (1985) Allograft renal vein thrombosis. *Transplant Proc* 17:1746–1750.

Miller A, Marsh CL, Stanson AW et al (1989) Treatment of transplant renal artery stenosis: experience and reassessment of therapeutic options. *Clin Transplant* 3:101–109.

Morse SS, Sniderman KW, Strauss EB, Bia MJ (1985) Post biopsy renal allograft arteriovenous fistula: therapeutic embolization. *Urol Radiol* 7:161–164.

Newman-Sanders APG, Gedroyc WG, Al-Kutoubi MA et al (1994) The use of expandable metal stents in transplant renal artery stenosis. *Clin Radiol* 50:245–250.

O'Brien DP III, Parrott TS, Walton KN, Lewis EL (1974) Renal arteriovenous fistulas. *Surg Gynecol Obstet* 139:739–743.

Palleschi J, Novick A, Braun W, Magnusson MO (1990) Vascular complications of renal transplantation. *Urology* 16:61–67.

Roberts JP, Hocher NL, Fryd DS et al (1989) Transplant renal artery stenosis. *Transplantation* 48:580–583.

Schiff M, Rosenfield AT, McGuire EJ (1979) The use of percutaneous antegrade renal perfusion in kidney transplant recipients. *J Urol* 122:246–248.

Smith TP, Hunter DW, Letourneau JG et al (1988) Urinary obstruction of renal transplants: diagnosis by antegrade pyelography and results of percutaneous treatment. *Am J Roentgenol* 151:507–510.

Stratemeier E, Lee RG, Hill T, Clouse ME (1987) Delayed images of glucoheptonate distribution after renal transplants. *Clin Nucl Med* 10:357–360.

Teruel JL, Escobar EM, Querda C et al (1983) A simple and safe method for management of lymphocele after renal transplantation. *J Urol* 130:1058–1059.

Thomalla JV, Lingeman JE, Leapman SB, Filo RS (1985) The manifestation and management of late urological complications in renal transplant recipients: use of the urological armamentarium. *J Urol* 134:944–948.

Thrasher JB, Temple DR, Spees EK (1990) Extravesical versus Leadbetter–Politano ureteroneocystostomy: a comparison of urological complications in 320 renal transplants. *J Urol* 144:1105–1109.

Vidne BA, Leapman SB, Butt KM, Kountz SL (1976) Vascular complications in human transplantation. *Surgery* 79:77–81.

Warner JJ, Matalon TAS, Rabin DN et al (1987) Percutaneous interventional radiologic procedures for diagnosis and treatment of urologic complications in renal transplant patients. *Transplant Proc* 19:2203–2204.

Wilms GE, Peene PT, Baert AL et al (1991) Renal artery stent placement with use of the Wallstent endoprosthesis. *Radiology* 179:457–462.

Zincke H, Woods JE, Aguila JJ et al (1973) Experience with lymphoceles after renal transplantation. *Surgery* 77:444–450.

7 IMMUNOSUPPRESSIVE DRUGS: PHARMACOLOGY

In collaboration with P Kelly*

Pharmacokinetic concepts provide a basis for individualization of drug therapy to optimize outcomes. Most hospital laboratories routinely measure patient serum, plasma, or whole-blood concentrations of many drugs, including antibiotics (aminoglycosides, vancomycin), antiepileptics (phenytoin, phenobarbital), antiarrhythmics (lidocaine, procainamide, digoxin), and immunosuppressive agents (cyclosporine, CsA; tacrolimus, TRL). The therapeutic range of a drug is defined as the concentrations at which the desired pharmacological effect is produced and adverse effects prevented in most patients. The significant inter- and intrapatient variability of the effects of a given concentration of therapeutic agents causes substantial difficulty in achieving concentrations in the therapeutic range. In addition, the variable clinical responses of patients demand individualization of the drug regimen.

GENERAL PRINCIPLES OF PHARMACOKINETICS

The study of pharmacokinetics seeks to describe the absorption, distribution, metabolism, and elimination of drugs. Table 7.1 lists some of the terms, abbreviations, and equations commonly used to describe pharmacokinetic parameters. When administered orally, a drug must be absorbed across the biological membranes of the gastrointestinal tract to reach the systemic circulation, after which the drug leaves the vasculature to penetrate tissues and is distributed to sites of therapeutic or toxic effects.

The amount of drug that enters the systemic circulation is expressed as the area under the concentration-versus-time curve (AUC) profile. This profile depicts the drug concentrations in plasma, serum, or whole blood at various times after drug administration (Figure 7.1). The AUC, which is expressed in units of concentration multiplied by time (e.g. mg/l $\times$ hour, or, through rearrangement, mg $\times$ hour/l), is calculated mathematically by the trapezoidal rule. A trapezoid, as shown by the shaded area in Figure 7.1, is formed by the data points, namely, the two concentrations bounded by the time interval. The AUC is the sum of the areas of the individual trapezoids. The concentration

* Division of Immunology and Organ Transplantation, Department of Surgery,
University of Texas Medical School, Houston

Abbreviation	Definition	Equation
%CV	Percent coefficient of variation	Standard deviation $\div$ mean $\times$ 100
τ	Dosing interval	
AUC	Area under the curve	Trapezoidal rule
C_{av}	Average concentration	AUC $\div$ τ
CL/F	Apparent oral clearance	Dose $\div$ AUC
C_{max}	Maximum obtained concentration	
C_{min}/C_0	Minimum concentration/trough	
C_{ss}	Steady-state concentration	
D	Dose	
F	% bioavailability	$(AUC_{oral}) \div (AUC_{IV}) \times 100$
ka	Absorption rate constant	
ke	Elimination rate constant	$-2.303 \times$ slope of terminal elimination phase
LD	Loading dose	
MD	Maintenance dose	
$t_{1/2}$	Half-life	$0.693 \div$ ke
t_{max}	Time to maximum concentration	
V_d	Volume of distribution	CL $\div$ ke

Table 7.1 Pharmacokinetic abbreviations and equations

reflects the outcome of two opposing but simultaneous processes, namely, absorption, which increases the concentration, and elimination, which reduces it (Figure 7.2).

Rapid absorption of a drug results in a high initial blood concentration and a rapid fall during the elimination phase. When a drug is absorbed slowly, it is distributed during the absorption phase; the peak concentrations occur later and are lower due to the participation of elimination processes (Figure 7.3). The time to reach the concentration peak (C_{max}) is defined as the t_{max}; the period before C_{max} is broadly classified as the absorption phase; and the period thereafter, as the elimination phase (Figure 7.2). After administration of the same dose for a sufficient period, the amount of drug eliminated during the dosing interval equals the amount reaching the systemic circulation, and the patient is said to have reached a 'clinical steady-state' (ss). Thus, at steady-state, the AUC values during each dosing interval are relatively constant, and the concentration–time profiles, as indicated in Figure 7.4 by areas A, B, C, D, and E, can essentially be superimposed.

Most drugs obey 'linear' pharmacokinetics; that is, the AUC value is proportional to the administered dose. For instance, double the dose increases the AUC by a factor of two. However, when AUC values change disproportionately to the dose, the drug is said to obey 'nonlinear' (Michaelis–Menten) pharmacokinetics. The nonlinearity is displayed

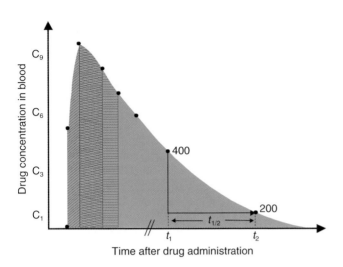

Figure 7.1. Area under the concentration-versus-time curve following oral administration of a drug. The shaded area (AUC) is calculated by the trapezoidal rule, as shown for the first three data points.

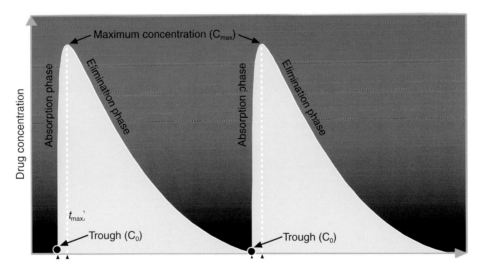

Figure 7.2. Concentration–time profiles depicting the absorption and elimination phases following oral administration of a drug. The maximum drug concentration (C_{max}), time to C_{max} (t_{max}), and trough concentrations (C_0) are defined on the figure.

as a rapid increase in drug concentration, usually due to drug saturation of hepatic metabolism, of protein binding, or of active renal transport mechanisms (Figure 7.5).

Two types of general mechanisms govern drug metabolisms. Phase I reactions include oxidation, hydrolysis, or reduction, thereby rendering the agent more polar and

253

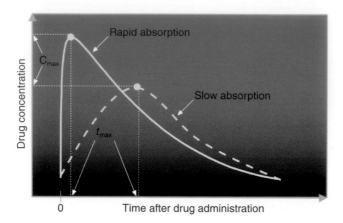

Figure 7.3. Concentration–time profiles of two drugs. One shows rapid (——), and the other, slow (- - - -), absorption following oral administration. Rapid absorption results in a higher C_{max} and shorter t_{max} compared to slow absorption, although the AUCs, indicating overall drug exposure, may be equivalent.

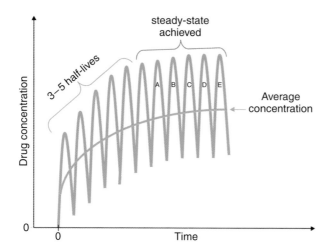

Figure 7.4. Pharmacokinetic profiles following multiple identical drug doses. After 3–5 half-lives, steady-state is achieved with both maximum (C_{max}) and minimum (C_0) drug concentrations, and the fluctuations between them remain essentially constant (areas A, B, C, D, and E).

increasing its propensity for elimination from the body. Phase II reactions conjugate drugs with glucuronide, acetate, or sulfate groups to form either inactive or active compounds. The parent drug, as well as its metabolites, is generally eliminated from the body via the urine, biliary tree, sweat, or exhalation.

A variety of physiological and pathophysiological variables can modify the pharmacokinetic behavior of drugs in individual patients. The three most important pharmacokinetic parameters that determine therapeutic effects are bioavailability (F), the fraction of absorbed drug that reaches the systemic circulation; clearance (CL), a measure of the ability of the body to eliminate the drug; and volume of distribution (Vd), a measure of the apparent space within the body that is available to contain the drug.

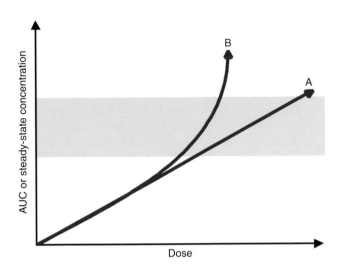

Figure 7.5. Relationship of drug dose to AUC (or a surrogate concentration) at steady-state. The shaded area shows the putative therapeutic range. The lines show the relation under linear (A) and nonlinear (B) pharmacokinetic behaviors.

Bioavailability

While absorption describes the rate and extent to which a drug leaves its site of administration and enters the circulation, bioavailability is of greatest concern to the clinician. Bioavailability is defined as the amount (or fraction) of administered drug that actually reaches the systemic circulation (Table 7.1). For example, an orally administered drug must first cross the stomach or intestinal mucosa, enter the portal blood, and pass through the liver before it reaches the systemic circulation. If a substantial portion of the drug undergoes destruction or transformation in the gut or liver prior to reaching the systemic circulation, its bioavailability is substantially reduced; the drug is said to display a 'first-pass' effect.

At least four factors influence the absorption of drugs. Since they must mix with the aqueous phase at the absorptive site, hydrophilic drugs soluble in aqueous solutions are more rapidly absorbed than those administered in an oily solution, suspension, or solid form. Furthermore, local production of gastrointestinal secretions may be necessary to prepare drugs for absorption, and intestinal diseases that reduce these secretions or interfere with the flow of bile or pancreatic juice may impair drug absorption. A third determinant of absorption is the surface area available: drug uptake may be attenuated after a small bowel resection. Finally, gastrointestinal motility is important, since many drugs are degraded in the acid environment of the stomach or during intestinal transit. Each factor, alone or in combination, influences absorption and helps to determine the clinical efficacy or toxicity of a drug.

Clearance

Clearance rates express the volume of biological fluid per unit of time that must be completely freed of drug to account for the elimination phase of decrease in drug concentra-

255

tion. Thus, clearance rates do not directly indicate the amount of drug eliminated from the body, but rather the volume of biological fluid that corresponds to that concentration of drug (Table 7.1). For a given patient and for the majority of drugs that display linear pharmacokinetics, clearance rates are usually constant over the range of concentrations encountered in clinical settings: a constant fraction of drug is eliminated per unit of time. For agents that show 'complete' bioavailability, that is, 100% delivery of drug into the systemic circulation, clinical steady-state is achieved once the rate of drug elimination equals the rate of drug administration. However, once the elimination mechanisms for a drug are saturated, the kinetics become nonlinear; despite the increased concentration, only a constant amount of drug is eliminated per unit of time. Under such circumstances, clearance rates become variable.

Volume of distribution

Similarly, the volume of distribution does not necessarily refer to an identifiable physiological space, but merely to the fluid volume that would be required to contain all the drug in the body at the same concentration as it is present in the blood or plasma (Table 7.1). The volume of distribution varies widely among drugs, depending on the degree of association with plasma proteins; the hydrophobicity, which determines the drug's partition coefficient in fat; and the avidity of the agent to bind to tissues. The volume of distribution for any given drug shows interindividual variations, as well as intraindividual variations as a function of age, gender, disease state, and body composition.

Half-life

The drug half-life ($t_{1/2}$) is the time required for the concentration in the blood, as an estimate of the amount of drug in the body, to decrease by 50% (Table 7.1). A derived parameter, the half-life changes as a function of both the clearance and the volume of distribution: as the clearance decreases, the half-life would be expected to increase; as the volume of distribution increases, the half-life would be expected to increase. Half-life estimates provide an index of the time required to reach steady-state after initiation of or a dose change in the drug regimen, and also indicate the time for the drug to be removed from the body. Thus, the half-life provides a means to estimate the appropriate dosing interval. After four half-lives, the observed concentration of drug reaches approximately 95% of the steady-state value. While half-life may easily be determined for some drugs, other agents follow a multiexponential pattern that includes two or more elimination phases, each with a distinct half-life value. The value that is usually reported is the terminal elimination phase. As analytical methods of greater sensitivity become available, lower concentrations can be measured, and thus the estimates of drug half-life are lengthened.

Variability

The variability of pharmacokinetic parameters is expressed as the percent coefficient of variation (%CV). Figure 7.6 shows the broad %CV of pharmacokinetic values among patients (inter individual) treated with a given dose of CsA by either the intravenous or the oral route. To compensate for this variability, one must adjust drug doses based upon concentration measurements in each patient (i.e. 'concentration control'). Of even greater interest is the intraindividual %CV. For example, one can discriminate cohorts of patients wherein each patient displays either a low or a high value of %CV over time (Figure 7.7). Cyclosporine intraindividual variability has been implicated as a cause of

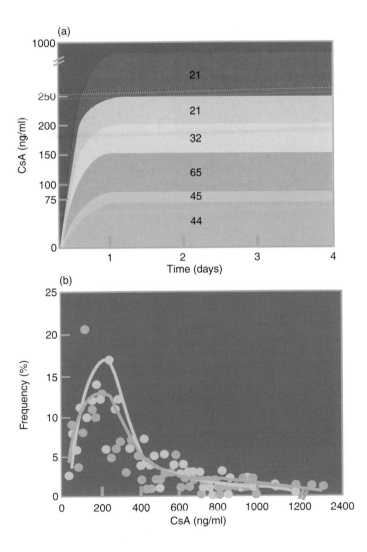

Figure 7.6. Interindividual pharmacokinetic differences among CsA concentrations. (a) Steady-state concentrations (C_{ss}) during 4 days of continuous administration of CsA. The numbers within each curve show the number of patients with C_{ss} values less than 75 ng/ml, green; 76–100 ng/ml, blue; 101–150 ng/ml, orange; 151–200 ng/ml, yellow; 201–250 ng/ml, pink; and more than 251 ng/ml, red. (b) The frequency distribution of CsA concentrations measured by the TDx (orange) versus a nonselective radioisotope (RIA; IncStar; green) assays after 7 days of twice-daily dosing of 7 mg/kg Sandimmune.

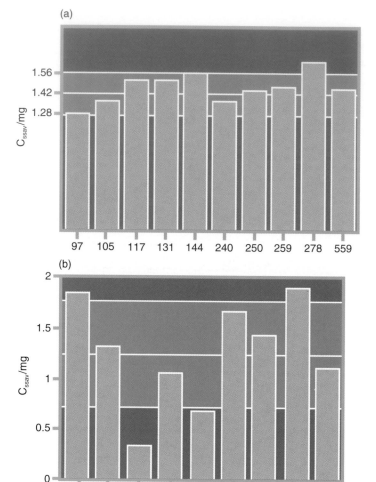

Figure 7.7. Distinct profiles of intraindividual variability over time. The values of the dose-corrected average CsA concentration (C_{ssav}/mg) at different times for a patient with (a) a %CV = 10% versus (b) %CV >40%. (Adapted from Kahan BD, Welsh M, Schoenberg L et al. Variable oral absorption of cyclosporine. A biopharmaceutical risk factor for chronic renal allograft rejection. *Transplantation* 1996; **62**:599–606. © 1996 Lippincott Williams & Wilkins. All rights reserved.)

acute (Holt et al 1986; Inoue et al 1994) and of chronic (Kahan et al 1996) allograft rejection.

Factors influencing pharmacokinetic parameters

Metabolism

The cytochrome P450 superfamily of heme proteins includes components of the mixed function oxidase system. The hepatic microsomal P450 system catalyzes the metabolism of a large number of lipophilic endogenous and exogenous compounds. Among the 27 identified P450 gene families, only three, CYP1, CYP2, and CYP3, are currently believed to be responsible for the majority of hepatic drug metabolism in humans (Wrighton and Stevens 1992). The metabolites formed by the action of P450 enzymes are more hydrophilic than the parent compound and are thus more readily excreted from the body. In some cases, however, drug metabolites react with cellular components, resulting in toxicity (Nebert et al 1987; Guengerich 1988).

The human cytochrome P450 enzyme CYP3A4, comprising approximately 30% of the total hepatic P450 system (Shimada et al 1994), is responsible for the metabolism of a large number of structurally diverse exogenous and endogenous compounds, including the xenobiotics CsA (Kronbach et al 1988), TRL (Sattler et al 1992), and sirolimus (SRL) (Sattler et al 1992). Other xenobiotics metabolized by CYP3A4 include erythromycin, dihydropyridine calcium channel blockers, lidocaine, midazolam, triazolam, and the 3-hydroxy-3-methylglutaryl coenzyme A (HMG-CoA) inhibitors such as lovastatin (Wrighton and Stevens 1992). Endogenous compounds metabolized by CYP3A4 include steroids such as testosterone, progesterone, cortisol, and estradiol (Wrighton and Stevens 1992). CYP3A4 activity appears to be inducible, that is, capable of being augmented, by administration of glucocorticoids, phenobarbital, phenytoin, and rifampin (Wrighton and Stevens 1992). In contrast, CYP3A4 activity may be inhibited by imidazole antifungals, macrolide antibiotics, verapamil, diltiazem, and 17α-ethinyl estradiol, many of which compete for the active site (Table 7.2).

At concentrations encountered under physiologic conditions, each drug is typically metabolized by a single isozyme of the P450 system. The individual phenotypes as well as disease states involving the liver or the gut P450 seem to determine the rate and pathway of metabolic clearance. For example, induction of CYP3A4 activity by phenytoin overwhelms other factors, leading to increased clearance that decreases concentrations; in contrast, inhibition of CYP3A4 activity by ketoconazole reduces drug clearance, with elevated concentrations of CsA or TRL. Similarly, hepatic insufficiency decreases the metabolic and/or elimination rates, increasing CsA or TRL concentrations. The concentration and activity of hepatic CYP3A4 display marked interindividual differences (Guengerich et al 1986; Wrighton et al 1987; Lown et al 1994; Shimada et al 1994). For example, differences in content of CYP3A4 within the liver result in a 66% interpatient variation in the clearance of intravenously administered CsA (Thummel et al 1994).

P-glycoprotein

Differences among the CYP3A4 activities in the liver do not appear to account for the majority of the interpatient variations observed after oral administration of CsA (Turgeon et al 1992). While one possible cause of this discrepancy is an abundant but variable expression of CYP3A4 in small bowel epithelial cells (Watkins et al 1987, Kolars et al 1992), another reason is the variable expression of intestinal P-glycoprotein. This multidrug resistance-1 (mdr-1) gene product is a versatile transporter that exports a wide variety of xenobiotics, including CsA (Schinkel and Borst 1991; Gottesman and Pastan 1993; Saeki et al 1993), TRL (Saeki et al 1993) and SRL (Arceci et al 1992), out of the cell. P-glycoprotein is located almost exclusively within the brush border on the

Substrates	Inhibitors	Inducers
Alfentanil	Clarithromycin	Carbamazepine
Alprazolam	Clotrimazole	Glucocorticoids
Amlodipine	Danazol	Phenobarbital
Astemizole	Dexamethasone	Phenytoin
Atorvastatin	Diltiazem	Rifabutin
Cisapride	Erythromycin	Rifampin
Clarithromycin	Fluconazole	Troglitazone
Cortisol	Grapefruit juice	
Cyclosporine	Itraconazole	
Diazepam	Ketoconazole	
Diltiazem	Miconazole	
Erythromycin	Quinidine	
Ethinyl estradiol	Ranitidine	
Felodipine	Troleandomycin	
Fentanyl	Verapamil	
Gemfibrozil		
Hydrocortisone		
Lidocaine		
Lovastatin		
Miconazole		
Midazolam		
Nicardipine		
Nifedipine		
Progesterone		
Simvastatin		
Sirolimus		
Sufentanil		
Tacrolimus		
Terfenadine		
Testosterone		
Triazolam		
Troleandomycin		
Verapamil		

Table 7.2 Substrates for inhibitors and inducers of the cytochrome P450 enzyme CYP3A4

apical or luminal surface of the enterocyte, where it pumps xenobiotics from the cytoplasm into the intestinal lumen (Thiebaut et al 1987; Hsing et al 1992; Penny and Campbell 1994; Saitoh and Aungst 1995).

CYP3A4 and P-glycoprotein play complementary roles in the pharmacokinetics of drug absorption and elimination. For instance, there is a striking overlap between the substrates of CYP3A4 and the inhibitors of P-glycoprotein: CsA, TRL, diltiazem, verapamil, and erythromycin are all CYP3A4 substrates and P-glycoprotein inhibitors (Hofsli and Nissen-Meyer 1989; Yusa and Tsuruo 1989; Holt et al 1992). Due to its transport function and high levels of expression in intestinal cells, P-glycoprotein reduces drug absorption, thereby contributing to variations in pharmacokinetics of CsA, TRL, and SRL (Lown et al 1997; Figure 7.8).

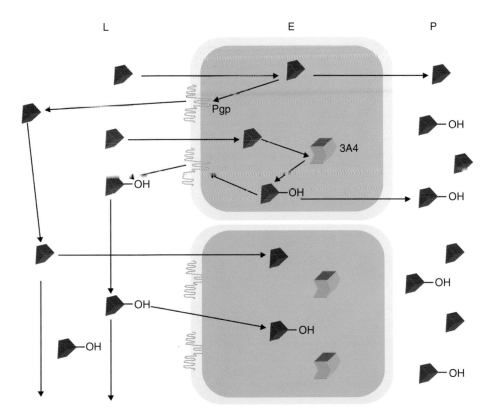

Figure 7.8. Interaction of the substrate CsA, cytochrome P450 3A4 (3A4), and p-glycoprotein (Pgp) in the intestine. After absorption from the lumen (L) into the enterocyte (E), CsA (▷) can either (1) enter the portal circulation (P); (2) be extruded back into the intestinal lumen via Pgp, where it can be absorbed further down the intestine; or (3) be metabolized by 3A4 to a metabolite (▷-OH) that can be either absorbed into the portal circulation or extruded into the intestinal lumen by Pgp.

THERAPEUTIC DRUG MONITORING

Therapeutic drug monitoring (TDM) seeks to provide a surrogate marker for therapeutic versus toxic effects (Table 7.3). TDM has been advocated for critical dose drugs, which display (1) a narrow therapeutic window; (2) high intra- and interpatient pharmacokinetic variability in absorption, distribution, metabolism, and elimination; (3) an inconsistent relation of drug dose to blood concentration; and (4) the potential for life-threatening events as a result of these variabilities. TDM strategies seek to provide guidelines for the individualized selection of drug doses utilizing serial measurements of a pharmacokinetic or pharmacodynamic parameter. The measurement of the particular parameter must be reproducible, easy to perform, rapid, and predictive of clinical outcome (Awni 1992).

The blood concentrations of immunosuppressants are usually measured in whole blood. The methods display reasonable selectivity for the active moiety, and satisfactory intra- and interday reproducibility. The appropriate concentration index to estimate drug exposure depends on the immunosuppressive agent.

In contradistinction to pharmacokinetics, which assesses the effects of the body on the drug, pharmacodynamics is the study of the effects of a drug on the body to produce the clinical response. For immunosuppressive drugs, the ideal pharmacodynamic index would be an in vitro surrogate of allograft rejection. Several markers have been advocated as surrogates: namely, enumeration of peripheral blood lymphocyte subpopulations (Kerman and Geis 1976); dampened mixed lymphocyte cultures or mitogen-driven lymphocyte proliferation indices (Rogers et al 1984); transferrin receptor expression on mononuclear cells (Mohanakumar et al 1986; Mooney et al 1990); or measurements of cytokine product (Yoshimura and Kahan 1985; Yoshimura et al 1991) or mRNA concentrations (interleukin-1, interleukin-2, and interferon-γ; Yoshimura et al 1988) in either unstimulated or mitogenic or alloantigenic stimulated lymphocytes. Unfortunately, none of these pharmacodynamic methods shows a clear correlation with clinical outcomes (Awni 1992).

Drug	Therapeutic C_0 (ng/ml)	Toxic C_0 (ng/ml)	Therapeutic AUC (ng $\times$ hour/ml)
Cyclosporine	250–350	>400	3600–6000
Tacrolimus	5–20	>25	NR
Sirolimus	5–10	>15	200–450
Mycophenolate mofetil	$>3 \times 10^3$	NR	$>40 \times 10^3$

NR, not reported.

Table 7.3 Therapeutic immunosuppressive versus toxic concentrations for maintenance immunosuppressive agents during the first 3 months posttransplant

CYCLOSPORINE

Drug measurement

Five methods are widely utilized to measure CsA concentrations in blood samples (Table 7.4). The original method, high-performance liquid chromatography (HPLC), specifically detects the parent CsA compound and remains the gold standard for other analytical methods (Kahan et al 1990). However, automated techniques have superseded this method for routine clinical monitoring because of the cumbersome nature of HPLC, which requires a high level of technical skill, expensive equipment, relatively long turnaround times, and extensive extraction procedures. The most popular automated procedure is a fluorescence polarization immunoassay (FPIA, TDx analyzer, Abbott Diagnostics, Chicago, IL), which utilizes a monoclonal antibody (MAb) relatively specific for parent CsA. The TDx system requires little technical expertise; has a rapid turnaround time of about 2 hours for 60 samples; and shows good sensitivity, with lower and upper limits of detection (25 and 1500 ng/ml, respectively) within the general clinical range (Napoli and Kahan 1990). However, the assay shows cross-reactivities with CsA metabolites, namely, 8.5% and 2.5% for AM1 and AM4N, respectively (vide infra for CsA metabolism; Wang et al 1991). Indeed, the FPIA may display concentrations 12–67% higher than HPLC estimates, depending on whether the patient has received a renal, liver, or heart transplant (Yatscoff et al 1990; Moyer et al 1991; Rogers et al 1991; Schroeder et al 1991a; Dusci et al 1992; Salm et al 1993; LeGatt et al 1994). The monoclonal FPIA CsA assay has been adapted by an improved method of sample pretreatment and by a rapid organic extraction (Wallemacq and Alexandre 1999) in the new AxSYM immunoanalyzer (Abbott). The FPIA CsA assay method is claimed to reduce metabolite cross-reactivity by 50%, despite the use of the same MAb as the TDx. The decreased cross-reaction improves the correlation with results of HPLC (Steimer 1999). The AxSYM assay uses 184 µl of each sample and analyzes 59 samples per hour. The analytical range of the assay is 25–800 µg/l, with intra- and interday variability ranging from 6% to 8.2% and from 4% to 5.8%, respectively (Schutz et al 1998; Wallemacq and Alexandre 1999).

The third method, Cyclo Trac (Diasorin, Stillwater, MN), is a whole-blood radioimmunoassay (RIA) that detects CsA over a concentration range of 25–1200 µg/l (Holt et al 1994). The CsA in the patient sample competes with a ^{125}I-labeled CsA tracer for binding to a mouse anti-CsA specific MAb different from that used in the TDx (Lee et al 1991). Compared with HPLC, the RIA overestimates CsA concentrations by 22–30%, due to cross-reactivity with the metabolites AM9 (2.2–15%), AM4N (1.7–4.4%), and AM1 (0.7–5.7%) (Wallemacq et al 1990; Wong and Ma 1990; Tredger et al 1992). Because the RIA assay is labor intensive, requires more time than FPIA (20 samples and controls performed in approximately 3.5–4 hours; Holt et al 1994), exposes laboratory technicians to low levels of γ-radiation, and generates a low-level radiation waste, it is not widely employed in TDM laboratories.

The fourth method, the enzyme-multiplied immunoassay (EMIT, Syva Company,

Assay	Detection range (ng/ml)	Turnaround time (hours)	Metabolite cross-reactivity (%)	Advantages*	Disadvantages*
HPLC	25–1500	24	0	1	4, 7
FPIA					
TDx	25–1500	2 (60 samples)	12–67	2, 3, 5, 6	1
AxSYM	25–800	1 (60 samples)	6–35	3, 5, 6	1, 2
RIA	25–1200	3–4 (20 samples)	22–30	1	3, 7
EMIT	25–500	2–3 (40 samples)	8–30	1	2
CEDIA	25–620	NR	18–23	5	1

NR, not reported.

*1 = specificity; 2 = precision; 3 = sensitivity; 4 = technical expertise needed; 5 = technical expertise not needed; 6 = fast sample turnaround time; 7 = slow sample turnaround time.

Table 7.4 Comparison of assays for cyclosporine whole-blood concentrations

San Jose, CA), uses a specific mouse MAb in a CobasMira (Roche Diagnostic Systems, Indianapolis, IN) chemistry system. The EMIT is a binding assay in which CsA in the sample competes with a conjugate of CsA-bacterial glucose 6-phosphate dehydrogenase for binding to a MAb. When the CsA conjugate binds to antibody, the residual glucose 6-phosphate dehydrogenase activity free in the supernatant decreases. Therefore, the CsA concentration in the patient sample is directly proportional to the enzyme activity detected by spectrophotometry. The assay range has been reported to be 25–500 μg/l CsA in whole blood, but the measurements may be accurate to 12.5 μg/l (Morris et al 1992). The assay is useful for the measurement of trough (C_0) concentrations, but cannot be applied to AUC estimates, wherein peak concentrations are generally at or above the upper limit of detection. The EMIT assay contains a unique monoclonal anti-CsA antibody that displays little overall cross-reactivity with the CsA metabolites AM9 (4–9%), AM4N (<1%), and AM1 (<1%) (Dasgupta et al 1991; Rosano et al 1991). The mean overestimates of CsA concentrations, compared to HPLC measurements, range from 8% to 30% (Oellerich et al 1995). Assays of 20 samples (and controls) require approximately 75 min, and 40 samples can be analyzed in 2–2.5 hours (Holt et al 1994).

Finally, a cloned enzyme donor immunoassay (CEDIA, F. Hoffman-La Roche Ltd, Basel, Switzerland) for CsA quantifies CsA in whole blood samples based on the spontaneous association of a short recombinant β-galactosidase fragment and a recombinant β-galactosidase monomer to form an active enzyme tetramer. Cyclosporine chemically attached to the fragment competes with CsA in the patient sample to bind an anti-CsA antibody, thereby interfering with the formation of tetramer. The CsA concentration in the sample is directly proportional to the residual enzyme activity (Schutz et al 1998). The lower limit of detection is 25 μg/l, with intra- and interday variability of 7.8–8.2% and 5.5–11%, respectively (Schutz et al 1998). Cross-reactivities with CsA metabolites are 5.4–6.5%, 27.7–29.3%, and 5.6% for AM1, AM9, and AM4n, respectively (Schutz et al 1998; Steimer 1999). Compared to HPLC, the CEDIA assay produces an 18–23% overestimation of whole blood CsA concentrations (Schutz et al 1998; Steimer 1999).

Drug formulations

Three formulations of CsA are currently available for administration to transplant patients: Sandimmune, Neoral, and SangCya. Sandimmune is an olive- (liquid) or corn oil- (gel cap) based product that shows tremendous intra- and interindividual variations in absorption, distribution, metabolism, and elimination. This variability complicates its safe and effective use (Kahan 1985). The variability in Sandimmune pharmacokinetic parameters may be due to differences in the rate of gastric emptying (Drewe et al 1992); the amount and/or composition of biliary, pancreatic, and duodenal/small bowel secretions; the function and motility of the small bowel; and the degree of intestinal cytochrome P450 metabolism (Tjia et al 1991) and p-glycoprotein activity (Lown et al 1997). The Sandimmune formulation must be digested by pancreatic enzymes and emulsified by bile into hydrophilic particles prior to CsA absorption (Mehta et al 1988).

In the oral formulation, Neoral, CsA is incorporated into a microemulsion preconcentrate, which contains surfactant, lipophilic and hydrophilic solvents, and ethanol. Neoral forms a homogeneous, macroscopically transparent and thermodynamically stable monophasic solution of droplets, the individual diameters of which are less than 100 nm (Vonderscher and Meinzer 1994). The ready dissolution of Neoral upon contact with aqueous fluids without requiring the actions of bile, enzymes, or small intestinal secretions produces an increased bioavailability (Mueller et al 1994a). Although Neoral shows better correlations of dose to AUC as well as to trough concentrations (Kahan et al 1994), two pharmacokinetic parameters that show poor correlations with Sandimmune doses, the associations are not sufficiently robust to overcome the need for TDM.

SangCya is the first generic formulation of CsA to be approved for use in the United States. In an aqueous environment, this liquid forms a microdispersion, as opposed to the microemulsion of Neoral. The United States Food and Drug Administration has given the drug an AB rating, determining that SangCya is therapeutically equivalent to the Neoral oral solution. However, SangCya is neither bioequivalent nor interchangeable with Sandimmune (Schroeder et al 1998).

Pharmacokinetic properties

CsA is slowly, incompletely, and variably absorbed from the gastrointestinal tract, predominantly from the small intestine (Drewe et al 1992). Sandimmune absorption is highly variable, reaching a maximum blood concentration at 1–4 hours, with an absorption half-life ranging from 0.5 to 3 hours (Grevel 1986; Lindberg et al 1986). Patients treated with Sandimmune display a variety of absorption profiles, including rapid or slow as well as biphasic absorption profiles. As a consequence of the physical and chemical limitations of Sandimmune, the bioavailability of CsA in this formulation varies from 1% to 89% (Kahan 1985; Kahan and Grevel 1988) with a mean value of about 30% (Kahan 1985; Vonderscher and Meinzer 1994). Table 7.5 shows the pharmacokinetic parameters for the most commonly used immunosuppressants.

The relationship between Sandimmune dose and CsA blood concentrations is nonlinear and unpredictable. Indeed, an 80-fold variation in trough CsA concentrations has been reported among transplant recipients treated with the same dose of Sandimmune for 1 week (Figure 7.6; Kahan 1994). Trough (C_0) or minimum (C_{min}) concentrations of CsA after administration of Sandimmune display little value to predict systemic exposure as estimated by the AUC (Kahan and Grevel 1988; Kovarik et al 1994b; Kahan et al 1995a; Figure 7.9).

In contrast, CsA in the Neoral formulation is absorbed more quickly than in the Sandimmune formulation, as evidenced by a shorter (1–2 hours) t_{max} (Figure 7.10; Kovarik et al 1994a, b; Mueller et al 1994b). Furthermore, among healthy volunteers, CsA C_{max} and AUC values of Neoral are approximately 70–135% higher than those of Sandimmune (Kovarik et al 1994b; Mueller et al 1994b). Also, Neoral displays a higher

Drug	Relative bioavailability (%)	Clearance (ml/min per kg)	Volume of distribution (l/kg)	Half-life (hours)
Cyclosporine				
Sandimmune*	30 ± 13	5.7 ± 1.8	3.6 ± 1.4	11.4 ± 4.4
Neoral[†,‡]	73 ± 22	4.9 ± 1.5	NR	7.3 ± 1.6
SangCya[§]	NR	8.2 ± 1.6	8.1 ± 1.9	11.5 ± 1.8
Tacrolimus[¶]	19.7 ± 10.4	1.5 ± 0.8	1.0 ± 0.7	18.9 ± NR
Sirolimus**,[††]	15 ± NR	3.5 ± 1.6	12 ± 5	62 ± 16

NR, Not reported.
*Frey et al 1988.
[†]Chueh and Kahan 1998.
[‡]Kovarik et al 1994b.
[§]Schroeder et al 1998.
[¶]Fitzsimmons et al 1998.
**Zimmerman and Kahan 1997.
[††]Yatscoff et al 1995.

Table 7.5 Pharmacokinetic parameters (mean ± SD)

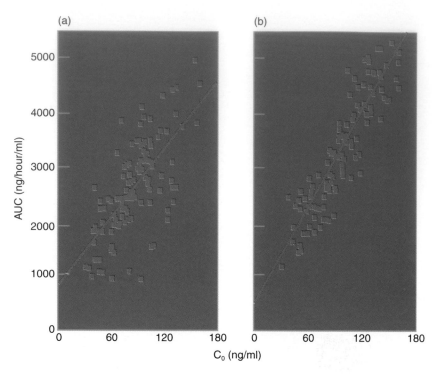

Figure 7.9. Lack of robust correlation between CsA trough concentrations and AUC during steady-state oral treatment. (a) Sandimmune: $r^2 = 0.49$. (b) Neoral: $r^2 = 0.81$. (Kovarik JM, Mueller EA, van Bree JB et al. Reduced inter- and intraindividual variability in cyclosporine pharmacokinetics from a microemulsion formulation. *J Pharmacol Sci* 1994; **83**:444–446. © 1994 Lippincott Williams & Wilkins. All rights reserved.)

correlation between dose and AUC, compared with Sandimmune ($r = 0.61$–0.7 versus 0.5–0.52, respectively; Kahan et al 1995a).

After 1:1 conversion from Sandimmune to Neoral, renal transplant recipients showed greater overall CsA exposure, as indicated by increased AUC and C_{max} (Kovarik et al 1994a; Kahan et al 1995a). The CsA trough concentrations were 22% greater when the drug was administered in the fasting, rather than in the fed, state (Kovarik et al 1994a; Kahan et al 1995a; Figure 7.11). Intra- and interpatient coefficients of variation for AUC, C_{max}, t_{max}, C_0, and C_{12} CsA concentrations were all significantly lower among patients treated with Neoral versus Sandimmune (Figure 7.12; Kovarik et al 1994a; Kahan et al 1995a). Although compared with Sandimmune the Neoral formulation displays a better correlation between trough CsA concentrations and drug exposure (AUC; Figure 7.9), the correlation between dose and blood concentration is not reliable (Kovarik et al 1994a; Kahan et al 1995a), due to the immense interpatient variability.

Following absorption, CsA is distributed in blood primarily in red blood cells (60–70%), leukocytes (9%), and plasma (4%). In the last compartment, 21% is bound to lipoproteins and 8% to other plasma proteins (Lemaire and Tillement 1982; Kahan

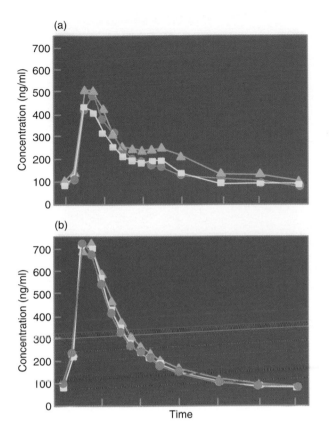

Figure 7.10. Mean CsA concentration-versus-time curves from patients receiving the same dose of either (a) Sandimmune or (b) Neoral at week 8 (■), week 12 (●), and 1 year (▲). Values for t_{max} are 1.9, 2.4, and 2.5 hours for Sandimmune and 1.4, 1.3, and 1.4 hours for Neoral, respectively. (Wahlberg J, Wilczek HE, Fauchald P et al. Consistent absorption of cyclosporine from a microemulsion formulation assessed in stable renal recipients over a one-year study period. *Transplantation* 1995; **60**:648–652. © 1995 Lippincott Williams & Wilkins. All rights reserved.)

1989; Gupta and Benet 1990; Urien et al 1990; Kolansky et al 1992). CsA uptake by and binding within erythrocytes becomes saturated at drug concentrations above 3–5 mg/l (Akagi et al 1991). The majority of CsA is distributed outside the blood compartment. Due to the hydrophobicity of the drug, it displays a large apparent volume of distribution (4–8 l/kg), which varies according to body weight and which may be significantly increased in children (Misteli et al 1990; Hoyer et al 1991; Fahr 1993). Tissue levels of CsA appear to correlate with cyclophilin levels and lipid content. The major drug depots, which may contain up to 10-fold higher concentrations than blood, include the leukocyte-rich thymus, spleen, and lymph nodes, as well as the fat-rich organs—liver, pancreas, kidneys, thyroid, lungs, and skin (Kahan et al 1983; Reid et al 1983; Lensmeyer et al 1991).

Despite extensive (>99%) conversion of CsA into more than 30 metabolites by CYP3A4 via hydroxylation, demethylation, sulfation, and position 1 cyclization (Christians 1988; Lucey et al 1990; Christians and Sewing 1993), the cyclic structure of CsA is preserved (Figure 7.13). The conversion products are designated based upon CsA being cyclosporin A, followed by an M designating a metabolite, and a number indicating the

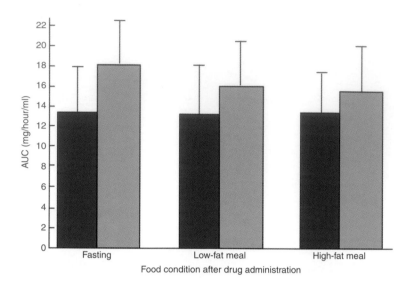

Figure 7.11. Mean CsA AUCs for various food conditions after administration of Sandimmune (dark red) or Neoral (pink) in renal transplant recipients converted from Sandimmune to the microemulsion formulation Neoral. Each error bar represents one standard deviation ($P < 0.01$ Sandimmune versus Neoral for each food condition). (Kahan BD, Dunn J, Fitts C et al. Reduced inter- and intrasubject variability in cyclosporine pharmacokinetics in renal transplant recipients treated with a microemulsion formulation in conjunction with fasting, low-fat meals, or high-fat meals. *Transplantation* 1995; **59**:505–511. © 1995 Lippincott Williams & Wilkins. All rights reserved.)

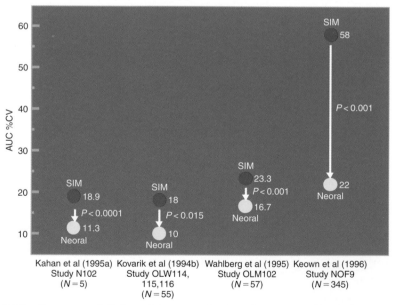

Figure 7.12. Summary of clinical trials comparing Sandimmune and Neoral. Neoral (yellow) demonstrates a significantly lower intrasubject variability (% coefficient of variability, %CV) of CsA AUC than Sandimmune (SIM; red). The numbers represent the %CV and the 'P' value is calculated by an analysis of variance.

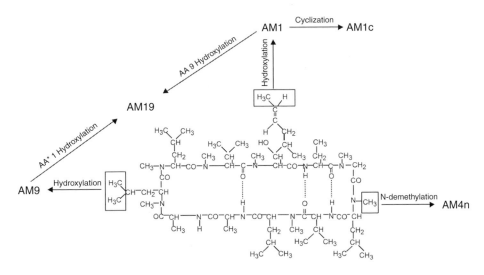

Figure 7.13. Metabolic pathway of CsA. AM1, AM9, and AM4n are the predominant metabolites found in human blood and urine. Other metabolites of CsA result from further metabolism of the primary metabolites. (*AA = amino acid.)

amino acid position of the conversion. The use of two numbers indicates transformations at two positions. Unless designated by an 'n' to signify demethylation or a 'c' to signify cyclization, all other metabolites represent hydroxylations (Kahan et al 1990). Although metabolism occurs mainly in the liver, CYP3A4 also is present in the gastrointestinal mucosa (Hoppu et al 1991; Kolars et al 1991; Webber et al 1992) and kidney (Haehner et al 1996). The most active metabolites—AM1, followed by AM9 (Figure 7.13)—display only 10–20% of the immunosuppressive activity of the parent drug (Copeland et al 1990; Rosano et al 1990; Radeke et al 1992). At the trough time point, AM1 constitutes approximately 27% of the total concentration of CsA and its metabolites in blood (Lensmeyer et al 1991). AM1 and AM9 also show the highest degree of cross-reactivity in polyclonal radioimmunoassay (RIA) kits for CsA concentration determinations.

The clearance rates of CsA show a wide interpatient variation. Children display higher rates, and, conversely, patients with either reduced levels of low-density serum lipoproteins or hepatic impairment, decreased clearance (Kahan 1989). The elimination of CsA follows linear kinetics, with an apparent terminal half-life of about 19 hours (Yee 1991). More than 90% of a CsA dose is excreted in bile, of which less than 1% is excreted as unchanged drug. Six percent of an oral dose is excreted in the urine, with only 0.1% as parent drug (Venkataramanan et al 1985; Maurer and Lemaire 1986).

CsA passes through the placenta and appears to concentrate there, with levels approaching 4–6 times that of maternal peripheral blood (Flechner et al 1985). Random peripheral whole blood CsA concentrations in infants being breast fed by mothers under CsA therapy were less than 30 ng/ml (Nyberg et al 1998); corresponding trough CsA concentrations in the mothers ranged from 50–227 ng/ml. Serum creatinine levels remained normal following 4–12 months breast feeding in these infants, despite the fact that breast milk CsA concentrations were nearly equal to those found in the blood of the mothers. The calculated dose of CsA received by the infants was less than 0.1 mg/kg body weight per day.

Therapeutic drug monitoring

Although the trough concentration or C_0—the blood drug level measured on samples obtained immediately prior to the next dose—represents a suitable measure of exposure for some drugs, such as SRL (Kahan et al 1995b), this measurement displays a poor correlation with drug exposure for CsA, whether delivered in the oil-based (Kahan and Grevel 1988) or microemulsion formulation (Kahan et al 1995a). Within the therapeutic range 175–350 ng/ml during the critical first 3 months posttransplantation, CsA concentrations show no relationship to episodes of either acute rejection or nephrotoxicity (Klintmalm et al 1985; Henry et al 1988; Sommer et al 1988; Uchida et al 1988; Stiller and Keown 1990); indeed, CsA trough concentrations within the target range have been found among patients displaying frank evidence of these two complications (Bowers et al 1986; Stiller and Keown 1990; Nankivell et al 1994). Outside the therapeutic range, CsA concentrations clearly correlate with both occurrences (Irschik et al 1984; Kahan et al 1984; Holt et al 1986; Holt et al 1989; Martinez et al 1989): low concentrations are associated with rejection episodes, and high concentrations with toxicity (Figure 7.14).

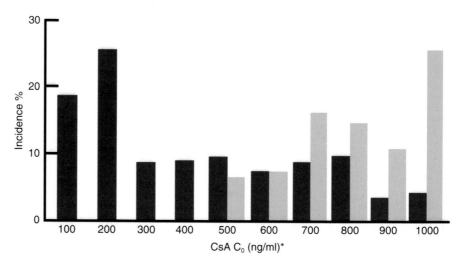

Figure 7.14. Lack of utility of trough (C_0) measurements of CsA concentrations: percentage of patients diagnosed as having either rejection (dark green) or nephro- or hepatotoxicity (light green) as a function of CsA trough concentration measured in serum by a polyclonal radioimmunoassay. A significant overlap between toxicity and rejection is shown in the 300–800 μg/l therapeutic range. (Bowers LD. Therapeutic monitoring for cyclosporine: difficulties in establishing a therapeutic window. *Clin Biochem* 1991 Feb; **24**(1):81–87. © 1991 Canadian Society of Clinical Chemists. Reprinted with permission.)

Since most centers utilize trough level monitoring and maintain patients in a putative therapeutic range, more sensitive methods of drug monitoring have been investigated to optimize CsA therapy, including AUC monitoring either as full profiles or as limited sampling estimates. Individual patient AUC determinations not only provide the only reliable estimates of CsA exposure, but also predict the occurrence of acute rejection episodes (Kasiske et al 1988; Lindholm and Kahan 1993), and possibly acute and subacute nephrotoxicity (Meyer et al 1993).

AUC monitoring seeks to estimate total CsA exposure during the dosing interval, thereby providing an individualized profile of CsA pharmacokinetics. AUC estimates provide pharmacokinetic parameters to predict starting doses or to adjust maintenance oral doses of the drug (Kahan et al 1990; Chueh and Kahan 1998). In an initial study, Lindholm and Kahan (1993) observed that neither the occurrence of acute rejection episodes nor the 1-year graft survival rates correlated with the dose, but rather with the average concentration (C_{av}), the quotient of the AUC, and the dosing interval (in hours; Figure 7.15). Furthermore, in pharmacokinetic analysis, low oral bioavailability was a more important predictor of rejection than was a rapid clearance rate (Figure 7.16). In addition, the degree of intraindividual variability of AUC values correlates with the development of chronic rejection in renal transplant recipients (Kahan et al 1996; Figure 7.17).

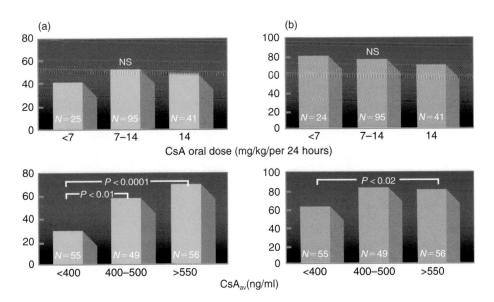

Figure 7.15. Therapeutic effect of CsA therapy stratified by dose or concentration. (a) The percentage of patients who were free of an acute rejection episode. (b) The 1-year graft survival rates. The upper panels show data stratified by dose (mg/kg per day) and the lower panels, by C_{av} (ng/ml). (Lindholm A, Kahan BD. Influence of cyclosporine pharmacokinetics, trough concentrations, and AUC monitoring on outcome after kidney transplantation. *Clin Pharmacol Ther* 1993 Aug; **54**(2):205–218. © Mosby, Inc. Reprinted with permission.)

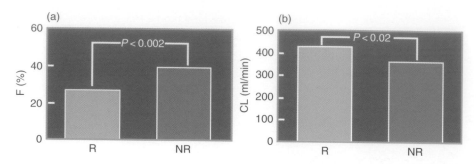

Figure 7.16. Comparison of the impact of pharmacokinetic parameter differences among rejector (R) versus nonrejector (NR) patients. (a) Comparison of the relative oral bioavailability, and (b) clearance between the two cohorts of patients treated with a CsA–prednisone dual-drug regimen. '*P*' values were determined by analysis of variance.

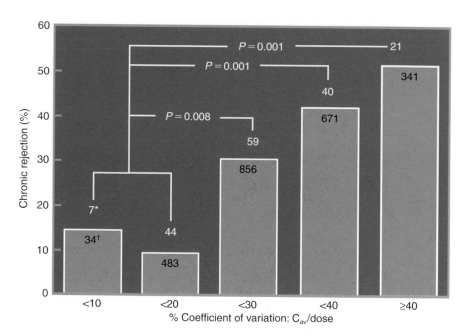

Figure 7.17. Association between the intrapatient percentage coefficient of variation (%CV) of the dose-corrected average CsA concentration (AUC/dosing interval in hours, C_{av}) with the incidence of chronic rejection. Serial pharmacokinetic profiles were performed in 179 patients to select Sandimmune (CsA) doses that would produce target C_{av} of 350 μg/l. An intraindividual variability greater then 20% correlated with an increased risk of chronic rejection. *Number of patients in cohorts stratified by the particular %CV range; †number of pharmacokinetic profiles performed in each cohort. (Adapted from Kahan BD, Welsh M, Schoenberg L et al. Variable oral absorption of cyclosporine. A biopharmaceutical risk factor for chronic renal allograft rejection. *Transplantation* 1996; **63**:599–606. © 1996 Lippincott Williams & Wilkins. All rights reserved.)

An obvious disadvantage of AUC monitoring is the requirement for numerous, precisely timed blood samples. To at least partially alleviate this problem, abbreviated kinetic profiles, utilizing a 'limited sampling' strategy, have been applied to predict the full AUC value (Table 7.6; Johnston et al 1990; Grevel and Kahan 1991). Two-sample estimates, namely, at 2 and 6 hours (Amante and Kahan 1996) or 0 and 2 hours (Keown et al 1996; Primmett et al 1998) post-Neoral dosing, have shown reasonable correlations with full AUC estimates obtained with six blood samples taken over a 12-hour dosing interval. Still other workers recommend a three-sample strategy using measurements at trough as well as at 1 and 3 hours postdosing (Gaspari et al 1998), or a five-sample method calculating a 0–4-hour AUC (Mahalati et al 1999). A single sample at C_2, as opposed to C_0, has been advocated for monitoring Neoral therapy in liver transplant patients (Cantarovich et al 1998; Grant et al 1999). Not only was the C_2 level shown to correlate with both AUC_{0-4} ($r^2 = 0.85$; Cantarovich et al 1998) and AUC_{0-6} ($r^2 = 0.93$; Grant et al 1999), but also monitoring of patients with the C_2 level resulted in lower average doses yet greater clinical benefit (Cantarovich et al 1998). Unfortunately, these abbreviated strategies reflect the absorption phase of drug pharmacokinetics and provide no information about drug clearance unless the patient consistently takes the drug at the same time each day, in which case C_0 reflects the drug elimination rate. For patients with rapid clearance, particularly children, who are administered Neoral using an 8-hour dosing regimen, a limited sampling strategy including 2- and 4-hour postdosing samples shows an excellent correlation with the AUC (Meier-Kriesche et al 1998). The limited sampling strategy represents a compromise with AUC monitoring, while still providing more information than a single trough concentration measurement.

Sampling times	Equation	Correlation with full AUC (r^2)
12-hour AUC		
C_0, C_1*	$422.17 + 15.22(C_0) + 1.3(C_1)$	0.856
C_0, C_2	$441.42 + 12.34(C_0) + 2.48(C_2)$	0.90
C_2, C_6	$195.8 + 2.4(C_2) + 7.7(C_6)$	0.96
C_0, C_1, C_2	$112.07 + 9.55(C_0) + 0.96(C_1) + 12.05(C_2)$	0.97
C_0, C_2, C_3	$30.51 + 5.06(C_0) + 1.25(C_1) + 4.11(C_3)$	0.96
C_0, C_1, C_3	$135.79 + 5.189(C_0) + 1.267(C_1) + 4.15(C_3)$	0.98
8-hour AUC		
C_2, C_4	$129 + 1.84(C_2) + 4.39(C_4)$	0.96

*All whole-blood concentrations were obtained at the given time point after dose administration.

Table 7.6 Abbreviated sampling strategies for estimating the full Neoral AUC

Therapeutic target concentrations

The therapeutic target concentration range for any drug represents the range wherein there is an increased probability of obtaining the desired clinical response with a relatively low risk of unacceptable toxicity. The marked intra- and interindividual variations in CsA pharmacokinetics proffer strong arguments to prevent over- or underimmunosuppression. Most transplant centers utilize a higher range of target concentrations during the early postoperative period. Thereafter, the drug dose is tapered to a lower maintenance concentration range, with adjustments for evidence of nephro- or other toxicities (Table 7.7; Oellerich et al 1995).

However, in many centers, kidney transplant recipients are treated with individualized drug regimens that affect the choice of the suitable target concentrations. While we tend to prefer a double-drug regimen with CsA and steroids, other centers utilize triple-drug regimens with CsA, steroids, and azathioprine (AZA) or mycophenolate mofetil (MMF). Although these centers may tend to reduce the CsA exposure, relying on the immunosuppressive effects of the nucleoside inhibitor, this unwise strategy may result in an increased incidence of rejection episodes (Wrenshall et al 1990). In contrast, the use of a CsA, steroid, and SRL combination permits marked reduction of CsA exposure, at least among patients other than African-Americans (Kahan et al 1999b). When quadruple induction treatment protocols are used, CsA is introduced slowly under the cover of antilymphocyte antibodies. Routine CsA monitoring is particularly valuable during the first 3 months, when kidney transplant recipients may experience increasing serum creatinine as a result of either rejection or nephrotoxicity. Pharmacokinetic monitoring procedures such as AUC monitoring (Kahan and Grevel 1988; Phillips et al 1988) not only

Drug	Starting oral dose	Target trough concentration range (ng/ml)	
		Initial (First 90 days)	Maintenance (Thereafter tapering)
Cyclosporine			
Sandimmune	8–17 mg/kg per day	250–350	150–250
Neoral	8–12 mg/kg per day	250–350	150–250
SangCyA	8–15 mg/kg per day	250–375	150–250
Tacrolimus	0.3 mg/kg per day	10–20	5–15
Sirolimus	5–15 mg/day	10–15	5–10
Mycophenolate mofetil	2–3 mg/day	$>3 \times 10^3$	$>3 \times 10^3$

Table 7.7   Usual immunosuppressive therapeutic regimens

can resolve this issue (Lindholm and Kahan 1993), but also can yield improved long-term kidney allograft function (Awni et al 1990; Grevel et al 1990) through more effective dosing of CsA (Kahan et al 1992; Lindholm et al 1993).

FK506/TACROLIMUS/PROGRAF

Drug measurement

No assay specific for the parent tacrolimus (TRL) compound is presently available for use in the clinical setting. Due to the lack of a strong chromophore, the chemical structure of TRL does not permit traditional HPLC analysis by ultraviolet detection without sacrificing sensitivity (Kobayashi et al 1991). An HPLC-mass spectroscopy (MS) method that is sensitive and specific for the identification of TRL and its metabolites in whole blood, plasma, and urine has been developed by Christians et al (1991a), but, due to its high technical demands, has not been utilized in routine clinical laboratories. Rather, this method represents a standard against which other assays are compared, and a means to estimate concentrations of drug metabolites.

The majority of clinical trials studying TRL have used an enzyme-linked immunosorbent assay (ELISA), in which a first, nonspecific mouse MAb is used to bind drug, and a second, rabbit antimouse IgG antibody is used to amplify the detection (Wallemacq et al 1993). The assay is linear over the range of 0.1–10 ng/ml for plasma and 1–80 ng/ml for whole blood, with intra-assay coefficients of variation ranging from 3 to 8% in whole blood. The turnaround time is 6 hours. An automated whole blood microparticle enzyme immunoassay (MEIA) developed for use on the IMx analyzer (Abbott) uses the same nonspecific MAb as the ELISA assay. However, the MEIA assay offers the advantages of automation and rapid turnaround of 23 samples in approximately 30 min. The detection limit is 5–60 ng/ml, which is considered adequate for most clinical situations, except for pharmacokinetic studies or when low TRL doses are used (Grenier et al 1991). Thus, the methodology provides little useful information except to detect unexpectedly low (or high) drug concentrations.

Pharmacokinetic behavior

The absorption profile of TRL is quite variable. In some patients, the drug is absorbed rapidly, reaching peak concentrations within 0.5 hours; in other patients, it is absorbed slowly over a prolonged period, yielding a flat profile (Jain et al 1990, 1991a). The oral bioavailability of TRL ranges from 5 to 67%, with a mean value of 29% in liver, small bowel, and kidney transplant patients (Venkataramanan et al 1991). The rate and extent of TRL absorption are highly variable, regardless of the type of organ transplanted. Although pediatric and adult patients show similar TRL absorption, the higher clearance displayed by pediatric patients requires that larger doses be administered (Furukawa et al 1992). The poor bioavailability of TRL necessitates the use of 3–4 times higher oral than intravenous doses to obtain similar blood concentrations.

Clamping of the T-tube in liver transplant patients increases the absorption of Sandimmune (Mekki et al 1993), but not Neoral (Levy et al 1994) or TRL (Jain et al 1991a; Warty 1991b). This finding suggests that TRL, like Neoral, does not require the participation of bile for absorption.

Preliminary studies indicate an effect of food on absorption. Administration of TRL with a low-fat breakfast, consisting of toast, muffin, orange juice, and coffee, had little effect on TRL plasma concentrations compared with the fasting state. However, coadministration with meals containing a moderate content of fat seemed to reduce the extent and rate of absorption of orally administered TRL (Beysens et al 1991).

Distribution

The partitioning of TRL between erythrocytes and plasma is dependent upon drug concentration, hematocrit, temperature, and plasma protein concentration (Ericzon et al 1991; Jusko and D'Ambrosio 1991; Kay et al 1991; Machida et al 1991). The blood concentration of TRL is 10–30 times higher than the corresponding plasma concentrations (Jain et al 1990; Jusko and D'Ambrosio 1991; Kobayashi et al 1991; Machida et al 1991; Habucky 1992). In blood, TRL is primarily associated with erythrocytes, wherein an intracellular protein with a molecular weight range corresponding to FK binding proteins (FKBP) appears to be primarily responsible for drug binding. When high concentrations of TRL saturate uptake by erythrocytes, the blood/plasma ratios decrease (Kay et al 1991; Kobayashi et al 1991). However, the increase in hematocrit that occurs among renal transplant recipients with time after transplantation tends to increase the blood/plasma ratio of TRL (Machida et al 1991). In plasma, TRL is associated with an α_1-acid glycoprotein, an acute phase protein (Kay et al 1991; Warty et al 1991a), the concentration of which increases in plasma with time posttransplant, thereby decreasing the blood/plasma ratio of TRL (Kay et al 1991). Unlike CsA, TRL does not significantly associate with plasma lipoproteins (Christians et al 1991b; Ericzon et al 1991; Jain et al 1991a).

Animal studies indicate that TRL accumulates in the lung, spleen, heart, kidney, pancreas, brain, muscle, and liver tissue relative to blood or plasma (Venkataramanan et al 1990; Ericzon et al 1991). The presence of TRL in cerebrospinal fluid has not been documented, even among patients with TRL-induced neurotoxicity. To reach the fetal circulation, TRL must pass through the placenta, which displays concentrations that are on average four times greater than maternal plasma concentration. The concentration of TRL in cord plasma is about 35% of the corresponding maternal concentration (Wijnen et al 1991). TRL concentrations in breast milk are similar to the plasma concentrations.

Metabolism

Tacrolimus is primarily eliminated from the body by metabolism. At least nine metabolites have been either isolated from in vivo sources of human and rat bile, or generated in vitro by human, rat, or rabbit liver microsomes (Christians et al 1990, 1991a, 1992; Kay et al 1991; Jain et al 1993a). The major metabolite generated by liver microsomes in vitro is a demethylated TRL (13-desmethyl-FK506) of molecular weight (MW) 790 (Christians et al 1990, 1991a). Additional metabolic pathways include hydroxylation (MW 820), a combination of hydroxylation and demethylation (MW 804), double demethylation (MW 776), double demethylation and hydroxylation (MW 792), and double demethylation and dihydroxylation (MW 808; Christians et al 1991a, 1992a, Jain et al 1991a; Figure 7.18).

Numerous observations suggest that CYP3A4 is primarily responsible for the metabolism of TRL (Christians et al 1990; Sattler et al 1992; Vincent et al 1992): (1) there is a significant correlation between TRL metabolism and nifedipine oxidation by human liver microsomes (Vincent et al 1992); (2) TRL metabolism is inhibited by anti-CYP3A4 antibodies (Christians et al 1990; Vincent et al 1992) and by the specific CYP3A4 blockers troleandomycin and gestodene (Sattler et al 1992; Vincent et al 1992); (3) dexamethasone (Sattler et al 1992; Vincent et al 1992) induced TRL metabo-

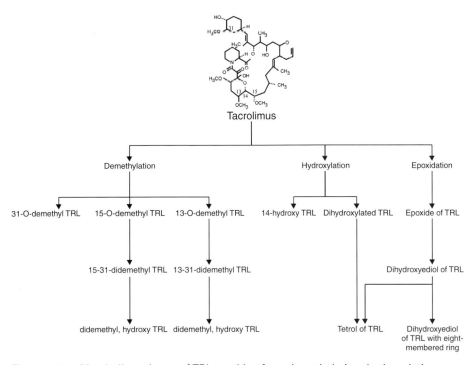

Figure 7.18. Metabolic pathway of TRL resulting from demethylation, hydroxylation, or epoxidation of the parent molecule. Metabolites have been identified in the bile, blood, and urine of transplant recipients. (Venkataramanan R, Swaminathan A, Prasad T et al. Clinical pharmacokinetics of tacrolimus. *Clin Pharmacokinet* 1995 Dec; **29**(6).404–430. © Adis International Limited. Reprinted with permission.)

lism but neither phenobarbital nor 3-methylcholanthrene (Sattler et al 1992); and (4) TRL metabolism may be reconstituted by addition of human CYP3A4 (Vincent et al 1992). However, additional components of the cytochrome P450 system also may metabolize TRL based on the only partial inhibition by (1) anti-CYP3A4 antibodies (Christians et al 1990); (2) anti-CYP1A antibodies (Christians et al 1990); or (3) 7,8-benzoflavone (Christians et al 1990). In addition, there is a significant correlation between TRL metabolism in vitro and chlorzoxazone hydroxylation (CYP2E1) or 7-ethoxycoumarin demethylation (CYP2A6; Vincent et al 1992).

Since TRL is primarily eliminated by metabolism, it is subject to alterations in hepatic function. Patients with impaired liver function display higher trough TRL concentrations, decreased clearance rates, and longer half-lives (Warty et al 1991b). The oral bioavailability of TRL is increased in dogs by experimental induction of cholestasis (Stiff et al 1992). Liver transplant recipients with significant perioperative graft dysfunction tend to display higher TRL plasma concentrations in spite of dose reduction, in comparison to liver transplant recipients, who display relatively normal graft function despite receiving the same or lower doses of TRL (Abu-Elmagd et al 1991a, b). Thus, patients with impaired hepatic function are vulnerable to drug-induced toxicities due to TRL overdose. Due to the contribution of gastrointestinal mucosa to TRL metabolism, impaired gut metabolism increases drug bioavailability. Because pediatric patients appear to clear TRL more rapidly than adults, they require weight-corrected doses that are 2–4 times higher than those of adults to maintain therapeutic drug concentrations (Jain et al 1993b; McDiarmid et al 1993).

Excretion

The renal contribution to TRL clearance as unchanged drug (or metabolites that cross-react with the antibody used in the ELISA assay) represents less than 1% of the total (Jain et al 1991a). HPLC-MS analysis of bile from liver transplant patients indicates the presence of a large amount of TRL that is not reactive in the ELISA assay. Thus, biliary obstruction is expected to increase TRL metabolite concentrations in the blood. However, in bile, neither unchanged TRL nor metabolites with MW 790—namely, 13-, 15-, or 31-O-demethyl TRL—is found (Christians et al 1991a). Among these metabolites, 13-O-demethyl TRL shows no, and 15- and 31-O-demethyl TRL, approximately 100%, cross-reactivity in the ELISA assay. Only 31-O-demethyl TRL seems to possess significant immunosuppressive activity; indeed, it may be equal to that of the parent compound (Iwasaki et al 1993, 1995).

Therapeutic drug monitoring

Trough concentration monitoring of TRL is the most commonly used clinical tool to guide TRL therapy, since C_0 shows a reasonable correlation with AUC (Figure 7.19).

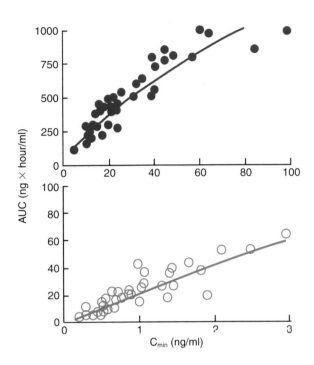

Figure 7.19. Relationship between TRL AUC and 12-hour trough values in whole blood (●) and plasma (○) in liver transplant patients ($r^2 = 0.89$ for whole blood; $r^2 =$ not reported for plasma). (Jusko WJ, Piekoszewski W, Klintmalm GB et al. Pharmacokinetics of tacrolimus in liver transplant patients. *Clin Pharmacol Ther* 1995 Mar; **57**(3):281–290. © Mosby, Inc. Reprinted with permission.)

Unfortunately, due to the broad cross-reactivities of the antibodies used in the assays, there have been greater difficulties in establishing useful relationships between trough concentrations and clinical outcomes for TRL than for CsA. Although several studies suggest a lack of correlation between plasma or whole blood TRL trough concentrations and the occurrence of acute rejection episodes (Jain et al 1991b; Japanese FK 506 Study Group 1991; Backman et al 1994; Erden et al 1994; Winkler et al 1995), there appears to be a stronger correlation between drug-induced toxicity and TRL trough concentrations (Japanese FK 506 Study Group 1991; Winkler et al 1991; Backman et al 1994). While either rejection or drug-induced toxicity may occur within the therapeutic whole blood C_0 range of 5–20 µg/l TRL, extremely low or high concentrations may forecast rejection or toxic events, respectively (Japanese FK 506 Study Group 1991; Alessiani et al 1993). Therefore, trough concentration monitoring seems to be a valid tool for neither TRL nor CsA.

RAPAMYCIN/SIROLIMUS/RAPAMUNE

Measurement techniques

HPLC methods using ultraviolet (UV) or mass spectroscopy (MS) are currently the methods of choice for determining sirolimus (SRL) concentrations in patient whole blood samples, which should be collected in tubes containing EDTA as an anticoagulant and protected from light at all times to minimize drug deterioration (Napoli and Kahan 1994; Yatscoff et al 1995a). HPLC-UV analysis of SRL whole-blood samples has a sensitivity of 1 μg/l, and a less than 12% CV over the concentration range of 2.5–100 μg/l (Yatscoff et al 1992, 1995a). In EDTA-treated blood, SRL has been reported to be stable for 24 hours at room temperature, up to 7 days at 2–8°C, and up to 3 months at −20°C (Yatscoff et al 1992, 1995a). An immunoassay (IMx) currently in development for measurement of SRL whole-blood concentrations overestimates parent compound concentrations by at least 25% due to cross-reactivity with drug metabolites.

Absorption

In the initial clinical trials, SRL was administered orally as an oil-based solution that displays an apparent oral bioavailability of about 15% (Yatscoff et al 1995b; Yatscoff 1996). Single doses of drug, ranging from 1 to 34 mg/m^2, were rapidly absorbed by stable renal transplant recipients, with a mean t_{max} ranging from 0.8 to 3 hours and dose-proportionate C_{max} and AUC values (Yatscoff et al 1995b; Johnson et al 1996; Brattstrom et al 1997; Ferron et al 1997) over the range 3–15 mg/m^2.

Following administration of multiple doses ranging from 0.5 to 6.5 mg/m^2 per 12 hours for at least 14 days, the t_{max} was 1.4 ± 1.2 hours, with a good correlation between the AUC and the C_0 ($r^2 = 0.94$; Napoli and Kahan 1996; Zimmerman and Kahan 1997). Figure 7.20 illustrates the good correlation between AUC and C_0 among renal transplant patients treated with SRL at our center. Although initial studies suggested that African-American patients displayed a two-fold increase in t_{max} from 1.1 to 2.0 hours and a 45% increase in oral clearance compared to patients of other ethnic backgrounds (Zimmerman and Kahan 1997), an expanded data set from analysis of pharmacokinetic profiles among 120 patients treated de novo with SRL failed to reveal an impact of ethnicity on SRL absorption or oral clearance rates (Kahan et al 1999a).

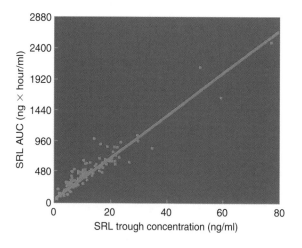

Figure 7.20. Relation between SRL AUC and trough whole-blood concentrations from 115 pharmacokinetic studies ($r^2 = 0.95$) in stable renal transplant recipients receiving the liquid formulation. (Napoli KL, Kahan BD. Routine clinical monitoring of sirolimus (rapamycin) whole-blood concentrations by HPLC with ultraviolet detection. *Clin Chem* 1996 Dec; **42**(12): 1943–1948. © American Association for Clinical Chemistry. Reprinted with permission.)

Pharmacokinetic profiling to estimate drug exposure, for example among subjects treated with drugs that also affect the cytochrome P450 system, may utilize a limited sampling strategy, including samples at 0, 2, and 6 hours (Kaplan et al 1997), that provides a reasonable estimate of AUC using the equation:

$$AUC_{0-24} = \{-15.2 + [5.9 \times (C_0)] + [2.9 \times (C_2)] + [13 \times (C_6)]\} \times 24.$$

The value calculated from this limited sampling protocol predicts a value that is 86% of the AUC calculated by the trapezoidal rule from a full set of seven samples, namely, less than a 15% difference (Kaplan et al 1997). However, this equation has only been shown to predict AUC values for patients receiving the liquid formulation of SRL. Studies are needed to identify situations wherein an AUC estimate is warranted in lieu of a trough concentration.

A solid formulation of SRL was more recently developed to improve palatability. Conversion of stable renal transplant recipients from the oil-based liquid to the tablet form of SRL is not only safe and well tolerated, but also results in similar AUC values. The tablet SRL formulation shows lower C_{max} values and a prolonged t_{max}, indicating that the rates of absorption of the two formulations are not identical. However, an equivalent extent of absorption was documented by comparisons using similar 0–12 hour AUC values for the liquid versus the tablet when measured prior to and 2, 4, and 8 weeks postconversion (Kelly et al 2000; Figure 7.21).

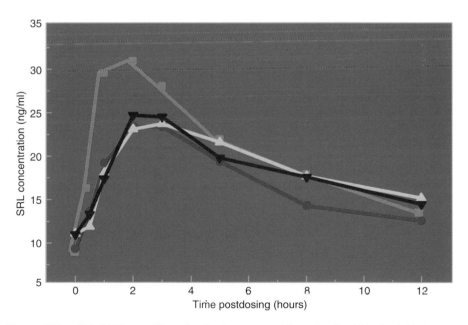

Figure 7.21. SRL AUC_{0-12} profiles of patients converted from the liquid to the tablet formulation. AUC profiles were obtained at the time of the last dose of liquid SRL (■) and then at 2 (●), 4 (▲), and 8 (▼) weeks post-conversion to the tablet form.

Distribution

In human whole blood, SRL is primarily sequestered among cellular components, particularly red blood cells (95%)—possibly related to their high content of FKBP12, an immunophilin binding protein (Kay et al 1991)—as well as 1% in lymphocytes, 1% in granulocytes, and 3% in plasma (Yatscoff et al 1993). This distribution is similar to that of TRL, but differs substantially from that of CsA, which is relatively less sequestered in red blood cells (60%). Approximately 40% of SRL in the plasma fraction is associated with lipoproteins; the remaining 60% presents as free or unbound drug, which represents 0.175% of the total drug in whole blood (Yatscoff et al 1993). In contrast to CsA, which shows clinical toxicities as a result of abnormal serum triglyceride or cholesterol concentrations (Verrill et al 1987; de Groen et al 1988), lipoprotein abnormalities appear to have little impact on SRL distribution in whole blood (Yatscoff et al 1993).

Sirolimus is extensively distributed among body tissues, with an apparent volume of distribution of 5.6–16.7 l/kg in stable renal transplant recipients (Yatscoff et al 1995b; Ferron et al 1997; Zimmerman and Kahan 1997). Analysis of the tissue distribution of SRL in rats supports these clinical observations. Following gavage of 0.4–1.6 mg/kg per day for 14 days, the drug was extensively distributed in the rat heart, intestine, kidney, liver, lung, muscle, spleen, and testes, usually at tissue-to-blood partition coefficients of less than 20 (Napoli et al 1997). The extravascular distribution of SRL in humans has not been formally quantified.

Metabolism

The metabolic pathway of SRL has only been postulated from in vitro studies. The drug appears to be metabolized by the cytochrome P450 CYP3A enzymes in both humans and rats. Human liver microsomes show a correlation between the metabolism of either SRL or TRL and CYP3A4 activity, as estimated by nifedipine oxidation, or inhibition with specific pharmacologic agents (triacetyl oleandomycin or gestodene) or by preincubation with anti-CYP3A4 antibodies (Sattler et al 1992). In contrast, the cytochrome P450 enzymes, CYP1A2, CYP2E1, CYP2D1, and CYP2A6, do not seem to mediate SRL metabolism (Sattler et al 1992). In vitro incubation of human liver microsomes with SRL yielded two metabolites: 41-O-demethyl-sirolimus and hydroxy-sirolimus, each of which displayed less than 10% of the immunosuppressive activity of the parent drug (Christians et al 1992b). Approximately 10 metabolites have been identified in the bile of rats receiving SRL, but the immunosuppressive activity of these metabolites has not been determined (Yatscoff et al 1995b).

SRL metabolites account for as much as 56% of all SRL derivatives measured in trough whole blood samples from kidney graft recipients (Streit et al 1996). Hydroxy-SRL concentrations can reach 71% of the total SRL concentration, while demethyl-, dihydroxy-, and didemethyl-SRL may reach approximately 35, 20, and 20%, respectively, of the remainder. Indeed, trough blood samples contain a higher content of SRL metabolites than of unchanged drug. These findings contrast with those for the structural analog TRL, for which the drug metabolites comprise only 20% of the total content in blood (Streit et al 1996).

Elimination

SRL concentration–time curves exhibit two or three phases of exponential decay after reaching the C_{max}. Apparent total body clearance and elimination half-life estimates range from 127 to 240 ml/hour per kg and from 57 to 63 hours, respectively, in stable kidney transplant patients receiving single oral doses ranging from 1 to 34 mg/m^2. Neither parameter seemed to be related to dose (Yatscoff et al 1995b; Yatscoff 1996). Following multiple doses, the apparent average clearance of SRL was 208 ml/hour per kg, with an elimination half-life of 62 hours (Zimmerman and Kahan 1997). In contrast to CsA and TRL, SRL is suitable for once-daily dosing, due to the long elimination half-life. Early data from kidney transplant patients receiving SRL suggest that steady-state drug concentrations are established within 5–7 days after initiation or alteration of the dose.

Therapeutic drug monitoring

Formal prospective studies to examine the impact of SRL concentrations to predict allograft outcomes were not conducted within the phase III development program. However, retrospective analysis of blood samples drawn on days 1–5 and months 1, 2, 3, 4, 6, and 12 from renal transplant recipients in the United States and in the global multicenter phase III trials suggest that SRL C_0 values below 10 ng/ml, as measured by the IMx method, were associated with an increased risk of allograft rejection. Furthermore, the SRL C_0 value appeared to have at least a 10-fold greater predictive value for the occurrence of rejection compared to the CsA C_0.

In contrast, an initial phase I/II study of renal transplant recipients treated de novo with SRL combined with CsA and prednisone suggested that C_0 values above 15 ng/ml, as measured with the specific HPLC-UV assay, were associated with an increased risk of thrombocytopenia, hypertriglyceridemia, or leukopenia (Kahan et al 1998a).

SDZ RAD

SDZ RAD, a hydroxyethyl derivative of SRL (Figure 7.22), is a new hydrophilic derivative that shows immunosuppressive effects slightly less potent than those of SRL (Schuler et al 1997). SDZ RAD displays synergy with CsA in vitro in two-way murine

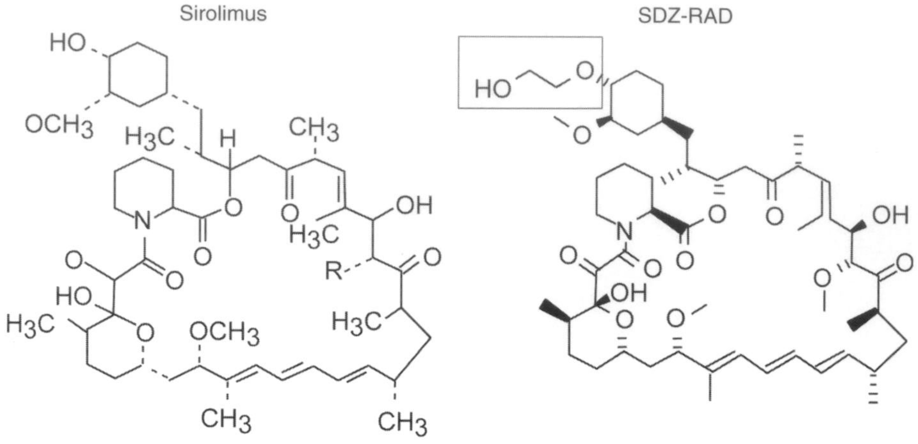

Figure 7.22. Chemical structures of SRL and SDZ RAD. SDZ RAD is a 40-O-(2-hydroxyethyl) derivative of SRL (area shown in box).

mixed lymphocyte reactions, and in vivo using rat orthotopic kidney and heterotopic heart allotransplantation models (Schuurman et al 1997). Initial pharmacokinetic studies in stable renal transplant recipients administered with 0.25, 0.75, 2.5, or 7.5 mg SDZ RAD as daily oral single or multiple doses showed a dose-dependent increase in C_{max}, C_0, and AUC (Appel et al 1997, Kahan et al 1999c). Single oral doses of 0.25, 0.75, 2.5, and 7.5 mg yielded SDZ RAD C_{max} concentrations of 2.6, 14, 46, and 86 ng/ml, and AUC values of 22, 91, 221, and 477 ng × hour/ml, respectively. The half-life of SDZ RAD decreased from 78 to 32 hours, with increasing doses of 0.75–7.5 mg (Appel et al 1997).

Following multiple daily doses of 0.75, 2.5, and 7.5 mg, the pharmacokinetics of SDZ RAD were linear in kidney transplant recipients. C_{max} and AUC values were 8.3, 33, and 79 ng/ml, and 67, 211, and 497 ng × hour/ml, respectively (Table 7.8; Kahan et al 1999c). Coadministration of SDZ RAD with CsA for a period of 1 month did not affect the steady-state pharmacokinetics of CsA following single or multiple dosing (Appel et al 1997; Kahan et al 1999c). TDM considerations for SDZ RAD in humans should be similar to those of RAPA. The clinical efficacy of SDZ RAD is presently under investigation in phase III multicenter trials.

| Parameter | Mean value (SD) | | | |
| | Sirolimus* | SDZ RAD† | | |
	(0.5–6.5 mg/m² per 12 hours)	0.75 mg/day	2.5 mg/day	7.5 mg/day
t_{max} (hours)	1.4 (1.2)	2.0 (0.3)	1.8 (0.8)	1.5 (0.3)
Half-life (hours)	62 (16)	19.2 (3.4)	18.1 (7.6)	16.0 (5.6)
CL/F (ml/hour per kg)	208 (95)	129 (NR)	138 (NR)	193 (NR)
Vd/F (l/kg)	12 (5)	3.6 (NR)	3.6 (NR)	4.5 (NR)

NR, not reported.
*From Kahan et al 1998a.
†From Kahan et al 1999c.

Table 7.8 Pharmacokinetic parameters of the target of rapamycin (TOR) inhibitors, sirolimus and SDZ RAD, following multiple dosing

MYCOPHENOLATE MOFETIL

Drug measurement

Mycophenolate mofetil (MMF) is a 2-morpholinoethyl ester prodrug of mycophenolic acid (MPA). After gastrointestinal absorption, MMF is rapidly hydrolyzed by widely distributed esterases to MPA, its active form (Figure 7.23), and transformed to the glucuronide MPAG. For the therapeutic monitoring of MMF therapy, HPLC is considered the reference measurement method, and plasma, the matrix of choice since the majority of drug is found therein (Shaw et al 1995). HPLC assays can determine the content of

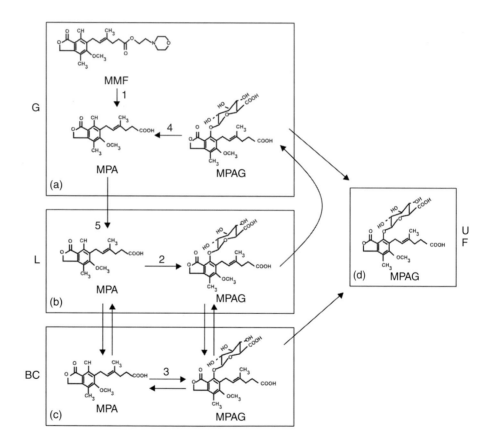

Figure 7.23. Pharmacologic model of MMF elimination. (a) Upon gastrointestinal (G) absorption, MMF is rapidly converted by esterases to the active moiety MPA (1). (b) Hepatic (L) glucuronidation of MPA to MPAG (2) is the predominant metabolic route. (c) In the circulating blood compartment (BC), dynamic equilibrium (3) occurs between MPA and MPAG concentrations. (d) MPAG is primarily eliminated in the urine (U) and to a lesser extent in the feces (F). Some of the MPAG that is not eliminated in the feces (F) undergoes enterohepatic recirculation (ER), and is converted in the gut back to MPA (4), which can then be absorbed and returned to the systemic circulation (5).

MMF, MPA, and MPAG (Tsina et al 1996a, b). After administration of doses of 100–3500 mg/day, plasma concentrations of MPA range from 2–18 µg/l (Chou 1993; Wolfe et al 1997).

MMF parent drug cannot be detected in plasma after oral administration, but is measurable after intravenous infusion (Bullingham et al 1996a), indicating almost complete first-pass de-esterification of the drug. Following termination of intravenous administration, the MMF concentration declines rapidly and the drug cannot be detected in plasma 10 min after cessation of the infusion (Bullingham et al 1996a). Since degradation of MMF by isolated blood or plasma is relatively slow, tissue de-esterification must be widespread and rapid (Tsina et al 1996b). MMF is not quantifiable in plasma samples of patients experiencing kidney impairment, indicating that renal failure has little effect on the process of de-esterification of MMF to MPA (Shah et al 1995).

Absorption

Plasma concentration-versus-time profiles of MPA following oral administration of MMF are characterized by an initial C_{max} at about 1 hour and a second peak between 6 and 12 hours postdose (Bullingham et al 1996a; Figure 7.24a). Plasma mycophenolic acid glucuronide, the phenolic glucuronide metabolite of MPA, also shows secondary peaks, which are less pronounced and more delayed relative to the MPA peaks (Bullingham et al 1996a, b; Parker et al 1996; Figure 7.24b). Enterohepatic cycling appears to

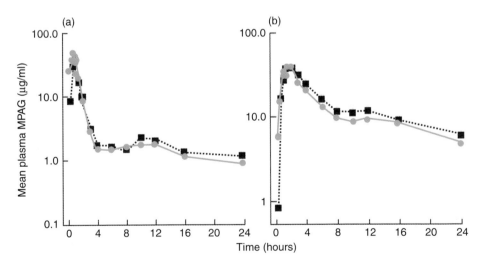

Figure 7.24. Pharmacokinetic profiles of MPA and MPAG after administration of a single 1.5 g dose of MMF to 12 healthy volunteers. (a) Mean plasma concentrations of MPA versus time after intravenous (●) versus oral (■) delivery. (b) Mean plasma concentrations of MPAG versus time after intravenous (●) versus oral (■) delivery. (Bullingham R, Monroe S, Nicholls A, Hale M. *J Clin Pharmacol* **36**(4), pp. 315–324, © 1996 by *J Clin Pharmacol*. Reprinted by permission of Sage Publications, Inc.)

be responsible for the occurrence of the secondary peaks, with reabsorption of MPA following deglucuronidation of MPAG by gut flora (Figure 7.23; Bullingham et al 1998). A significant proportion of the plasma AUC for MPA derives from this enterohepatic cycling, resulting in an apparent oral MPA bioavailability of approximately 95% in both healthy individuals and renal transplant recipients (Bullingham et al 1996c).

During the early posttransplant period, the mean plasma MPA AUC is about 30–50% lower than that observed when the same dose is administered 3 months later. The increase in the mean AUC of MPA occurs slowly over a period of several months (Bullingham et al 1998). The increase in AUC of MPA and MPAG is most evident among hepatic, and less pronounced for cardiac than for renal, transplant recipients (Bullingham et al 1998).

Distribution

In the whole-blood compartment, more than 99% of the MPA is found in the plasma, with only 0.1% in cellular elements (Langman et al 1994; Nowak and Shaw 1995). Mycophenolate mofetil is avidly bound to human serum albumin (HSA), but not to α_1-acid-glycoprotein, with an average of 2.5% of MPA free in the plasma of patients with normal renal function (Bullingham et al 1996c). While the binding of MPA to HSA is not altered by therapeutic plasma concentrations of CsA, TRL, or prednisone (Nowak and Shaw 1995), the free MPA fraction increases 6–8-fold in the presence of escalating sodium salicylate concentrations, presumably due to competition for HSA binding. Free MPA seems to be the pharmacologically active fraction, based upon the selective in vitro pharmacodynamic assay of the drug to inhibit the activity of purified human inosine monophosphate dehydrogenase (IMPDH) after phytohemagglutin A-induced proliferation of human peripheral blood mononuclear cells (Nowak and Shaw 1995).

The free fraction of MPA increases as much as three-fold when MPAG concentrations exceed 475 mg/l (Shaw et al 1998), presumably due to displacement from HSA binding sites. In vitro studies adding more than 100 mg/l MPAG to normal plasma revealed a progressive increase in the MPA concentration in the free fraction (Nowak and Shaw 1995). Renal transplant patients with delayed graft function display a three-fold increase in free MPA fraction by 7 days postoperatively (7.7 versus 2.5%), presumably due to either failure to excrete MPAG, or alteration in the binding of acidic drugs to HSA because of renal dysfunction (Shaw et al 1998). Indeed, the clearance of MPAG is highly correlated with the glomerular filtration rate ($r^2 = 0.91$; Johnson et al 1998). The free MPA fraction may also increase in the presence of low HSA concentrations, elevated serum bilirubin concentrations, or other drugs that interfere with protein binding (Shaw et al 1998).

Metabolism

MPAG, the primary metabolite of MPA, is produced via the glucuronyl transferase pathway, primarily in the liver and possibly in other tissues such as the gastrointestinal tract and the kidney (Figure 7.23). MPAG is excreted by the renal route; an average of 96% of the MMF dose is recovered in the urine as MPAG, together with small amounts of nonconjugated MPA (0.5%), but not MMF (Bullingham et al 1998).

Therapeutic drug monitoring

The regimen of twice-daily administration of MMF is suggested by the observed MPA half-life of about 16 hours (Bullingham et al 1996a, 1998). Low MPA exposure, as estimated by the AUC, demonstrates a significant association with an increased risk of an acute renal transplant rejection episode (Figure 7.25). MPA AUC_{0-12} values above 40 mg $\times$ hour/l provide effective immunosuppression, in contrast to the 68% incidence associated with values below this threshold (Japan Investigation Committee 1995; Hale et al 1998). Trough plasma MPA concentrations greater than 3 μg/ml were not, and values below 1 μg/ml were, associated with an increased risk of acute rejection episodes among cardiac transplant recipients (Meiser et al 1999a). Trough MPA concentrations may not solely reflect the immunosuppressive efficacy. Cardiac transplant recipients receiving more than 2250 mg or less than 1250 mg of MMF daily displayed similar 8-hour MPA concentrations despite significantly different C_{max} values (Meiser et al 1999b). Identification of the importance of AUC versus C_0 values for prediction of proclivity to rejection episodes may be facilitated by a limited sampling strategy that

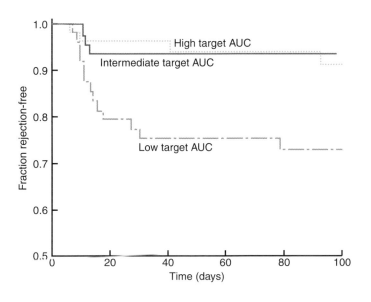

Figure 7.25. Kaplan–Meier curves for freedom from rejection for patients maintained on a MMF concentration-controlled regimen. Target mycophenolic acid AUC values (mg $\times$ hour/l) were 16.1 (low), 32.2 (intermediate), and 60.6 (high). The dotted line (- - - - - -) shows the high target AUC, the solid line (———), the intermediate target AUC; and the dash-dotted line (- — - —), the low target AUC. (Hale MD, Nicholls AJ, Bullingham RE et al. The pharmacokinetic-pharmacodynamic relationship for mycophenolate mofetil in renal transplantation. *Clin Pharmacol Ther* 1998 Dec; **64**(6): 672 683. © Mosby, Inc. Reprinted with permission.)

includes concentrations measured predose, as well as 20, 40, 75, and 120 min postdose. This AUC_{0-2} estimate of MPA shows good agreement with the 12-hour AUC estimate from samples obtained during entire dosing interval (Hale et al 1998).

The use of TRL concurrently with MMF therapy may augment MPA blood levels in comparison to CsA therapy. Renal transplant recipients displayed 92% and 30% increases in MPA trough levels and AUC_{0-12}, respectively, following conversion from CsA to TRL therapy while maintaining the same MMF dose. Additionally, MPAG C_{max} and AUC_{0-12} were lower following the conversion to TRL. It has been suggested that TRL displays an inhibitory effect on the conversion of MPA to MPAG and affects the enterohepatic recirculation of MPAG, resulting in increased MPA and decreased MPAG levels (Zucker et al 1999). Conversely, MPA trough levels increased by 70% 3 months following CsA discontinuation in renal transplant recipients (Smak Gregoor et al 1999). Additional studies will need to be performed to ascertain the exact mechanism of these changes and to separate the effect of withdrawing CsA versus that of adding TRL.

The active moiety of MMF, MPA, is a potent, selective, and reversible inhibitor of IMPDH, thereby blocking de novo synthesis of the purine guanosine (Figure 7.26). Lymphocytes are particularly sensitive to the effects of MPA, since they are incapable of utilizing the purine salvage pathway (Allison et al 1993). Thus, measurement of IMPDH activity (Langman et al 1995) may provide a pharmacodynamic monitoring tool to assess the biological activity of MPA in individual transplant patients. During chronic MMF therapy, there appears to be an inverse relationship between MPA concentrations and IMPDH activity. Peak MPA concentrations display approximately 40%

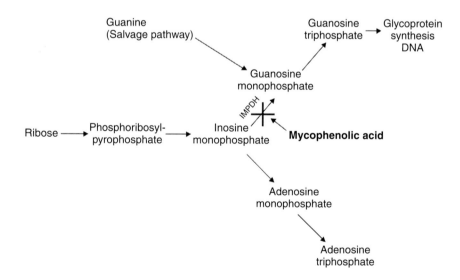

Figure 7.26. The de novo pathway for generation of guanosine monophosphate is dependent upon the conversion of inosine monophosphate by inosine monophosphate dehydrogenase (IMPDH), the site of inhibition by mycophenolic acid.

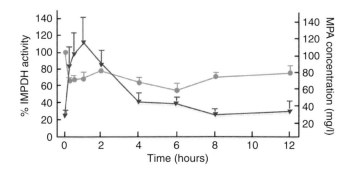

Figure 7.27. Correlation of IMPDH activity and mycophenolic acid concentration throughout a 12-hour dosing interval after administration of MMF. ●, % IMPDH activity; ▼, MPA concentration.

inhibition of IMPDH activity (Figure 7.27; Langman et al 1996), suggesting that only a partial as opposed to a complete blockade of IMPDH is required for immunosuppression. Unfortunately, clinical trials have not been conducted to assess the correlation of pharmacodynamic monitoring of IMPDH activity with the outcome of MMF therapy.

AZATHIOPRINE

To avoid hydrolysis and inactivation of the unshielded mercapto- group on 6-mercaptopurine (6-MP) in the gut, a prodrug, azathioprine (AZA), was synthesized by conjugation via the sulfur atom to an imidazole ring (Elion 1972). Nucleophilic attack in the liver cleaves the imidazole bond, releasing 6-MP. Despite extensive clinical experience with AZA, the frequent occurrence of myelotoxicity, especially leukopenia and thrombocytopenia, remains the single most reliable pharmacodynamic surrogate and dose-limiting factor (Haesslein et al 1972).

Drug measurement

Sensitive and specific HPLC assays are available to measure AZA, 6-MP, and the inactive metabolite 6-thiouric acid (6-TU) in plasma or serum (Lin et al 1980; Erdmann et al 1988; Liliemark et al 1990; El-Yazigi and Wahab 1993). These assays display linearity and reproducibility throughout the concentration ranges 5–2000 ng/ml for AZA, 10–500 ng/ml for 6-MP, and 10–2500 ng/ml for 6-TU (Erdmann et al 1988; El-Yazigi and Wahab 1993). The active metabolites of 6-MP are the 6-thioguanine nucleotides (6-TGN), which may be quantitated using HPLC in 100 μl samples of packed red blood cells (Lennard 1987; Erdmann et al 1990) and are believed to reflect the concentration of 6-TGN in other, less accessible cells and tissues.

Absorption

After oral administration, the bioavailability of unchanged AZA is about 15% (Ohlman et al 1993), with an additional 40% detected as 6-MP (Lin et al 1980; Odlind et al 1986). After administration of AZA, both the parent compound and its 6-MP product appear only transiently in the plasma, namely, half-lives of approximately 10 min and 2 hours, respectively (Lin et al 1980; Odlind et al 1986; Salemans et al 1987; Chan et al 1990). Based on the findings of rapid elimination of AZA and of 6-MP, it would seem preferable to utilize regimens of more frequent dosing. However, treatment with six-times-daily dosing of AZA failed to yield better therapeutic results than a twice-daily regimen (Lennard et al 1982). Indeed, clinical experience indicates that once-daily administration of AZA is adequate, suggesting that as yet unidentified pharmacologically active metabolites of AZA persist much longer than either the parent compound or 6-MP.

Metabolism

The metabolism of AZA is complex and incompletely understood. The drug is rapidly converted in vivo to 6-MP, which is further metabolized to 6-TU or, alternatively, to thioinosinic acid and 6-TGN (Figure 7.28). These intracellular metabolites are thought to be largely responsible for the immunosuppressive and myelotoxic activities of AZA (Brockman 1963; Tidd and Paterson 1974b). For example, clinical studies suggest that intracellular TGN concentrations are associated with bone marrow toxicity (Lennard et al 1983, 1984).

Elimination

The elimination of AZA and 6-MP is rapid, usually resulting in undetectable plasma levels within 3 hours for AZA and 6 hours for 6-MP. In contrast, red blood cell levels of TGN remain relatively unchanged during the entire dosing interval. In a single patient, the half-life of TGN was reported to be 13 days (Tidd and Paterson 1974a). Although the interpatient variability in intracellular TGN levels is quite high (94%), the intraindividual variability is only 15% (Chan et al 1990; Bergan et al 1994a).

Approximately 1% of the AZA dose is excreted in the urine as 6-MP, but parent compound is not detectable in the urine (Salemans et al 1987; Bergan et al 1994a). Although there is no apparent correlation between renal function and elimination of AZA, 6-MP, or TGN (Lin et al 1980; Salemans et al 1987; Chan et al 1990), Bergan et al (1994b) observed a correlation between high 6-TGN concentrations and increased levels of serum creatinine. The apparently long elimination half-life of TGN may predispose renal failure patients to excessive accumulation of the active metabolite in body tissues over time, resulting in myelosuppression.

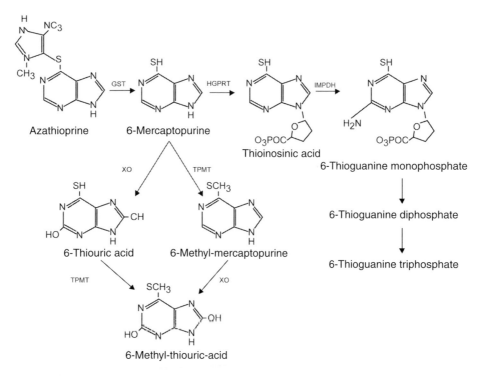

Figure 7.28. The metabolic pathway of AZA conversion, showing the alternate pathway of TPMT versus 6-thioguanine nucleotides. GST, glutathione S-transferase; HGPRT, hypoxanthine-guanine phosphoribosyltransferase; XO, xanthine oxidase; TPMT, thiopurine methyltransferase; IMPDH, inosine monophosphate dehydrogenase.

Therapeutic drug monitoring

The standard of care for more than 30 years has been to base initial AZA doses on body weight, making adjustments thereafter according to the myelotoxic pharmacodynamic indices of leukocyte and/or platelet counts. Thus, the monitoring of complete blood counts remains routine even among patients receiving stable drug doses long term. Unfortunately, the effect on bone marrow seems to be independent of the immunosuppressive efficacy; the induction of leukopenia is not required for the therapeutic effect (Swanson and Schwartz 1967; Schutz et al 1995). Neither AZA nor 6-MP plasma concentrations seem to be practical or useful; both parent compound and its major metabolite are eliminated rapidly from the circulation, and neither concentration correlates with the therapeutic effects (Lennard et al 1984, 1986; Ohlman et al 1993). In contrast, two monitoring techniques have been proposed to correlate with clinical events, and provide guides to clinical therapy: AZA intracellular metabolites (6-TGN) and measurement of thiopurine methyltransferase (TPMT) activity.

The 6-TGN family, which represents the major metabolites of AZA, is believed to mediate both the immunosuppressive and myelotoxic activities of the drug. Erythrocyte concentrations, which are measured by HPLC as an index of tissue concentrations (Lennard 1987; Erdmann et al 1990), seem to correlate with drug-induced toxicities. In contradistinction to values between 30 and 425, 6-TGN concentrations greater than 425 pmol/8×10^8 red blood cells have been associated both with a lower value of, and a shortened time to, the nadir neutrophil count (Lennard et al 1984).

There appears to be a reciprocal relationship between TPMT activity and the formation of 6-TGN. The TPMT activity appears to be controlled at least in part by a genetic polymorphism. Approximately 0.3% of the population display a deficiency of this enzyme activity; 11% show intermediate activity; and 89%, high activity (Weinshilboum and Sladek 1980). Estimates of TPMT activity in red blood cells may provide an individualized profile of drug metabolism, thereby identifying patients who may be at risk for drug-induced toxicity (low TPMT activity) or for allograft rejection due to inadequate AZA immunosuppression (high TPMT activity).

BASILIXIMAB

The chimeric mouse–human anti-interleukin-2 receptor (IL-2R) MAb basiliximab (Simulect, Novartis, Basle, Switzerland), is administered at a dose of 20 mg just prior to and 4 days after renal transplantation. Basiliximab binds with high specificity and affinity to the α-subunit (CD25) on activated T-lymphocytes (Amlot et al 1995). When complexed with basiliximab, the IL-2R is not available for ligand binding, thereby inhibiting the generation of proliferative responses to this cytokine (Amlot et al 1995). Serum basiliximab concentrations may be estimated by a two-step competitive ELISA that quantitates basiliximab in patient sera versus standard amounts of biotinylated basiliximab using a polyclonal rabbit anti-idiotypic antibody. The sensitivity limit of the assay is 0.05 mg/l, and the precision ranges from 7% to 20% (Kovarik et al 1997).

After a single infusion of 15–20 mg basiliximab to renal transplant recipients, serum concentrations generally range from 5 to 10 mg/l (Kovarik et al 1996). In vitro experiments demonstrate that concentrations of at least 1 mg/l inhibit more than 90% of the binding of IL-2 to an IL-2 R-expressing T-lymphocyte line (Amlot et al 1995). Within 24 hours after a single intravenous dose of 2.5–25 mg, basiliximab quickly saturates the IL-2R, namely, 90% of receptor sites on peripheral lymphocytes are not available for ligand binding (Amlot et al 1995; Kovarik et al 1996). When serum basiliximab concentrations exceed 0.2 mg/l as measured by ELISA, or 0.7–1 mg/l by RIA (Amlot et al 1995; Kovarik et al 1996), IL-2R saturation is achieved in adult or pediatric renal transplant recipients.

The elimination half-life of basiliximab is 7–13 days in adult renal transplant recipients who receive either 15 or 20 mg doses 2 hours before, as well as one or two doses within 10 days after, transplant surgery (Kovarik et al 1996, 1999), and 9 days in children given 12 mg/m^2 before as well as on day 4 after surgery (Kovarik et al 1998). In adults, administration of basiliximab is followed by 90% saturation of IL-2R on peripheral lymphocytes for 4–6 weeks (Kahan et al 1998b; Kovarik et al 1999), the period during which the majority of acute rejections occur (Basadonna et al 1993). Pediatric transplant recipients treated with 12 mg/m^2 2 hours before and on day 4 after transplant surgery display IL-2R saturation for 29 days. However, the mean duration of IL-2R saturation following basiliximab administration failed to correlate with either the occurrence of an acute rejection episode or the severity of the episode as graded by the Banff classification (Kovarik et al 1999). Because the significance of the concentration of or the degree of IL-2R saturation by antibody is uncertain, these measurements seem to be neither necessary nor beneficial to optimize results with this MAb.

DACLIZUMAB

Daclizumab is a humanized-mouse anti-IL-2R MAb directed against the CD25 α-chain of the IL-2R (Waldmann and O'Shea 1998). Similar to basiliximab, daclizumab treatment renders T-lymphocytes unavailable for IL-2 binding, which is required for proliferation in response to this ligand. The humanized reagent daclizumab displays a 10-fold lower avidity and affinity for CD25 than basiliximab and is thus used at approximately 10-fold higher doses. Serum daclizumab concentrations may be estimated by ELISA testing, wherein wells coated with CD25 bind circulating daclizumab in the patient serum sample, thereby preventing adherence of biotinylated CD25 that is conjugated to peroxidase-labeled streptavidin and serves as the quantitation standard. The working range of the assay is 25–400 mg/l, with an overall precision of 5% (Fayer et al 1995).

In a phase I trial in stable renal transplant recipients, the 11-day half-life of daclizumab (Vincenti et al 1997) was longer than the 4 days observed among patients treated for graft-versus-host disease (Anasetti et al 1994), but shorter than the 20-day half-life reported in a subsequent phase III clinical trial using de novo administration (Vincenti et al 1998). The US FDA-approved dosing regimen stipulates intravenous delivery of 1 mg/kg of daclizumab every other week, starting at 0–12 hours prior to transplantation and continuing for five total doses. This regimen yields sustained serum concentrations of and IL-2R saturation by the antibody for 12 weeks after transplantation (Vincenti et al 1997). At 4 weeks after the last dose of daclizumab, 74% of the IL-2R remains saturated with antibody (Vincenti et al 1997).

As in the case of basiliximab, daclizumab displays an uncertain relation between dose (or serum concentrations) and the pharmacodynamic effects of either IL-2R saturation or interruption of IL-2-mediated immune effects. Lower concentrations of daclizumab are required to saturate the IL-2R α-subunit (0.5–1.0 mg/l) than either to downregulate mixed lymphocyte responses (1–10 mg/l; Stock et al 1996) or to suppress T-cell proliferation by 90% (3–5 mg/l; Junghans et al 1990). The pharmacodynamic findings that administration of five doses of daclizumab at 2-week intervals provides saturation for up to 12 weeks posttransplant are consistent with the results of extrapolation of serum concentrations, suggesting that the corresponding value at 12 weeks would be 4 mg/l (Vincenti et al 1997).

ANTI-CD3 MONOCLONAL ANTIBODY

The murine MAb muromonab CD3 (OKT3, Ortho, N. Raritan, NJ) directed against the CD3 antigen blocks T-cell activation. Serum concentrations may be estimated by ELISA. Plates precoated with a polyclonal serum containing goat antimouse IgG-antibodies are incubated with serum from a patient treated with OKT3. Thereafter, a second goat antimouse IgG-antibody conjugated to alkaline phosphatase is added to the reaction. Binding of conjugate to OKT3 trapped on the wells by the original xenoantibody triggers a color change in added substrate that is directly proportionate to the OKT3 concentration. Serum OKT3 levels are quantitated by comparison of the absorbance values of the patient's sample to standards of known concentration. The ELISA displays a precision of 4–8% for OKT3 concentrations between 500 and 1200 ng/ml (Schroeder et al 1994).

A single dose of 2.5 mg OKT3 administered 12–24 hours before renal transplantation results in peak serum concentrations at 1 hour postdosing, followed by a rapid decrease thereafter to undetectable amounts by 12 hours (Madden et al 1994). Trough plasma OKT3 concentrations increase gradually during a 10–14-day course of administration, decreasing rapidly after discontinuation of treatment (Schroeder et al 1989; Norman 1990; Hesse et al 1991). After 2–4 days of antibody administration, mean steady-state trough serum concentrations range from 500 to 1000 μg/l, approaching the threshold of 1000 μg/l that is required to block cytotoxic T cell function in vitro (Goldstein et al 1986, 1988).

OKT3 is eliminated via binding to lymphocytes. Coated cells may be removed by the reticuloendothelial system (Schroeder et al 1994), but additionally the antigen–antibody complexes may be either shed into the serum or endocytosed into the cells. An initial rapid clearance of antibody from the serum occurs, but decreases concentrations by 60% within the first 4 hours and makes them undetectable by 12 hours (Goldstein et al 1988; Madden et al 1994). The half-life of OKT3 in serum is approximately 18 hours during treatment of acute rejection episodes, versus 36 hours when administered for induction prophylaxis immediately posttransplant (Goldstein et al 1988; McDiarmid et al 1990). In the presence of human antimouse OKT3 antibodies, OKT3 disappears more rapidly (Hammond et al 1990; Abramowicz et al 1994).

Mean serum OKT3 concentrations are higher among women than men, among liver compared to renal or cardiac recipients during the first 7–10 days of therapy, and among renal compared with cardiac patients during the latter phase of therapy (Schroeder et al 1994). OKT3 concentrations also are higher among patients aged less than 10 years and in hosts displaying only low titers or an absence of human antimouse antibodies compared to subjects who display seroconversion (Schroeder et al 1994).

Low plasma OKT3 concentrations have been not only associated with failure of therapy (McDiarmid et al 1990; Schroeder et al 1991b; Abramowicz et al 1994), but also seem to represent a better pharmacodynamic index than enumeration of CD3$^+$ cells, which by itself fails to reliably indicate plasma OKT3 concentrations or evidences of early sensitization (Gebel et al 1989; Shaefer et al 1990; McCarthy et al 1993; Broughan et al 1994). However, due to the lack of a readily available assay to monitor serum OKT3 concentrations, and the proposed restriction of the sale of reagents to detect human antimonoclonal OKT3 antibody titers (Gebel et al 1989; Moore et al 1991; Ryckman et al 1991; Schroeder et al 1991b; Hammond et al 1993; Abramowicz et al 1994; Toyoda et al 1995), clinicians must depend upon continued clinical surveillance and follow-up transplant biopsies to assess the antirejection effects of therapy. Thus, unanticipated increases in serum creatinine levels after 7 days of therapy or abrupt increases in the percentage of CD3$^+$ T lymphocytes in the patient's circulation suggest refractoriness to therapy and the need for a transplant biopsy to evaluate the progression of the alloimmune response.

USE OF PHARMACOKINETICS IN THE DEVELOPMENT OF DRUGS FOR IMMUNOSUPPRESSION

Pharmacokinetics and therapeutic drug monitoring represent essential components of rational immunosuppressive therapy, providing guidelines for initial regimens and subsequent adjustments of drug doses. The difficulties encountered during the development of optimal CsA therapy underscore the need to prospectively address the pharmacokinetic characteristics and variability of new immunosuppressive agents to guide TDM strategies. These data are necessary not only for approval and registration of new drugs, but also for the safe and effective use of a new drug by a physician. Thus, incorporation of pharmacokinetic and kinetic/dynamic analyses within each phase of drug development expedites identification of optimal dosing regimens and provides an essential framework to refine and improve therapeutic outcomes among unique populations, such as the pediatric age group.

Preclinical pharmacokinetic studies seek to interpret toxicity/safety evaluations in animals as well as humans. These preclinical data on drug kinetics and drug–drug interactions guide study design. Initial human studies of tolerance to and pharmacokinetics of ascending drug doses in stable transplant patients seek to establish dose–concentration–effect relations for subsequent studies using de novo drug administration. Furthermore, these phase I studies in stable recipients assess the drug delivery formulation and may also identify patient subpopulations displaying special characteristics, such as drug–disease interactions, that may perturb the pharmacokinetic/dynamic relationship.

The principal goal of phase II clinical trials is to provide evidence of the desired therapeutic effect and, by virtue of dose–effect relations, guide the design of the larger and longer phase III clinical trials. In addition, to determine the best dose range and optimal dosing interval, phase III trials provide information about adjustments for patients suffering organ dysfunction or treated with concomitant medications. The dose–concentration response relations estimate both the lowest effective and also the optimal drug concentration. The phase III concentration data seek to explain the lack of efficacy, unusual responses, drug–drug and drug–disease interactions, as well as inter- and intrapatient variability among large data sets of patients. In summary, efficient and rational drug development demands well-designed clinical trials that not only establish long-term safety and effectiveness in relevant populations, but also identify the optimal dosing interval and dose adjustment algorithms.

CONCLUSION

Pharmacologic investigations have become critical for rational immunosuppressive drug therapy. Measurement of blood concentrations of CsA, TRL, SRL, and MMF is relatively simple and reproducible, albeit that automated techniques specific for the active drug are not yet available. Emerging evidence suggests that, despite their nonselective nature, these drug concentrations proffer intermediate endpoints that can predict the patient's proclivity to adverse events. For example, there is an increased risk of an acute allograft rejection episode when a patient displays trough values below the recognized limits of 250 ng/ml for CsA, 5 ng/ml for TRL, 10 ng/ml for SRL, and 3 μg/ml for MPA. Conversely, patients who display values above the toxic thresholds have a greater incidence of adverse reactions. As more information is gathered, it should be possible to determine the role of pharmacokinetic profiling rather than merely trough concentration measurements for optimal therapy with TRL, SRL, or MMF, as has now gained increased acceptance for CsA. Thus, an understanding of pharmacokinetic principles, coupled with the use of concentration–time profiles in selected cases, can guide clinicians to individualize drug therapy for optimal results.

REFERENCES

Abramowicz D, Goldman M, Mat O et al (1994) OKT3 serum levels as a guide for prophylactic therapy: a pilot study in kidney transplant recipients. *Transplant Int* 7:258–263.

Abu-Elmagd K, Fung JJ, Alessiani M et al (1991a) The effect of graft function on FK506 plasma levels, dosages, and renal function, with particular reference to the liver. *Transplantation* 52:71–77.

Abu-Elmagd KM, Fung JJ, Alessiani M et al (1991b) Strategy of FK 506 therapy in liver transplant patients: effect of graft function. *Transplant Proc* 23:2771–2774.

Akagi H, Reynolds A, Hjelm M (1991) Cyclosporin A and its metabolites, distribution in blood and tissues. *J Int Med Res* 19:1–18.

Alessiani M, Cillo U, Fung JJ et al (1993) Adverse effects of FK506 overdose after liver transplantation. *Transplant Proc* 25:628–634.

Allison AC, Kowalski WJ, Muller CD, Eugui EM (1993) Mechanism of action of mycophenolic acid. *Ann NY Acad Sci* 696:63–87.

Amante AJ, Kahan BD (1996) Abbreviated area-under-the-curve strategy for monitoring cyclosporine microemulsion therapy in immediate post-transplant period. *Clin Chem* 42:1294–1296.

Amlot PL, Rawlings E, Fernando ON et al (1995) Prolonged action of a chimeric interleukin-2 receptor (CD25) monoclonal antibody used in cadaveric renal transplantation. *Transplantation* 60:748–756.

Anasetti C, Hansen JA, Waldmann TA et al (1994) Treatment of acute graft-versus-host disease with humanized anti-Tac: an antibody that binds to the interleukin-2 receptor. *Blood* 84:1320–1327.

Appel S, Paradis K, Kom A et al (1997) Safety, tolerability, and pharmacokinetics of the new immunosuppressant SDZ RAD in stable renal transplant recipients (abstract). *American Society of Transplant Physicians 16th Annual Meeting*, Chicago, May 1997.

Arceci RJ, Stieglitz K, Bierer BE (1992) Immunosuppressants FK506 and rapamycin function as reversal agents of the multidrug resistance phenotype. *Blood* 80:1528–1536.

Awni WM (1992) Pharmacodynamic monitoring of cyclosporin. *Clin Pharmacokinet* 23:428–448.

Awni W, Heim-Duthoy K, Kasiske BL (1990) Monitoring of cyclosporine by serial post-transplant pharmacokinetic studies in renal transplant patients. *Transplant Proc* 22:1343–1344.

Backman L, Nicar M, Levy M et al (1994) FK506 trough levels in whole blood and plasma in liver transplant recipients. *Transplantation* 57:519–525.

Basadonna GP, Matas AJ, Gillingham KJ et al (1993) Early versus late acute renal allograft rejection: impact on chronic rejection. *Transplantation* 55:993–995.

Bergan S, Rugstad HE, Bentdal O et al (1994a) Kinetics of mercaptopurine and thioguanine nucleotides in renal transplant recipients during azathioprine treatment. *Ther Drug Monit* 16:13–20

Bergan S, Rugstad HE, Bentdal O, Stokke O (1994b) Monitoring of azathioprine treatment by determination of 6-thioguanine nucleotide concentrations in erythrocytes. *Transplantation* 58:803–808.

Beysens AJ, Wijnen RM, Beuman GH et al (1991) FK506: monitoring in plasma or in whole blood? *Transplant Proc* 23:2745–2747.

Bowers LD (1991) Therapeutic monitoring for cyclosporine: difficulties in establishing a therapeutic window. *Clin Biochem* 24:81–87.

Bowers LD, Canafax DM, Singh J et al (1986) Studies of cyclosporine blood levels: analysis, clinical utility, pharmacokinetics, metabolites, and chronopharmacology. *Transplant Proc* 18(Suppl 5):137–143.

Brattstrom C, Sawe J, Tyden G et al (1997) Kinetics and dynamics of single oral doses of sirolimus in sixteen renal transplant recipients. *Ther Drug Monit* 19:397–406.

Brockman RW (1963) Biochemical aspects of mercaptopurine inhibition and resistance. *Cancer Res* 23:1191–1201.

Broughan TA, Valenzuela R, Escorcia E et al (1994) Mouse antibody-coated lymphocytes during OKT3 therapy in liver transplantation. *Clin Transpl* 8:488–491.

Bullingham R, Monroe S, Nicholls A, Hale M (1996a) Pharmacokinetics and bioavailability of mycophenolate mofetil in healthy subjects after single-dose oral and intravenous administration. *J Clin Pharmacol* 36:315–324.

Bullingham R, Shah J, Goldblum R, Schiff M (1996b) Effects of food and antacid on the pharmacokinetics of single doses of mycophenolate mofetil in rheumatoid arthritis patients. *Br J Clin Pharmacol* 41:513–516.

Bullingham RE, Nicholls A, Hale M (1996c) Pharmacokinetics of mycophenolate mofetil (RS61443): a short review. *Transplant Proc* 28:925–929.

Bullingham RE, Nicholls AJ, Kamm BR (1998) Clinical pharmacokinetics of mycophenolate mofetil. *Clin Pharmacokinet* 34:429–455.

Cantarovich M, Barkun JS, Tchervenkov JI et al (1998) Comparison of neoral dose monitoring with cyclosporine trough levels versus 2-hour postdose levels in stable liver transplant patients. *Transplantation* 66:1621–1627.

Chan GL, Erdmann GR, Gruber SA et al (1990) Azathioprine metabolism: pharmacokinetics of 6-mercaptopurine, 6-thiouric acid and 6-thioguanine nucleotides in renal transplant patients. *J Clin Pharmacol* 30:358–363.

Chou D (1993) Therapeutic drug monitoring (immunosuppressive drugs). *Anal Chem* 65:412R–415R.

Christians U (1988) Measurement of CsA and 18 metabolites in blood, bile, and urine by high-performance liquid chromatography. *Transplant Proc* 20(Suppl 2):609–613.

Christians U, Sewing KF (1993) Cyclosporin metabolism in transplant patients. *Pharmacol Ther* 57:291–345.

Christians U, Kruse C, Kownatzki R et al (1990) Measurement of FK506 by HPLC and isolation and characterization of its metabolites. *Transplant Proc* 23:940–941.

Christians U, Braun F, Kosian N et al (1991a) High-performance liquid chromatography/mass spectrometry of FK506 and its metabolites in blood, bile, and urine of liver grafted patients. *Transplant Proc* 23:2741–2744.

Christians U, Radeke HH, Kownatzki R et al (1991b) Isolation of an immunosuppressive metabolite of FK506 generated by human microsome preparations. *Clin Biochem* 24:271–275.

Christians U, Braun F, Schmidt M et al (1992a) Specific and sensitive measurement of FK506 and its metabolites in blood and urine of liver graft recipients. *Clin Chem* 38:2025–2032.

Christians U, Sattler M, Schiebel HM et al (1992b) Isolation of two immunosuppressive metabolites after in vitro metabolism of rapamycin. *Drug Metab Dispos* 20:186–191.

Chueh SC, Kahan BD (1998) Pretransplant test-dose pharmacokinetic profiles: cyclosporine microemulsion versus corn oil-based soft gel capsule formulation. *J Am Soc Nephrol* 9:297–304.

Copeland KR, Yatscoff RW, McKenna RM (1990) Immunosuppressive activity of cyclosporine metabolites compared and characterized by mass spectroscopy and nuclear magnetic resonance. *Clin Chem* 36:225–229.

Dasgupta A, Saldana S, Desai M (1991) Analytical performance of EMIT cyclosporin assay evaluated. *Clin Chem* 37:2130–2133.

de Groen PC, Wiesner RH, Krom RA (1988) Cyclosporin A induced side effects related to a low serum cholesterol level: an indication for a free cyclosporin A assay. *Transplant Proc* 20 (Suppl 2):374–376.

Drewe J, Beglinger C, Kissel T (1992) The absorption site of cyclosporine in the human gastrointestinal tract. *Br J Clin Pharmacol* 33:39.

Dusci LJ, Hackett LP, Chiswell GM, Ilett KF (1992) Comparison of cyclosporine measurement in whole blood by high performance liquid chromatography, monoclonal fluorescence polarization immunoassay, and monoclonal enzyme-multiplied immunoassay. *Ther Drug Monit* 14:327–332.

Elion GB (1972) Significance of azathioprine metabolites. *Proc R Soc Med* 65:257–260.

El-Yazigi A, Wahab FA (1993) Pharmacokinetics of azathioprine after repeated oral and single intravenous administration. *J Clin Pharmacol* 33:522–526.

Erden E, Warty V, Magnone M et al (1994) Plasma FK506 levels in patients with histopathologically documented renal allograft rejection. *Transplantation* 58:397–398.

Erdmann GR, Chan GLC, Canafax DM (1988) HPLC determination of 6-thiouric and 6-mercaptopurine in organ transplant serum. *J Liq Chromatogr* 11:971–981.

Erdmann GR, France LA, Bostrom BC, Canafax D (1990) A reversed phase high performance liquid chromatography approach to determining total red blood cell concentrations of 6-thioguanine, 6-mercaptopurine, methylthioguanine, and methylmercaptopurine in a patient receiving thiopurine therapy. *Biomed Chromatogr* 4:47–51.

Ericzon BG, Ekqvist B, Groth CG, Sawe J (1991) Pharmacokinetics of FK506 during maintenance therapy in liver transplant patients. *Transplant Proc* 23:2775–2776.

Fahr A (1993) Cyclosporin clinical pharmacokinetics. *Clin Pharmacokinet* 24:472–295.

Fayer BE, Soni PP, Binger MH et al (1995) Determination of humanized anti-tac in human serum by a sandwich enzyme linked immunosorbent assay. *J Immunol Methods* 186:47–54.

Ferron GM, Mishina EV, Zimmerman JJ, Jusko WJ (1997) Population pharmacokinetics of sirolimus in kidney transplant patients. *Clin Pharmacol Ther* 61:416–428.

Fitzsimmons WE, Bekersky I, Dressler D et al (1998) Demographic considerations in tacrolimus pharmacokinetics. *Transplant Proc* 30:1359–1364.

Flechner BD, Gorski JC, Vandenbranden M et al (1985) The presence of cyclosporine in body tissues and fluids during pregnancy. *Am J Kidney Dis* 5:60–63.

Frey FJ, Horber FF, Frey BM (1988) Trough levels and concentration time curves of cyclosporine in patients undergoing renal transplantation. *Clin Pharmacol Ther* 43:55–62.

Furukawa H, Imventarza O, Venkataramanan R et al (1992) The effect of bile duct ligation and bile diversion on FK506 pharmacokinetics in dogs. *Transplantation* 53:722–725.

Gaspari F, Perico N, Signorini O et al (1998) Abbreviated kinetic profiles in area-under-the-curve monitoring of cyclosporine therapy. *Kidney Int* 54:2146–2150.

Gebel HM, Lebeck LL, Jensik SC et al (1989) Discordant expression of CD3 and T cell receptor antigens on lymphocytes from patients treated with OKT3. *Transplant Proc* 21:1745–1746.

Goldstein G, Fuccello AJ, Norman DJ et al (1986) OKT3 monoclonal antibody plasma levels during therapy and the subsequent development of host antibodies to OKT3. *Transplantation* 42:507–511.

Goldstein G, Norman DJ, Henell KR, Smith IL (1988) Pharmacokinetic study of Orthoclone OKT3 serum levels during treatment of acute renal allograft rejection. *Transplantation* 46:587–589.

Gottesman MM, Pastan I (1993) Biochemistry of multidrug resistance mediated by the multidrug transporter. *Ann Rev Biochem* 62:385–427.

Grant D, Kneteman N, Tchervenkov J et al (1999) Peak cyclosporine levels (C_{max}) correlate with freedom from liver graft rejection: results of a prospective, randomized comparison of neoral and sandimmune for liver transplantation (NOF-8), *Transplantation* 67:1133–1137.

Grenier FC, Luczkiw JI, Bergmann M et al (1991) A whole blood FK 506 assay for the IMx analyzer. *Transplant Proc* 23:2748–2749.

Grevel J (1986) Absorption of cyclosporine A after oral dosing. *Transplant Proc* 18(Suppl 5):9–15.

Grevel J, Kahan BD (1991) Abbreviated kinetic profiles in area-under-the-curve monitoring of cyclosporine therapy. *Clin Chem* 37:1905–1908.

Grevel J, Napoli KL, Kahan BD (1990) Steady state concentrations of cyclosporine for therapeutic monitoring. *Transplant Proc* 22:1339–1342.

Guengerich FP (1988) Roles of cytochrome P-450 enzymes in chemical carcinogenesis and cancer chemotherapy. *Cancer Res* 48:2946–2954.

Guengerich FP, Martin MV, Beaune PH et al (1986) Characterization of rat and human liver microsomal cytochrome P-450 forms involved in nifedipine oxidation, a prototype for genetic polymorphism in oxidative drug metabolism. *J Biol Chem* 261:5051–5060.

Gupta SK, Benet LZ (1990) High-fat meals increase the clearance of cyclosporine. *Pharmacol Res* 7:46–48.

Habucky K (1992) FK506: its pharmacokinetics and interactions with other drugs. PhD thesis, University of Pittsburgh.

Haehner BD, Gorski JC, Vanderbranden M et al (1996) Bimodal distribution of renal cytochrome P450 3A activity in humans. *Mol Pharmacol* 50:52–59.

Haesslein HC, Pierce JC, Lee HM, Hume DM (1972) Leukopenia and azathioprine management in renal homotransplantation. *Surgery* 71:598–604.

Hale MD, Nicholls AJ, Bullingham RES et al (1998) The pharmacokinetic–pharmacodynamic relationship for mycophenolate mofetil in renal transplantation. *Clin Pharmacol Ther* 64:672–683.

Hammond EA, Yowell RL, Greenwood J et al (1993) Prevention of adverse clinical outcome by monitoring of cardiac transplant patients for murine monoclonal CD3 antibody (OKT3) sensitization. *Transplantation* 55:1061–1063.

Hammond EH, Wittwer CT, Greenwood J et al (1990) Relationship of OKT3 sensitization and vascular rejection in cardiac transplant patients receiving OKT3 rejection prophylaxis. *Transplantation* 50:776–782.

Henry ML, Bowers VD, Fanning WJ et al (1988) Cyclosporine levels are not helpful. *Transplant Proc* 20(Suppl 2):419–421.

Hesse CJ, Heyse P, Stolk B et al (1991) Immune monitoring of heart transplant patients receiving either one or two cycles of OKT3 prophylaxis. Induced anti-idiotypic and anti-isotypic anti-OKT3 antibodies do not prohibit depletion of peripheral T cells due to second OKT3 treatment. *Clin Transplant* 5:446–455.

Hofsli E, Nissen-Meyer J (1989) Reversal of drug resistance by erythromycin: erythromycin increases the accumulation of actinomycin D and doxorubicin in multidrug-resistant cells. *Int J Cancer* 44:149–154.

Holt DW, Marsden JT, Johnston A et al (1986) Blood cyclosporin concentrations and renal allograft dysfunction. *BMJ* 293:1057–1059.

Holt DW, Marsden JT, Johnston A, Taube DH (1989) Cyclosporine monitoring with polyclonal and specific monoclonal antibodies during episodes of renal allograft dysfunction. *Transplant Proc* 21:1482–1484.

Holt DW, Johnston A, Roberts NB et al (1994) Methodological and clinical aspects of cyclosporine monitoring: report of the Association of Clinical Biochemists' task force. *Ann Clin Biochem* 31:420–446.

Holt V, Kouba M, Bietel M, Voght G (1992) Stereoisomers of calcium antagonists which differ markedly in their potencies as calcium blockers are equally effective in modulating drug transport by p-glycoprotein. *Biochem Pharmacol* 43:2601–2608.

Hoppu K, Koskimies O, Holmberg C et al (1991) Evidence for pre-hepatic metabolism of oral cyclosporine in children. *Br J Clin Pharmacol* 32:477–481.

Hoyer PF, Brodehl J, Ehrich JH, Offner G (1991) Practical aspects in the use of cyclosporin in paediatric nephrology. *Pediatr Nephrol* 5:630–638.

Hsing S, Gatmaitan Z, Arias IM (1992) The function of Gp170, the multidrug-resistance gene product, in the brush border of rat intestinal mucosa. *Gastroenterology* 102:879–885.

Inoue S, Beck Y, Nagao T, Uchida H (1994) Early fluctuation in cyclosporine A trough levels affects long-term outcome of kidney transplants. *Transplant Proc* 26:2571–2573.

Irschik E, Tilg H, Niederwieser D et al (1984) Cyclosporin blood levels do correlate with clinical complications. *Lancet* ii:692–693.

Iwasaki K, Shiraga T, Nagase K et al (1993) Isolation, identification and biological activities of oxidative metabolites of FK506, a potent immunosuppressive macrolide lactone. *Drug Metab Dispos* 21:971–977.

Iwasaki K, Shiraga T, Matsuda H et al (1995) Identification and biological activities of the metabolites oxidized at multiple sites of FK506. *Drug Metab Dispos* **23**:28–34.

Jain AB, Venkataramanan R, Cadoff E et al (1990) Effect of hepatic dysfunction and T-tube clamping on FK506 pharmacokinetics and trough concentrations. *Transplant Proc* **22**:57–59.

Jain AB, Fung JJ, Tzakis AG et al (1991a) Comparative study of cyclosporine and FK506 dosage requirements in adult and pediatric orthotopic liver transplant patients. *Transplant Proc* **23**:2763–2766.

Jain AB, Todo S, Fung JJ et al (1991b) Correlation of rejection episodes with FK506 dosage, FK506 level, and steroids following primary orthotopic liver transplantation. *Transplant Proc* **23**:3023–3025.

Jain A, Venkataramanan R, Lever J et al (1993a) FK506 and pregnancy in liver transplant patients. *Transplantation* **56**:1588–1589.

Jain AB, Abu-Elmagd K, Abdallah H et al (1993b) Pharmacokinetics of FK 506 in liver transplant recipients following continuous intravenous infusion. *J Clin Pharmacol* **33**:606–611.

Japan RS-61443 Investigation Committee (1995) Pilot study of mycophenolate mofetil (RS-61443) in the prevention of acute rejection following renal transplantation in Japanese patients. *Transplant Proc* **27**:1421–1424.

Japanese FK506 Study Group (1991) Japanese study of FK506 on kidney transplantation: the benefit of monitoring the whole blood FK506 concentrations in patients. *Transplant Proc* **23**:3085–3088.

Johnson EM, Zimmerman J, Duderstadt K et al (1996) A randomized, double-blind, placebo-controlled study of the safety, tolerance, and preliminary pharmacokinetics of ascending single doses of orally administered sirolimus (rapamycin) in stable renal transplant recipients. *Transplant Proc* **28**:987.

Johnson H, Swan SK, Heim-Duthoy KL et al (1998) The pharmacokinetics of a single oral dose of mycophenolate mofetil in patients with varying degrees of renal function. *Clin Pharmacol Ther* **63**:512–518.

Johnston A, Sketris I, Marsden JT et al (1990) A limited sampling strategy for the measurement of cyclosporine AUC. *Transplant Proc* **22**:1345–1346.

Junghans RP, Waldmann TA, Landolfi NF et al (1990). Anti-Tac-H, a humanized antibody to the interleukin 2 receptor with new features for immunotherapy in malignant and immune dis orders. *Cancer Res* **50**:1495.

Jusko WJ, D'Ambrosio R (1991) Monitoring FK506 concentrations in plasma and whole blood. *Transplant Proc* **23**:2732–2735.

Jusko WJ, Piekoszewski W, Klintmalm GB et al (1995) Pharmacokinetics of tacrolimus in liver transplant patients. *Clin Pharmacol Ther* **57**:281–290.

Kahan BD (1985) Overview: individualization of cyclosporine therapy using pharmacokinetic and pharmacodynamic parameters. *Transplantation* **40**:457–476.

Kahan BD (1989) cyclosporine. *N Engl J Med* **321**:1725–1738.

Kahan BD (1994) *Neoral: A New Formulation of cyclosporine.* New York: World Medical Press, pp. 12–19.

Kahan BD, Grevel J (1988) Optimization of cyclosporine therapy in renal transplantation by a pharmacokinetic strategy. *Transplantation* **46**:631–644.

Kahan BD, Ried M, Newburger J (1983) Pharmacokinetics of cyclosporine in human renal transplantation. *Transplant Proc* **15**:446–453.

Kahan BD, Wideman CA, Reid M et al (1984) The value of serial serum trough cyclosporine levels in human renal transplantation. *Transplant Proc* **16**:1195–1199.

Kahan BD, Shaw LM, Holt D et al (1990) Consensus document: Hawk's Cay meeting on therapeutic drug monitoring of cyclosporine. *Clin Chem* **36**:1510–1516.

Kahan BD, Welsh M, Rutzky L et al (1992) The ability of pre-transplant test-dose pharmacokinetic profiles to reduce early adverse events after renal transplantation. *Transplantation* 53:345–351.

Kahan BD, Dunn J, Fitts C et al (1994) The Neoral formulation: improved correlation between cyclosporine trough levels and exposure in stable renal transplant recipients. *Transplant Proc* 26:2940–2943.

Kahan BD, Dunn J, Fitts C et al (1995a) Reduced inter- and intrasubject variability in cyclosporine pharmacokinetics in renal transplant recipients treated with a microemulsion formulation in conjunction with fasting, low-fat meals, or high-fat meals. *Transplantation* 59:505–511.

Kahan BD, Murgia MG, Slaton J, Napoli K (1995b) Potential applications of therapeutic drug monitoring of sirolimus immunosuppression in clinical renal transplantation. *Ther Drug Monit* 17:672–675.

Kahan BD, Welsh M, Rutzky LP (1995c) Challenges in cyclosporine therapy: the role of therapeutic monitoring by area under the curve monitoring. *Ther Drug Monit* 17:621–624.

Kahan BD, Welsh M, Schoenberg L et al (1996) Variable oral absorption of cyclosporine. A biopharmaceutical risk factor for chronic renal allograft rejection. *Transplantation* 62:599–606.

Kahan BD, Podbielski J, Napoli KL et al (1998a) Immunosuppressive effects and safety of a sirolimus/cyclosporine combination regimen for renal transplantation. *Transplantation* 66:1040–1046.

Kahan BD, Rajagopalan PR, Hall ML, Kovarik JM (1998b) Basiliximab (Simulect™) is efficacious in reducing the incidence of acute rejection episodes in renal allograft patients: results at 12 months (abstract). *Transplantation* 65:S189.

Kahan BD, Napoli KL, Mosheim M et al (1999a) Pharmacokinetic and pharmacodynamic correlations of cyclosporine (cyclosporine) and rapamycin (RAPA) in 120 patients treated for at least 2 years at a single center (abstract 788), American Society of Transplantation, Chicago. *Transplantation* 67:S203.

Kahan BD, Julian BA, Pescovitz MD et al for the Rapamune Study Group (1999b) Sirolimus reduces the incidence of acute rejection episodes despite lower cyclosporine doses in Caucasian recipients of mismatched primary renal allografts: a phase II trial. *Transplantation* 68:1526–1532.

Kahan BD, Wong RL, Carter C et al (1999c) A phase I study of a 4-week course of the rapamycin analogue SDZ-RAD (RAD) in quiescent cyclosporine–prednisone-treated renal transplant recipients. *Transplantation* 68:100–1106

Kaplan B, Meier-Kriesche HU, Napoli K, Kahan BD (1997) A limited sampling strategy for estimating sirolimus area-under-the-concentration curve. *Clin Chem* 43:539–540.

Kasiske BL, Heim-Duthoy K, Rao KV, Awni WM (1988) The relationship between cyclosporine pharmacokinetic parameters and subsequent acute rejection in renal transplant recipients. *Transplantation* 46:716–722.

Kay JE, Kwateng SE, Geraghty F, Morgan GY (1991) Uptake of FK506 by lymphocytes and erythrocytes. *Transplant Proc* 23:2760–2762.

Kelly PA, Napoli KL, Kahan BD (2000) Conversion from liquid to solid rapamycin formulations in stable renal allograft transplant recipients. *Biopharm Drug Dispos* 20:249–253.

Keown P, Landsberg D, Holloran P et al (1996) A randomized, prospective multicenter pharmacoepidemiologic study of cyclosporine microemulsion in stable renal recipients. Report of the Canadian Neoral Renal Transplantation Study Group. *Transplantation* 62:1744–1752.

Kerman RH, Geis WP (1976) Total and active T cell dynamics in renal allograft recipients. *Surgery* 79:398–407.

Klintmalm G, Sawe J, Fingden O et al (1985) Cyclosporine plasma levels in renal transplant patients. *Transplantation* 39:132–137.

Kobayashi M, Tamura K, Katayama N et al (1991) FK506 assay past and present—characteristics of FK506 ELISA. *Transplant Proc* 23:2725–2729.

Kolansky G (1992) Cyclosporine formulary considerations. *Pharmacy and Therapeutics* 17:494–504.

Kolars JC, Awni WM, Merion RM, Watkins PB (1991) First-pass metabolism of cyclosporin by the gut. *Lancet* 338:1488–1490.

Kolars JC, Schmiedlin-Ren P, Schuetz JD et al (1992) Identification of rifampin-inducible P450IIIA4 (CYP3A4) in human small bowel enterocytes. *J Clin Invest* 90:1871–1878.

Kovarik J, Mueller EA, van Bree JB et al (1994a) Cyclosporine pharmacokinetics and variability from a microemulsion formulation—a multicenter investigation in kidney transplant patients. *Transplantation* 58:658–663.

Kovarik JM, Mueller EA, van Bree JB et al (1994b) Reduced inter- and intraindividual variability in cyclosporine pharmacokinetics from a microemulsion formulation. *J Pharmacol Sci* 83:444–446.

Kovarik JM, Rawlings E, Sweny P et al (1996) Prolonged immunosuppressive effect and minimal immunogenicity from chimeric (CD25) monoclonal antibody SDZ CHI 621 in renal transplantation. *Transplant Proc* 28:913–914.

Kovarik J, Wolf P, Cisterne JM et al (1997) Disposition of basiliximab, an interleukin-2 receptor monoclonal antibody, in recipients of mismatched cadaver renal allografts. *Transplantation* 64:1701–1705.

Kovarik J, Menster M, Broyer P et al (1998) Disposition of basiliximab, a chimeric IL-2 receptor (CD25) monoclonal antibody, in pediatric renal transplant patients (abstract). *Transplantation* 65:S66.

Kovarik JM, Moore R, Wolf P et al (1999) Screening for basiliximab exposure-response relationships in renal allotransplantation. *Clin Transplant* 13:32–38.

Kronbach T, Fischer V, Meyer UA (1988) Cyclosporine metabolism in human liver: identification of a cytochrome P 450III gene family as the major cyclosporine-metabolizing enzyme explains interactions of cyclosporine with other drugs. *Clin Pharmacol Ther* 43:630–635.

Langman LJ, LeGatt DF, Yatscoff RW (1994) Blood distribution of mycophenolic acid. *Ther Drug Monit* 16:602–607.

Langman LJ, LeGatt DF, Yatscoff RW (1995) Pharmacodynamic assessment of mycophenolic acid-induced immunosuppression by measuring IMP dehydrogenase activity. *Clin Chem* 41:295–299.

Langman LJ, LeGatt DF, Halloran PF, Yatscoff RW (1996) Pharmacodynamic assessment of mycophenolic acid-induced immunosuppression in renal transplant recipients. *Transplantation* 62:666–672.

Lee SC, Brudzinski AM, Yaswineli JL et al (1991) Measurement of cyclosporin A by a specific radioimmunoassay with a monoclonal antibody and ^{125}I tracer. *Clin Biochem* 24:43–48.

LeGatt DF, Coates JE, Simpson AI et al (1994) A comparison of cyclosporine assays using sequential samples from selected transplant patients. *Clin Biochem* 27:43–48.

Lemaire M, Tillement JP (1982) Role of lipoproteins and erythrocytes in the in vitro binding and distribution of cyclosporine A in the blood. *J Pharm Pharmacol* 34:715–718.

Lennard L (1987) Assay of 6-thioinosinic acid and 6-thioguanine nucleotides, active metabolites of 6-mercaptopurine in human red blood cells. *J Chromatogr* 423:169–178.

Lennard L, Brown CB, Fox M, Maddocks JL (1982) Azathioprine dosage schedule and rejection episodes in renal transplant recipients. *Br J Clin Pharmacol* 14:567–569.

Lennard L, Rees CA, Lilleyman JS, Maddocks JL (1983) Childhood leukemia: a relationship between intracellular 6-mercaptopurine metabolites and neutropenia. *Br J Clin Pharmacol* 16:359–363.

Lennard L, Brown CB, Fox M, Maddocks JL (1984) Azathioprine metabolism in kidney transplant recipients. *Br J Clin Pharmacol* 18:693–700.

Lennard L, Keen D, Lilleyman JS (1986) Oral 6-mercaptopurine in childhood leukemia: Parent drug pharmacokinetics and active metabolite concentrations. *Clin Pharmacol Ther* 40:287–292.

Lensmeyer GL, Wiebe DA, Carlson IH, Subramanian R (1991) Concentrations of cyclosporin A and its metabolites in human tissues postmortem. *J Anal Toxicol* 15:110–115.

Levy G, Rochon J, Freeman D et al (1994) Cyclosporine Neoral in liver transplant recipients. *Transplant Proc* 26:2949–2952.

Liliemark J, Pettersson B, Lafolie P et al (1990) Determination of plasma azathioprine and 6-mercaptopurine in patients with rheumatoid arthritis treated with oral azathioprine. *Ther Drug Monit* 12:339–343.

Lin SN, Jessup K, Floyd M et al (1980) Quantitation of plasma azathioprine and 6-mercaptopurine levels in renal transplant patients. *Transplantation* 29:290–294.

Lindberg A, Odlind B, Tufveson G et al (1986) The pharmacokinetics of cyclosporine A in uremic patients. *Transplant Proc* 18(Suppl 5):144–152.

Lindholm A, Kahan BD (1993) Influence of cyclosporine pharmacokinetics, trough concentrations, and AUC monitoring on outcome after kidney transplantation. *Clin Pharmacol Ther* 54:205–218.

Lindholm A, Welsh M, Rutzky L, Kahan BD (1993) The adverse impact of high cyclosporine clearance rates on the incidence of acute rejection and graft loss. *Transplantation* 55:985–993.

Lown KS, Kolars JC, Thummel KE et al (1994) Interpatient heterogeneity in expression of CYP3A4 and CYP3A5 in small bowel. Lack of prediction by the erythromycin breath test. *Drug Metab Dispos* 22:947–955.

Lown KS, Mayo RR, Leichtman AB et al (1997) Role of intestinal P-glycoprotein (mdr1) in interpatient variation in the oral bioavailability of cyclosporine. *Clin Pharmacol Ther* 62:248–260.

Lucey MR, Kolars JC, Merion RM et al (1990) Cyclosporin toxicity at therapeutic blood levels and cytochrome P-450 IIIA. *Lancet* 335:11–15.

Machida M, Takahara S, Ishibashi M et al (1991) Effect of temperature and hematocrit on plasma concentration of FK506. *Transplant Proc* 23:2753–2754.

Madden RL, Schroeder TJ, Alexander JW, First MR (1994) Single dose OKT3: adverse effects, pharmacokinetics, and anti-OKT3 antibody response. *Transplant Sci* 4:111–114.

Mahalati K, Belitsky P, Sketris I et al (1999) Neoral monitoring by simplified sparse sampling area under the concentration–time curve: its relationship to acute rejection and cyclosporine nephrotoxicity early after kidney transplantation. *Transplantation* 68:55–62.

Martinez L, Foradori A, Vaccarezza A et al (1989) Monitoring of cyclosporine blood levels with polyclonal and monoclonal assays during episodes of renal graft dysfunction. *Transplant Proc* 21:1490–1491.

Maurer G, Lemaire M (1986) Biotransformation and distribution in blood of cyclosporine and its metabolites. *Transplant Proc* 18(Suppl 5):25–34.

McCarthy C, Light JA, Aquino A et al (1993) Correlation of CD3[+] lymphocyte depletion with rejection and infection in renal transplants. *Transplant Proc* 25:2477–2478.

McDiarmid S, Millis M, Terashita G et al (1990) Low serum OKT3 levels correlate with failure to prevent rejection in orthotopic liver transplant patients. *Transplant Proc* 22:1774–1776.

McDiarmid SV, Colonna JO 2d, Shaked A et al (1993) Differences in oral FK 506 dose requirements between adult and pediatric liver transplant patients. *Transplantation* 55:1328–1332.

Mehta M, Venkataramanan R, Burckart GJ et al (1988) Effect of bile on cyclosporine absorption in liver transplant patients. *Br J Clin Pharmacol* 25:579–584.

Meier-Kriesche HU, Kaplan B, Brannan P et al (1998) A limited sampling strategy for the estimation of eight-hour Neoral areas under the curve in renal transplantation. *Ther Drug Monit* 20:401–407.

Meiser BM, Pfeiffer M, Schmidt D et al (1999a) Combination therapy with tacrolimus and mycophenolate mofetil following cardiac transplantation: importance of mycophenolic acid therapeutic drug monitoring. *J Heart Lung Transplant* 18:143–149.

Meiser BM, Schmidt D, Pfeiffer M et al (1999b) MMF-dose adjustments based on MPA-trough levels after heart transplantation: difference between high and low dose pharmacokinetics (abstract). *Transplantation* **67**:S110.

Mekki Q, Lee C, Carrier S et al (1993) The effect of food on oral bioavailability of tacrolimus (FK506) in liver transplant patients (abstract). *Clin Pharmacol Ther* **53**:229.

Meyer MM, Munar M, Udeaja J, Bennett W (1993) Efficacy of area under the curve cyclosporine monitoring in renal transplantation. *J Am Soc Nephrol* **4**:1306–1315.

Misteli C, Rey E, Pons G et al (1990) Pharmacokinetics of oral cyclosporin A in diabetic children and adolescents. *Eur J Clin Pharmacol* **38**:181–184.

Mohanakumar T, Hoshinaga K, Wood NL et al (1986) Enumeration of transferrin-receptor-expressing lymphocytes as a potential marker for rejection in human cardiac transplant recipients. *Transplantation* **42**:691–694.

Mooney ML, Carlson P, Hastillo A et al (1990) Transferrin receptors and CD4/CD8 lymphocyte ratios in rejection and infection in cardiac transplantation recipients. *Transplant Proc* **22**:2389–2393.

Moore CK, O'Connell JB, Renlund DG et al (1991) Cardiac allograft cellular rejection during OKT3 prophylaxis in the absence of sensitization. *Transplant Proc* **23**:1055–1058.

Morris RG, Saccoia NC, Ryall RG (1992) Specific enzyme-multiplied immunoassay and fluorescence polarization immunoassay for cyclosporin compared with Cyclotrac [^{125}I] radioimmunoassay. *Ther Drug Monit* **14**:226–2233.

Moyer TP, Winkels J, Krom R, Wiesner R (1991) Evaluation of Abbott TDx monoclonal assay of cyclosporine in whole blood. *Clin Chem* **37**:1120–1121.

Mueller EA, Kovarik JM, van Bree JB et al (1994a) Influence of a fat-rich meal on the pharmacokinetics of a new oral formulation of cyclosporine in a cross-over comparison with the market formulation. *Pharm Res* **11**:151–155.

Mueller EA, Kovarik JM, van Bree JB et al (1994b) Improved dose linearity of cyclosporine pharmacokinetics from a microemulsion formulation. *Pharm Res* **11**:301–304.

Nankivell BJ, Hibbins M, Chapman JR (1994) Diagnostic utility of whole blood cyclosporine measurements in renal transplantation using triple therapy. *Transplantation* **58**:989–989.

Napoli KL, Kahan BD (1990) Nonselective measurement of cyclosporine for therapeutic drug monitoring by fluorescence polarization immunoassay with a rabbit polyclonal antibody. I: Evaluation of the serum methodology and comparison with a sheep polyclonal antibody in an 3H tracer mediated radioimmunoassay. *Transplant Proc* **22**:1175–1180.

Napoli KL, Kahan BD (1994) Sample clean-up and high performance liquid chromatography techniques for measurement of whole blood rapamycin concentrations. *J Chromatogr Biomed Appl* **654**:111–120.

Napoli KL, Kahan BD (1996) Routine clinical monitoring of sirolimus (rapamycin) whole-blood concentrations by HPLC with ultraviolet detection. *Clin Chem* **42**:1943–1948.

Napoli KL, Wang M, Stepkowski SM, Kahan BD (1997) Distribution of sirolimus in rat tissue. *Clin Biochem* **30**:135–142.

Nebert DW, Jaiswal AK, Meyer UA, Gonzalez FJ (1987) Human P-450 genes: evolution, regulation and possible role in carcinogenesis. *Biochem Soc Trans* **15**:586–589.

Norman DJ (1990) The clinical role of OKT3. *Cardiol Clin* **8**:97–105.

Nowak R, Shaw LM (1995) Mycophenolic acid binding to human serum albumin: characterization and relation to pharmacodynamics. *Clin Chem* **41**:1011–1017.

Nyberg G, Haljamae U, Frisenette-Fich C et al (1998) Breast-feeding during treatment with cyclosporine. *Transplantation* **65**:253–255.

Odlind B, Hartvig P, Lindstrom B et al (1986) Serum azathioprine and 6-mercaptopurine levels and immunosuppressive activity after azathioprine in uremic patients. *Int J Immunopharmacol* **8**:1–11.

Oellerich M, Armstrong VW, Kahan BD et al (1995) Lake Louise consensus conference on cyclosporine monitoring in organ transplantation: report of the consensus panel. *Ther Drug Monit* 17:642–654.

Ohlman S, Lafolie P, Lindholm A et al (1993) Large interindividual variability in bioavailability of azathioprine in renal transplant recipients. *Clin Transplant* 7:65–70.

Parker G, Bullingham R, Kamm B, Hale M (1996) Pharmacokinetics of oral mycophenolate mofetil in volunteer subjects with varying degrees of hepatic oxidative impairment. *J Clin Pharmacol* 36:332–344.

Penny JI, Campbell FC (1994) Active transport of benzo[a]pyrene in apical membrane vesicles from normal human intestinal epithelium. *Biochem Biophys Acta* 1226:232–236.

Phillips TM, Karmi SA, Frantz SC, Henriques HF (1988) Absorption profiles of renal allograft recipients receiving oral doses of cyclosporine: a pharmacokinetic study. *Transplant Proc* 20(Suppl 2):457–461.

Primmett DR, Levine M, Kovarik JM et al (1998) Cyclosporine monitoring in patients with renal transplants: two- or three-point methods that estimate area under the curve are superior to trough levels in predicting drug exposure. *Ther Drug Monit* 20:276–283.

Radeke HH, Christians U, Sewing KF, Resch K (1992) The synergistic immunosuppressive potential of cyclosporin metabolite combinations. *Int J Immunopharmacol* 14:595–604.

Ried M, Gibbons S, Kwork D et al (1983) Cyclosporine levels in human tissues of patients treated for one week to one year. *Transplant Proc* 15(Suppl 1):2434–2437.

Rogers AJ, Yoshimura N, Kerman RH, Kahan BD (1984) Immunopharmacodynamic evaluation of cyclosporine-treated renal allograft recipients. *Transplantation* 38:657–664.

Rogers LC, Smith FA, Jamero A (1991) Evaluation of the Abbott TDx monoclonal cyclosporine A assay in pediatric cardiac transplant patients (abstract). *Clin Chem* 37:1014.

Rosano TG, Brooks CA, Dybas MT et al (1990) Selection of an optimal assay method for monitoring CsA therapy. *Transplant Proc* 22:1125–1128.

Rosano T, Brooks C, Dybas M (1991) EMIT monoclonal antibody assay evaluated for cyclosporin monitoring in whole blood. *Clin Chem* 37:989.

Ryckman FC, Schroeder TJ, Pedersen SH et al (1991) Use of monoclonal antibody immunosuppressive therapy in pediatric renal and liver transplantation. *Clin Transplant* 5:186–190.

Saeki T, Ueda K, Tanigawara Y et al (1993) Human P-glycoprotein transports cyclosporin A and FK506. *J Biol Chem* 268:6077–6080.

Saitoh H, Aungst BJ (1995) Possible involvement of multiple P-glycoprotein-mediated efflux systems in the transport of verapamil and other organic cations across rat intestine. *Pharm Res* 12:1304–1310.

Salemans J, Hoitsma AJ, De Abreu RA et al (1987) Pharmacokinetics of azathioprine and 6-mercaptopurine after oral administration of azathioprine. *Clin Transplant* 1:217–221.

Salm P, Norris RLG, Taylor PJ et al (1993) A reliable high-performance liquid chromatography assay for high-throughput routine cyclosporin A monitoring in whole blood. *Ther Drug Monit* 15:65–69.

Sattler M, Guengerich FP, Yun CH et al (1992) Cytochrome P-450 enzymes are responsible for biotransformation of FK506 and rapamycin in man and rat. *Drug Metab Dispos* 20:753–761.

Schinkel AH, Borst P (1991) Multidrug resistance mediated by P-glycoproteins. *Semin Cancer Biol* 2:213–226.

Schroeder TJ, First MR, Hurtubise PE et al (1989) Immunologic monitoring with Orthoclone OKT3 therapy. *J Heart Transpl* 8:371–380.

Schroeder T, Vine W, Ruckrigi D et al (1991a) Evaluation of the new cyclosporine monoclonal antibody fluorescent polarization immunoassay in cardiac and renal transplants (abstract). *Clin Chem* 37:990.

Schroeder TJ, Ryckman FC, Hurtubise PE et al (1991b) Immunological monitoring during and following OKT3 therapy in children. *Clin Transplant* 5:191–196.

Schroeder TJ, Michael AT, First MR et al (1994) Variations in serum OKT3 concentration based upon age, sex, transplanted organ, treatment regimen, and anti-OKT3 antibody status. *Ther Drug Monit* 16:361–367.

Schroeder TJ, Cho MJ, Pollack GM et al (1998) Comparison of two cyclosporine formulations in healthy volunteers: bioequivalence of the new Sang-35 formulation and neoral. *J Clin Pharmacol* 38:807–814.

Schuler W, Sedrani R, Cottens S et al (1997) SDZ RAD, a new rapamycin derivative. Pharmacological properties in vitro and in vivo. *Transplantation* 64:36–42.

Schutz E, Gummert J, Mohr FW et al (1995) Azathioprine myelotoxicity related to elevated 6-thioguanine nucleotides in heart transplantation. *Transplant Proc* 27:1298–1300.

Schutz E, Svinarov D, Shipkova M et al (1998) Cyclosporine whole blood immunoassays (AxSYM, CEDIA, and Emit): a critical overview of performance characteristics and comparison with HPLC. *Clin Chem* 44:2158–2164.

Schuurman HJ, Cottens S, Fuchs S et al (1997) SDZ RAD, a new rapamycin derivative. Synergism with cyclosporine. *Transplantation* 64:32–35.

Shaefer MS, Stratta RJ, Pirruccello SJ et al (1990) Peripheral CD3 lymphocyte monitoring of liver transplant recipients being treated with OKT3 for rejection or induction immunosuppression (abstract). *Pharmacotherapy* 10:248.

Shah J, Bullingham R, Rice P et al (1995) Pharmacokinetics of oral mycophenolic mofetil (MMF) and metabolites in renally impaired patients (abstract). *Clin Pharmacol Ther* 57:149.

Shaw LM, Sollinger HW, Halloran P et al (1995) Mycophenolate mofetil: a report of the consensus panel. *Ther Drug Monit* 17:690–699.

Shaw LM, Mick R, Nowak I et al (1998) Pharmacokinetics of mycophenolic acid in renal transplant patients with delayed graft function. *J Clin Pharmacol* 38:268–275.

Shimada T, Yamazaki H, Mimura M et al (1994) Interindividual variations in human liver cytochrome P-450 enzymes involved in the oxidation of drugs, carcinogens and toxic chemicals: studies with liver microsomes of 30 Japanese and 30 Caucasians. *J Pharmacol Exp Ther* 270:414–423.

Smak Gregoor PJH, de Sevaux RGL, Hene RJ et al (1999) Effect of discontinuing cyclosporine on mycophenolic acid trough levels in kidney transplant recipients. (abstract). American Society of Transplant Physicians 18th Annual Meeting, Chicago, May 1999.

Sommer BG, Sing DE, Henry ML et al (1988) Serum cyclosporine kinetic profile. Failure to correlate with nephrotoxicity or rejection episodes following sequential immunotherapy for renal transplantation. *Transplantation* 45:86–90.

Steimer W (1999) Performance and specificity of monoclonal immunoassays for cyclosporine monitoring: how specific is specific? *Clin Chem* 45:371–381.

Stiff DD, Venkataramanan R, Prasad TNV (1992) Metabolism of FK506 in differentially induced rat liver microsomes. *Res Commun Chem Pathol Pharmacol* 78:121–124.

Stiller C, Keown P (1990) Failure of ^{125}I-tracer selective monoclonal antibody levels on a whole blood matrix to predict rejection or nephrotoxic episodes in renal transplant patients under anti-lymphocyte globulin and prednisone therapy. *Transplant Proc* 22:1253–1254.

Stock PG, Lantz M, Light S, Vincenti F (1996) In vivo (phase I) trial and in vitro efficacy of humanized anti-TAC for the prevention of rejection in renal transplant recipients. *Transplant Proc* 28:915–916.

Streit F, Christians U, Schiebel HM et al (1996) Sensitive and specific quantification of sirolimus (rapamycin) and its metabolites in blood of kidney graft recipients by HPLC/electrospray-mass spectrometry. *Clin Chem* 42:1417–1425.

Swanson MA, Schwartz RS (1967) Immunosuppressive therapy: the relation between clinical response and immunologic competence. *N Engl J Med* 277:163–170.

Thiebaut F, Tsuruo T, Hamada H et al (1987) Cellular localization of the multidrug-resistance gene product P-glycoprotein in normal human tissues. *Proc Natl Acad Sci USA* 84:7735–7738.

Thummel KE, Shen DD, Podoll TD et al (1994) Use of midazolam as a human cytochrome P450 3A probe: I. In vitro-in vivo correlations in liver transplant patients. *J Pharmacol Exp Ther* 271:549–556.

Tidd DM, Paterson AR (1974a) Distinction between inhibition of purine nucleotide synthesis and the delayed cytotoxic reaction of 6-mercaptopurine. *Cancer Res* 34:733–737.

Tidd DM, Paterson AR (1974b) A biochemical mechanism for the delayed cytotoxic reaction of 6-mercaptopurine. *Cancer Res* 34:738–746.

Tjia JF, Webber IR, Back DJ (1991) CsA metabolism by the gastrointestinal mucosa. *Br J Clin Pharmacol* 31:344–346.

Toyoda M, Galfayan K, Wachs K et al (1995) Immunologic monitoring of OKT3 induction therapy in cardiac allograft recipients. *Clin Transplant* 9:472–480.

Tredger JM, Gonde CE, Williams R (1992) Monitoring cyclosporin in liver transplant recipients: effects of clinical status on the performance of two monoclonal antibody-based methods. *Clin Chem* 38:108–113.

Tsina I, Chu F, Hama K et al (1996a) Manual and automated (robotic) high-performance liquid chromatographic methods for the determination of mycophenolic acid and its glucuronide conjugate in human plasma. *J Chromatogr Biomed Appl* 675:119–129.

Tsina J, Kaloostian M, Lee R et al (1996b) High-performance liquid chromatographic method for the determination of mycophenolate mofetil in human plasma. *J Chromatogr Biomed Appl* 681:347–353.

Turgeon DK, Normolle DP, Leichtman AB et al (1992) Erythromycin breath test predicts oral clearance of cyclosporine in kidney transplant recipients. *Clin Pharmacol Ther* 52:471–478.

Uchida K, Yamada N, Orihara A et al (1988) Minimal low dosage of cyclosporine therapy in renal transplantation by careful monitoring of high-performance liquid chromatography whole blood levels. *Transplant Proc* 20(Suppl 2):394–401.

Urien S, Zini R, Lemaire M, Tillement JP (1990) Assessment of cyclosporine A interactions with human plasma lipoproteins in vitro and in vivo in the rat. *J Pharmacol Exp Ther* 253:305–309.

Venkataramanan R, Starzl TE, Yang S et al (1985) Biliary excretion of cyclosporine in liver transplant patients. *Transplant Proc* 17:286–289.

Venkataramanan R, Jain A, Cadoff E et al (1990) Pharmacokinetics of FK506: preclinical and clinical studies. *Transplant Proc* 22:52–56.

Venkataramanan R, Jain A, Warty VS et al (1991) Pharmacokinetics of FK 506 in transplant patients. *Transplant Proc* 23:2736–2740.

Venkataramanan R, Swaminathan A, Prasad T et al (1995) Clinical pharmacokinetics of tacrolimus *Clin Pharmacokinet* 29:404–430.

Verrill HL, Girgis RE, Easterling RE et al (1987) Distribution of cyclosporine in blood of renal transplant recipient with type V hyperlipoproteinemia. *Clin Chem* 33:423–428.

Vincent SH, Karanam BV, Painter SK, Chiu SH (1992) In vitro metabolism of FK506 in rat, rabbit, and human liver microsomes: identification of a major metabolite and of cytochrome P450-3A as the major enzymes responsible for its metabolism. *Arch Biochem Biophys* 294:454–460.

Vincenti F, Lantz M, Birnbaum J et al (1997) A phase I trial of humanized anti-interleukin 2 receptor antibody in renal transplantation. *Transplantation* 63:33–38.

Vincenti F, Kirkman R, Light S et al (1998) Interleukin-2-receptor blockade with daclizumab to prevent acute rejection in renal transplantation. Daclizumab Triple Therapy Study Group. *N Engl J Med* 338:161–165.

Vonderscher J, Meinzer A (1994) Rationale for the development of Sandimmune Neoral. *Transplant Proc* 26:2925–2927.

Wahlberg J, Wilczek HE, Fauchald P et al (1995) Consistent absorption of cyclosporine from a microemulsion formulation assessed in stable renal transplant recipients over a one-year study period. *Transplantation* 60:648–652.

Waldmann TA, O'Shea J (1998) The use of antibodies against the IL-2 receptor in transplantation. *Curr Opin Immunol* 10:507–512.

Wallemacq PE, Alexandre K (1999) Evaluation of the new AxSYM cyclosporine assay: comparison with TDx monoclonal whole blood and EMIT cyclosporine assays. *Clin Chem* 45:432–435.

Wallemacq PE, Lee SC, Lhoest G, Hassoun A (1990) Cross-reactivity of cyclosporin metabolites in two different radioimmunoassays in which the same specific antibody is used. *Clin Chem* 36:385.

Wallemacq PE, Firdaous I, Hassoun A (1993) Improvement and assessment of enzyme-linked immunosorbent assay to detect low FK 506 concentrations in plasma or whole blood within 6 hours. *Clin Chem* 39:1045–1049.

Wang PP, Simpson E, Meucci V et al (1991) Cyclosporine monitoring by fluorescence polarization immunoassay. *Clin Biochem* 24:55–58.

Warty V, Venkataramanan R, Zendehrouh P et al (1991a) Distribution of FK 506 in plasma lipoproteins. *Transplant Proc* 23:954–955.

Warty VS, Venkataramanan R, Zendehrouh P, Mehta S, McKaveney T et al (1991b) Practical aspects of FK 506 analysis (Pittsburgh experience). *Transplant Proc* 23:2730–2731.

Watkins PB, Wrighton SA, Schuetz EG et al (1987) Identification of glucocorticoid-inducible cytochromes P-450 in the intestinal mucosa of rats and man. *J Clin Invest* 80:1029–1036.

Webber IR, Peters WH, Back DJ (1992) Cyclosporin metabolism by human gastrointestinal mucosal microsomes. *Br J Clin Pharmacol* 33:661–664.

Weinshilboum RM, Sladek SL (1980) Mercaptopurine pharmacogenetics: monogenic inheritance of erythrocyte thiopurine methyltransferase activity. *Am J Hum Genet* 32:651–662.

Wijnen RMH, Ericzon BG, Tiebosch AT et al (1991) Toxicity of FK 506 in the cynomolgus monkey: noncorrelation with FK506 serum levels. *Transplant Proc* 23:3101–3104.

Winkler M, Jost U, Ringe B et al (1991) Association of elevated FK 506 plasma levels with nephrotoxicity in liver-grafted patients. *Transplant Proc* 23:3153–3155.

Winkler M, Wonigeit K, Undre N et al (1995) Comparison of plasma versus whole blood as matrix for FK 506 drug level monitoring. *Transplant Proc* 27:822–825.

Wolfe EJ, Mathur V, Tomlanovich S et al (1997) Pharmacokinetics of mycophenolate mofetil and intravenous ganciclovir alone in and in combination renal transplant recipients. *Pharmacotherapy* 17:591–598.

Wong PY, Ma J (1990) Specific and non-specific ^{125}I-Incstar assays. *Transplant Proc* 22:1166–1170.

Wrenshall LE, Matas AJ, Canafax DM et al (1990) An increased incidence of late acute rejection episodes in cadaver renal allograft recipients given azathioprine, cyclosporine, and prednisone. *Transplantation* 50:233–237.

Wrighton SA, Stevens JC (1992) The human hepatic cytochromes P450 involved in drug metabolism. *Crit Rev Toxicol* 22:1–21.

Wrighton SA, Thomas PE, Willis P et al (1987) Purification of a human liver cytochrome P-450 immunochemically related to several cytochromes P-450 purified from untreated rats. *J Clin Invest* 80:1017–1022.

Yatscoff RW (1996) Pharmacokinetics of rapamycin. *Transplant Proc* 28:970–973.

Yatscoff RW, Copeland KR, Faraci CJ (1990) Abbott TDx monoclonal antibody assay evaluated for measuring cyclosporine in whole blood. *Clin Chem* 36:123–126.

Yatscoff RW, Faraci C, Bolingbroke P (1992) Measurement of rapamycin in whole blood using reverse-phase high performance liquid chromatography. *Ther Drug Monit* 14:138–141.

Yatscoff RW, LeGatt D, Keenan R, Chackowsky P (1993) Blood distribution of rapamycin. *Transplantation* 56:1202–1206.

Yatscoff RW, Boeckx R, Holt DW et al (1995a) Consensus guidelines for therapeutic drug monitoring of rapamycin: report of the consensus panel. *Ther Drug Monit* 17:676–680.

Yatscoff RW, Wang P, Chan K et al (1995b) Rapamycin: distribution, pharmacokinetics, and therapeutic range investigations. *Ther Drug Monit* 17:666–671.

Yee GC (1991) Recent advances in cyclosporine pharmacokinetics. *Pharmacotherapy* 11:130S-134S.

Yoshimura N, Kahan BD (1985) Pharmacodynamic assessment of in vivo cyclosporine effect on interleukin-2 production by lymphocytes of kidney transplant recipients. *Transplantation* 40:661–666.

Yoshimura N, Kahan BD, Matsui S et al (1988) Cyclosporine effect on immunoregulatory cells in kidney transplant recipients: suppression of gamma-interferon and interleukin production. *Transplant Proc* 20(Suppl 2):69–74.

Yoshimura N, Oka T, Kahan BD (1991) Sequential determinations of serum interleukin 6 levels as an immunodiagnostic tool to differentiate rejection from nephrotoxicity in renal allograft recipients. *Transplantation* 51:172–176.

Yusa K, Tsuruo T (1989) Reversal mechanism of multidrug resistance by verapamil: direct binding of verapamil to P-glycoprotein on specific sites and transport of verapamil outward across the plasma membrane of K562/ADM cells. *Cancer Res* 49:5002–5006.

Zimmerman JJ, Kahan BD (1997) Pharmacokinetics of sirolimus in stable renal transplant patients after multiple oral dose administration. *J Clin Pharmacol* 37:405–415.

Zucker K, Rosen A, Nichols A et al (1999) A definitive effect of administration of tacrolimus on the pharmacokinetics of mycophenolate mofetil in renal transplant patients (abstract). American Society of Transplant Physicians 18th Annual Meeting, Chicago, May 1999.

8 IMMUNOSUPPRESSIVE DRUGS: MOLECULAR AND CELLULAR MECHANISMS OF ACTION

The development of immunosuppressive agents parallels the progress in our understanding of the cellular and molecular mechanisms that mediate allograft rejection. Initial approaches in this century sought to dampen the immune response using nonselective cytotoxic agents, benzene and toluene, which kill elements of host resistance (Murphy 1914). Based upon the recognition of the importance of lymphocyte proliferation to the development of immunity, the relatively nonselective antimetabolite azathioprine (AZA) and the alkylating agent cyclophosphamide were utilized, followed recently by the more potent drug mycophenolate mofetil (MMF). These agents are nonselective, affecting the proliferation of virtually all cells—a shortcoming that has been remedied in the last two decades by the development of selective T-cell inhibitors that block the synthesis (cyclosporine, CsA, and tacrolimus, TRL), the reception (antiCD25 monoclonal antibodies, MAbs), and the transduction (sirolimus, SRL) of signals generated by cytokine humoral mediators critical to the immune response.

Immunosuppressive agents may be classified based upon their site of action in the cell cycle (Figure 8.1, Table 8.1). Corticosteroids exert a variety of actions, but those most important to transplantation include generalized anti-inflammatory effects, as well as the disruption of antigen presenting cell (APC) functions that are necessary for the initial recognition functions of the immune system. After antigen signal reception, transduction of the message to produce cellular activation during the G_0 to the G_1 phase of the cell cycle is disrupted by the binding of antiCD3 MAb. Thereafter, CsA (or TRL) disrupts the progression of the activation cascade by dampening T-cell production of proinflammatory lymphokines. During the G_1 build-up, antiCD25 MAbs block the binding of interleukin-2 (IL-2) to the α-chain of its heterotrimeric receptor, and SRL (or SDZ RAD) blocks the signal transduction cascade after signal reception. A variety of antiproliferative agents, including AZA and MMF, disrupt nucleoside synthesis required for proliferation, clonal expansion, as well as generation of memory cells. The entire army of T cells may be reduced by monoclonal or polyclonal reagents directed toward surface markers that are relatively restricted to elements of the immune system.

Site	Immunosuppressive agents
Antigen presentation	Steroids
G_0 to G_1	
Signal one	CsA, TRL
Signal two	SRL
G_1 buildup	
Cytokine reception	Anti-IL-2R
Cytokine signal transduction	SRL, SDZ RAD
S	AZA, MMF
Global	ATGAM, thymoglobulin

Table 8.1. Sites of action of immunosuppressive drugs in the cycle of T cell activation

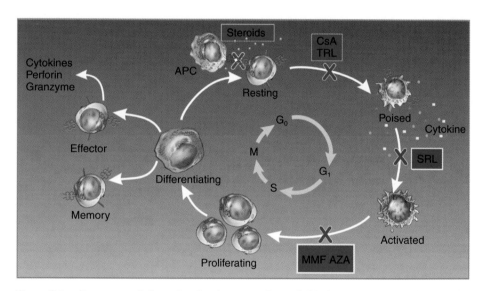

Figure 8.1. Summary of sites of action in presently available immunosuppressive agents.

INHIBITORS OF ANTIGEN RECOGNITION: STEROIDS

Table 8.2 shows three of the autoinflammatory mechanisms of maintenance corticosteroid therapy: namely, to dampen IL-1 and IL-6 costimulatory activity; to dampen the synthesis of proinflammatory molecules—platelet activating factor (PAF), prostaglandins, leukotrienes—as well as the release of tumor necrosis factor-α (TNF-α); to dampen chemotactic, oxygen burst and cytotoxic activities of elements of nonspecific resistance; and to stabilize the membranes of cells regarded as targets of ischemic or immune responses.

Figure 8.2 shows one generally recognized mechanism of action of steroids in all tissues: namely, to stabilize the inhibitory factor IκB, thereby blocking generation of NF-κB, a proinflammatory regulatory factor for cytokine gene transcription. Cortisol binds to cytosolic receptors that are present in variable amounts in different cell types, producing complexes that migrate into the nucleus, therein interacting with specific DNA sequences in a glucocorticoid receptor element (GRE)—that is, a promoter region of specific target genes—thereby modulating their transcription. Head-to-head dimers of steroid–receptor complexes form a loop via a zinc finger binding at one end to the DNA sequence and at the other end to another copy of the receptor (Torchia et al 1997). Three types of interactions can occur between DNA and receptor complexes (Karin 1998): upregulation of gene expression; downregulation of gene expression; or interference with the binding of specific regulatory molecules, such as Jun-Fos, which form the activator protein-1 (AP-1) transcription element. The last mechanism explains the inhibitory effect of steroids on genes that have no obvious GRE regulatory element. Following corticoid binding to receptor, the complex enters the nucleus and interacts with the transcription factor AP-1, preventing its association with nuclear factor of activated T cells (NF-AT) and Oct-1, and thereby deterring promoter functions for proinflammatory cytokines.

As shown in Figure 8.3, glucocorticoids also favor inhibition of NF-κB generation by promoting the induction and stability of IκB. During T-cell activation, IκB kinase

Anti-inflammatory effects on antigen presenting cells (APCs)
I. $\downarrow$ Costimulation factors: IL-1 and IL-6
II. $\downarrow$ Synthesis of platelet activating factor (PAF), prostaglandins, leukotrienes; $\downarrow$ Release of TNF-α
III. $\downarrow$ Chemotactic, O$^-$ burst and cytotoxic response
IV.   Stabilization of target cells

Table 8.2. Corticosteroids: maintenance therapy

317

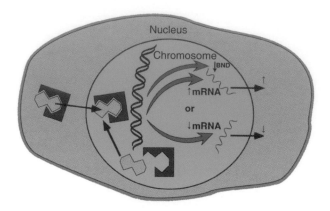

Figure 8.2. Mechanisms of action of steroids on DNA transcription. The steroid binds to a receptor, and the complexes either bind to DNA, enhancing or inhibiting mRNA transcription, or prevent binding of other regulatory proteins (BND).

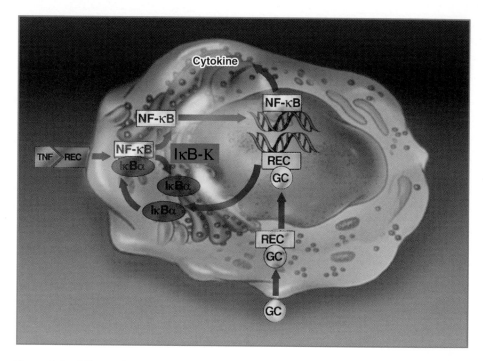

Figure 8.3. Effects of steroids to induce and stabilize IκB, thereby inhibiting the effects of IκB kinase.

phosphorylates IκB, which is ubiquinated and then degraded, thereby releasing NF-κB to migrate into the nucleus. The nuclear localization sequence of NF-κB p65 is masked by its association with IκB or similar sequences (Baeuerle and Baltimore 1996). Proteolytic processing of either IκB or the ankyrin-repeat-containing regions of the p105 precursor allows nuclear entry. The effects of steroids on NF-κB dampen the CD28 costimulation pathway (Fessler et al 1996). Furthermore, steroids inhibit phorbol myristate/ionomycin induction of upregulated expression of CD40 ligand (CD40L), possibly also by interfering with NF-AT generation and binding to DNA sites (Bischof and Melms 1998).

Thus, steroids in maintenance doses exert both transcriptional and nontranscriptional effects. In addition, bolus administration of high doses of steroids alters lymphocyte trafficking, promoting emigration of these cells from the circulation—an effect that, at the time of and shortly after transplantation, is useful to decrease diapedesis into the graft and to direct antigen recognition. In a recent paper, Schmidt et al (1999) found that glucocorticoids promote apoptosis in human monocytes by downregulation of IL-1β and TNF-α.

INHIBITORS OF SIGNAL ONE: T-CELL ACTIVATION AND PROGRESSION FROM G_0 TO G_1

The activation of T cells requires three signals (Figure 8.4). Alloreactive T cells bear specific receptors (TCRs) that bind to a narrow spectrum of antigenic peptides on the surface of APCs. The distinctive variable regions formed by the membrane distal portions of the α- and β-chains provide recognition units that trigger specific T cell clonal proliferation and differentiation (Figure 8.5). The recognition event is transferred from the cell membrane to the cell interior by pertubation of the CD3 membrane complex that comprises five membrane-spanning proteins designated $\gamma\delta\varepsilon\zeta\eta$- or $\zeta\zeta$-chains that initiate a programmed series of phosphorylations of membrane-associated and cytoplasmic kinases. One principal group of enzymes catalyzes the phosphorylation of inositols, leading to a rapid increase in cytosolic calcium via influx through surface channels and via release from intracellular membrane stores. The calcium current activates calmodulin

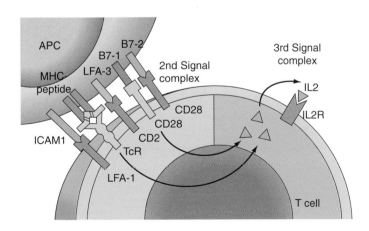

Figure 8.4. Three signals of the immune response: signal one delivered by MHC-peptide to TCR, complemented by ICAM-1/LFA-1 and LFA-3/CD2 co-receptors; signal two by B7–1 and B7–2 to CD28; and signal three by cytokine (IL-2) to its receptor (IL-2R).

319

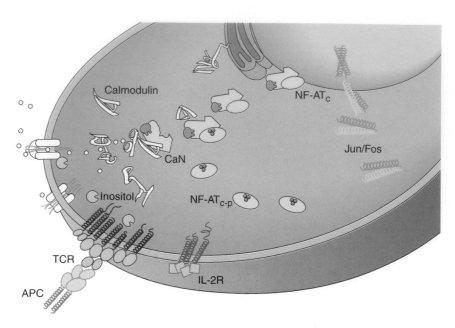

Figure 8.5. T cell receptor (TCR)-mediated signal transduction to generate regulatory proteins.

(CaM), thereby releasing the regulatory activity of the B subunit (CNB) on the catalytic activity of the A subunit (CNA) of the phosphatase calcineurin (CaN).

Among the numerous substrates of CaN is the phosphate-bonded, inactive form of NF-AT. NF-AT, a multimeric complex, promotes the transcription of the cytokine genes encoding IL-2, IL-3, IL-4, IL-5, granulocyte-macrophage-CSF, TNF-α, CD40L, and Fas ligand (FasL) (Crabtree and Clipstone 1994) via cis-acting elements (Crabtree and Clipstone 1994; Rao 1994). Calcium mobilization activates pre-existing cytoplasmic NF-AT proteins. The NF-AT family comprises at least four members: NF-ATp; NF-ATc; NF-AT3; and NF-AT4, all of which interact with the same IL-2 NF-AT binding site (Northrop et al 1994). Members of this family show a conserved, 300-residue NF-AT homology region that mediates DNA binding and protein–protein interactions with AP-1 factors. Specific serine residues in the homology region must be dephosphorylated by CaN. The DNA binding loop is bounded on the N-terminus by a region of moderate homology, and on the C-terminus by a region of minimal homology among the NF-AT family members. At the level of DNA binding, the cytoplasmic NF-AT component interacts with an inducible nuclear component composed of members of the AP-1 family (Jain et al 1992) to produce the effective regulatory complex (Masuda et al 1997). A 15-amino-acid C-terminal sequence flanking the conserved region regulates the trans-activator function of NF-AT (Imamura et al 1998). The N-terminus of NF-AT contains a Ca^{2+}-sensitive inhibitory domain (CRI sequence) at which CaN binds to multiple residues of NF-AT. Interestingly, the binding of NF-AT to CaN is necessary but not sufficient for its transcriptional activation, but is essential for NF-AT

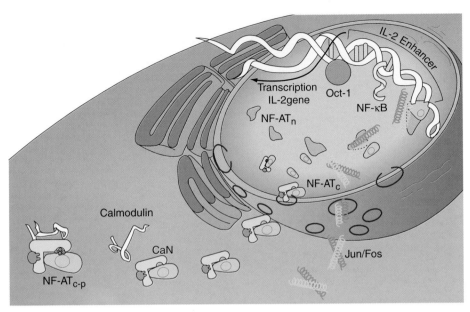

Figure 8.6. The action of NF-AT on the IL-2 gene as an example of the role of regulatory proteins.

nuclear translocation via an amino acid sequence that encodes a nuclear localization signal (Ruff and Leach 1995; Beals et al 1997), which is presumably mediated by the CRI and unmasked by CaN. In both the cytoplasm and the nucleus, CaN remains physically associated with substrate NF-AT, even after dephosphorylation, presumably to prevent enzymatic reversal by the constitutive NF-AT kinase (Shibasaki et al 1996). Genes that encode some isoforms of NF-AT are also present in testis, ovary, skeletal muscle, and kidney, possibly regulating IL-15 generation.

In addition, at least one member of the family—NF-AT4—also bears a nuclear export signal, at which site it is rephosphorylated, triggering an active export process (Kehlenbach et al 1998) that is mediated by Crm-1, an export receptor, via a sequence rich in leucine. Zhu and McKeon (1999) have shown that CaN antagonizes Crm-1-mediated nuclear export by binding to the export site. Whether CaN is necessary to promote DNA binding or to further dephosphorylate NF-AT to maintain its transcriptional activity is uncertain.

Following dephosphorylation of NF-AT, the CNA/B carries the product through the nuclear membrane (Figure 8.6), protecting it from the action of a kinase that actively seeks to rephosphorylate NF-AT. NF-AT serves as the primary regulatory protein, in concert with Oct-1, NF-κB, AP-1, CD28 regulatory sequences, DAP40, and a number of as yet unidentified factors that promote the transcription of proinflammatory cytokines (Figure 8.7). In addition to its critical role in NF-AT activation, CaN activates

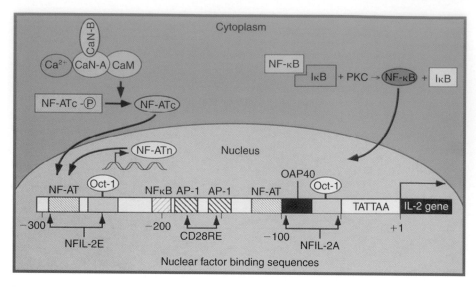

Figure 8.7. The sequence of regulatory binding sequences that promote IL-2 expression.

Jun kinase (Su et al 1994) and AP-1 regulatory proteins (Rincon and Flavell 1994). Two general types of immunosuppressive agents are presently available to disrupt the signal one cascade: the anti-CD3 murine MAb (OKT3), and the CaN inhibitors CsA and TRL.

Anti-CD3 monoclonal antibody

MAbs are produced by hybridomas generated from the fusion of two types of mouse cells: nutrient-dependent plasmacytoma cells and splenic cells that produce an antibody reactive with a specific marker on human lymphocytes. The former cells contribute immortality, and the latter elements, the synthesis of a single antibody of defined specificity.

Muromonab CD3 (Orthoclone OKT3, Ortho Pharmaceutical, Raritan, NJ), a murine MAb of the immunoglobulin (Ig) G_{2a} class, binds to the ε-chain of the CD3 receptor, inducing modulation and immunological inactivation of T cells (Cosimi 1987). The effect is selective, since the CD3 complex serves as a distinctive signal transduction unit, primarily localized on thymus-derived (T) lymphocytes (Hayes 1993). Thus, within minutes of delivery, this MAb produces marked and selective reduction in the numbers of cells displaying CD3, but neither the pan T-cell marker CD2 nor the T-cell subset markers CD4/CD8 (Figure 8.8). The expression of CD3 markers on patient peripheral blood lymphocytes is sought using in vitro addition of fluorescein-conjugated (F*) antiCD3 antibodies. The finding of an only transient decrease in total T cells is

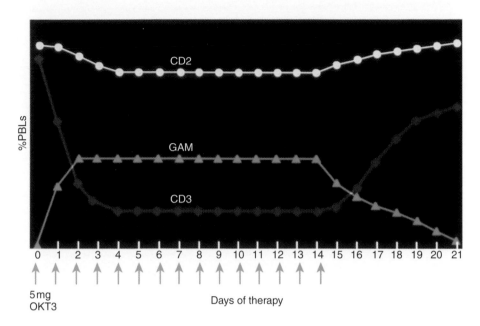

Figure 8.8. Serial enumeration of surface components on the peripheral blood T cells from patients treated with OKT3: CD2 (white line), CD3 (red line), goat anti-mouse antibodies (GAM, green line).

consistent with the hypothesis of CD3 modulation. This modulation phenomenon may be due to antibody-mediated covering of the epitope ('blindfolding'), or to shedding of CD3/OKT3 antigen–antibody complexes into the circulation or their endocytosis into the cell (Figure 8.9a). Following cessation of therapy at day 14, the number of accessible CD3 markers gradually returns toward the baseline value.

A second tool to assess the therapeutic effects of OKT3 is a goat antimouse antibody (GAM) that detects T cells bearing surface complexes of CD3 with mouse OKT3. The difference between the number of CD2$^+$ lymphocytes and the number of GAM-positive cells represents the fraction of 'nude' elements, displaying an absence of surface CD3 markers. This population may reflect cells that have shed or endocytosed OKT3/CD3 complexes, as well as those that display impaired synthesis of or altered expression of CD3-ε (Figure 8.9a).

Calcineurin inhibitors

Figure 8.10 depicts the structures of the drugs that block either the synthesis (CsA and TRL) or the signal transduction (SRL and SDZ RAD) of proinflammatory cytokines. Although CsA ($C_{62}H_{111}O_{112}$, molecular weight 1203) and TRL (molecular weight 729)

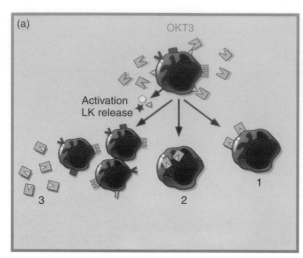
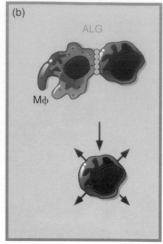

Figure 8.9. Mechanisms of action of various antilymphocyte antibodies. (a) OKT3-(Ⓜ) mediated modulation of CD3 (△) expression: (1) binding producing blindfolding; (2) endocytosis of CD3/OKT3 complexes; (3) shedding of complexes (▨) after activation and lymphokine release. (b) Antilymphocyte globulin (ALG) action to coat host T cells with antibody produces adherence via their Fc receptors, resulting in opsonization by macrophages and T cell digestion.

are structurally distinct, they share a common mechanism of action. CsA, a fungal product of *Tolypocladium inflatum Gams*, which was discovered in a soil sample from Hardanger Vidda in southern Norway, is a cyclic, highly hydrophobic endecapeptide that contains an array of unusual amino acids, including D-alanine at position 8, sarcosine at position 3, and the unique N-methyl-(4R)-4-butenyl-4-methylthreonine at position 1 (Figure 8.10a). Among the 11 amino acids in CsA, seven are N-methylated and 10 are aliphatic, namely, α-aminobutyric acid (position 2), sarcosine (position 3), N-methyl-leucine (positions 4, 6, 9, and 10), valine (position 5), alanine (position 7), D-alanine (position 8), and N-methyl-valine (position 11). TRL (Figure 8.10b), an actinomycete product discovered on Mount Fuji, is a macrocyclic lactone bearing a picolinic structure that is also shared by both SRL (Figure 8.10c) and SDZ RAD (Figure 8.10d). Although their mechanisms of action differ, TRL is structurally related to SRL (or SDZ RAD), since these agents are macrocyclic lactones.

CsA, TRL, and SRL are in fact prodrugs; that is, to gain pharmacologic activity, they must bind to cytoplasmic components termed immunophilins. After binding to the corresponding immunophilin, the agents undergo at least some minor structural conversion (Table 8.3). The immunophilins are cytoplasmic cis-trans prolyl-peptidyl isomerases, namely, cyclophilin (CyP), which binds to CsA, and FK-binding proteins (FKBPs), which bind to TRL and SRL. The drugs seem to enhance the capacity of the immunophilin to bind to and thereby inhibit CaN (Cardenas et al 1994). The CsA-CyP

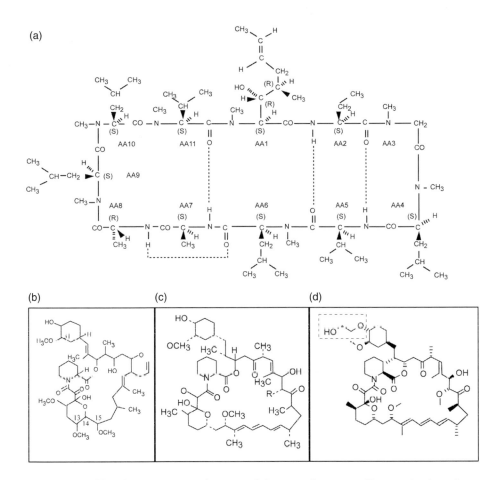

Figure 8.10. Chemical structures of approved drugs to disrupt cytokine synthesis and signal transduction. (a) CsA; (b) TRL; (c) SRL; (d) SDZ RAD. The dotted structure in (d) represents the difference between SDZ RAD and SRL.

(or TRL-FKBP) complexes block T-cell activation by binding to the heterotrimeric association of the phosphatase CNA/B, Ca^{2+}, and CaM 8, forming an inhibitory CyP/CsA/CNA/B, Ca^{2+}, CaM pentameric association (Figure 8.11), which thereby dampens the dephosphorylation (Figure 8.12), transport, and release of NF-AT in the nucleus (Johansson and Moller 1990; Henderson et al 1991).

Other CsA-sensitive CaN substrates include IκB (Frantz et al 1994) Na^+/K^+ ATPase (Apcria et al 1992; Tumlin and Sands 1993), and nitric oxide synthase (Dawson et al 1993). In contrast to their apparent inhibitory effects on the transcription of mRNAs encoding proinflammatory interleukins, CsA and TRL both seem to enhance the expression of transforming growth factor-β (TGF-β), a cytokine that has not only immuno-

325

	CsA	TRL	SRL
Structure	Endecapeptide	Macrocyclic lactone	Macrocyclic lactone
Binding protein	CyP	FKBP12	FKBP12
Enzyme target	CaN	CaN	mTOR
Site of action	G_0 to G_1	G_0 to G_1	G_1 build-up (and G_0 to G_1)

Table 8.3. Comparison of mechanisms of action: cyclosporine, tacrolimus, sirolimus (SDZ RAD)

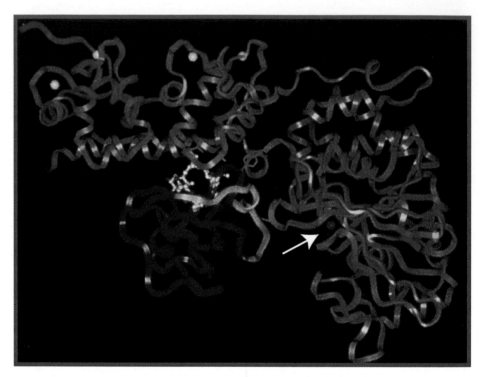

Figure 8.11. Ribbon diagram showing interaction of FKBP12/TRL/CaN. Brown ribbon: calcineurin A; blue ribbon: calcineurin B; red ribbon: FKBP; white structure: TRL; arrow shows the phosphorylation site. (Griffith JP, Kim JL, Kim EE et al. X-ray structure of calcineurin inhibited by the immunophilin-immunosuppressant FKBP12-FK506 complex. *Cell* 1995; **82**(3):507–522. © Cell Press. Reprinted with permission.)

suppressive effects—possibly at least in part mediated by cell cycle arrest in the G_1 phase via upregulated p21 activity (Khanna and Hosenspud 1999)—but also a proclivity to cause renal allograft fibrosis (Suthanthiran et al 1996; Shin et al 1998; Khanna et al 1999). TGF-β stimulates the production of matrix proteins, as well as inhibitors of

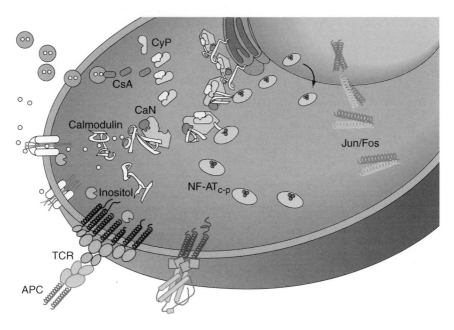

Figure 8.12. Site of action of the calcineurin (CaN) inhibitor CsA.

matrix degradation. In a clinical study, Shihab et al (1996) found increased TGF-β in renal allografts that experienced either acute or chronic rejection. Cuhaci et al (1999) found that 72% of CsA-treated patients displayed high intragraft levels of TGF-β, and that these patients showed a more rapid decline in renal function than patients who displayed low levels.

Attention continues to focus on new formulations to enhance tolerability and activity of CaN inhibitors, including liposomal (Moffat et al 1999) and topical (Tran et al 1999) preparations. The nephrotoxicity of CaN inhibitors has raised intense interest in molecular analogs displaying reduced toxicity.

INHIBITORS OF SIGNAL THREE: CYTOKINE STIMULATION FOR THE G_1 BUILD-UP

Following reception of the signal delivered by immunostimulatory cytokines, T cells progress through the G_1 build-up, a process that includes protein synthesis, further DNA transcription of mRNAs encoding activation factors, and preparation for nucleoside synthesis in the S-phase. The cytokine IL-2 provides a model to understand cytokine-mediated events. IL-2 ligand binds to IL-2 receptors (IL-2R), particularly the

327

(a)

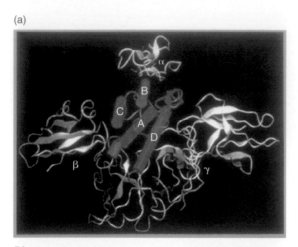

(b)

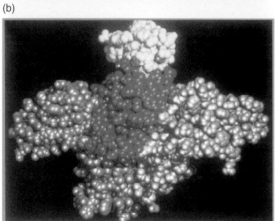

Figure 8.13. Interaction between IL-2 and IL-2R. (a) Ribbon diagram showing α-chain (yellow) binding to the four helices of the IL-2 ligand. (b) Space filling diagram. IL-2 is red; IL-2Rα, yellow; IL-2R β-chain, green; and IL-2R γ-chain, blue.

high-affinity form that includes an α-chain (p55, CD25) bearing a short cytoplasmic tail, a β-chain (p75, CD122) bearing a long tail, and a γ-chain (p65, CD132) bearing a signaling portion of intermediate length (Figure 8.13; Taniguchi and Minami 1993; Sugamura et al 1996).

Interleukin-2 receptor MAb reagents

Expression of the α-chain (CD25) following activation of T lymphocytes produces rapid formation of αβγ heterotrimers, markedly increasing the affinity of the constitutive βγ ligand receptor complexes. Since IL-2Rα is present on only activated and not resting T cells, anti-IL-2R MAbs proffer a more selective class of immunosuppressive agents than antilymphocyte globulins or OKT3, both of which bind to surface markers present on both resting and activated T cells. Furthermore, because the IL-2R α-chain is a polypeptide with only a short cytoplasmic tail, it cannot trigger cellular activation and thus does not elicit the cytokine release syndrome.

Basiliximab (CHI 621, Simulect, Novartis, East Hanover, NJ) and daclizumab (Zenapax, Hoffman-LaRoche, Nutley, NJ) are two anti-IL-2R MAb reagents recently approved by the US Food and Drug Administration (FDA) for prophylaxis of acute rejection episodes in renal transplant recipients. Figure 8.14 compares the structures of the fully xenogeneic mouse parent MAb, of the mouse-human chimeric MAb (basiliximab), and of the humanized MAb (daclizumab). In the chimeric form, the variable portion of the light chains of the antibodies is of murine origin; the remainder of the structure is derived from the constant region of human IgG_1. In contrast, the structure of daclizumab is almost entirely stipulated by human IgG_1, except for the limited murine

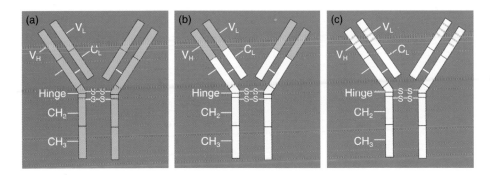

Figure 8.14. Diagrammatic representation of MAbs. (a) Native murine antihuman IL-2R MAb. (b) Chimeric mouse-human MAb. (c) Humanized anti-IL-2R MAb. The orange sections show the murine components, and the white sections, the human components, of the MAbs.

Antibody properties	Basiliximab (Amlot et al 1995)	Daclizumab (Queen et al 1989)
Mouse MAb (isotype; % structure)	RFT2 (2a) 25%	Anti-Tac (2a) 10%
Human backbone (% structure)	IgG_1 (75%)	IgG_1 (90%)
Affinity kD (nM)	0.1	1.0–3.0
MLR IC_{50} (nM)	0.03	0.2
Plasma concentration IL-2R blockade (μg/mL)	0.2	1.0–5.0
% Anti-idiotypic sensitization	0.4	8.4

Table 8.4. Comparison of basiliximab and daclizumab

sequences that encode the three complementary determining regions in the variable portion. Both the chimeric and the humanized IL-2R MAbs display prolonged serum half-lives (Nashan et al 1997; Vincenti et al 1998a), and only rarely evoke neutralizing antibodies (Hakimi et al 1991), probably due to the extensive portion of the structure that is human. However, the two preparations display an important difference: The chimeric antibody is about 10-fold more potent than the humanized one, as shown both by the concentrations necessary to inhibit lymphocyte proliferation in vitro, and by the doses required in vivo to achieve therapeutic effects (Table 8.4; Vincenti et al 1998b; Kahan et al 1999; Nashan et al 1999).

Mammalian target of rapamycin (mTOR) inhibitors

Following membrane reception of the ligand signal, cellular activation in the G_1 phase is mediated by a cascade of kinases (Figure 8.15). Among these enzymes is the phosphatidyl-inositol kinase mTOR, which regulates the phosphorylation status of several sarcoma (src)-like, receptor-type, and cell-cycle-dependent kinases, as well as intracellular phosphatases. One important molecular target of mTOR is the $p70^{S6}$ (but not the $p85^{S6}$) mitogen-activated protein kinase (MAPK). Both the $p70^{S6}$ and the $p85^{S6}$ MAPKs hyperphosphorylate the 40S ribosomal protein S6, an essential step in G_1 progression. Inhibition of this hyperphosphorylation occurs at the same concentrations as those required for SRL to block cell proliferation (Brown et al 1994, 1995; Figure 8.16). A probable second target of mTOR is $p27^{kip}$, the degradation of which activates downstream serine-threonine protein kinases ($p34^{cdc2}$) and generates two factors that control the rate of T cell progression into the S-phase of the cell cycle: namely, the active $p34^{cdc2}$-cyclin D heterodimers that form the critical 'maturational promoting factor', and the cyclin-dependent kinase cdk2, which is the catalytic partner of cyclin E. Third, mTOR triggers degradation of PHAS-1, releasing the elongation factor EIF4, which is necessary for protein translation on ribosomes. Interestingly, mTOR seems to have a fourth target: namely, c-Rel activity, which thereby activates NF-κB in the costimulatory pathway of G_0 to G_1 activation.

Sirolimus

Sirolimus (SRL, $C_{51}H_{79}NO_{13}$, rapamycin, RAPA, Rapamune; Wyeth-Ayerst, Princeton, NJ) is a macrocyclic lactone product of *Streptomyces hygroscopicus*, which was discovered in the soil of the Vai Atari region of Rapa Nui (Easter Island; Sehgal et al 1975; Vezina et al 1975; Figure 8.10c). Sirolimus not only prolongs allograft survival in animal models (Calne et al 1989; Morris et al 1990; Stepkowski et al 1991), but also interacts synergistically with CsA (Kahan et al 1991). SDZ RAD (Figure 8.10d), 40-O-(2-hydroxyethyl)-rapamycin ($C_{531}H_{83}NO_{14}$, SDZ RAD, Novartis, East Hanover, NJ), is a structural analog of SRL that also displays a synergistic interaction with CsA, both in

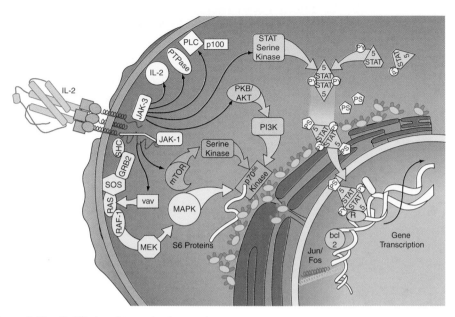

Figure 8.15. IL-2R signal transduction pathways.

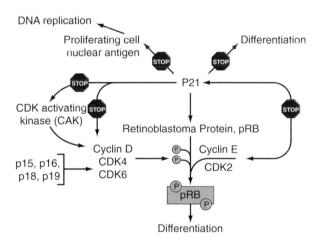

Figure 8.16. Effects of SRL to disrupt G_1 cell cycle progression.

vitro and in vivo, in animal models (Schuurman et al 1997). However, SDZ RAD seems to display a two- to three-fold lower immunosuppressive potency than SRL in vitro and in heart transplant models, possibly due to a lower affinity of SDZ RAD for FKBP12, a difference that may be at least partially offset by the improved absorption of the more hydrophilic analog SDZ RAD (Schuler et al 1997).

331

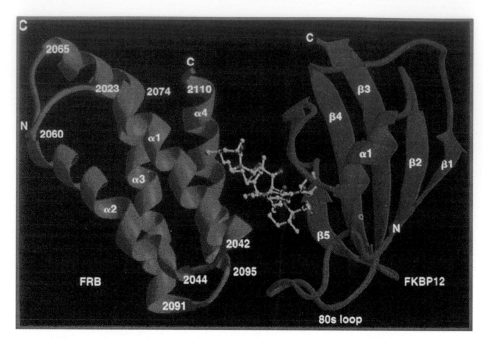

Figure 8.17. Ribbon diagram showing SRL as a bridge between FKBP12 and the mammalian target of rapamycin (mTOR). The FKBP12 is shown in blue; SRL, green; and mTOR (FRB, FK-RAPA binding protein), red.

SRL blocks both Ca^{2+}-dependent and Ca^{2+}-independent events, including transduction of signals delivered by the lymphokines IL-2, IL-4, IL-7, and IL-15, as well as, to a lesser degree, by the nonlymphoid cytokines fibroblast growth factor (FGF), stem cell factor, platelet-derived growth factor (PDGF), colony stimulating factor (CSF), and insulin growth factor (IGF). SRL undergoes little modification in the cytoplasm upon forming the inhibitory drug–immunophilin complexes with FKBP12 (Kuo et al 1992), and thereafter crosslinking to mTOR (Figure 8.17), thus blocking activation of p70[S6] kinase, increasing the stability of p27[kip], and inhibiting generation of the elongation factor EIF4 in T cells. In addition to its multiple effects on T-cell maturation, SRL exerts unique actions on B cells, including inhibition of Ig isoform switching (Ferraresso et al 1994).

The combination of CsA to inhibit cytokine synthesis, anti-IL-2R MAbs to block IL-2 reception, and SRL to inhibit signal transduction forms the cytokine paradigm (Figure 8.18). While the interaction of CsA with anti-IL-2R seems to be only additive, that between CsA and SRL is synergistic. Hitchings (1973) convincingly demonstrated the principle of therapeutic synergism using the combination of sulfa, which blocks the conjugation by microorganisms of pteridine and para-amino benzoic acid to form dihydrofolate, and trimethoprim, which inhibits the action of folate reductase to form

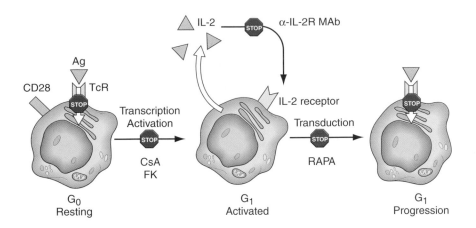

Figure 8.18. The cytokine paradigm.

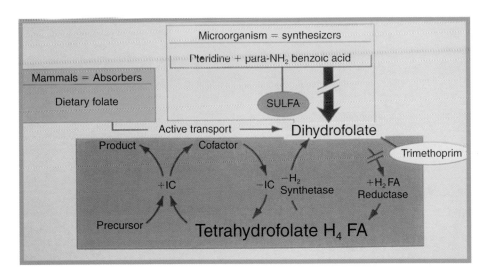

Figure 8.19. Molecular mechanism of synergy of the sulfa-trimethoprim combination.

tetrahydrofolate (Figure 8.19). The synergistic interaction not only broadened the therapeutic spectrum of the combination, but also permitted the use of reduced amounts of each drug, thereby mitigating the toxicity. Using the rigorous median effect analysis (Chou 1991), SRL and CsA were shown to display a synergistic interaction both in vitro, providing inhibition of mitogen- or alloantigen- or cytokine-driven lymphoprolif-

(a)

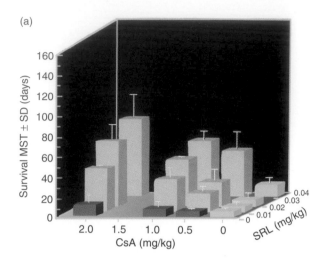

(b)

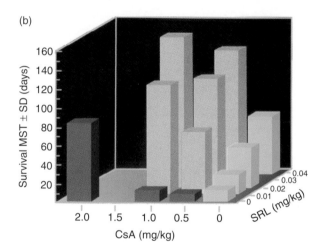

Figure 8.20. Synergistic interaction between CsA and SRL. (a) Effects on heart allografts. (b) Effects on kidney allografts. Red bars indicate effects of CsA alone; blue bars, SRL alone; yellow bars, the CsA plus SRL combination groups. (Stepkowski SM, Tian L, Napoli KL et al. Synergistic mechanisms by which sirolimus and cyclosporin inhibit rat heart and kidney allograft rejection. *Clin Exp Immunol* 1997 Apr; **108**(1):63–68. © 1997 Blackwell Science Ltd. Reprinted with permission.)

eration (Kahan et al 1991), and in vivo, markedly prolonging the survival of cardiac, renal, small bowel, liver, and pancreatico-duodenal allografts (Stepkowski et al 1991). Figure 8.20 illustrates two sets of in vivo data documenting the synergistic interaction between CsA and SRL (Stepkowski et al 1997). A 14-day course of gavage administration of CsA alone (0.5, 1.0, or 2.0 mg/kg) or SRL alone (0.01, 0.02, 0.04 mg/kg per day) only modestly prolonged the mean survival times of cardiac allografts exchanged between histoincompatible rats, namely, from 7 to 13 days. In contrast, combination of the two agents (Figure 8.20a) markedly accentuated the effect, providing a 93-day survival. Similar results were obtained with kidney allografts (Stepkowski et al 1997; Figure 8.20b).

This synergistic effect seems to occur due to both pharmacokinetic and pharmaco-

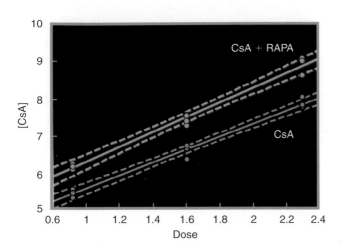

Figure 8.21. Impact of SRL coadministration on whole blood CsA concentrations. CsA concentrations as a function of dose in hosts treated with CsA alone (green line) or with CsA-SRL combination (orange line).

dynamic interactions of SRL and CsA. The pharmacokinetic interaction, which is probably due to mutual inhibition of cytochrome P450 3A4 activity (Figure 8.21; Stepkowski et al 1997), occurs most conspicuously at high concentrations and may be offset by expressing the exposure to each drug not as the dose, but as the whole blood drug concentration. Thus, the rational use of the CsA-SRL combination demands concentration measurements.

Even after compensating for the pharmacokinetic interaction by concentration control, it is possible to demonstrate a pharmacodynamic interaction, which is due to at least two components. First, the actions of CsA to interrupt the generation of NF AT-mediated cytokine gene transcription complement the effects of SRL to inhibit the co-stimulation cascade of c-Rel activity necessary to generate NF-κB, thereby potentiating the inhibitory effect of CsA on cytokine mRNA expression (Figure 8.22; Tian et al 1997). Since concordant action of signal one and signal two is essential for full activation in the G_0 to G_1 transition, the inhibitory effects of SRL on signal two enhance CsA-mediated inhibition of the signal one cascade. Second, the action of CsA to reduce the synthesis of proinflammatory cytokines (particularly IL-2, but also IFN-γ, IL-10, or IL-4) complements the sequential action of SRL to inhibit signal transduction during the G_1 build-up. (Figure 8.23).

In contrast to the uniformly synergistic interactions between CsA and SRL, coadministration of the two macrocyclic lactones TRL and SRL yields inconsistent results. In vitro assays suggest an antagonistic interaction (Dumont et al 1990), while in vivo studies claim that the effects are more than additive, based upon prolongation of the survival of rat or mouse heart tissue allografts (Vu et al 1997; Chen et al 1998), and of human liver allografts. Unfortunately, these studies did not combine simultaneous parent drug concentration measurements to assess the contribution of pharmacokinetic interactions to the apparent prolongation of graft survival. Clearly, a final assessment

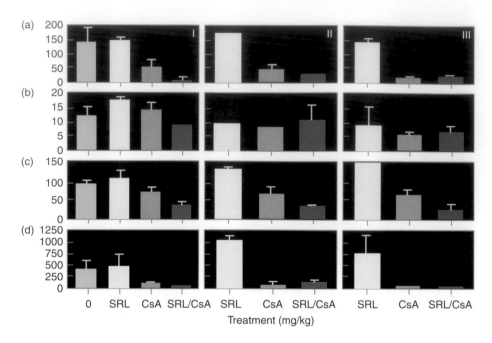

Figure 8.22. Cytokine mRNA transcription by lymphocytes derived from hosts treated with different immunosuppressive regimens. The measured cytokines (in fentograms) included (a) IL-10, (b) IL-4, (c) IL-2, and (d) IFN-γ. Host treatment regimens for 2 weeks were no drug(s) (blue); SRL 0.02 mg/kg per day (yellow); CsA 1.0 mg/kg per day (orange); and SRL 0.02 mg/kg per day plus CsA 1.0 mg/kg per day (red) in panel I. The same SRL doses with CsA 2.0 mg/kg per day are shown in panel II, and with CsA 4.0 mg/kg per day in panel III. (Reprinted from *Transpl Immunol* **5**, Tian L, Stepkowski SM, Qu X, Wang ME, Wang M, Yu J, Kahan BD, Cytokine mRNA expression in tolerant heart allografts after immunosuppression with cyclosporine, sirolimus or brequinar, pages 189–198. © 1997, with permission from Elsevier Science.)

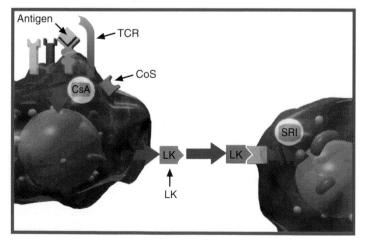

Figure 8.23. Sequential actions of CsA in the G_0 to G_1 transition and of SRL in the G_1 build-up.

must await clinical trials comparing a TRL–SRL regimen to the well-documented effects of the synergistic CsA–SRL combination. Of some concern is the fact that Vu et al (1998) also claimed a synergistic interaction between SRL and MMF (without drug measurements to compensate for a likely pharmacokinetic interaction). A recent European multicenter study contradicted this finding, showing better rejection prophylaxis with the combination of SRL–AZA–prednisone (Pred) than with SRL-MMF-Pred (H Kreis, unpublished work).

INHIBITORS OF THE S-PHASE: ANTIPROLIFERATIVE AGENTS

One of the first observed characteristics of alloimmune responses was marked lymphocyte proliferation, which increases the number of specifically reactive cells. The first therapeutic strategy to interrupt cell proliferation in the immune cascade was thus sublethal total-body irradiation (TBI), which damages the DNA of rapidly dividing tissues. Although a few kidneys from nonidentical twins were successfully engrafted using TBI, as reported by Hamburger (1959) in Paris and by Merrill et al (1960) in Boston, the procedure was rapidly abandoned due to its irreversible effects and high rates of morbidity and mortality (Hamburger et al 1959). Conditioning of the recipient by total lymphoid irradiation—a modified strategy that focuses treatment on lymphoid elements as opposed to bone marrow—showed encouraging results in a single-center trial (Levin et al 1985); however, the technique is too cumbersome for routine application, due to the needs both for fractionated treatments, and for completion of the treatment prior to transplant with only a 2-week window of immunosuppression.

The modern era of immunosuppression began with the use of the antiproliferative drug, 6-mercaptopurine (6-MP; Purinethol, Burroughs-Wellcome, UK; Figure 8.20a). In 1959, Schwartz and Damashek (1959) demonstrated that 6-MP inhibited antibody production by rabbits injected with bovine serum albumin. The nitroimidazole-derivative of 6-MP, AZA, was developed by Hitchings and Elion to avert the susceptibility of the unshielded mercapto-group to gut hydrolysis. AZA displays a more consistent bioavailability than the parent compound, yielding more-reproducible immunosuppression (Calne et al 1962). On the one hand, attempts to improve immunosuppressive efficacy with the alkylating agent cyclophosphamide (Fox 1964; Starzl et al 1971) or the pyrimidine synthesis inhibitor brequinar (Joshi et al 1997) have realized only a low level of efficacy relative to the toxicity of these drugs. On the other hand, more selective inhibitors of the purine synthesis, MMF and its mechanistic analog, mizorbine (MZB), have proved useful in clinical practice.

Figure 8.24 shows the sites of action of the five antiproliferative immunosuppressive agents that interrupt the S-phase of cell-cycle progression. AZA blocks steps both before and after generation of inosinic acid monophosphate (IMP), whereas MPA acts selectively to inhibit IMP dehydrogenase (IMPDH), thus reducing production of xanthylic

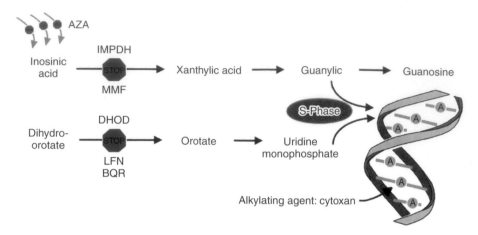

Figure 8.24. Sites of action of antiproliferative immunosuppressive agents.

acid, and, subsequently, guanylic acid (GA) and guanosine monophosphate (GMP). In the biosynthetic pathway for pyrimidines, two drugs that have not been approved by the US FDA, namely, leflunomide and brequinar, inhibit dihydro-orotate dehydrogenase (DHOD) conversion of dihydro-orotic acid to orotic acid and, subsequently, to uridine monophosphate. Another agent that disrupts the S-phase is the alkylating agent cyclophosphamide, which crosslinks and thereby prevents the separation of DNA strands, a step that is necessary for cell replication.

Azathioprine

The nitroimidazole derivative of 6-MP, azathioprine (AZA, Imuran, Glaxo-Wellcome, Greenford, UK) acts as a competitive inhibitor of both the de novo and salvage pathways of nucleoside synthesis (see Chapter 7). Within the cell, AZA is converted by hypoxanthine-guanine phosphoribosyl transferase (HGPRT) to 6-thioinosinic acid monophosphate (TIMP; Winkelstein 1979), which is metabolized to 6-thioxanthylic acid by inosine monophosphate dehydrogenase. Thioxanthylic acid is then converted to thioguanine monophosphate by GMP synthetase (Bertino 1973). Furthermore, the presence of TIMP, an analog of IMP, activates a negative feedback circuit that limits additional production of IMP from its precursors. In addition to the effects on IMPDH, TIMP inhibits phosphoribosyl-pyrophosphate aminotransferase, the first step in the de novo synthesis of purines, thereby reducing the synthesis of adenyl-succinic acid monophosphate and xanthylic acid monophosphate, which are precursors of adenine monophosphate and guanidine monophosphate, respectively. Thiopurine methyl transferase activity displays a negative correlation with erythrocyte 6-thioguanine (TGN) levels (Lennard et al 1987). Similar to other purines, the thiopurine intermediates are converted by xanthine oxidase, which is present in many tissues, particularly the liver, to 6-thiouric acid, which is eliminated in the urine. Also, methylation of 6-MP or of 6-thioinosinic acid by TPMT produces 6-methyl-mercaptopurine, as well as small amounts of TGN, the primary active metabolite of AZA (Lennard and Maddocks 1983). Both of these products may be directly incorporated into nucleic acids as fraudulent bases (Chan et al 1987), leading to chromosomal breakage, nucleic acid distortion, interference with DNA repair (Elion 1967; Tidd and Paterson 1974), and an increased proclivity to malignant cell transformation as well as to benign papillomatosis.

Mycophenolate mofetil

Mycophenolate mofetil (MMF, CellCept, RS-61443; Roche Laboratories, Nutley, NJ) is a synthetic derivative of mycophenolic acid (MPA), which is produced by the mold *Penicillium glaucum*. Although initially studied for its antibiotic and antiviral properties, MPA (Figure 8.25c) was later shown to display immunosuppressive activity in experimental (Mitsui and Suzuki 1969; Morris et al 1991) as well as clinical (Sollinger 1995) transplantation. In a canine model, the combination of MMF with CsA prolonged allograft survival more potently than either agent alone (Platz et al 1991), although the interaction between CsA and MMF has been subsequently shown both in vitro and in vivo to be only additive. In 1995, the US FDA approved MMF as an agent superior to AZA for adjunctive use with CsA for the prevention of acute renal allograft rejection episodes.

MMF interferes with purine synthesis by acting as a noncompetitive, reversible inhibitor of IMPDH (allegedly specific for the type II isoform) and of guanylate synthetase (Allison and Eugui 1996; Lowe et al 1997). MMF binds to the site designated for the oxidized form of nicotinamide adenine dinucleotide (NAD$^+$), thereby preventing conversion of inosine monophosphate (IMP) to xanthine monophosphate (XMP; Fleming et al 1996; Makara et al 1996). This inhibition results in intracellular depletion of guanosine, but not adenosine, nucleotides, thereby halting the progression of activated T and B cells during the S-phase of the cell cycle (Natsumeda and Carr 1993; Allison and Eugui 1996).

GLOBAL AGENTS FOR IMMUNODEPRESSION: DEPLETING ANTIBODIES

The depletion paradigm is based upon the basic science observations that T lymphocytes play a critical role in the development of both cellular and antibody-mediated alloimmune responses. Xenogeneic polyclonal horse and rabbit antihuman lymphocyte sera

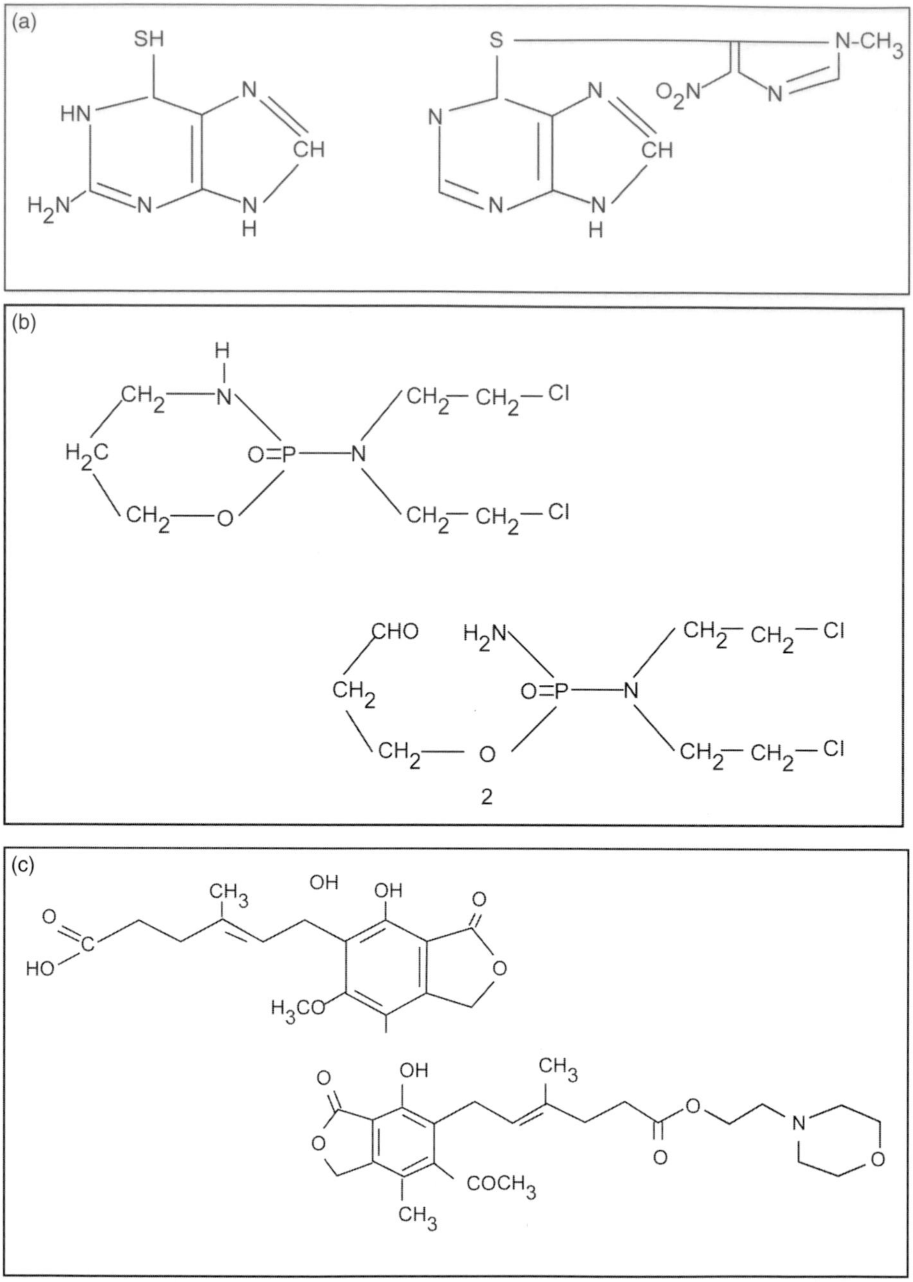

Figure 8.25. Structures of antiproliferative agents. (a) 6-MP (left) and AZA (right). (b) Cyclophosphamide (top) and its active intermediate aldophosphamide (bottom) generated by hepatic cytochrome p450 metabolism. (c) MPA (top) and MMF (bottom).

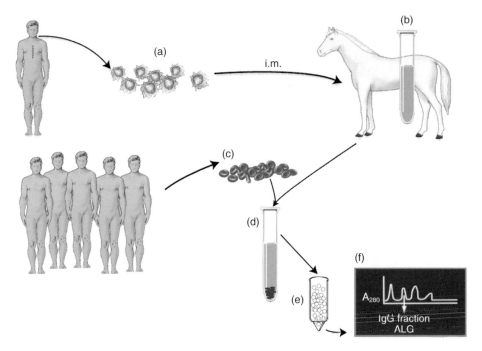

Figure 8.26. Production of equine antihuman lymphocyte globulin. (a) Human thymocytes are harvested from thymus samples at the time of cardiac surgery. (b) Production of crude antiserum in horses. (c) Adsorption of serum with erythrocytes from a panel of donors. (d) Elution from ion exchange chromatography. (e) Elution profile showing IgG fraction (f).

(ALS) have been used to deplete T and/or B cells (Anderson et al 1967; Russell and Monaco 1967; Starzl et al 1967; Najarian et al 1970) in the fashion originally described by Metchnikoff (1899) a century ago. While particularly useful to reverse acute rejection episodes (Starzl et al 1967; Najarian et al 1970), these agents display a narrow therapeutic window and a proclivity toward intense T-cell inhibition. This excessive immunosuppression increases the incidence and severity of opportunistic infections, particularly cytomegalovirus (CMV) infections and lymphomas, far beyond those observed under maintenance drug regimens.

Antihuman polyclonal antibodies were first prepared for clinical use in horses (Figure 8.26; Starzl et al 1967) and were followed by the development of more potent preparations in rabbits. The two polyclonal antibody preparations currently available in the US are ATGAM (Pharmacia-Upjohn, Kalamazoo, MI), a horse antihuman thymocyte globulin, and the recently approved thymoglobulin (Sangstat, Menlo Park, CA), a rabbit antihuman thymocyte globulin. The antibody moieties within the preparations bind to a variety of lymphocyte cell surface receptors (Figure 8.9b). This coating of the cell

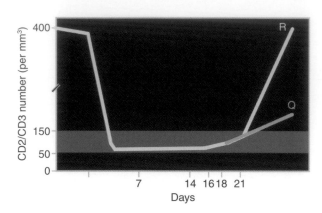

Figure 8.27. Profile of peripheral blood lymphocyte markers during ATGAM therapy. The number of CD2$^+$ or CD3$^+$ cells is determined using a fluoresceinated antibody; the blue band shows the therapeutic range, 50–150 T cells/mm^3. Upon completion of treatment, the cell counts during the recovery phase may forecast a recurrent rejection (R) or a quiescent course (Q).

prepares it for digestion (opsonization) via complement-mediated lysis or reticulo-endothelial cell-dependent phagocytosis. The therapeutic effect of profound immunosuppression is achieved when the T-lymphocyte count is reduced to 150 T cells/mm^3, as evidenced by enumeration of CD2$^+$ lymphocytes using a fluoresceinated antibody in the flow cytometer. Reduction of peripheral T-cell counts to no more than 50 cells/mm^3 is accompanied by the side-effects associated with severe immunosuppression. During antilymphocyte therapy, the number of peripheral blood leukocytes markedly decreases. Upon completion of the course, serial measurements of total T cells can be used to identify patients likely to experience recurrent rejection versus those likely to follow a quiescent course (Figure 8.27).

CONCLUSION

The array of available immunosuppressive agents provides a battery to attack the immune system at several sites. Steroids disrupt antigen recognition and provide a general dampening of the immune response. While no approved agent is presently available to block T-cell receptor function, the transduction of the membrane signal to produce cytoplasmic activation is inhibited by OKT3 binding of CD3ε. The activation pathway generated by antigen (signal one) is disrupted by inhibition of CaN either by CsA or TRL). The costimulatory activation (signal two) is dampened by SRL. Critical signal three stimulation by cytokines may be blockaded by anti-CD25 MAbs and interrupted by mTOR inhibition by SRL (or SDZ RAD). The use of global immunodepressants, specifically polyclonal antilymphocyte antibodies, seeks to harness the immune response at both ends of the therapeutic spectrum: induction therapy and anti-rejection treatment.

REFERENCES

Allison AC, Eugui EM (1996) Purine metabolism and immunosuppressive effects of mycophenolate mofetil (MMF). *Clin Transplant* **10**:77.

Amlot PL, Rawlings E, Fernando ON et al (1995) Prolonged action of a chimeric interleukin-2 receptor (CD25) monoclonal antibody used in cadaveric renal transplantation. *Transplantation* **60**:748–756.

Anderson NF, James K, Woodruff MF (1967) Effect of antilymphocytic antibody and antibody fragments on skin-homograft survival and the blood-lymphocyte count in rats. *Lancet* **i**:1126–1128.

Aperia A, Ibarra F, Svensson LB et al (1992) Calcineurin mediates a-adrenergic stimulation of Na$^+$, K$^+$-ATPase activity in renal tubule cells. *Proc Natl Acad Sci USA* **89**:7394–7397.

Baeuerle PA, Baltimore D (1996) NF-κB: ten years after. *Cell* **87**:13–20.

Beals CR, Clipstone NA, Ho SN, Crabtree GR (1997) Nuclear localization of NF-ATc by a calcineurin-dependent, cyclosporin-sensitive intramolecular interaction. *Gene Dev* **11**:824–834.

Bertino JR (1973) Chemical action and pharmacology of methotrexate, azathioprine, and cyclophosphamide in man. *Arthritis Rheum* **16**:79–83.

Bischof F, Melms A (1998) Glucocorticoids inhibit CD40 ligand expression of peripheral CD4$^+$ lymphocytes. *Cell Immunol* **187**:38–44.

Brown EJ, Albers MW, Shin TB et al (1994) A mammalian protein targeted by G1-arresting-rapamycin-receptor complex. *Nature* **369**:756–758.

Brown EJ, Beal PA, Keith CT et al (1995) Control of p70 s6 kinase by kinase activity of FRAP in vivo. *Nature* **377**:441–446.

Calne RY, Alexandre GP, Murray JE (1962) A study of the effects of drugs in prolonging survival of homologous renal transplants in dogs. *Ann NY Acad Sci* **99**:743–7461.

Calne RY, Collier DS, Lim S et al (1989) Rapamycin for immunosuppression in organ allografting. *Lancet* **ii**:227.

Cardenas ME, Hemenway C, Muir RS et al (1994) Immunophilins interact with calcineurin in the absence of exogenous immunosuppressive ligands. *EMBO J* **13**:5944–5957.

Chan GLC, Canafax DM, Johnson CA (1987) The therapeutic use of azathioprine in renal transplantation. *Pharmacotherapy* **7**:165–177.

Chen H, Qi S, Xu D et al (1998) Combined effect of rapamycin and FK506 in prolongation of small bowel graft survival in the mouse. *Transplant Proc* **30**:2579–2581.

Chou T-C (1991) The median-effect principle and the combination index for quantitation of synergism and antagonism. In: Chou T-C, Rideout DC (eds). *Synergism and Antagonism in Chemotherapy*. San Diego: Academic Press, pp. 61–102.

Cosimi AB (1987) Clinical development of orthoclone OKT3. *Transplant Proc* **14**(Suppl 1):7–16.

Crabtree GR, Clipstone NA (1994) Signal transmission between the plasma membrane and nucleus of T lymphocytes. *Ann Rev Biochem* **63**:1045–1083.

Cuhaci B, Kumar MSA, Bloom RD et al (1999) Transforming growth factor-β levels in human allograft chronic fibrosis correlate with rate of decline in renal function. *Transplantation* **68**:785–780.

Dawson TM, Steiner JP, Dawson VL et al (1993) Immunosuppressant FK506 enhances phosphorylation of nitric oxide synthase and protects against glutamate neurotoxicity. *Proc Natl Acad Sci USA* **90**:9808–9812.

Dumont FJ, Melino MR, Staruch MJ et al (1990) The immunosuppressive macrolides FK506 and rapamycin act as reciprocal antagonist in murine T cells. *J Immunol* **144**:1418–1424.

Elion GB (1967) Biochemistry and pharmacology of purine analogs. *Fed Proc* **26**:898–904.

Ferraresso M, Tian L, Ghobrial R et al (1994) Rapamycin inhibits production of cytotoxic but not noncytotoxic antibodies and preferentially activates TH2 cells that mediate long-term survival of heart allografts in rats. *J Immunol* 153:3307–3318.

Fessler BJ, Paliogianni F, Hama N et al (1996) Glucocorticoids modulate CD28 mediated pathways for interleukin 2 production in human T cells: evidence for posttranscriptional regulation. *Transplantation* 62:1113–1118.

Fleming MA, Chambers SP, Connelly PR et al (1996) Inhibition of IMPDH by mycophenolic acid: dissection of forward and reverse pathways using capillary electrophoresis. *Biochemistry* 35:6990–6997.

Fox M (1964) Suppression of tissue immunity by cyclophosphamide. *Transplantation* 2:475–486.

Frantz B, Nordby EC, Bren G et al (1994) Calcineurin acts in synergy with PMA to inactivate IκB/MAD3, an inhibitor of NF-κB. *EMBO J* 13:861–870.

Griffith JP, Kim JL, Kim EE et al (1995) X-ray structure of calcineurin inhibited by the immunophilin-immunosuppressant FKBP12-FK506 complex. *Cell* 82:507–522.

Hakimi J, Chizzonite R, Luke DR et al (1991) Reduced immunogenicity and improved pharmacokinetics of humanized anti-Tac in cynomolgus monkeys. *J Immunol* 147:1352–1359.

Hamburger J, Vayesse J, Crosnier J (1959) Transplantation of kidney between nonhomozygotic twins after irradiation of the recipient. *Presse Med* 67:1771.

Hayes JM (1993) The immunobiology and clinical use of current immunosuppressive therapy for renal transplantation. *J Urol* 149:437–448.

Henderson DJ, Naya I, Bundick RV et al (1991) Comparison of the effects of FK506, cyclosporine A, and rapamycin on IL-2 productions. *Immunology* 73:316–321.

Hitchings GH (1973) Biochemical background of trimethoprim-sulphamethoxazole. *Med J Aust* 1(Suppl):5–9.

Imamura R, Masuda ES, Naito Y et al (1998) Carboxyl-terminal 15-amino acid sequence of NFATx1 is possibly created by tissue-specific splicing and is essential for transactivation activity in T cells. *J Immunol* 161:3455–3463.

Jain J, McCaffrey PG, Valge AV, Rao A (1992) Nuclear factor of activated T cells contains Fos and Jun. *Nature* 356:801–804.

Johansson A, Moller E (1990) Evidence that the immunosuppressive effects of FK506 and cyclosporine are identical. *Transplantation* 50:1001–1007.

Joshi AS, King SYP, Zajac BA et al (1997) Phase I safety and pharmacokinetic studies of brequinar sodium after single ascending oral doses in stable renal, hepatic and cardiac allograft recipients. *J Clin Pharmacol* 37:1121–1128.

Kahan BD, Gibbons S, Tejpal N et al (1991) Synergistic interactions of cyclosporine and rapamycin to inhibit immune performances of normal human peripheral blood lymphocytes in vitro. *Transplantation* 51:185–191.

Kahan BD, Rajagopalan PR, Hall ML, for the United States Simulect Renal Study Group (1999) Reduction of the occurrence of acute cellular rejection among renal allograft recipients treated with basiliximab, a chimeric anti-interleukin-2-receptor monoclonal antibody. *Transplantation* 67:276–284.

Karin M (1998) New twists in gene regulation by glucocorticoid receptor: is DNA binding dispensable? *Cell* 93:487–490.

Kehlenback RH, Dickmanns A, Gerace L (1998) Nucleocytoplasmic shuttling factors including Ran and CRM1 mediate nuclear export of NFAT in vitro. *J Cell Biol* 141:863–874.

Khanna AK, Hosenspud JD (1999) Cyclosporine induces the expression of the cyclin inhibitor p21. *Transplantation* 67:1262–1268.

Khanna A, Cairns V, Hosenspud JD (1999) Tacrolimus induces increased expression of transforming growth factor-b1 in mammalian lymphoid as well as nonlymphoid cells. *Transplantation* 67:614–619.

Kuo CJ, Chung J, Fiorentino DF et al (1992) Rapamycin selectively inhibits interleukin-2 activation of p70 S6 kinase. *Nature* 358:70–73.

Lennard L, Maddocks JL (1983) Assay of 6-thioguanine nucleotide, a major metabolite of aza-thioprine, 6-mercaptopurine and 6-thioguanine in human red blood cells. *J Pharmacol* **35**:15–18.

Lennard L, Van Loon JA, Lilleyman JS, Weinshilboum RM (1987) Thiopurine pharmacogenetics in leukemia: correlation of erythrocyte thiopurine methyltransferase activity and 6-thioguanine nucleotide concentrations. *Clin Pharmacol Ther* **41**:18–25.

Levin B, Hoppe RT, Collins G et al (1985) Treatment of cadaveric renal transplant recipients with total lymphoid irradiation, antithymocyte globulin, and low-dose prednisone. *Lancet* **ii**:1321–1325.

Lowe JK, Brox L, Henderson JF (1997) Consequences of inhibition of guanine nucleoside synthesis by mycophenolic acid and virazole. *Cancer Res* **37**:736–743.

Makara GM, Keseru GM, Katjar-Peredy M, Anderson WK (1996) Nuclear magnetic resonance and molecular modeling study on mycophenolic acid: implications for binding to inosine monophosphate dehydrogenase. *J Med Chem* **30**:1236–1242.

Masuda ES, Liu J, Imamura R et al (1997) Control of NFATx1 nuclear translocation by a calcineurin-regulated inhibitory domain. *Mol Cell Biol* **17**:2066–2075.

Merrill JP, Murray JE, Harrison H et al (1960) Successful homotransplantation of the kidney between nonidentical twins. *N Engl J Med* **262**:1251–1260.

Metchinkoff E (1899) Etude sur la resorption des cellules. *Ann Inst Pasteur* **13**:737–769.

Mitsui A, Suzuki S (1969) Immunosuppressive effect of mycophenolic acid. *J Antibiot (Tokyo)* **22**:358–363.

Moffat SD, McAlister V, Calne RY, Metcalfe SM (1999) Potential for improved therapeutic index of FK506 in liposomal formulation demonstrated in a mouse cardiac allograft model. *Transplantation* **67**:1205–1208.

Morris RE, Wu J, Shorthouse R (1990) A study of the contrasting effects of cyclosporine, FK 506, and rapamycin on the suppression of allograft rejection. *Transplant Proc* **22**:1638–1641.

Morris RE, Wang J, Blum JR et al (1991) Immunosuppressive effects of the morpholinoethyl ester of mycophenolic acid (RS-61443) in rat and nonhuman primate recipients of heart allografts. *Transplant Proc* **23**(Suppl 2):19–25.

Murphy JB (1914) Heteroplastic tissue grafting effected through roentgen ray lymphoid destruction. *JAMA* **62**:1459.

Najarian JS, Simmons RL, Gewurz H et al (1970) Anti-human lymphoblast globulin. *Fed Proc* **29**:197–201.

Nashan B, Moore R, Amlot P et al (1997) Randomized trial of basiliximab versus placebo for control of acute cellular rejection in renal allograft recipients. *Lancet* **350**:1193–1198.

Nashan B, Light S, Hardie IR et al (1999) Reduction of acute renal allograft rejection by daclizumab. Daclizumab Double Therapy Study Group. *Transplantation* **67**:110–115.

Natsumeda Y, Carr SF (1993) Human type I and II IMP dehydrogenase as targets. *Ann NY Acad Sci* **696**:88–93.

Northrop JP, Ho SN, Chen L et al (1994) NF-AT components define a family of transcription factors targeted in T-cell activation. *Nature* **369**:497–502.

Platz KP, Sollinger HW, Hullett DA et al (1991) RS-61443—a new, potent immunosuppressive agent. *Transplantation* **51**:27–31.

Queen C, Schneider WP, Selick HE et al (1989) A humanized antibody that binds to the interleukin 2 receptor. *Proc Natl Acad Sci USA* **86**:10029–10033.

Rao A (1994) NF-ATp: a transcription factor required for the co-ordinate induction of several cytokine genes. *Immunol Today* **15**:274–281.

Rincon M, Flavell RA (1994) AP-1 transcriptional activity requires both T-cell receptor-mediated and co-stimulatory signals in primary T lymphocytes. *EMBO J* **13**:4370–4381.

Ruff VA, Leach KL (1995) Direct demonstration of NFATp dephosphorylation and nuclear localization in activated HT-2 cells using a specific NFATp polyclonal antibody. *J Biol Chem* **270**:22602–22607.

Russell PS, Monaco AP (1967) Heterologous anti-lymphocyte sera and some of their effects. *Transplantation* 5:1086–1099.

Schmidt M, Pauels H-G, Lügering N et al (1999) Glucocorticoids induce apoptosis in human monocytes: potential role of IL-1b. *J Immunol* 163:3484–3490.

Schuler W, Sedrani R, Cottens S et al (1997) SDZ RAD, a new rapamycin derivative: pharmacological properties in vitro and in vivo. *Transplantation* 64:36–42.

Schuurman HJ, Cottens S, Fuchs S et al (1997) SDZ RAD, a new rapamycin derivative: synergism with cyclosporine. *Transplantation* 64:32–35.

Schwartz RS, Damashek DW (1959) Drug-induced immunological tolerance. *Nature* 183:1682.

Sehgal SN, Baker H, Vezina C (1975) Rapamycin (AY-22,989), a new antifungal antibiotic: II. Fermentation, isolation and characterization. *J Antibiot (Tokyo)* 28:727–732.

Shibasaki F, Price ER, Milan D, McKeon F (1996) Role of kinases and the phosphatase calcineurin in the nuclear shuttling of transcription factor NF-AT4. *Nature* 382:370–373.

Shihab FS, Tanner AM, Shao Y, Weffer MI (1996) Expression of TGF-beta 1 and matrix proteins is elevated in rats with chronic rejection. *Kidney Int* 50:1904–1913.

Shin GT, Khana A, Ding R et al (1998) In vivo expression of transforming growth factor beta 1 in humans. *Transplantation* 65:313–318.

Sollinger HW (1995) Mycophenolate mofetil for the prevention of acute rejection in primary cadaveric renal allograft recipients. U.S. Renal Transplant Mycophenolate Mofetil Study Group. *Transplantation* 60:225–232.

Starzl TE, Marchioro TL, Porter KA et al (1967). The use of heterologous antilymphoid agents in canine renal and liver homotransplantation and in human renal transplantation. *Surg Gynecol Obstet* 124:301–308.

Starzl TE, Halgrimson CG, Penn I et al (1971) Cyclophosphamide and human organ transplantation. *Lancet* ii:70–74.

Stepkowski SM, Chen H, Daloze P, Kahan BD (1991) Rapamycin, a potent immunosuppressive drug for vascularized heart, kidney, and small bowel transplantation in the rat. *Transplantation* 51:22–26.

Stepkowski SM, Tian L, Napoli KL et al (1997) Synergistic mechanisms by which sirolimus and cyclosporin inhibit rat heart and kidney allograft rejection. *Clin Exp Immunol* 108:63–68.

Su B, Jacinto E, Hibi M et al (1994) JNK is involved in signal integration during costimulation of T lymphocytes. *Cell* 77:727–736.

Sugamura K, Asao H, Kondo M et al (1996) The interleukin-2 receptor gamma chain: its role in the multiple cytokine receptor complexes and T cell development in XSCID. *Ann Rev Immunol* 14:179–205.

Suthanthiran M, Morris RE, Strom TB (1996) Immunosuppressants: cellular and molecular mechanisms of action. *Am J Kidney Dis* 28:159–172.

Taniguchi T, Minami Y (1993) The IL-2/IL-2 receptor system: a current overview. *Cell* 73:5–8.

Tian L, Stepkowski SM, Qu X et al (1997) Cytokine mRNA expression in tolerant heart allografts after immunosuppression with cyclosporine, sirolimus or brequinar. *Transpl Immunol* 5:189–198.

Tidd DM, Paterson AR (1974) Distribution between inhibition of purine nucleotide synthesis and the delayed cytotoxic reaction of 6-mercaptopurine. *Cancer Res* 34:733–737.

Torchia J, Rose DW, Inostroza J et al (1997) The transcriptional co-activator p/CIP binds CBP and mediates nuclear-receptor function. *Nature* 387:677–684.

Tran HS, Malli D, Chrzanowski FA et al (1999) Site-specific immunosuppression using a new formulation of topical cyclosporine A with polyethylene glycol-8 glyceryl caprylate/caprate. *J Surg Res* 83:136–140.

Tumlin JA, Sands JM (1993) Nephron segment-specific inhibition of $Na^{(+)}/K^{(+)}$-ATPase activity by cyclosporin A. *Kidney Int* 43:246–251.

Vezina C, Kudelski A, Sehgal SN (1975) Rapamycin (AY-22,989), a new antifungal antibiotic: I. Taxonomy of the producing streptomycete and isolation of the active principle. *J Antibiot (Tokyo)* **28**:721–726.

Vincenti F, Kirkman R, Light S et al (1998a) Interleukin-2 receptor blockade with daclizumab to prevent acute rejection in renal transplantation. *N Engl J Med* **338**:161–165.

Vincenti F, Nashan B, Light S (1998b) Daclizumab: outcome of phase III trials and mechanism of action. Double Therapy and the Triple Therapy Study Groups. *Transplant Proc* **30**:2155–2158.

Vu MD, Qi S, Xu D et al (1997) Tacrolimus (FK506) and sirolimus (rapamycin) in combination are not antagositic but produce extended graft survival in caridac transplantation in the rat. *Transplantation* **64**:1853–1856.

Vu MD, Qi S, Xu D et al (1998) Synergistic effects of mycophenolate mofetil and sirolimus in prevention of acute heart, pancreas, and kidney allograft rejection and in reversal of ongoing heart allograft rejection in the rat. *Transplantation* **66**:1575–1580.

Winkelstein A (1979) The effect of azathioprine and 6-MP on immunity. *J Immunopharmacol* **1**:429–454.

Zhu J, McKeon F (1999) NF-AT activation requires suppression of Crm1-dependent export by calcineurin. *Nature* **398**:256–260.

9 ESTABLISHED IMMUNOSUPPRESSIVE DRUGS: CLINICAL AND TOXIC EFFECTS

INTRODUCTION

Optimal immunosuppression must harness three principles: the three 'S's (Table 9.1). The first principle, selectivity, is defined as the enhanced activity of an immunosuppressive agent toward T and B cell alloimmune as opposed to nonspecific (monocyte, granulocyte, macrophage, and natural killer (NK) cell) elements of host resistance. The second essential property of optimal immunosuppression is that the agents act in synergy, or in supra-additive fashion. Specificity, the third property of an optimal regimen, is the ultimate goal of therapy, namely, the induction of donor-specific tolerance achieving allograft acceptance with the smallest, strictly donor-specific, defect in the host's immune repertoire.

Established immunosuppressive agents used alone or in combination display these properties to varying degrees. For example, the first generation of selective immunosuppressive agents—cyclosporine (CsA), tacrolimus (TRL), and sirolimus (SRL)—act primarily on T lymphocytes. However, achieving adequate immunosuppression requires that each agent be used at doses that cause appreciable morbidity. Moreover, while the combination of CsA and SRL displays synergy, markedly decreasing the rate of acute rejection episodes while permitting CsA and SRL dose reduction, the ongoing need for antimicrobials and the partially overlapping toxicity profiles of the two drugs limit this therapeutic regimen. None of the established regimens achieves specificity, or tolerance induction, which remains the ultimate goal of transplant therapy. This chapter describes the current state of transplant immunosuppression, reviewing general concepts as well as the efficacy and toxicity of agents used in various combinations.

- Selectivity
- Synergy
- Specificity

Table 9.1. Three 'S's of Immunosuppression

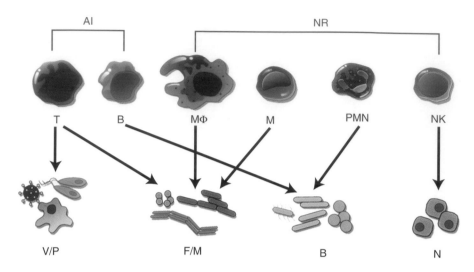

Figure 9.1. Elements of host resistance. The immune response includes adaptive immunity (AI) and nonspecific responses (NR), including macrophages (MΦ), monocytes (M), polymorphonuclear leukocytes (PMN), and natural killer cells (NK). These elements are responsible for the control of viral (V), protozoan (P), fungal (F), mycobacterial (M), bacterial (B) and neoplastic (N) invaders.

GENERAL CONCEPTS OF IMMUNOSUPPRESSION

Immunosuppressive therapy for transplantation seeks to selectively disrupt the activation of B and T cells, which are the major vectors of immune responses to foreign antigens, including proliferation, production of mediators, maturation, and generation of memory cells that are specifically reactive to donor tissue. In contrast, elements of non-specific host resistance, such as polymorphonuclear leukocytes (PMNs), monocytes/macrophages, and NK cells, mediate immune effects in response to a variety of inflammatory stimuli regardless of the specific antigen (Figure 9.1). The goal of immunosuppressive treatment is to achieve a state of stable tolerance, wherein the host accepts the parasitism of the graft while resisting infections and neoplastic invaders.

Immunosuppressive efficacy index

The immunosuppressive efficacy index seeks to express selectivity, namely, the relative potency of an agent to inhibit B and T cells of the specific adaptive response as opposed to elements of the nonspecific response. This index is defined as the ratio of the concentration necessary to paralyze nonspecific resistance versus that to alter specific resistance (Figure 9.2). Because of their poor therapeutic window, chemical toxins and other substances that nonselectively paralyze or kill B cells, T cells, and elements of nonspecific

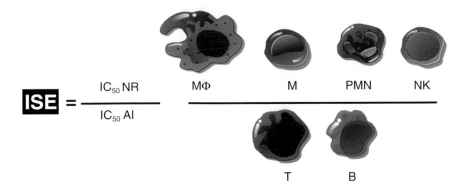

$$ISE = \frac{IC_{50} \, NR}{IC_{50} \, AI}$$

MΦ   M   PMN   NK

T   B

Figure 9.2. Immunosuppressive efficacy (ISE) index: an expression of the ratio of concentrations to inhibit the nonspecific responses (NR) versus adaptive immunity (AI).

resistance are not useful for clinical therapy. The original antiproliferative drug azathioprine (AZA), which shows an immunosuppressive index of less than 1.0, more effectively blocks the proliferation of bone marrow cells that mediate nonspecific resistance than it blocks lymphoid B or T cells. Similarly, steroids more effectively inhibit a variety of phagocytic, chemotactic, and antigen presentation functions of monocytes and macrophages than they alter cytokine production by T cells. Therefore, the combination of AZA and steroids displays a low immunosuppressive efficacy index: a high incidence of serious infections, particularly of bacterial origins, and an only modest degree of immunosuppression.

In contrast, CsA displays a high index of immunosuppressive efficacy, acting relatively selectively to dampen the initial activation phase, including the synthesis of cytokines by T cells, with little effect on nonspecific resistance (Drath et al 1983). Another reagent with a high index is the anti-CD3 monoclonal antibody (MAb), which is directed toward cell surface molecules that are primarily displayed on lymphocytes. Thus, these agents fulfill the first of the three 'S's' of immunosuppression—selectivity (Table 9.1). Other potent selective drugs include TRL and SRL.

Therapeutic toxicities of immunosuppressive agents

Aggressive therapy with reagents that display a high efficacy index may, as a result of excessive inhibition of T and B cells, produce immunosuppressive toxicities, namely, the emergence of viral, protozoan, or fungal infections and/or the development of neoplasms, particularly posttransplant lymphoproliferative disorder (PTLD). The mildest form of infection, an increased incidence of herpes simplex virus (HSV) with involvement of mucocutaneous junctions, generally responds to acyclovir chemotherapy. However, severe cases of herpetic pneumonitis or encephalitis may be life-threatening. Similarly, infections with another DNA virus, cytomegalovirus (CMV), may produce a broad spectrum of disease. Although frequently presenting as a mild constitutional syndrome of fever and malaise, moderate-to-severe infections may evolve to injure the bone marrow, liver, kidney, lung, pancreas, or gastrointestinal tract. Indeed, chronic CMV infections may cause proteinuria and may contribute to graft vascular disease. Another not uncommon outcome of excessive T cell inhibition is the emergence of oncogenic viruses, such as Epstein–Barr virus (EBV), which has been associated with PTLD and which primarily involves B but on occasion T cells (Berg et al 1992). Another important oncogenic infection, Kaposi's sarcoma, may be caused by human herpes virus 8 (Oksenhendler et al 1998; Regamey et al 1998; Jaffe and Pellett 1999).

The first clinical trial of CsA, using doses of 24 mg/kg (which are now recognized to be more than three times the necessary amount) in combination with a variety of other agents caused several recipients to display malignancies and virtually all patients to experience infections, many of which were lethal (Calne et al 1978). Similarly, the early experience with TRL, the mechanistic analog of CsA, was fraught with a high incidence of neoplasia (Starzl et al 1989). This form of comorbidity is not uncommon. Thus, for patients at high risk for viral infections—for example, a seronegative recipient of a seropositive organ—both prophylactic treatment with antiviral agents (such as gancyclovir or acyclovir and/or immune globulin) and posttransplant surveillance for viral detection are compulsory, including blood tests for viral products by polymerase chain reaction or serologic detection of early antigen.

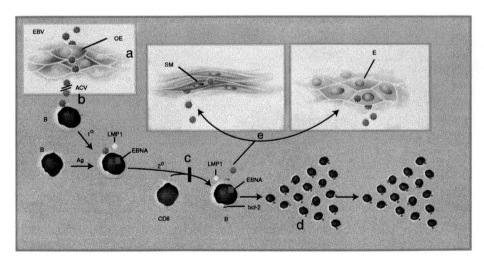

Figure 9.3. Morphogenetic results of Epstein–Barr viral (EBV) infection. (a) EBV (red particles) infects oral epithelium (OE). The proliferation of virus may be dampened by acyclovir (ACV) treatment. (b) Lysis of infected OE-releases EBV particles that infect B lymphocytes, which, in the presence of antigen (Ag) stimulation, express EBV nuclear antigen (EBNA) and surface marker (LMP1). (c) In the absence of CD8[+] T lymphocyte control owing to inhibition by immunosuppressants, viral proliferation is unencumbered. (d) B lymphocytes undergo polyclonal and later monoclonal proliferation, producing posttransplant lymphoproliferative disease (PTLD). The cells may undergo a cytogenetic event, evolving to malignant monoclonal proliferation. (e) Dissemination of EBV to other tissues—smooth muscle (SM) and epithelial (E) cells—potentially leading to tumors.

Epstein–Barr virus remains dormant in the B lymphocytes of nonimmunosuppressed patients, owing to the capacity of T cells to suppress infection. However, inception of intense immunosuppression releases this control, permitting viral outgrowth (Figure 9.3). In mild cases, this viral proliferation resembles infectious mononucleosis; in more serious cases, an initial proliferation of polyclonal B cells progresses to a monoclonal neoplasm that does not display genetic abnormalities. These infections can be controlled by intense and long-term acyclovir therapy (Figure 9.4). However, monoclonal tumors that display gene rearrangements demand intense chemotherapy. Another outcome of excessive immunosuppression is Kaposi's sarcoma, which frequently presents initially as punctate, hemorrhagic skin lesions on the legs (Figure 9.5), and which may progress to ulcerating or fungating lesions (Figure 9.6) and eventually to systemic involvement (Figure 9.7).

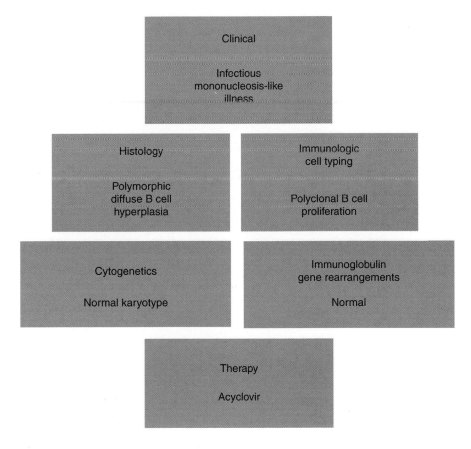

Figure 9.4. Characteristics of benign lymphoproliferation. Clinical syndrome of an infectious mononucleosis illness with histologic appearance of a polymorphic diffuse B cell hyperplasia and polyclonal immunoglobulin phenotype with normal cytogenetics and without gene rearrangement. This illness responds to acyclovir.

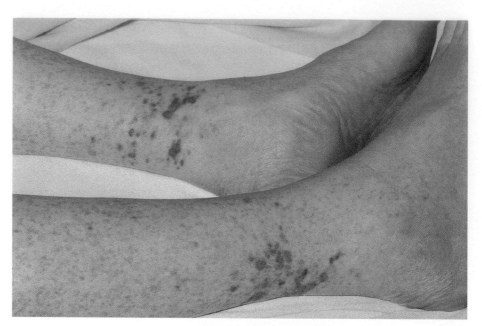

Figure 9.5. Bilateral punctate hemorrhagic lesions of Kaposi's sarcoma

(a) (b)

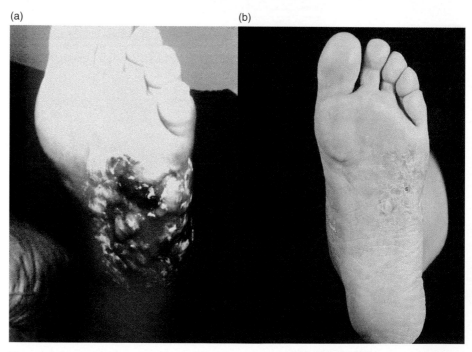

Figure 9.6. Involution of Kaposi's sarcoma of the foot after withdrawal of immunosuppression. (a) Fungating Kaposi's sarcoma appearing within 3 months posttransplant in a patient of Mediterranean descent treated with CsA, AZA, and Pred. (b) Resolution of lesion within 9 months after cessation of immunosuppressive therapy and radiation treatments.

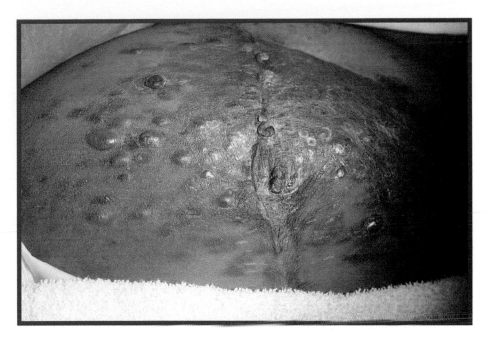

Figure 9.7. Kaposi's sarcoma of the abdominal wall. Appearance of bulbous lesions over the pannus of a 52-year-old woman on AZA-Pred therapy for 7 years. The patient succumbed to the disease despite cessation of immunosuppressive therapy.

The frequency of PTLD varies considerably among transplant centers, ranging from 0.4 to 25% of recipients, depending upon the intensity of the immunosuppressive regimen (Boubenider et al 1997). Birkeland et al (1999) reported that, compared to a combination of antilymphocyte globulin (ALG), CsA and prednisone (Pred), prophylactic treatment with high doses of acyclovir combined with a steroid-free regimen reduced the incidences of PTLD and of EBV serologic conversion. In contrast, the advent of intense immunosuppression with mycophenolate mofetil (MMF) and TRL therapy has decreased the time to development of PTLD (Alfrey et al 1992). In addition to the likely effects of immunosuppressants to promote viral infections, Hojo et al (1999) found that increased production of transforming growth factor-β (TGF-β) expression induced by CsA (or TRL) altered the morphology and reduced adhesion to the matrix of neoplastic cells, events that could accelerate the spread of neoplastic cells.

Another form of immunologic toxicity, aberrant T-cell maturation, may advance to autoimmune disease, possibly by disruption of thymic processes to eliminate rogue clones reactive toward autologous tissues. Thus, patients chronically treated with immunosuppressants may display an augmented incidence of Psoriasis vulgaris. Figure 9.8 shows an immunoelectrophoretic pattern of polyclonal κ gammopathy in the serum of a patient who presented with polyarteritis nodosum 7 years posttransplant.

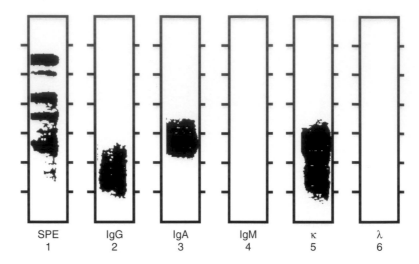

| SPE | IgG | IgA | IgM | κ | λ |
| 1 | 2 | 3 | 4 | 5 | 6 |

Figure 9.8. Autoimmune disease in a renal transplant patient. A 56-year-old man, 7-year status post-renal transplant, presented with polyarteritis nodosum and displayed a monoclonal IgA [κ] gammopathy, as seen by the prominent immunoprecipitate in Lanes 3 and 5.

Nontherapeutic toxicities of immunosuppressive agents

Immunosuppressants are also associated with a variety of nontherapeutic toxicities. Although AZA had infrequently induced a form of hepatitis, the first significant nontherapeutic toxicity to be encountered was the nephrotoxicity caused by CsA (and later shown to be shared by TRL). Although initial preclinical work in animal models failed to reveal the effect, CsA-induced dysfunction was evident among the first cohort of de novo renal transplant patients tested with the drug (Calne et al 1978). Indeed, the nephrotoxicity appears to be inextricably tied to the immunosuppressive effects, since Wenger (1986) was unable to identify an active structural analog free of this complication. Both immunosuppression and nephrotoxicity seem to result primarily, at least in the early phases, from inhibition of the cytoplasmic phosphatase calcineurin, and, in the later period, from possible upregulated synthesis of TGF-β. In addition to nephrotoxicity, TRL displays a prominent neurotoxicity that presumably reflects an exquisite drug sensitivity of the calcineurin isozyme expressed in the brain. Further structure/function investigations will be necessary to determine whether the hyperlipidemic and/or myelosuppressive toxicities of the macrocyclic lactone SRL are inextricably tied to its immunosuppressive effects on the mammalian target of rapamycin (mTOR). However, it is clear that the structural analog of SRL, SDZ RAD, shares a similar adverse reaction profile.

Window of immunosuppressive versus nonimmunosuppressive toxicities

The therapeutic window of a drug seeks to express the relation of the drug doses (or whole blood concentrations) that produce immunosuppressive effects versus those associated with toxic reactions. Figure 9.9 shows that virtually any effective concentration of CsA (or TRL) incurs a concomitant penalty of nephrotoxicity. For example, 80% of patients afflicted with *Psoriasis vulgaris* that had been resistant to other therapies displayed a therapeutic benefit upon treatment with 5 mg/kg CsA (Figure 9.10a), whereas this dose produced a doubling of the serum creatinine value in almost 40% of patients (Figure 9.10b). In the renal transplant setting, physicians have accepted the trade-off of a 20–30% reduction in allograft renal function in exchange for a 50–60% reduction in the incidence of acute rejection episodes. Unfortunately, the therapeutic window of CsA is not only relatively narrow, but also varies among individual patients. Since it is not possible to predict the effects of a given drug dose (or blood concentration) on the immunosuppressive versus the toxic outcomes in a single patient, robust therapeutic recommendations for dose/concentration are impossible, and treatment depends upon physician acumen. The narrow therapeutic windows characteristic of CsA and TRL, and probably of SRL, are typical of 'critical dose drugs'. These drugs require concentration

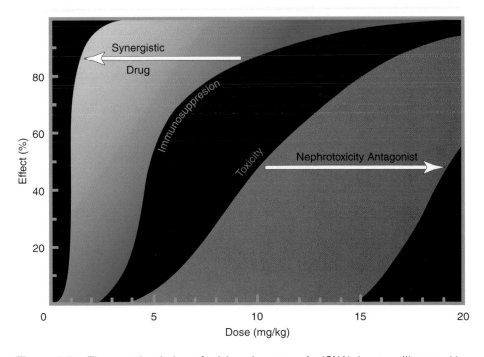

Figure 9.9. Therapeutic window of calcineurin antagonist (CNA) drugs, as illustrated by cyclosporine (CsA). The shaded area shows the window between immunosuppression and toxicity. The area to the right shows potential broadening with a drug that ameliorates nephrotoxicity; the area to the left, with a synergistic immunosuppressant.

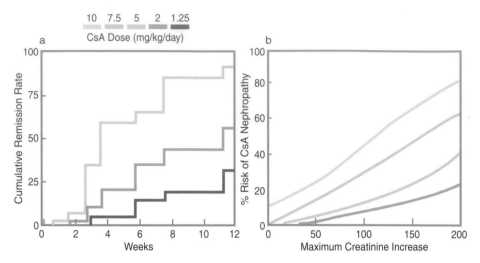

Figure 9.10. Therapeutic window of CsA treatment in *Psoriasis vulgaris*. (a) Cumulative success rate during the first 3 months of treatment with CsA: 1.25 mg/kg per day (red line); 2.5 mg/kg per day (blue line); or 5 mg/kg per day (brown line). (Reprinted with permission from Timonen et al, *Br J Dermatol* **122**(Suppl 36):33–39, © 1990 Blackwell Science Ltd.) (b) Estimated risk of developing CsA nephropathy based upon dose: 2 mg/kg per day (blue line); 5 mg/kg per day (brown line), 7.5 mg/kg per day (green line); or 10 mg/kg per day (pink line). (Feutren G, Mihatsch MJ. Risk factors for cyclosporine-induced nephropathy in patients with autoimmune diseases. International Kidney Biopsy Registry of Cyclosporine in Autoimmune Diseases. *N Engl J Med* 1992 Jun 18; **326**(25):1654–1660. © 1992 Massachusetts Medical Society. All rights reserved.)

monitoring, although it is recognized that the variable dynamic sensitivity of the enzymes that represent the pharmacologic target renders this strategy imprecise (Kahan 1999).

Two strategies employing adjunctive drugs might broaden the narrow therapeutic-to-toxic window (Figure 9.9). The first strategy is to administer an agent that enhances immunosuppression synergistically, thereby augmenting the therapeutic effect achieved by a given concentration of the reference drug. The second strategy is to administer an agent that mitigates or counteracts the toxicity, thereby reducing the incidence or extent of adverse reaction to the reference drug. Because there is no available strategy to ameliorate CsA, TRL, or SRL toxicity, recent progress has depended upon the development of drugs that display synergistic therapeutic effects. Thus, administration of SRL in combination with CsA has been clearly shown to produce drug synergy (the second 'S' of the goals for immunosuppressants (Table 9.1)) and to mutually broaden the therapeutic windows of both the calcineurin antagonist (CNA) and the mTOR inhibitor.

INDICATIONS FOR IMMUNOSUPPRESSIVE THERAPY

Induction therapy

Immunosuppression for transplantation may be divided into five settings: induction, acute rejection prophylaxis, maintenance, antirejection, and refractory rejection therapies. The 'induction' strategy seeks to utilize an intense initial immunosuppressive regimen to avert the occurrence or to delay the onset of an acute rejection episode. This strategy is based upon the belief that accelerated or early acute rejection episodes have a more pernicious outcome than do later episodes. However, clinical data have not confirmed this theory: induction therapy using either antilymphocyte sera or OKT3 has not been shown to improve 1-year graft survival rates. Indeed, only a few studies suggest that induction therapy reduces the incidence, although it does delay the onset, of acute rejection episodes.

A second and more tenable basis for the use of induction therapy with antilymphocyte preparations is to avert the de novo use of CNAs, which, due to their proclivity to produce renal dysfunction, may impair the recovery of the allograft from the ischemia–reperfusion events associated with organ harvest, storage, and revascularization (discussed in Chapter 10). The acute nephrotoxic injury has been associated with high concentrations of CNAs, especially when delivered by intravenous infusion (Novick et al 1986). However, the adoption of more-moderate CNA dosage regimens has diminished this problem, and induction therapy with antilymphocyte sera, which was popular between 1985 and 1995, has widely been abandoned due to its toxicity and expense. A 7-day course of ATGAM (Pharmacia & Upjohn Co., Kalamazoo, MI, USA) costs approximately US$ 3000, and of OKT3, US$ 2500.

Not only have the recently introduced anti-interleukin-2 receptor (IL-2R) MAbs been demonstrated to reduce acute rejection rates when used in combination with CsA, but also they are less toxic, only slightly less potent, and somewhat less costly. A full course of basiliximab costs US$ 2000, and daclizumab, US$ 6000. In CNA-free regimens, the anti-IL-2R reagents combined with MMF produced only limited therapeutic effects: Vincenti et al (1999) found that nearly 50% of patients treated with daclizumab and MMF induction therapy experienced acute rejection episodes. In contrast, Hong and Kahan (1999) observed that therapy with anti-IL-2R MAbs in combination with SRL and delayed introduction of CsA conferred protection against an acute rejection episode among six recipients of grafts at low risk for delayed graft function, as well as among 82% of a general transplant population that included retransplant, African-American, and pediatric patients.

Acute rejection prophylaxis and maintenance therapy

The maintenance immunosuppressive regimen includes the agents used indefinitely to prevent the emergence of allograft rejection. Typically, patients are treated with one baseline agent that acts as the cornerstone of their chronic immunosuppressive therapy. Present practice adds other agents to the regimen, sometimes to enhance the potency of the baseline drug for prophylaxis prior to rejection, sometimes to intensify the therapy in response to evidence of rejection, and sometimes to allow dose reduction of the baseline agent to mitigate a toxicity. In most cases, the doses of the maintenance agent(s) are reduced over time, based on the concept of 'graft accommodation', the gradual acceptance of the graft by the host. This phenomenon has been attributed to a reduced release of foreign histocompatibility antigens or pro-inflammatory materials from the stable, nonischemic graft, and/or, less likely, to the repopulation of the graft vasculature with host elements.

Although the presently established agents have all been shown to be effective for prophylaxis of acute rejection, none displays a documented effect against the occurrence or progression of chronic rejection. Therefore, the physician has considerably more confidence in the rational administration of drugs during the early posttransplant period, when the focus is on acute rejection, than during the later phase of chronic allograft attrition, when adequate drug doses must be counterbalanced by considerations of morbidities caused by adverse reactions. The dilemma is heightened by the observation that CsA, TRL, SRL, and MMF, potential maintenance agents, all show greater inhibitory effects on T than on B cells. This shortcoming may account for the failure of existing regimens to dampen the emergence of chronic rejection, which is due, at least in part, to alloantibody-mediated damage.

Anti-rejection therapy

Histopathologic evidences of the presence and severity of the host response typically guide the choice of agents for, and the length of treatment of acute rejection episodes. Mild rejection episodes (Banff grade 1) are characterized by 'tubulitis', namely, infiltration of proximal tubules with lymphocytes. These episodes generally respond to corticosteroid therapy. Moderate rejection episodes (Banff grade 2), characterized by a more violent histopathologic response, less frequently respond to corticosteroids, particularly in those patients who display evidence of endovasculitis, including lymphocyte adhesion to, and reactive swelling or disruption of, endothelium. These patients generally require treatment with antilymphocyte antibodies. Severe rejection episodes (Banff grade 3), which show hemorrhage, arterial disruption, and/or parenchymal necrosis, are rarely entirely reversible, despite the use of combinations of antirejection agents. When drug regimens fail, addition of plasmapheresis may be undertaken if the patient's condition can tolerate this measure, and particularly if the presence of antidonor-specific antibodies can be demonstrated (Pascual et al 1998).

Refractory rejection therapy

The definition of 'refractory' rejection is highly controversial. Some workers define a rejection episode as refractory if it does not reverse after steroid treatment and suggest a benefit from TRL or MMF in this setting (Sollinger et al 1992; Fung and Starzl 1995). A more rigorous definition of a refractory rejection episode is one that is both steroid- and antilymphocyte antibody-resistant, as documented by the presence of a positive kidney biopsy (Slaton and Kahan 1996). In this setting, addition of SRL to a CsA-Pred or a TRL-Pred regimen has been shown to ameliorate renal function.

AGENTS AFFECTING ANTIGEN PRESENTATION

Steroids

Therapeutic effects

Steroids were first introduced into the transplant clinic by Hamburger (Starzl 1993) and rapidly adopted in combination regimens with AZA. After intraoperative treatment with high intravenous doses (pulses) in an attempt to drive lymphocytes from the circulation, steroids are administered in a regimen of tapering drug doses. Virtually all renal transplant patients are presently maintained indefinitely on 'low-dose' steroid, primarily because withdrawal of this agent has been associated with a 30% incidence of acute rejection episodes and/or premature graft attrition.

When used to treat acute rejection episodes, steroids tend to produce only a modest therapeutic effect that requires several days to be realized, but is frequently sufficient to reverse mild cases. Because of the low potency of steroids, some physicians question even an initial trial of steroid therapy and recommend the immediate use of antilymphocyte preparations (Ferguson 1994). Other physicians debate the appropriate length of a trial period before a rejection episode is deemed 'steroid-resistant'. The factors that influence a decision to withhold or prematurely abandon an attempt to reverse a rejection episode with steroid therapy include: the presence or progression of clinical signs of rejection (fever, increasing graft swelling or tenderness, and oliguria); a rapidly rising serum creatinine; intolerance to the regimen, owing to the induction or exacerbation of posttransplant diabetes mellitus (PTDM); as well as onset of psychosis, profound myopathy, or gastrointestinal bleeding. However, the most objective criterion of failure, steroid resistance, is a transplant biopsy showing progression of the rejection lesion despite at least a few days of treatment.

Dosage regimens

While no clinical trials have established the benefit of a tapering schedule from high doses to modest amounts of steroids for maintenance therapy, the practice is now firmly entrenched in transplant pharmacotherapy. After an intraoperative dose of methylprednisolone 250 mg, the steroid dose is rapidly tapered from 30 mg every 6 hours to 15 mg twice daily over 7 days, and subsequently to 15 mg daily by 2–3 months. Dose targets are 10 mg by 6 months, 7.5 mg at 12 months, and 5 mg at 24 months. Some physicians have advocated an alternate-day instead of a daily regimen of drug dosing in an attempt to mitigate toxicity; however, this strategy has not yielded consistent clinical benefits. Thus, most patients are maintained on a daily regimen.

Total avoidance of steroid treatment de novo is rarely utilized by transplant centers. Although the initial European trials utilized CsA monotherapy (no concomitant steroids), 50% of patients required steroid institution due to the occurrence of a rejection episode (Anonymous 1983). In another study, the patients under a steroid aversion protocol showed a significantly higher rate of acute rejection episodes than those treated de novo with steroids (Bry et al 1991). However, greater success of steroid avoidance was reported by Birkeland (1998) in a group of Danish patients, probably as a result of good HLA-matching and low immune responder status.

The usual strategy is rather to initiate steroid therapy, with attempts at withdrawal depending upon patient request, good HLA matching, or evidence of drug-induced morbidities. The clinicians' decisions must be based upon their perception of the safety of steroid withdrawal. A delay in withdrawal may compromise some of the potential benefits to be gained from a steroid-free regimen, specifically—prevention of cataract formation (Matsunami et al 1994), amelioration of diabetes mellitus (Hricik et al 1991), and mitigation of bone destruction.

Flechner et al (1985) reported upon 2-year data that recipients whose lymphocytes failed to display a proliferative response upon in vitro challenge with cells from either HLA-identical or -haploidentical donors could be withdrawn from steroids at 6 months. A subsequent report (Kahan et al 1989) confirmed these observations at a 5-year time point. Independent of any immunologic test, Stratta et al (1988) reported successful early steroid withdrawal among 89% of patients who received HLA-identical grafts and among 58% of recipients who had received pretransplant donor-specific transfusions. Using a quadruple induction regimen, Schulak et al (1990) reported that 40% of cadaveric-donor and 60% of living-related donor kidney transplants tolerated withdrawal of steroids at 1 week after inception of CsA. Although Grinyó et al (1997) observed that 26 Spanish patients receiving a CsA-MMF regimen successfully underwent steroid withdrawal without acute rejection episodes within 10 months, a US multicenter trial showed an increased rate of rejection among withdrawn patients, leading to cessation of the trial. In contrast, patients tolerate withdrawal of steroids from a CsA-SRL regimen (Kahan et al 1998a).

Steroid withdrawal after 6 months seems safer than after 3 months. At 6 months posttransplant, 80% of patients were successfully withdrawn, with only a 29% incidence of acute rejection episodes (Hricik et al 1992b). A meta-analysis of randomized, prospective trials (Hricik et al 1993) confirmed a 48% rate of acute rejection episodes among CsA-treated patients withdrawn from steroids, compared to 30% among patients maintained on steroids. Despite an initial enthusiasm for steroid withdrawal from a TRL-based regimen, the long-term results suggest little benefit over that already demonstrated using CsA, namely, a successful outcome among 66% of pediatric renal transplantation patients restored to normal growth (Shapiro et al 1999b).

Although this analysis did not reveal a hazard for long-term graft survival, both the placebo-controlled trial organized by the Canadian Multicentre Transplant Study Group (Sinclair et al 1992) and a recent analysis by Ratcliffe et al (1996) document this complication of withdrawal. Compared to steroid-treated controls, patients not receiving steroids displayed greater rates of sclerosing arteriopathy (Offermann et al 1993) and interstitial fibrosis (Isoniemi et al 1992). However, it remains unclear whether this risk applies only to patients who, after steroid withdrawal, suffer an obvious or a subclinical acute rejection episode (Hricik et al 1995).

The presence of a biopsy-confirmed rejection episode that shows either grade I (mild) or grade II cellular score by the Banff criteria demands expeditious therapy. The steroid regimen may use boluses of 250, 500, or 1000 mg of methylprednisolone, without or with a recycling of oral steroids from about 200 mg in divided doses, followed by a taper schedule. At the University of Texas at Houston, three boluses of 500 mg methylprednisolone are delivered intravenously on the day of diagnosis. Beginning on the next day, 200 mg oral Pred (50 mg four times within 1 day) is administered, followed by a tapering schedule to 30 mg by 1 week and 15 mg by 2 months.

Toxicities

Because of their prominent effects on monocytes, granulocytes, and macrophages, steroids display a poor immunosuppressive efficacy index. Treatment with high doses of steroids, particularly for prolonged periods, markedly increases the patient's proclivity to bacterial and fungal infections.

These effects on the nonspecific immune system eclipse the action of steroids to block the generation of NF-κβ. Most recipients attribute their major posttransplant complaints—Cushingoid appearance, friable skin, weight gain, muscle weakness, and buffalo hump—to steroids. In addition, steroids produce laboratory findings that are potentially debilitating. Steroids increase the level of blood lipids, a finding that may owe, at least in part, to induction of insulin resistance; to an augmented activity of acetyl CoA carboxylase, which thereby increases the production of low- and high-density lipoproteins (LDL and HDL); to decreased triglyceride clearance; to inhibition of 26-hydroxylase; and to altered binding kinetics of LDL to the LDL receptor. By causing islet cell toxicity, CsA may facilitate the development of steroid-induced diabetes in some patients.

In addition to augmented hyperlipidemia and diabetogenicity, steroids share other adverse reactions with CsA, particularly effects to promote bone resorption and to exacerbate hypertension. Generally, steroids are believed to be the primary inciting factor for avascular necrosis, osteomalacia, and/or osteoporosis, diseases that can be markedly accelerated by the concomitant presence of hyperparathyroidism. Adverse effects on bone may be produced by as little as one 5-day course of steroids.

The benefits of steroid withdrawal have been documented in the pediatric population by accelerated growth (Tejani et al 1989) and in the adult group by an increase in bone density (Julian et al 1991), an amelioration of hypertension (Hricik et al 1992a), a 20% decrease in serum cholesterol and triglyceride concentrations (Kupin et al 1988), and an improved glycemic control (Schulak and Hricik 1994).

AGENTS AFFECTING SIGNAL ONE RECEPTION: G_0 TO G_1 TRANSITION IN THE CYTOKINE PARADIGM

Anti-CD3 monoclonal antibody

Therapeutic effects

Currently, OKT3, an immunoglobulin (Ig) G_{2a} murine MAb directed against the ε-chain of CD3, is used for induction (Millis et al 1989; Shield et al 1996), as well as for anti-rejection therapy (Friedman et al 1987; Solomon et al 1993). On the one hand, OKT3 induction therapy has been claimed to delay the onset and, possibly, to decrease the incidence of acute rejection episodes. However, 1-year patient and/or graft survival rates are not improved by this therapy. On the other hand, OKT3 therapy plays an established role in the reversal of steroid-resistant acute rejection episodes; treatment with this MAb reverses 80% of episodes in which steroid therapy failed to resolve the elevated serum creatinine (Ortho Multicenter Transplant Study Group 1985).

The beneficial effects of treatment with OKT3 may not appear until 4–7 days after initiation, a delay that has been attributed to the transient activation of T cells within the graft, producing a nephropathic syndrome. Occasionally, OKT3 therapy provides only transient improvement. A subsequent deterioration in renal function during the course of OKT3 therapy has been attributed in some cases to the presence of host human antimurine antibodies (HAMA) that neutralize the therapeutic agent. However, in most instances, the OKT3 resistance can be attributed to a pharmacodynamic resistance caused by the emergence of immune mechanisms not susceptible to the modulation of T cell function. Some physicians advocate a switch to polyclonal xenogeneic antibody in an attempt to obtain a depletion therapy; however, because of the limited possibility of therapeutic success, the morbidity associated with an additional course of treatment is rarely justified. 'Refractory' rejection episodes that fail to respond to a 14- (or preferably 21-) day course of an antilymphocyte antibody place the patient at high risk for graft loss.

Dosage regimens

The usual dose of OKT3 to obtain rejection reversal is 5 mg once daily for 14 days. If a posttreatment transplant biopsy shows persistent rejection, an additional 7-day course is recommended. To reduce the proclivity of patients to viral infections or to the cytokine release syndrome, some workers have advocated either an abbreviated 7–10-day course or reduced 2.5 mg doses. Although it is theoretically appealing to use the number of peripheral blood $CD3^+$ T cells as an indicator of therapeutic efficacy, this parameter correlates imperfectly with the clinical outcome.

Toxicities

The first obstacle to therapy using anti-CD3 MAb is the cytokine release syndrome, which is caused by T-cell activation following antibody binding to surface CD3 markers. Within 1 hour after the administration of the first and, to a lesser extent, subsequent doses, the MAb transiently stimulates T cells, which thereby release pro-inflammatory cytokines, including tumor necrosis factor-α (TNF-α), IL-2, and interferon-γ (IFN-γ). The patient may manifest a pleiotropic array of symptoms, including fever (73%), chills (57%), tremors (10%), dyspnea (21%), chest pain/tightness (14%), wheezing (11%), nausea (11%), and/or vomiting (13%) (Ortho Multicenter Transplant Study Group 1985). One adverse reaction of great concern is OKT3-induced nephropathy, which presumably results from local release of cytokines within the kidney allograft.

In addition to the possibility of using only low (2 mg) doses, strategies to decrease the occurrence and severity of the cytokine release syndrome include obtaining a chest X-ray to minimize the risk of severe pulmonary edema; premedicating the patient with a cocktail of methylprednisolone (5–8 mg/kg), diphenhydramine hydrochloride (25–50 mg intravenously), and acetaminophen (500 mg by mouth); and/or using a low initial OKT3 dose (1 mg) followed by slow escalation of the next two doses that day (2 mg and 2 mg) and the next day (2.5 mg and 2.5 mg) before reaching the prescribed full therapeutic dose of 5 mg. Several toxicities represent indications to abandon OKT3 therapy: aseptic meningitis with obtundation, nuchal rigidity, and/or headache; appearance of CMV early antigen, particularly with fever, pneumonitis, cytopenias, or stigmata of visceral disease; or failure to show a therapeutic effect, particularly in the presence of a positive test for HAMA. Immunobiological research is currently striving to overcome the cytokine release syndrome by developing MAbs that block critical surface markers but are incapable of producing T-cell activation.

The second obstacle to therapy is the production of neutralizing HAMA, an event that occurs in nearly 50% of patients following the initial course of treatment. The presence of HAMA may render a patient resistant to a second course of OKT3 treatment. Thus, before initiating repeat treatment with OKT3, it is useful to rule out the presence of HAMA. The laboratory at The University of Texas at Houston currently uses OKT3 covalently bound to tosylated dynabeads (M-280) to test for the presence of HAMA. The binding of patient serum to the coated beads is evaluated by flow cytometry after incubation with a fluorescein-conjugated goat anti-human antibody (Jackson ImmunoResearch Laboratories, West Grove, PA, USA). The obstacle of HAMA is being addressed by engineering antibodies that contain a majority of human amino acid sequences, with only limited regions of the xenogenic sequences in the complementarity-determining regions (see Chapter 10). In addition to these short-term obstacles, administration of doses of OKT3 over 75 mg has been associated with the development of PTLD among cardiac transplant recipients (Swinnen et al 1990).

Calcineurin antagonists

Calcineurin antagonists (CNA) serve as the cornerstone of current immunosuppressive maintenance therapy. The short- and long-term results of renal transplantation among patients under maintenance treatment with CsA or TRL, alone or in combination with MMF, are similar (Yang et al 1999). Thus, the selection of a CNA is generally based on physician preference, on patient intolerance to one of the alternate drugs (for example, due to the cosmetic side-effects of CsA or the neurotoxicity of TRL), on ill-defined pharmacodynamic resistance, and/or on idiopathic nephrotoxic sensitivity.

Therapeutic effects

Cyclosporine (CsA) was discovered in 1968 and developed as an immunosuppressive agent by Borel et al (1976). CsA represented the first T-cell selective pharmacologic agent free of the myelodepressive complications associated with the antiproliferative agents. Following its introduction by Calne et al (1978), CsA treatment in combination with steroids was shown to dramatically improve cadaveric renal allograft survival rates from 50 to 80% at 1 year, and from 25 to 60% at 5 years, compared with previous experience using the AZA-steroid combination (Starzl et al 1982; Kahan et al 1985). A major reason for the improvement was the capacity of CsA to mitigate immunologic risk factors, particularly immune responder status, HLA mismatch, lack of pretransplant transfusions, retransplant, or the presence of a spleen, an immunopotentiating organ, in the host (Figure 9.11) (Kahan et al 1995). Figure 9.12 shows the impact of CsA to

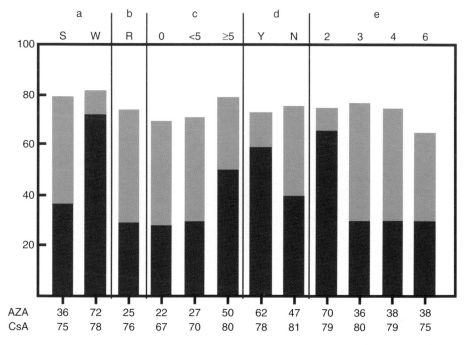

Figure 9.11. Impact of CsA to mitigate immunologic risk factors. The letters in the top row represent the risk factors, the bottom numbers, the 1-year graft survival corresponding to CsA or AZA treatment. (a) Immune responder status strong (S) versus weak (W). (b) Retransplant (R). (c) Number of pretransplant transfusions 0 versus <5 versus ≥5. (d) Splenectomy yes (Y) or no (N). (e) HLA-A, -B, -DR mismatches 2, 3, 4, or 6. Dark red bars show 1-year graft survival under AZA-Pred treatment; pink bars, under CsA-Pred treatment. (Adapted from Kahan BD, Van Buren CT, Flechner SM et al. Clinical and experimental studies with cyclosporine in renal transplantation. *Surgery* 1985; **97**:125–40.)

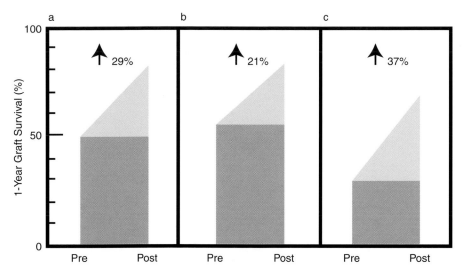

Figure 9.12. Comparison of 1-year graft survival rates immediately post-introduction of CsA therapy. (a) Kidney. (From Rosenthal et al 1983.) (b) Heart. (From Shumway and Kaye 1988.) (c) Liver. (Starzl et al 1982.)

Treatment[a]	N[b]	Incidence[c]		Mortality[d]	
		N (%)[e]	P[f]	N (%)[e]	P[f]
Azathioprine (AZA)	222	31 (14)		20 (64)	
			<0.05		<0.01
Cyclosporine (CsA)	231	19 (8)		3 (16)	

[a]Baseline treatment in conjunction with steroid therapy. AZA initiated at 3 mg/kg and titered to maintain white blood cell count above 5000/mm³; CsA initiated at 14 mg/kg and tapered progressively to 5–7 mg/kg at 1 year. Steroids rapidly tapered from 120 to 30 mg/day by 10 days, 25 mg/day at 1 month, 15 mg/day by 6 months, and 10 mg/day by 12 months.

[b]Number of patients in each treatment group.

[c]Incidence of various infections that produced generalized sepsis.

[d]Mortality rate within 1 year of presentation of the infection.

[e]Number of patients (N) and fraction of overall cohort (%).

[f]P-values by Fisher's exact test.

Table 9.2. Outcome of serious infections as a function of the primary immunosuppressant

increase renal, hepatic, and cardiac allograft survival at 1 year. Table 9.2 illustrates the higher selectivity for alloimmune responses of a CsA-Pred over an AZA-Pred regimen. CsA treatment was associated with a decreased incidence of (8 versus 14%, respectively, $P < 0.05$) and mortality rate (16 versus 64%, respectively, $P < 0.01$) from serious infections following renal transplant (Kahan et al 1985).

The original olive oil-based formulation of CsA, Sandimmune (Novartis, Basle, Switzerland), was approved by the US Food and Drug Administration (FDA) in 1983. The recently introduced microemulsion formulation (Neoral, Novartis, Basle, Switzerland), approved by the US FDA in 1995, addressed the highly variable, partial, and bile-dependent gastrointestinal absorption of the original preparation (Kahan 1985a, b), resulting in a modest, albeit significant, reduction in the incidence of acute rejection episodes (Niese and Keown 1998; Pollard et al 1999). Neoral displays excellent general safety and tolerability, either as de novo therapy (Barone et al 1996; Pescovitz et al 1997) or upon conversion from Sandimmune (Kahan et al 1995). However, due to the greater bioavailability of Neoral, some workers have reported that conversion from Sandimmune to Neoral generally requires dose reduction to avert exacerbation of nephrotoxicity (Bennett et al 1996a; Khajehdehi et al 1999). Preliminary experience has suggested that conversion from Neoral to the third available form of CsA, the generic brand SangCya (SangStat, Menlo Park, CA, USA) was not associated with a high risk of complications (First et al 1998); however, wider experience will be needed before safety is assured in all patient subgroups.

Interestingly, a growing literature suggests other possible uses of CNAs in diseases caused by excessive stimulation of calcineurin activity. For example, upregulated synthesis of insulin-like growth factor (IGF-1) activates calcineurin-mediated calcium signaling, leading to myocardial hypertrophy caused by the expression of muscle-specific genes and the augmented content of the marker GATA-2 (Musaró et al 1999). CNA action may block these processes (Semsarian et al 1999).

Tacrolimus (TRL) was discovered in 1984 by Goto et al (1987). TRL (Prograf, Fujisawa USA, Inc., Deerfield, IL, USA) was approved by the US FDA in 1994 for use in liver transplantation and in 1997 for kidney transplantation. Although the original report on TRL therapy described the 'salvage' of liver allografts in patients suffering ongoing rejection despite CsA-based immunosuppression (Starzl et al 1989), numerous studies now suggest beneficial immunosuppressive effects of TRL as a de novo agent for acute rejection prophylaxis in a variety of solid organ transplants.

In vitro experiments and in vivo animal transplant models suggest that TRL displays a 25–50-fold greater immunosuppressive effect than CsA; however, this benefit has been difficult to document in humans due to the equally narrow therapeutic window of the two agents. Tables 9.3 and 9.4 compare the efficacy of TRL- versus (Sandimmune) CsA-based immunosuppressive therapy, in conjunction with AZA-Pred, among renal (Mayer et al 1997; Pirsch et al 1997) or liver recipients (European FK506 Multicentre Liver Study Group 1994; US Multicenter FK506 Liver Study Group 1994; Jonas et al 1995; Fung et al 1996; Wiesner 1998). Although the incidence of acute rejection episodes was significantly reduced among renal transplant recipients treated with TRL compared with Sandimmune (30.7 versus 46.6%, $P = 0.001$ in the US and 25.9 versus 45.7%, $P = 0.001$ in the European multicenter trials) the overall patient and graft survival rates were similar. Rejection episodes resistant to increased doses of steroids occurred in 11.3% of TRL and 21.6% of CsA recipients ($P = 0.001$). However, the rates of occurrence of chronic allograft rejection did *not* differ significantly

Trial	No. of patients	1-year survival rates (%)						Acute rejection episodes (%)		
		Patient			Graft					
		TRL	CsA	P	TRL	CsA	P	TRL	CsA	P
US multicenter[a]	412	95.6	96.6	NS	91.2	87.9	NS	30.7	46.6	0.001
European multicenter[b]	448	93	96.5	NS	82.5	86.2	NS	25.9	45.7	0.001

NS: not significant.

[a]Pirsch et al 1997.

[b]Mayer et al 1997.

Table 9.3. Randomized, controlled clinical trials on the efficacy of tacrolimus (TRL) versus Sandimmune cyclosporine (CsA)-based immunosuppressive therapy in conjunction with azathioprine (AZA) and prednisone (Prec) in renal transplantation

Trial	No. of patients	Duration (years)	Survival rates						Acute rejection episodes (%)[a]		
			Patient			Graft					
			TRL	CsA	P	TRL	CsA	P	TRL	CsA	P
US trials											
Multicenter[b]	529	1	88	88	NS	82	79	NS	59	65	0.002
Fung et al[c]	154	4	84	84	NS	ND	ND	ND	63.8	83	0.003
Wiesner multicenter[d]	529	5	79	73.1	NS	71.8	66.4	NS	68	76	<0.001
European trials											
Jonas et al[e]	121	1	90.2	96.7	NS	88.5	91.7	NS	34.4	33.3	NS
Multicenter[f]	545	1	82.9	77.5	NS	77.5	72.6	NS	40.5	49.8	0.04

NS: not significant; ND: no data reported.

[a]Acute rejection rates between 1 and 5 years' follow-up.

[b]US Multicenter FK506 Liver Study Group 1994.

[c]Fung et al 1996.

[d]Wiesner 1998.

[e]Jonas et al 1995.

[f]European FK506 Multicentre Liver Study Group 1994.

Table 9.4. Randomized, controlled clinical trials on efficacy of tacrolimus (TRL) versus Sandimmune cyclosporine (CsA)-based immunosuppressive therapy in liver transplantation

between TRL- and CsA-treated patients (5.2 and 9.3%, respectively; Mayer et al 1997).

Knoll and Bell (1999) performed a meta-analysis of randomized trials that fulfilled the requirements of the Jadad scale for inclusion. Among 1037 patients, the overall results showed no significant difference in patient or graft survival between TRL- and CsA-treated patients, but confirmed the apparently favorable effect of TRL on the occurrence of acute rejection episodes. Interestingly, a reduced rejection rate (8.9%) was encountered during the first month posttransplant using a 0.10 mg/kg dose of TRL (10–15 ng/ml whole blood concentration; Miller et al 1999) rather than the 0.15 mg/kg (15–20 ng/ml) previously recommended (Shapiro et al 1999a).

Size-limited and therefore anecdotal experiences in pancreas (Gruessner et al 1996), heart (Pham et al 1996; Tsamandas et al 1997; Reichart et al 1998), and lung (Keenan et al 1995) transplantation suggest that TRL and Sandimmune CsA display similar efficacy in preventing acute rejection episodes and improving graft survival. Using the combination of TRL, MMF, and Pred, Shapiro et al (1999a) recently observed a relatively high (27%) incidence of acute renal allograft rejection episodes. This result compares unfavorably with the 14% rate among patients in the pivotal trial treated with a combination regimen of SRL, CsA (Neoral), and Pred (Kahan et al 1998a), and with the 12% incidence among a small cohort treated with SRL, TRL, and steroids (MacDonald et al 1998). However, single-center reports from the University of Miami group (Roth et al 1998; Ciancio et al 1999) utilizing antibody induction combined with TRL, MMF, and steroids suggest that it may be possible to achieve results similar to those obtained using the CsA/SRL/Pred combination, albeit at far greater cost.

Two nonrandomized, open-label US trials using TRL for rescue therapy of kidney transplant rejection episodes refractory only to steroids yielded patient and graft survival rates of 94 and 93%, and 74 and 75%, respectively (Woodle et al 1996; Jordan et al 1997). These patients were converted from Sandimmune CsA to TRL at a median of 4.3 months, upon presumed 'unresponsiveness' to increased doses of steroids with or *without* administration of antilymphocyte antibody agents. Conversion tended to be 'successful', namely, 75% reversal, if the patient displayed a low serum creatinine value and if the maneuver was performed within 6 months posttransplant. Budde et al (1998) reported a successful outcome of conversion from Sandimmune to TRL in 50% of patients who showed histopathologic evidence of acute rejection, but no patient with the findings of chronic rejection on biopsy. Among hepatic allograft recipients, conversion to TRL in the settings of steroid-resistant acute or early chronic rejection processes was claimed to confer both histological and biochemical improvements (Fung et al 1991; Klintmalm et al 1993; Jain et al 1996; Sher et al 1997).

Benefits were also observed among pancreas graft recipients treated with TRL for refractory rejection (Hariharan et al 1995; Shaffer et al 1995; Teraoka et al 1995; Hariharan et al 1997). Gruessner et al (1996) reported 6-month data from a multicenter, open-label study of 154 pancreas allograft recipients treated with TRL de novo ($N = 82$), or converted from CsA to TRL for rescue therapy ($N = 61$) or for other reasons ($N = 11$). Among the de novo patients, 66% were simultaneous pancreas–kidney (SPK) transplant recipients, who collectively displayed a 6-month patient survival rate of 90% and a pancreas graft survival rate of 87%, results that were better than those obtained in an arbitrary post hoc matched-pair historical cohort of CsA recipients ($P = 0.04$). Within the first 6 months, the SPK group also showed a 35% rate of acute rejection episodes, all of which were reversible.

Dosage regimens

Both CsA and TRL are available for intravenous and oral administration. Because of their proclivity to produce a renal vasomotor injury, the intravenous formulations are rarely indicated for immunosuppressive therapy, particularly in the early posttransplant period. Continuous intravenous infusion seems to offer less toxicity, but also reduced efficacy compared with a bolus intravenous injection or even oral administration.

The initial dose of CsA delivered intravenously is 3 mg/kg per day; by the oral route, the recommended starting doses are 8–12 mg/kg per day CsA, usually administered in divided, twice-daily doses. The choice of the dose depends on whether the drug is delivered as the Sandimmune or as the better-absorbed Neoral formulation. Because of their propensity for greater rates of cytochrome P450 3A4 metabolism, children require higher doses (0.03–0.1 mg/kg per day intravenously or 0.15–0.3 mg/kg per day by mouth) and shorter dosing intervals to achieve whole blood concentrations similar to those of adults. Dose adjustment to achieve target concentrations is critical to avoid early acute rejection episodes (Lindholm and Kahan 1993). Furthermore, pediatric patients may benefit from an overlap of intravenous and oral drug administration to avoid suboptimal trough concentrations during the critical first 2 weeks posttransplantation. Similarly, because of their higher drug clearance rates and lower drug absorption than other ethnic groups, African-American patients seem to require larger drug doses than either Caucasian or Asian recipients (Lindholm et al 1992). Dose adjustments are generally performed based upon drug concentrations, as described in Chapter 7. Owing to the availability of reliable, automated methods and the understanding of drug pharmacokinetics, the relationships between concentration and effect of CsA are relatively well understood.

Tacrolimus is currently available for both intravenous (5 mg/ml in a 1 ml vial) and oral (1 mg and 5 mg capsules) administration. For continuous intravenous infusion, initial TRL doses are 0.01–0.1 mg/kg per day; when taken orally, a total of 0.1–0.3 mg/kg/day is administered in divided doses every 12 hours.

Unfortunately, the optimal therapeutic ranges for TRL drug concentrations during the induction, acute rejection prophylaxis, and maintenance phases of immunosuppression are unknown. The US multicenter study of the correlation between TRL concentrations and episodes of toxicity and rejection among 120 kidney transplant patients reported that optimal efficacy occurred with TRL trough concentrations of 5–15 μg/l (Laskow et al 1996). Concentrations below 5 μg/l were associated with a 30% incidence of acute rejection episodes, and those above 15 μg/l, with a 45% incidence of adverse events and a 3% incidence of rejection episodes. However, the enzyme-linked immunoassay to estimate TRL concentrations displays a high degree of crossreactivity between active parent and inactive metabolite compounds, and thus the kinetic–dynamic relations of the drug are less well understood than those for CsA.

Toxicities

Both CsA and TRL are associated with a major therapeutic limitation: renal dysfunction, which is believed to result from calcineurin inhibition (Bennett et al 1996a). The agents seem to produce similar degrees of clinical and histopathological evidence of nephrotoxicity that are proportionate to their therapeutic effects. Overall, the clinical findings suggest that CNAs induce a renal vasomotor effect that reduces creatinine clearance as one evidence of a generalized vasculopathy, as well as upregulating TGF-β, which may produce interstitial fibrosis.

Comparison of renal function among cardiac transplant recipients treated with high-dose CsA- versus AZA-based regimens documented specific reductions of glomerular filtration rate, renal plasma flow, and renal blood flow (Table 9.5). Figure 9.13 shows the plot of inverse creatinine values of cardiac recipients treated with a large dose of CsA versus those receiving an AZA-based regimen. Curtis et al (1986) reported similar findings in a study of renal allograft recipients converted from a CsA- to an AZA-based regimen. Even under optimal circumstances during treatment of renal allograft recipients with CsA or TRL-based regimens, the renal function usually declines by 25% during the first 6 months of therapy, followed thereafter by stabilization of the serum creatinine (Figure 9.14). Indeed, owing to the onset of rejection processes preceding renal compromise in AZA-treated transplant recipients, there is little difference at 5 years in the mean serum creatinine values of patients under an AZA- versus a CsA-based regimen (Figure 9.15). However, the longer-term results are not clear; the renal function in the CsA group may be inferior by 10 years.

Group	No. of patients	Glomerular filtration rate	Renal plasma flow[a]	Renal blood flow[a]
AZA	14	93 ± 3	480 ± 30	802 ± 52
CsA	17	51 ± 4[b]	320 ± 21[c]	501 ± 35[c]

[a]ml/min per 1.73 m^2.

[b]$P < 0.005$ versus AZA.

[c]$P < 0.001$ versus AZA.

Table 9.5. Comparison of renal function parameters among cardiac transplant patients treated with cyclosporine (CsA) versus azathioprine (AZA) immunosuppressive therapy (Myers et al 1984)

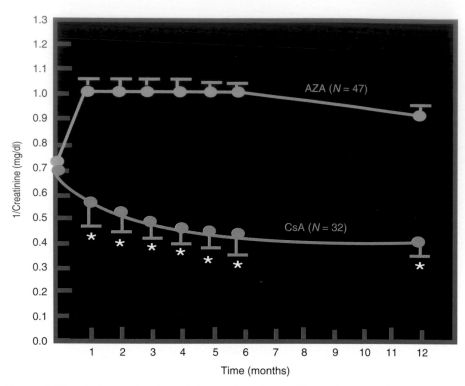

Figure 9.13. CsA-associated renal dysfunction observed in cardiac transplant recipients. Plot of inverse serum creatinine value among AZA-treated recipients ($N = 47$, green line) versus CsA-treated recipients ($N = 32$, red line). The difference between the determinations was significant at $P < 0.005$. (Myers BD, Ross J, Newton L, Luetscher J, Perlroth M. Cyclosporine-associated chronic nephropathy. *N Engl J Med* 1984 Sept 13; **311**(11):699–705. © 1984 Massachusetts Medical Society. All rights reserved.)

Pathophysiologic changes in preclinical models show that the afferent arteriole seems to be the primary target of CNA toxicity (Figure 9.16). The histologic findings of arteriolar hyalinosis (Figure 9.17) reflect endothelial and smooth muscle cell damage, producing vascular obliteration and striped interstitial fibrosis (Randhawa et al 1993; Katari et al 1997), changes that are more resistant to reversal, although some element of remodeling may occur. Calcineurin antagonists also seem to promote adhesion of platelets, particularly when the intima has been damaged and displays upregulated synthesis and/or release of endothelin and thromboxane A_2, as well as smooth muscle cell proliferation (Figure 9.18; Mason 1989). These effects alter blood flow and mesangial cell physiology, thereby enhancing the proclivity to hypertension and reducing the glomerular filtration rates (GFR). The reduced blood flow produces, at least initially, focal (Figure 9.19), later, striped (Figure 9.20), and eventually, more widespread interstitial fibrosis, which has been attributed to upregulated TGF-β synthesis (Yamamoto et al 1994; Sharma et al 1996).

Calcineurin antagonists alter the physiology of the distal segment of the proximal tubule, producing hyperuricemia, and of the loop of Henle, resulting in urinary wasting

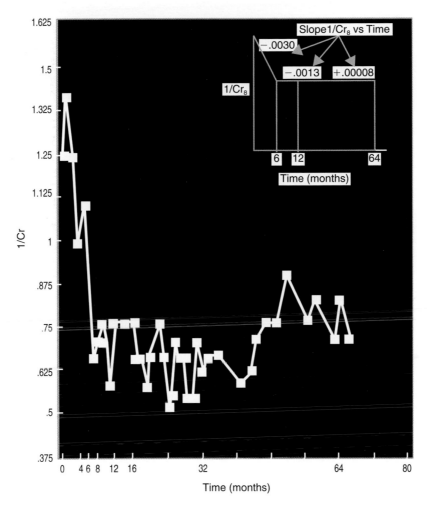

Figure 9.14. Plot of the inverse value of serum creatinine versus time in a CsA-treated renal transplant patient. Insert is a diagrammatic representation showing three phases of the nephrotoxic injury: the primary decrease during the first 6 months, a second phase of mild renal deterioration from 6 to 12 months, and a third phase of stabilization with modest improvement thereafter to 64 months upon slight CsA dose reduction.

of magnesium. The tubular effects cause hypomagnesemia, sodium retention, hyperkalemia, hyperuricemia, and hyperchloremic acidosis. The morphologic alterations that are most obvious in the distal segment of the proximal tubule include isometric vacuolization, giant mitochondria, and microcalcifications, changes that are generally reversible (Table 9.6).

Renal dysfunction appears to have a multifunctional expression, including an abnormal profile of local humoral mediators (Table 9.7). While few data support a reciprocal decrease in prostacyclin generation with an increase in thromboxane A_2 synthesis as the

Site	Largely reversible		Largely irreversible	
	Functional	Structural	Structural	
Afferent arterioles	↓ Glomerular filtration rate	Vasoconstriction	Endothelial cell injury	
	↑ Urea		Smooth muscle cell damage	
	↑ Blood pressure		Vascular obliteration	
Proximal tubule	Altered serum analytes	Isomeric vacuoles	Atrophy	
	↑ K⁺	Giant mitochondria	Striped interstitial fibrosis	
	↓ Mg	Microcalcification		
	↓ HCO_3			
	↑ Uric acid			

Table 9.6. Calcineurin antagonist (CNA)-induced renal changes

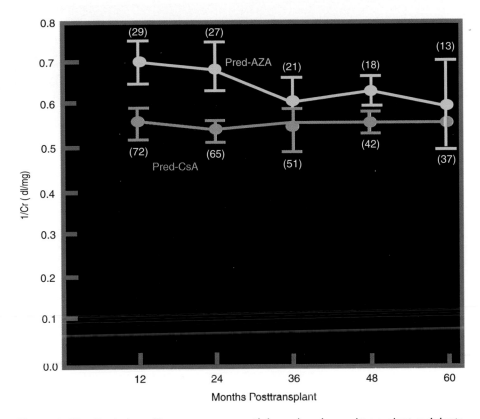

Figure 9.15. Evolution of inverse serum creatinine values in renal transplant recipients. Comparison of results using an AZA-Pred (N = 29, green line) versus a CsA-Pred (N = 72, red line) regimen over the period from 12 to 60 months. The differences in mean values were not significant.

seminal clinical event, considerable evidence suggests the roles of augmented local release of endothelin, TGF-β, and renin, possibly complemented by a decrease in endothelial-derived relaxation factor. In addition to the humoral mediators, several factors exacerbate the vasculopathic injury: augmented thrombogenicity by promoting ADP-stimulated platelet aggregation, thromboplastin generation, factor VII synthesis, thrombin release, and increased generation of platelet-derived growth factor. Calcineurin antagonists also seem to promote Ca^{2+} uptake into anoxic endothelium, to increase sympathetic tone, and to enhance atherogenicity related to hyper-cholesterolemia (Figure 9.18). Cyclosporine also promotes mitochondrial dysfunction, leading to the release of oxygen free radicals, with subsequent peroxidation of lipid membranes.

The three clinical forms of CNA-induced renal dysfunction are shown in Table 9.8. Acute nephrotoxicity occurs in the immediate postoperative period, particularly in marginal kidneys obtained from hypotensive or from pediatric or aged donors, all of which

377

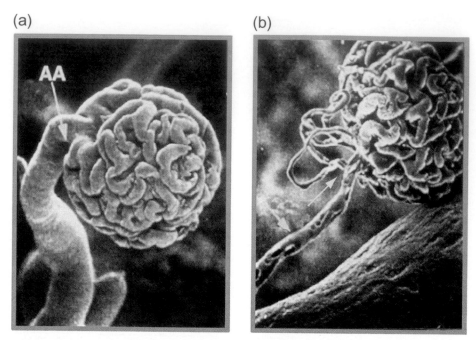

Figure 9.16. Constriction of the afferent arteriole (AA) in normal (a) versus CsA-treated (b) rat kidneys, as shown by the arrows. (English J, Evan A, Houghton DC, Bennett WM. Cyclosporine-induced acute renal dysfunction in the rat. Evidence of arteriolar vasoconstriction with preservation of tubular function. *Transplantation* 1987; **44**:135–141. © 1987 Lippincott Williams & Wilkins. All rights reserved.)

Reduced production of local vasodilators versus vasoconstrictors
    ↑ Endothelin
    ↑ TGF-β
    ↓ Endothelial-derived relaxation factor
    ↑ Local renin release
    ↓ Prostacyclin
    ↑ Thromboxane A_2
Increased generation of free oxygen radicals
Increased sympathetic tone
Increased Ca-dependent vasoconstrictor mechanisms
Increased thrombogenicity of blood
    ↑ ADP → platelet aggregation
    ↑ Thromboplastin
    ↑ Factor VII
    ↑ Thrombin → ↑ PDGF
Enhanced atherogenicity
    ↑ Cholesterol

Table 9.7. Vasculopathic components of the nephrotoxic injury induced by calcineurin antagonists (CNAs)

Type	Timing	Predisposing factors	Treatment
Acute	Days	Donor hypotension Pediatric-aged donor	CNA avoidance
Subacute	Days to months	High drug levels	CNA dose reduction
Chronic	Months	Chronic rejection	Switch to SRL?

Table 9.8. Forms of nephrotoxicity caused by calcineurin antagonists (CNAs)

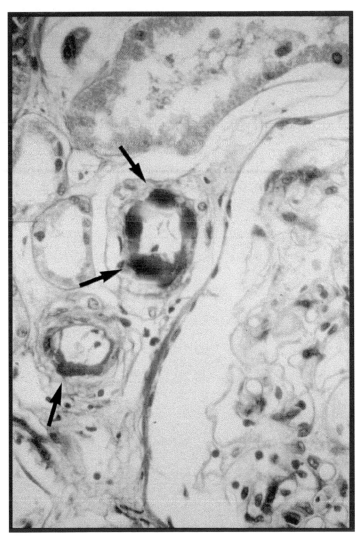

Figure 9.17. Arteriolar mucoid deposits in renal biopsy of CsA-treated patient (shown by arrows). (Alcian blue stain, ×42; micrograph courtesy of Dr Michael Mihatsch, Kanton Hospital, Basel, Switzerland.)

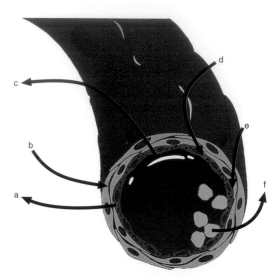

Figure 9.18. Diagrammatic representation of potential pathogenic mechanisms of CsA-induced arteriolar change. (a) Changes in endothelial cell physiology, including increased endothelin and thromboxane A_2 production, and/or decreased generation of prostacyclin and endothelial cell relaxation factor. (b) Increased sympathetic tone. (c) Increased serum cholesterol content, activation of intrinsic coagulation factors and platelet aggregation. (d) Prorenin granule invasion. (e) Promoted calcium ion uptake into anoxic endothelium. (f) Increased release of platelet-derived growth factor and of transforming growth factor-β (TGF-β).

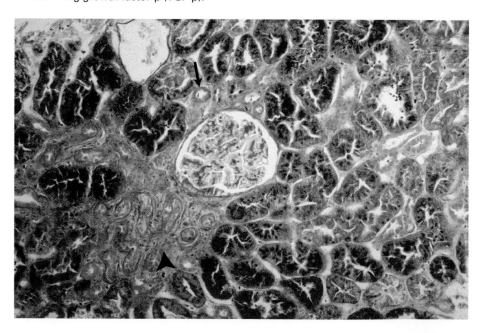

Figure 9.19. Fibrosis in a renal allograft in a CsA-treated patient. Arteriole demonstrating hyalinosis shown by arrow. Fibrotic area (shown by arrowhead) surrounded by relatively normal tubular cells. (Mallory Trichrome stain, ×24.)

(a)

(b)

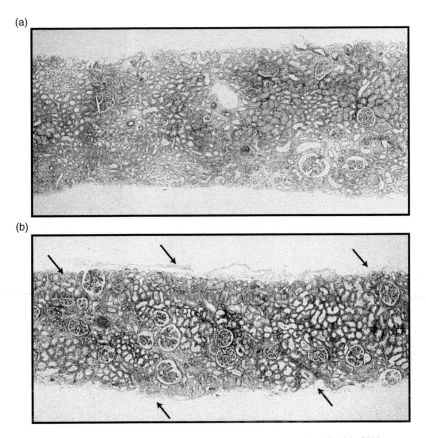

Figure 9.20. Striped interstitial fibrosis, an appearance associated with CNA nephrotoxicity. (a) Biopsy of a normal kidney. (b) Striped interstitial fibrosis (shown by arrows) separated by areas of normal renal parenchyma (hematoxylin and eosin [H&E] stain, ×10).

are highly vulnerable to adverse events. Because the 1-month serum creatinine value clearly correlates with 1-year graft survival (Figure 9.21), it is important to minimize the early injury to the allograft. The optimal therapeutic approach to protecting the allograft de novo is an induction regimen that avoids CNA drugs, yet is not associated with acute rejection episodes. However, this goal has been difficult to achieve in clinical practice. For example, the use of antilymphocyte antibodies, such as polyclonal equine antilymphocyte antibodies (Novick et al 1986), delays the occurrence but does not alter the incidence of acute rejection episodes. Use of MMF in combination with antithymocyte globulin (ATG) was associated with a substantial (25%) incidence of acute rejection episodes (Grinyó et al 1998). Zanker et al (1998) found that induction treatment with rabbit ATG and MMF did not substantially reduce the rate of delayed graft function, but was associated with a high incidence of CMV infections. The combination of MMF and anti-IL-2R was associated with a 50% incidence of acute rejection episodes

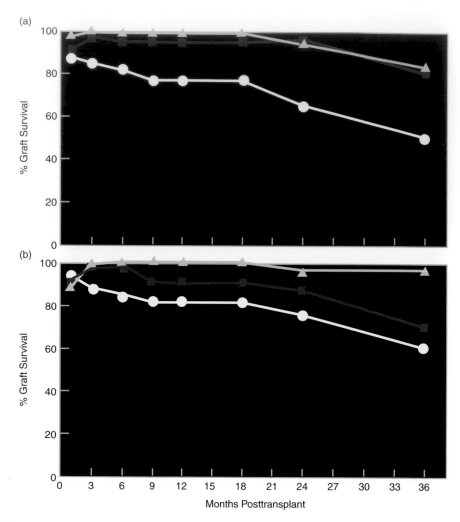

Figure 9.21. Impact of 1-month serum creatinine value or systolic blood pressure on 3-year graft survival. (a) Patients stratified by 1-month serum creatinine values less than 1.5 mg/dl (green line), 1.5–2.2 mg/dl (red line), or >2.2 (yellow line). The difference in graft survival between the >2.2 mg/dl versus the other groups was significant ($P < 0.0001$ by Fisher's exact test). (b) Patients stratified by 1-month reading of systolic blood pressure, <138 mmHg (green line), 139–152 mmHg (red line), or >152 mmHg (yellow line). The difference in graft survival between the >152 mmHg versus the other groups was significant ($P = 0.0002$ by Fisher's exact test). (Adapted from Kahan BD, Mickey R, Flechner SM et al. Multivariate analysis of risk factors impacting on immediate and eventual cadaver allograft survival in cyclosporine-treated recipients. *Transplantation* 1987; **43**:65–78.)

(Vincenti et al 1998), a rate that was only slightly improved with concomitant administration of reduced doses of CsA (Hueso et al 1998). Experience at The University of Texas at Houston demonstrated that patients treated de novo by elimination of CsA from a regimen of anti-IL-2R MAbs in combination with SRL showed superior renal function at 6 months compared to those treated with CsA exposures at values one-half those used in the absence of SRL.

Subacute nephrotoxicity is caused by, and reverses within 3–14 days upon reduction of, high levels of drug exposure. By definition, subacute nephrotoxicity is reversible. In contrast, chronic CNA-induced nephropathy is a progressive form of renal dysfunction. Figure 9.21 shows the impact of an elevated serum creatinine or systolic blood pressure value at 1 month to significantly decrease the probability of graft survival. Treatment of long-term CNA-induced nephrotoxicity by conversion to an AZA-based regimen has been associated with an increased risk of acute rejection episodes (Kasiske et al 1993; Hollander et al 1995). However, CsA dose reduction (Vianello et al 1993), especially with the addition of AZA (Lorber et al 1987; Mourad et al 1998), improves renal function among patients experiencing chronic toxicity, with less risk of an increased rate of acute rejection episodes. The risk of rebound rejection is further reduced when the CNA is combined either with MMF (Weir et al 1997) or, particularly, with SRL. However, the impaired renal function is only incompletely reversible, even upon conversion from CNA to SRL.

Non-renal toxicity with CsA therapy is well documented with adverse cosmetic effects, including hypertrichosis, lionization of the face of the pediatric patient, and, rarely, gingival hyperplasia (Kahan 1989) being shown. Hypertrichosis (or increased hair growth), which is distinguished from hirsutism (increased hair growth in the male pattern), tends to be mild, but can be exacerbated by concomitant treatment with minoxidil. The use of depilatories generally controls this problem. Similarly, the intensity of gingival hyperplasia, a condition that is seen rarely (<1% of patients), is mitigated by scrupulous dental hygiene (daily flossing and monthly scaling), as well as by the avoidance of concomitant phenytoin or nifedipine therapies. Gingivectomy is rarely required. The claim that, compared with TRL, CsA is associated with a greater degree of hypercholesterolemia has not been confirmed upon survey of the transplant literature. Furthermore, reports on differences in the incidences of hypertension with TRL versus CsA therapy have been inconsistent (Pirsch et al 1997; Radermacher et al 1998).

Non-renal toxicity of TRL therapy compared with CsA is more commonly associated with neurotoxicity, which may present as severe central nervous system disturbances including tremor, headache, seizures, and coma, necessitating conversion to CsA (Table 9.9, Figure 9.22). Furthermore, there is a question of impaired central nervous system function among TRL versus CsA patients, as evidenced upon psychologic and motor tests (DiMartini et al 1997). A second important toxicity of TRL compared with CsA is a significantly increased proportion of patients that experience new-onset PTDM, namely, 19 versus 4% ($P < 0.001$; Pirsch et al 1997). This complication is particularly common among African-American kidney transplant recipients (Neylan 1998). Although this phenomenon may result from the use of higher TRL doses needed to achieve target whole blood drug concentrations in this ethnic group (Andrews et al 1996; Radermacher et al 1998), African-American patients did not experience an increased incidence of other TRL-related adverse effects. In 80% of afflicted patients in this racial group, PTDM requires continuous insulin treatment beyond 2 years

Adverse event	TRL (N = 205)	CsA (N = 207)	P
Nephrotoxicity	45.5% (93)	41.5% (86)	NS
Neurotoxicity: tremor	53.6% (111)	33.8% (70)	0.001
Hypertension	49.8% (102)	52.2% (108)	NS
Posttransplant diabetes mellitus (PTDM)	19.9% (30)	2.90% (6)	0.001
Hyperlipidemia	30.7% (63)	38.2% (79)	NS
Hypercholesterolemia	7.80% (16)	14.5% (30)	NS
Alopecia	10.7% (22)	0.97% (2)	0.001
Hirsutism	0.49% (1)	8.7% (18)	0.001
Gingivitis	1.46% (3)	8.7% (18)	0.001

[a]From Pirsch et al 1997.

Table 9.9. Comparison of selected adverse events with tacrolimus (TRL) and cyclosporine (CsA)[a]

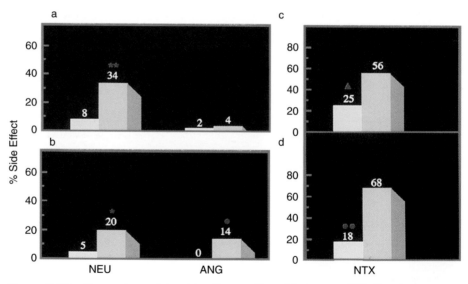

Figure 9.22. Comparison of the side-effect profiles of CsA versus TRL. Results in patients treated with CsA shown in yellow; TRL in green. (a) Comparison of incidence of neurotoxicity (NEU; **$P < 0.01$) and of angina (ANG) among liver transplant recipients. (b) Side-effects in renal transplant recipients (*$P < 0.05$), (•$P < 0.001$). (c) Percentage decline in glomerular filtration rate (▲$P < 0.05$). (d) Incidence of nephrotoxicity (••$P < 0.01$).

posttransplant. Upon microscopic examination of pancreatic graft biopsies from SPK transplant recipients, the Maryland group (Drachenberg et al 1999) observed a greater extent of islet cell damage among TRL- versus CsA-treated patients, a finding that was particularly exacerbated by the concomitant presence of steroids. Additionally, compared to those treated with CsA, TRL-treated patients experience an increased incidence of alopecia, nausea, and diarrhea (Table 9.9; Shapiro et al 1998).

AGENTS AFFECTING SIGNAL THREE RECEPTION

Anti-IL-2R monoclonal antibodies

Because of their proclivity to elicit HAMA, entirely murine anti-human IL-2R MAbs showed only modest clinical efficacy in the initial clinical experience. However, the new MAbs, which contain a preponderance of human structures, do not suffer this limitation and thus display considerable clinical benefit. A comparison of the potencies of the two types of reagents reveals a 10-fold-*lower* avidity for the IL-2R of the humanized MAb, daclizumab, than the chimeric MAb, basiliximab. (The structures of basiliximab and daclizumab are shown in Chapter 8.)

Therapeutic effects

Addition of five doses of daclizumab to a regimen of CsA, AZA, and steroids significantly reduced the incidence of biopsy-proven acute rejection within the first 6 months to 28%, compared to 43% for the placebo-treated group in the US trial (with AZA-Pred) and to 47% in the European cohort (without AZA; $P = 0.03$; Vincenti et al 1998; Nashan et al 1999). However, at 12 months, the CsA-AZA-Pred group displayed no benefit of daclizumab treatment (Daclizumab Product Insert). Two multicenter trials (US and worldwide) using the same protocol documented that administration of two 20 mg doses of basiliximab in combination with CsA and steroids decreased both the incidence (33% basiliximab group versus 48% placebo group, $P = 0.012$) and the severity of acute rejection episodes (Nashan et al 1997; Kahan et al 1999c; Table 9.10). Figure 9.23a shows that basiliximab-treated patients in the US trial displayed a significantly greater rate of freedom from occurrence of the composite index of an acute rejection episode, graft loss, or death. Furthermore, in this study, basiliximab-treated patients displayed better renal function during the first posttransplant year than placebo-treated patients (Kahan et al 1999c; Figure 9.23b).

The immunosuppressive activity of these reagents is limited by two shortcomings. First, the antibodies do not compete effectively with the IL-2 ligand for binding to the IL-2R. Thus, the present generation of anti-IL-2R MAbs cannot reverse acute rejection episodes. Second, the specificity of the antibodies for CD25 (IL-2Rα), while ensuring their reactivity with only activated T cells, does not prevent immune activation generated via other cytokines, such as IL-7 and IL-15, which can be recruited to mediate allorejection in IL-2 knockout animals. Despite these limitations, the anti-IL-2R MAbs represent important additions to the immunosuppressive arsenal, since they can be harnessed for induction therapy, thus reserving monoclonal OKT3 or polyclonal

| | Basiliximab | Daclizumab | |
	Kahan et al 1999c/ Nashan et al 1997[a]	Vincenti et al 1998[b]	Nashan et al 1999[c]
Number of patients	356/376	260	275
CsA + Pred+	—	AZA	—
Aggregate patient survival, 12 months (%)(P)	96%/97% (NS)[d]	98%/95% (NS)	99%/94% (0.01)
Aggregate graft survival, 12 months (%)(P)	91%/90% (NS)	91%/87% (NS)	83%/88% (NS)
Aggregate acute rejection episodes (%)(P)[e]	33%/48% (0.001)	28%/43% (0.001)	28%/47% (0.001)
Aggregate salvage treatment (%)(P)	15%/26% (0.001)	8%/15% (0.005)	8%/16% (0.02)

[a]Aggregate values from both studies combined using CsA-Pred comparator.

[b]Comparison to CsA-AZA-Pred baseline regimen.

[c]Comparison to CsA-Pred baseline regimen.

[d]Percentage of patients in MAb-treated group/percentage of patients in placebo group (P value).

[e]Biopsy-proved.

Table 9.10 Basiliximab versus daclizumab: 6-month results of pivotal trials

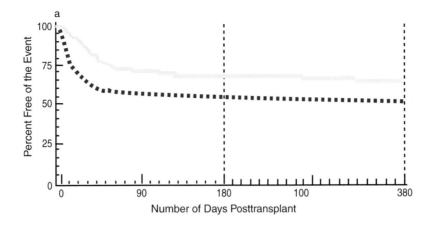

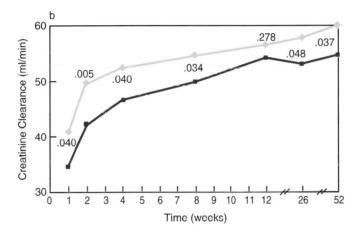

Figure 9.23. (a) Comparison of the percentage of patients free of the composite index of an acute rejection episode, graft loss, or death (Kaplan–Meier; $P = 0.002$). Patients treated with chimeric MAb shown by the yellow line; placebo, by the red, dotted line. (b) Comparison of calculated creatinine clearance values (ml/min) over the first year posttransplant among 308 patients receiving either chimeric anti-IL-2R MAb (yellow line) or placebo (red line). At each point, 'P' values represent the comparison of mean values by unpaired Student's t-test. (Both panels from Kahan BD, Rajagopalan PR, Hall M for the United States Simulect Renal Study Group. Reduction of the occurrence of acute cellular rejection among renal allograft recipients treated with basiliximab, a chimeric anti-interleukin-2-receptor monoclonal antibody. *Transplantation* 1999; **67**:276–284. © 1999 Lippincott Williams & Wilkins. All rights reserved.)

ATGAM/thymoglobulin antibody reagents for potential subsequent rejection episodes. While induction immunosuppression with daclizumab and MMF was attended by almost a 50% incidence of acute rejection episodes (Vincenti et al 1999), the combination of basiliximab with SRL has permitted extended periods (mean, 33 days) of freedom from concomitant CsA treatment. Only 18% of patients experienced acute rejection episodes, which occurred only in retransplant or African-American patients (Hong and Kahan 1999).

Dosage regimens

The FDA-approved regimen stipulates daclizumab administration intravenously at a dose of 1 mg/kg per dose beginning within 24 hours of transplant surgery, followed by four equal amounts every 14 days. For a 70 kg patient, 350 mg of antibody is administered. In contrast, the US FDA-approved regimen stipulates 20 mg basiliximab administered intravenously on day 0 and on day 4. Hence, the dose ratio of daclizumab to basiliximab is approximately 10:1. Anti-IL-2R MAbs produce a blockade of IL-2R, beginning at 10 hours after the initial dose and lasting as long as 4 months posttransplant, with an average period of effect lasting 60 days. As discussed in Chapter 7, there is no apparent benefit to monitoring either serum levels of antibody or the expression of CD25 on patient lymphocytes (Kovarik et al 1999).

Toxicities

In the randomized trials, patients treated with daclizumab or basiliximab showed no greater incidences of adverse reactions than those treated with placebo. Neither MAb elicited the cytokine release syndrome, since the CD25 polypeptide bears only a short cytoplasmic segment that does not perform a signal transduction function. Furthermore, the incidence of production of HAMA was modest, albeit about four-fold greater for daclizumab than for basiliximab.

Potential alternate agent

Although not presently US FDA-approved, the murine IgG_1 κ MAb (Biotest Pharma, Dreieich, Germany) directed against CD25 is undergoing initial trials for prophylaxis of organ transplant rejection. Prophylactic administration of 10 mg/day on alternate days for 10 days in combination with CsA and Pred was found to reduce the incidence of acute rejection episodes during the first month posttransplant (Van Gelder et al 1995b). Furthermore, continuous infusion of 10 mg/day for 10 days reversed steroid-resistant acute rejection episodes in 13 of 14 patients, with 12 of 14 patients displaying stable graft function at 1 year (Wiesel et al 1995). In another trial of 19 patients, 13 continued to bear functioning renal grafts at 3 years (Carl et al 1997). Successful treatment was associated with a decline in the serum levels of IL-2 and IL-6. Encouraging results with this MAb have also been reported in liver (Nashan et al 1996; Langrehr et al 1997), but not in cardiac (Van Gelder et al 1995a), allograft recipients. Although its administration does not elicit the cytokine release syndrome, this MAb readily provokes the production of HAMA and thus offers only limited clinical application.

mTOR INHIBITORS THAT BLOCK G_1 PROGRESSION

Sirolimus

Therapeutic effects

As a primary agent, SRL seems equipotent to CsA. A phase II open-label trial revealed that patients treated with a regimen of SRL-AZA-Pred showed an incidence of acute rejection rates at 6 months that was comparable to that of patients treated with a CsA-AZA-Pred regimen, namely, 41% and 38%, respectively (Groth et al 1999; Table 9.11).

However, the initial raison d'être for the clinical use of SRL was to potentiate the immunosuppressive effects of CsA in a dual-drug combination. The first phase II study, which was conducted at The University of Texas at Houston, demonstrated that addition of SRL to a CsA-Pred regimen reduced the incidence of acute rejection episodes from 35 to 7.5% (with two to three rejection episodes occurring in patients withdrawn from steroids; Table 9.11). Overall, the CsA-SRL combination permitted 78% of patients to be successfully withdrawn from steroid therapy at 2 years (Kahan et al 1998a). Similarly, a multicenter phase II trial showed that addition of SRL permitted a 40% reduction in Sandimmune CsA exposure among non-African-American patients, without increasing the incidence of acute rejection episodes from the 12% incidence observed with full doses of CsA (Kahan et al 1999b; Figure 9.24).

The pivotal phase III US and global trials showed that the efficacy failure rates (a composite of the occurrences of acute rejection episodes, graft loss, and/or death) at 6 months for treatment with SRL doses of 5 or 2 mg versus AZA (US trial) or placebo (global trial), respectively, were 16.8, 18.7, and 32.3% (US trial) versus 25.6, 30.0, and 47.7% (global trial), respectively ($P = 0.002$ and $P < 0.001$, respectively, for both studies). The incidences of acute rejection episodes in the two trials were 12.0 and 17.0% versus 29.8% ($P < 0.001$, $P = 0.002$), and 19.2 and 24.7% versus 41.5% ($P < 0.001$ and $P = 0.003$), respectively. Figure 9.25 shows that the overall rate of occurrence of the endpoint among patients in both studies (SRL 2 mg/day = 51, SRL

Phase	Site	Acute rejection incidence (%)	
		Experimental	Control
IIA[a]	Houston	SRL-CsA (7%)	CsA (35%)
IIB[b]	US/Europe	SRL-CsA (10%)	CsA (40%)
IIC[c]	Europe	SRL (41%)	CsA (38%)

[a]Kahan et al 1998a.
[b]Kahan et al 1999b.
[c]Groth et al 1999.

Table 9.11. Summary sirolimus (SRL) phase II open-label clinical trials

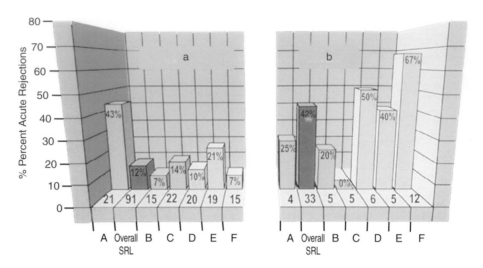

Figure 9.24. Results of phase IIB multicenter trial of SRL in combination with CsA and Pred, expressed as incidence of acute rejection episodes within 6 months. (a) Results in non-black patients. (b) Results in African-American patients. The cohorts include (A) full-dose CsA with no SRL; (B) full-dose CsA with 1 mg/m² SRL; (C) full-dose CsA with 3 mg/m² SRL; (D) reduced-dose CsA with 1 mg/m² SRL; (E) reduced-dose CsA with 3 mg/m² SRL; and (F) reduced-dose CsA with 5 mg/m² SRL. The pink bar represents the aggregate rate for all SRL groups. The number of patients in each cohort is indicated at the base of the panel, and the acute rejection rates are shown within the bars.

5 mg/day = 493, placebo = 130, AZA = 161) was significantly reduced and delayed ($P < 0.0001$). Furthermore, fewer patients treated with SRL displayed acute rejection episodes that were graded as moderate or severe by the Banff system (namely, 4.4, 8.12, and 17.4%, as well as 8.3, 12.4, and 25.4%, respectively) or required antibody therapy for reversal (namely, 2.9 and 5.6% versus 12.4%, $P < 0.001$ and $P = 0.017$; and 3.2 and 4.0% versus 8.5%, $P = 0.132$ and $P = 0.094$). Patient and graft survival rates were similar among all groups (Table 9.12). As is the case for other agents, higher (5 mg/day) doses of SRL were necessary to show a therapeutic effect in African-American patients (Kahan et al 1999a).

Preliminary findings among 18 adult patients suggest that SRL can reverse allograft rejection episodes that are refractory to both OKT3 and either ATGAM or MMF 'rescue', indeed permitting steroid withdrawal in some cases (Slaton and Kahan 1996; Kahan et al 1998b). The actuarial 2-year graft survival among these transplants destined for failure was about 80%. Furthermore, because SRL is *not* nephrotoxic, it represents a potent alternative to CNAs for use in induction immunosuppression. Figure 9.26a shows the protocol for patients to receive a course of an anti-IL-2R MAb together with SRL and steroids. Once the renal function has improved to a serum creatinine less than 3.0 mg/dl, which usually occurs within 7–150 days, CsA is initiated at low dose and gradually advanced. At 1 month after CsA inception, the steroids are withdrawn. Figure 9.26 illustrates the successful application of this strategy.

Outcome (%)	US trial[a]			Global trial[b]		
	Placebo/AZA	SRL 2 mg	SRL 5 mg	Placebo/AZA	SRL 2 mg	SRL 5 mg
Composite failure rate, 6 months	32.3	18.7	16.8	47.7	30.0	25.6
Acute rejection incidence, 6 months	24	15	11	42	25	19
Banff grade II or III severity	17.4	8.12	4.4	25.4	12.4	8.3
Antilymphocyte antibody	12.4	5.6	2.9	8.5	4.0	3.2
Graft survival						
6 months	94	98	93	88	93	93
12 months	94	95	92	NR[c]	NR[c]	NR[c]
Patient survival						
6 months	98	99	97	95	98	96
12 months	94	97	96	NR[d]	NR[d]	NR[d]

[a]Kahan et al 1999a.

[b]Data presented to the US Food and Drug Administration (FDA), 27 July 1999.

[c]NR: not reported; 12-month graft survival rates among the three groups ranged from 87.7% to 90.5% (P = NS; log rank).

[d]12-month patient survival rates among the three groups ranged from 94.6 to 96.5% (P = NS; log rank).

Table 9.12. Overall results of pivotal trials of sirolimus (SRL)

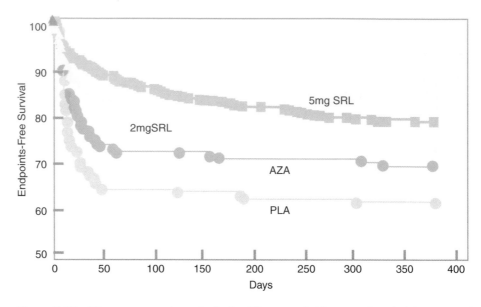

Figure 9.25. Time to composite endpoint for SRL groups in Phase III pivotal trials compared to AZA or placebo. The composite endpoint included an acute rejection episode, graft loss, or death. The treatment groups include SRL 5 mg (green), SRL 2 mg (yellow), AZA (purple), and placebo (blue). (Log-rank $P = 0.0001$ for the SRL groups versus the AZA + placebo groups.)

Chronic rejection currently represents the major obstacle to long-term renal allograft success. While this question has not been formally examined in a clinical trial, four observations suggest that SRL may be useful to prevent the occurrence or slow the progression of chronic rejection (Kahan 1998). First, SRL inhibits growth factor-driven proliferation of endothelial and smooth muscle cells in vitro (Akselband et al 1991; Graves et al 1995; Marx et al 1995; Obata et al 1996; Scott et al 1996; Mohacsi et al 1997; Simm et al 1997), presumably by blocking the action of cytokines critical to producing the immuno-obliterative vascular and bronchial lesions, the histologic hallmarks of chronic rejection. Second, SRL exerts a beneficial effect on the smooth muscle and endothelial cell responses to vascular injury provoked in vivo by balloon catheter injury or observed in aortic allografts (Geerling et al 1994; Gregory et al 1995). Third, SRL mitigates chronic rejection in rat renal allografts (Calne et al 1989; Meiser et al 1991; Morris et al 1995; Schmid et al 1997; Gallo et al 1999). Fourth, used in combination with CsA in humans, SRL reduces the incidence of acute rejection episodes, which are widely believed to forecast an increased risk of chronic rejection (Almond et al 1993; Kahan et al 1996). Furthermore, the administration of SRL permits either minimization or elimination of CsA, thereby promoting renal recovery during the early postoperative period and possibly mitigating CsA-induced renal dysfunction, which may exacerbate other processes that precipitate chronic graft failure. The potential effects of SRL on chronic rejection processes are being assessed by long-term surveillance of graft outcomes.

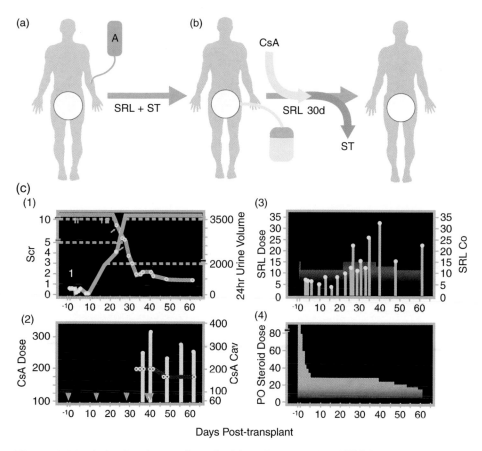

Figure 9.26. Induction therapy free of calcineurin antagonists (CNAs). (a) Protocol for initial treatment with anti-IL-2R MAbs (A) plus SRL and steroids (ST) for recipients of kidneys from marginal donors. When the serum creatinine value reaches 3.0 mg/dl, CsA therapy is initiated and steroids withdrawn 1 month later. (b) Clinical course of patient treated with induction protocol. (a) Evolution of serum creatinine (orange) showing the days of dialysis treatments with arrows and urine output (green line). (c1) Course of fall of serum creatinine (orange line) and increase in urine output (green line) shown together with timing of hemodialysis treatments (blue arrows). (c2) Zenapax treatments (1 mg/kg) shown by orange arrowheads. CsA therapy initiated at day 36 (purple line) with average concentration (C_{av}) values indicated by blue bars. (c3) SRL dose (mg/day) indicated in red with trough concentrations (ng/mL) shown as green bars. (c4) Steroid taper shown as total daily dose (in mg).

Dosage regimens

After a 15 mg loading dose, SRL monotherapy is initiated at 10 mg per day, with dose adjustments to achieve trough concentrations of 10–20 ng/ml. Because of its long half-life, SRL can be administered once daily (Zimmerman and Kahan 1997). If the patient experiences drug-induced toxicity, countermeasure therapy can be administered or the drug dose tapered. It is useful to use trough concentrations of SRL measured by high-performance liquid chromatography with ultraviolet detection (HPLC/UV; Napoli and Kahan 1996). However, if, during a monotherapy regimen, the tolerated daily dose is no more than 5 mg per day or the SRL trough concentration no more than 7.0 ng/ml, CsA (Neoral) must be initiated at about 100 mg twice daily, with adjustment to obtain the exposure necessary for adequate immunosuppression. When SRL is used in dual-drug therapy with CsA in Caucasians, the SRL dose is 2 mg per day, with a target trough concentration of 5–15 ng/ml, and CsA is administered twice daily at starting doses of 150–200 mg to obtain a target average blood drug concentration (C_{av}) of 350 ng/ml. After a 15 mg loading dose, African-Americans or other high-risk populations receive a 5 mg/day starting SRL dose, with CsA administered twice daily at 200–250 mg doses to obtain a target C_{av} of 400 ng/ml. The therapeutic window of trough concentrations for maintenance treatment with SRL is 5–15 ng/ml, and for CsA C_{av} values, 150 ng/ml.

Toxicities

Among the patients in the US and global pivotal phase III trials, the rate of malignancy at 1 year was 3.4% for the SRL 5 mg cohort, 3.1% for the placebo cohort, 1.8% for the AZA cohort, and 1.4% for the SRL 2 mg cohort. PTLD was the major cause of neoplasia among patients in the global trial. Only three cases of PTLD have occurred among the more than 400 patients treated with SRL at The University of Texas at Houston over a period of nearly 5 years. All three cases occurred within 90 days of transplantation and were associated with excessive immunosuppression: namely, an adolescent second-transplant recipient who was treated by a physician parent with doses that produced high levels of exposure of both SRL and CsA; an elderly man who experienced a severe CMV infection after treatment with OKT3 to provide a CsA holiday to facilitate renal allograft recovery; and a woman with renal allograft rejection that appeared to be refractory to murine OKT3, equine ATGAM, and rabbit thymoglobulin.

CsA and SRL appear to display few overlapping toxicities. In a phase I study, a 2-week treatment course failed to show a nephrotoxic or hypertensive interaction between SRL and CsA (Murgia et al 1996). The side-effect profile associated with SRL therapy included thrombocytopenia, leukopenia, and hyperlipidemia. In the phase III multicenter trial at the 6-month time point, changes in leukocyte count were less severe, but those in platelet count greater, among patients receiving SRL 5 mg or 2 mg than among those treated with AZA, namely, 7.6, 7.9, and $7.0 \times 10^3/mm^3$ ($P < 0.001$), and 216, 231, and $239 \times 10^3/mm^3$ ($P < 0.001$). Hemoglobin levels were 125.8, 130.1, and 130.6 g/l, respectively ($P < 0.001$).

Presently, it is not clear whether the decreases in platelet counts occur secondary to the direct effect of SRL on megakaryopoiesis by inhibition of stimulatory pathways (Quesniaux et al 1994) or as a result of enhanced platelet destruction by exaggerated clumping and aggregation. Both the thrombocytopenia and the leukopenia tend to occur during the first 4 weeks of therapy and appear to be concentration-dependent, particularly at SRL values higher than 16 ng/ml (Hong and Kahan 1999). Among patients who experience thrombocytopenia, 89% show a spontaneous resolution within 1–57 days (median 4 days). Among patients who display leukopenia, resolution occurs within 1–72 days (median 3 days) in 91% of patients. Sirolimus dose reduction was required in 5–8% of affected patients, while temporary drug suspension (ranging from 3 to 20 days) was required in an additional 4–5% of the patients. Refractory thrombocytopenia or leukopenia did not necessitate permanent drug cessation in any patient.

In cases of either extremely low peripheral blood cell counts or the need to continue SRL therapy in the face of decreased numbers of granulocytes, erythrocytes, or platelets, the drug-induced toxicity has been countered by administration of nonimmunostimulatory cytokines: granulocyte colony stimulating factor (G-CSF), erythropoietin, or IL-11, respectively. This strategy is based on the hypothesis that SRL crossinhibits the downstream signal pathways common to those transduced by the gp130 chain of hematologic growth factor receptors that is homologous to the β-chain of lymphokine receptors, the pharmacologic targets of drug action (Figure 9.27).

Addition of SRL to a CsA-based regimen did not significantly increase the incidence of bacterial, viral, or fungal infections in phase II studies in recipients of living- (Kahan

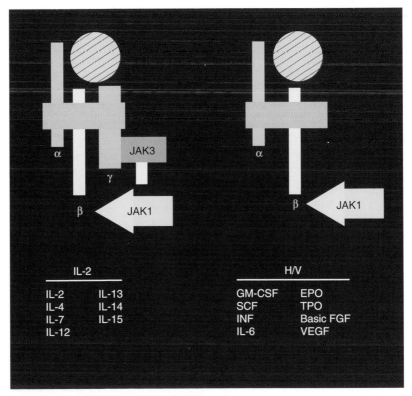

Figure 9.27. Components of the receptors of the IL-2 versus the hematologic/vascular (H/V) families of cytokines.

et al 1998a) or cadaveric- (Kahan et al 1999a) donor kidneys. In the two phase III trials, the overall incidence of CMV infection was 5%, with a 1% occurrence of the tissue-invasive form among all groups—SRL 2 and 5 mg, as well as the AZA and placebo cohorts. All four groups displayed similar incidences of herpes zoster and EBV, as well as *Pneumocystis carinii* infections. The SRL 5 mg daily dose group displayed an increased incidence of oral aphthous ulcers attributed to HSV infections, namely, 14.2% versus less than 7% for either the SRL 2 mg or the AZA and placebo groups. The four transplant groups—SRL 2 mg, SRL 5 mg, AZA, and placebo—displayed similar rates of bacterial sepsis (approximately 7%), pyelonephritis (22–28%), wound infections (5–8%), and pneumonia (3–7%). The major infectious complication observed in the phase II multicenter trial, *Pneumocystis carinii,* was avoided in subsequent studies by routine antimicrobial prophylaxis with sulfamethoxazole–trimethoprim.

SRL-treated (5 mg or 2 mg) patients in the phase III trials showed a modest but significant reduction in renal function compared to the AZA or the placebo cohorts, namely, respective serum values of 160, 155, 129, and 155 μM/l at 6 months, and 172, 158, 133, and 137 μM/l at 12 months (BD Kahan, unpublished work). There was no clear correlation of renal dysfunction to SRL concentrations. Preclinical work in salt-depleted rats failed to document a significant nephrotoxic effect of SRL alone (DiJoseph et al 1992; Andoh et al 1996); moreover, patients treated with SRL-AZA-Pred display significantly better renal function than those treated with CsA as the cornerstone of the regimen, namely, aggregate 12-month serum creatinine values of 117 among SRL versus 129 μM/l among CsA-treated patients ($P = 0.007$). Thus, it seems likely that the elevated values are not related to the SRL component of the regimen. Furthermore, patients treated with 1, 3, or 5 mg/m^2 SRL for *Psoriasis vulgaris* showed similar serum creatinine values as the placebo-treated cohort, namely, 85.2, 84.4, 85.7, and 86.5 μM/l, respectively. It therefore seems likely that SRL is not intrinsically nephrotoxic.

One explanation for the impaired renal function among SRL-CsA-Pred-treated patients is a pharmacokinetic interaction that increases CsA concentrations. Experimental animal data suggest that the interaction is primarily kinetic, namely, SRL inhibits CYP450 3A4 activity, thereby increasing the concentration of CsA in the blood and particularly in the kidney (Napoli et al 1998). Although Andoh and Bennett (1997) have proposed that the drug combination displays an additional mild, tubular effect that represents a dynamic component, the high CsA concentrations observed in their experimental group seem to proffer a more likely explanation for the renal dysfunction. While substitution of SRL for CsA may benefit at least a group of patients with persistent renal dysfunction despite an immunologically quiescent clinical course, large-scale clinical trials will be necessary to document amelioration of the nephrotoxicity.

Hyperlipidemia, the most serious side-effect of SRL, may exacerbate CsA-induced hypercholesterolemia, steroid-induced hypertriglyceridemia, as well as the dyslipidemias associated with renal disease (Keane 1999). SRL appears to interfere with lipid clearance from the blood, possibly by inhibiting lipoprotein lipase activity and/or by disrupting signal transduction by insulin or insulin-like growth factors, thereby retarding the uptake of fatty acids. SRL does not appear to have any toxic effect on the liver. Hyperlipidemia occurs in about 40% of renal transplant recipients, generally reaching its maximum values during the second posttransplant month. Thus, SRL-treated patients in the two pivotal trials showed significantly higher mean values of both triglycerides and cholesterol at 2, 3, 4, 6, and 9 but not 12 months for the 5 mg group, but only at 2 months for the 2 mg group. The incidence and severity of the hyperlipidemia was dose- and concentration-dependent. While patient instruction on a low-fat diet, progressive reduction in Pred dose, and increased exercise frequently ameliorates the condition, patients with triglyceride or cholesterol values above 300 mg/dl should receive counter-measure therapy.

The algorithm used to manage patients with elevated lipids at The University of Texas at Houston is based on whether elevations are observed in cholesterol or triglycerides only, or in both moieties. Patients with mild elevations of both levels are treated with atorvastatin (10 mg daily). Patients with more severe degrees of hypertriglyceridemia are treated with gemfibrozil (600 mg twice daily) and, in refractory conditions, with fish oil tablets (2 g four times daily). Patients with elevations in both triglycerides and cholesterol are treated with a combination of low doses of gemfibrozil (600 mg twice daily) and pravastatin (5–15 mg once daily). Only rarely do patients treated with this combination experience clinical symptoms of myopathy or laboratory evidence of an elevated creatine phosphokinase (CPK). Interestingly, at both 1 and 2 years, there was no significant difference in the incidence rates of conditions attributed to elevated blood lipids—pancreatitis, myocardial infarction, or stroke—between patients treated with SRL 2 or 5 mg daily versus AZA or placebo.

Diarrhea, delayed wound healing, and arthralgia represent less commonly observed toxicities of SRL. For the treatment groups in phase III pivotal trials (SRL 5 mg, SRL 2 mg, AZA, and placebo), the incidence rates of diarrhea were 39, 29, 28, and 27%, respectively. The condition did not appear to interfere with the absorption of SRL or other drugs and was rarely severe enough to require treatment. Because SRL inhibits signal transduction by a variety of growth factors, including epidermal growth factor and fibroblast-derived growth factor, it is not unexpected that the drug would retard wound healing and, presumably via similar mechanism(s), be associated with an increased incidence of lymphoceles. Impaired wound healing was reported in the pivotal trials at rates of 12, 10, 7, and 7%, respectively. Among patients in the US multicenter trial (Kahan et al 1999a), the incidences of infection in and the requirement for drainage of lymphoceles were similar among the treatment groups. Thus, despite the increased occurrences of lymphoceles encountered under SRL therapy, they did not display a more pernicious course.

SDZ RAD

SDZ RAD, a 25-hydroxy-ethyl derivative of SRL, is slightly more hydrophilic than the parent compound and displays a more rapid clearance rate. The analog drug is rapidly absorbed, reaching a maximum concentration (C_{max}) within 2 hours and displaying a half-life of 16–19 hours, which is significantly shorter than that of SRL (30 hours) and thus necessitates twice-daily dosing. SDZ RAD concentrations reach steady-state by 4 days, in contrast to 7 days for SRL. The pharmacokinetic parameters of SDZ RAD show dose-proportionality, with a good correlation between trough concentration and area-under-the-curve (AUC) concentrations (Kahan et al 1999d).

Little information is available on the immunosuppressive efficacy of the agent: preliminary data from a dose-escalation study suggest that doses of 2 and 4 mg SDZ RAD produce similar rates of acute rejection prophylaxis as 2 mg SRL (BD Kahan, unpublished work). Randomized, blinded multicenter trials are underway to assess the impact of addition to CsA and Pred of SDZ RAD compared to MMF. Future studies must gauge whether the SDZ RAD analog confers benefits beyond those achieved with SRL and whether these advantages are related to the hydrophilicity of the latter: namely, less time to attain steady state after administration, or, conversely, to dissipate its effects upon drug cessation. In a phase I study in stable renal transplant patients (Kahan et al 1999d), SDZ RAD displayed a similar spectrum of side-effects as that observed with SRL.

ANTIPROLIFERATIVE AGENTS FOR THE S-PHASE

Azathioprine

Therapeutic effects

Following the demonstration that AZA shows improved efficacy and reduced toxicity compared to 6-mercaptopurine (6-MP) in experimental renal transplantation in dogs (Calne 1960), administration of AZA to patients resulted in the first long-term survival of cadaveric kidney allografts in humans (Murray et al 1963). Subsequently, a number of studies reported beneficial effects of an AZA-Pred combination regimen (Goodwin et al 1963; Starzl et al 1964), which served as the 'conventional' immunosuppressive protocol from 1966 to 1983. However, this regimen displayed only a low immunosuppressive efficacy index: 85% of renal allograft recipients experienced acute rejection episodes, and only 50% of grafts survived 1 year. The limitations of AZA sparked an interest in the development of nucleoside synthesis inhibitors, which act noncompetitively to inhibit the synthesis of either purines (MMF and mizorbine) or pyrimidines (brequinar and leflunomide; Table 9.13).

Dosage regimens

Azathioprine therapy is generally initiated with a 5 mg/kg loading dose, followed by daily doses of 2–3 mg/kg. The dose is titered downward, based upon evidence of myelosuppression seeking to maintain the peripheral leukocyte count at $5000/mm^3$. Therapy

Property	AZA	MMF
Phase cell cycle	S	S
Synthesis inhibition	Purine de novo	Purine de novo
Molecular target(s)	Multiple	IMPDH
Type of inhibition	Competitive	Noncompetitive
Effective dose	50–300 mg	2000–3000 mg
Efficacy/toxicity ratio	1.0	3.0
Price per year	US $500	US $6000

Table 9.13. Comparison of the properties of antiproliferative agents azathioprine (AZA) versus mycophenolate mofetil (MMF)

is generally suspended if the granulocyte count is less than $750/mm^3$, in which case the patient is treated with parenteral granulocyte-stimulating factor. Attempts to use low-dose AZA (1–2 mg/kg) for CsA dose-sparing have proved unsuccessful, because the combination of AZA and CsA is only additive rather than synergistic (Vathsala et al 1990).

Toxicities

Azathioprine treatment is complicated by a dose-related side-effect: excessive myelosuppression. Generally, an AZA dose of 2–3 mg/kg is administered until the patient displays myelosuppression, based upon the assumption that the toxicity signifies significant inhibition of T cell proliferation. The major limitation of this strategy is the prolonged lag time between the discontinuation of AZA and the onset of bone marrow recovery, which is generally 5 days but may be as long as 1 month. Thus, administration of excessive drug doses poses the risk of severe myelosuppression (bone marrow 'wipeout') with susceptibility to invasive infection and proclivity to death. Other less frequent side-effects of AZA include drug-induced hepatitis, pancreatitis, and fever. Although skin rashes are only rarely observed, the disrupted DNA synthesis not infrequently results in papillomatosis (Figure 9.28).

Mycophenolate mofetil

Therapeutic effects

Randomized, double-blind, multicenter clinical trials conducted in the US, Canada, Europe, and Australia showed that addition to CsA and Pred of either 2 or 3 g daily doses of MMF, compared to AZA or placebo, significantly reduced the incidence and severity of acute renal allograft rejection episodes during the first 6 months (Sollinger et al 1995; Halloran et al 1997; Mathew et al 1998; Wiesel and Carl 1998; Table 9.14). However, addition of MMF showed less effect among African-American than among

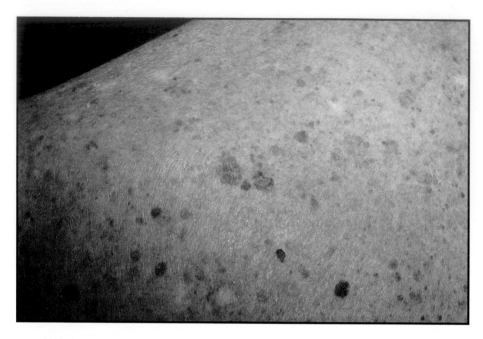

Figure 9.28. Papillomatosis on the back of a patient treated for 7 years with an AZA-steroid regimen.

Caucasian recipients (Schweitzer et al 1998). Furthermore, nonblinded studies reported that MMF provided better prophylaxis of acute rejection episodes than AZA in the settings of liver (Hebert et al 1999), SPK (Odorico et al 1998), heart (Kobashigawa et al 1998), and lung (Ross et al 1998) transplantations. However, MMF treatment did not improve patient or graft survivals at 1 or 3 years following cadaveric kidney transplantation (Sollinger et al 1995), suggesting that MMF did not impede the occurrence or the progression of chronic rejection—a clinical observation that does not support the preliminary findings claiming benefits in animal models (Morris et al 1991; Azuma et al 1995).

A randomized, double-blind study reported that, compared with an AZA-corticosteroid regimen, the combination of CsA, MMF, and corticosteroids displayed superior efficacy to reverse acute renal allograft rejection episodes refractory to conventional steroid-alone treatment regimens (Mycophenolate Mofetil Acute Renal Rejection Study Group 1998). However, 29.2% of MMF-treated patients required subsequent antilymphocyte antibody therapy.

Dosage regimens

MMF has generally been administered at a fixed dose: 2 g per day for all non-African-American patients and 3 g per day for African-American patients. Acute rejection rates

No. of patients	Duration (months)	Patient survival rates (%)				Graft survival rates (%)				Acute rejection episodes within 6 months (%)			
		AZA/Placebo	2 g MMF	3 g MMF	P	AZA/Placebo	2 g MMF	3 g MMF	P	AZA/Placebo	2 g MMF	3 g MMF	P
499[a]	6	97	96.4	94.5	NS	91.4	98.2	93.3	NS	47.6	31.1	31.3	0.0015[b] 0.0021[c]
491[d]	6	98.8	97.6	97.5	NS	91	95.7	93.7	NS	46.4	17	13.8	0.001 NR
1493[e]	12	95.3	96	95.3	NS	87.6	90.4	89.2	NS	40.8	19.8	16.5	0.0001 0.0001
503[f]	12	95.7	96.5	95.7	NS	88.8	91.2	92	NS	35.5	19.7	15.9	0.0287 0.0045
503[g]	36	91.4	95.3	90.9	NS	84.6	85.4	91.5	NS	35.5	19.7	15.9	0.0287 0.0045

NR: not reported; NS: not significant.
[a]Sollinger et al 1995.
[b]Comparison of AZA/placebo versus MMF 2 g.
[c]Comparison of AZA/placebo versus 3 gm MMF.
[d]European Mycophenolate Mofetil Cooperative Study Group 1995.
[e]Halloran et al 1997.
[f]Tricontinental Mycophenolate Mofetil Renal Transplantation Study Group 1996.
[g]Mathew et al 1998.

Table 9.14. Rates of patient survival, graft survival, and acute rejection under mycophenolate mofetil (MMF) therapy

among African-Americans treated with daily doses of 3 g versus 2 g MMF were 12.1% versus 31.8%, respectively (Neylan 1997).

MMF is generally administered in twice-daily divided doses. However, a significant proportion of patients cannot tolerate the full dose and thus require reduced amounts. Because the drug concentrations generated by the reduced doses may be insufficient to achieve a therapeutic effect, the incidence of acute rejection episodes may not be as low as was predicted by the clinical trials. Unfortunately, the HPLC method to measure mycophenolic acid (MPA) plasma concentrations is extremely cumbersome (Bullingham et al 1996), and automated techniques are not yet reliable.

Toxicities

Gastrointestinal complications (including diarrhea, esophagitis, gastritis, and gastrointestinal bleeding), as well as enhanced susceptibility to invasive forms of CMV, represent the most common adverse effects of MMF. Thus, the clinical observations are not consistent with the hypothesis that the drug's action to deplete endogenous dGTP pools would potentiate the inhibitory effect for viral prophylaxis of the triphosphate of acyclovir or gancyclovir (Allison and Eugui 1993). The frequent gastrointestinal intolerance encountered with the use of MMF may be overcome with a new enteric-coated formulation of mycophenolic acid (MPA; ERL080A, Novartis, Basle, Switzerland) that does not produce diarrhea (Schmouder et al 1999). A 720 mg dose of ERL080A resulted in an MPA exposure bioequivalent to that of 1000 mg of MMF (Schmouder et al 1999). ERL080A is currently being assessed for clinical efficacy in phase III trials.

GLOBAL AGENTS FOR IMMUNODEPRESSION

Polyclonal anti-T-cell antibodies

Following the seminal report of prolonged survival of rat skin allografts in response to administration of heterologous antisera to purified lymphoid cells (Woodruff and Anderson 1963), polyclonal antibodies were raised against human lymphocytes initially in equine (Iwasaki et al 1967) and more recently in rabbit hosts. The two polyclonal antibody preparations currently available in the US are ATGAM, a horse anti-human thymocyte globulin, and the recently approved thymoglobulin (Sangstat, Menlo Park, CA, US), a rabbit anti-human thymocyte globulin. In Europe, another rabbit preparation is marketed by Fresenius (Bad Homburg, Germany).

Therapeutic effects

Najarian and colleagues (Simmons et al 1972; Najarian et al 1976) reported that the addition of a polyclonal equine preparation both for induction and for antirejection therapy enhanced the efficacy of an AZA-Pred regimen, improving allograft survival from 51% to about 65%. However, this regimen markedly increased 1-year patient mortality rates from 7–10% to 15–20%. Furthermore, Sanchéz-Fructuoso et al (1998) found that induction therapy with rabbit ATG mitigated neither early renal dysfunction nor acute rejection episodes, but did augment the incidence of viral infections and PTLD. Therefore, most centers prefer to reserve the use of polyclonal antibodies to anti-rejection treatment, as documented by a multicenter study (Wechter et al 1979): compared to corticosteroids, ATGAM produced a higher rate of reversal of acute rejection episodes, although it did not improve graft survival. A multicenter, double-blind, randomized trial recently documented that thymoglobulin more frequently reversed steroid-resistant acute rejection episodes than did ATGAM (Gaber et al 1998). However, the adverse event, posttherapy infection, and 1-year patient/graft survival rates were similar in both groups (Table 9.15).

Dosage regimens

Although there are no absolute guidelines for the choice of an antilymphocyte preparation—ATGAM, thymoglobulin, or OKT3—the indications for inception of therapy are well established. In addition to failure of rejection to reverse after a course of steroids, other common indications for treatment with these preparations include a biopsy that shows vascular components of the rejection process (grade II or III), a rapid increase in serum creatinine value, or the development of oligoanuria.

A daily dose of 10–20 mg/kg of ATGAM is usually infused over 4 hours through an in-line filter into a central venous catheter or into the venous limb of an arteriovenous fistula, since delivery into a peripheral vein frequently causes thrombophlebitis. In contrast, thymoglobulin (1.5 mg/kg) is readily administered via a peripheral intravenous route using a 6-hour infusion. A therapeutic course of 7–14 days is usually sufficient to reverse rejection; extension of the course beyond 21 days is ill-advised, unless the patient is unable to tolerate the full dose. Morbid complications not infrequently include cytopenias, which prevent the delivery of a full antibody dose, and may require extension of the treatment course to achieve a therapeutic effect.

Clinical outcome	ATGAM	Thymoglobulin	P
Rejection reversal	76%	88%	0.027
Patient survival: 1 year	96.3%	92.8%	NS
Graft survival: 1 year	75%	83%	NS
Adverse events	93.8%	93.9%	NS
NS: not significant.			

Table 9.15. Comparison of rejection reversal with ATGAM versus thymoglobulin (Data from Gaber et al 1998).

Toxicities

Most of the adverse effects of polyclonal antibodies, namely, chills, fever, and arthralgia, owe to the large quantities of foreign protein contained in these preparations. Thrombocytopenia and leukopenia are not-uncommon side-effects during the period of administration, owing to the crossreactions of these antibodies with xenospecific markers on the surfaces of platelets and white blood cells. Furthermore, high doses or extended treatment periods markedly enhance the rates of CMV infections and PTLD.

CONCLUSION

The available matrix of immunosuppressive agents reflects the significant advances in therapy during the past 40 years. Cyclosporine, TRL, SRL, and OKT3 selectively blockade cells that mediate specific adaptive immune responses, while sparing elements of nonspecific host resistance. In contrast, both the specific and nonspecific components are inhibited by nucleoside synthesis inhibitors and by steroids. The recent development of the CsA-SRL combination, a regimen that displays a synergistic interaction, not only provides augmented immunosuppressive effects, but also permits marked reduction of the doses of each agent. While the overlapping hyperlipidemic tendencies of the two drugs render this combination less than ideal, it represents the best available therapy. The more potent maintenance immunosuppressive regimens have reduced the incidence of acute rejection episodes, particularly those that are steroid-resistant, and therefore markedly decreased the need for polyclonal or monoclonal antilymphocyte antibody therapy as well as the risks of CMV and PTLD. The future goal of immunosuppressive therapy, to produce only a narrow defect in the host repertoire and thus 'specificity'— the third 'S' in the therapeutic triumvirate—awaits the development of strategies that induce transplantation tolerance.

REFERENCES

Akselband Y, Harding MW, Nelson PA (1991) Rapamycin inhibits spontaneous and fibroblast growth factor B-stimulated proliferation of endothelial cells and fibroblasts. *Transplant Proc* 23:2833–2836.

Alfrey EJ, Friedman AL, Grossman RA et al (1992) A recent decrease in the time to development of monomorphous and polymorphous posttransplant lymphoproliferative disorder. *Transplantation* 54:250–253.

Allison AC, Eugui EM (1993) The design and development of an immunosuppressive drug, mycophenolate mofetil. *Semin Immunopathol* 14:353–380.

Almond PS, Matas A, Gillingham K et al (1993) Risk factors for chronic rejection in renal allograft recipients. *Transplantation* 55:752–756.

Andoh TF, Bennett WM (1997) The synergistic effects of cyclosporine and sirolimus. *Transplantation* 63:1703–1704.

Andoh TF, Burdmann EA, Fransechini N et al (1996) Comparison of acute rapamycin nephrotoxicity with cyclosporine and FK506. *Kidney Int* **50**:1110–1117.

Andrews PA, Sen M, Chang RW (1996) Racial variation in dosage requirements of tacrolimus. Letter. *Lancet* **348**:1446.

Anonymous (1983) Cyclosporin in cadaveric renal transplantation: 1-year follow-up of a multicentre trial. *Lancet* **ii**:986–989.

Azuma H, Binder J, Heeman V et al (1995) Effects of RS61443 on functional and morphological changes in chronically rejecting rat kidney allografts. *Transplantation* **59**:460–466.

Barone G, Chang CT, Choc MG Jr et al (1996) The pharmacokinetics of a microemulsion formulation of cyclosporine in primary renal allograft recipients. *Transplantation* **61**:875–880.

Bennett WM, DeMattos A, Meyer MM et al (1996a) Chronic cyclosporine nephropathy: the Achilles' heel of immunosuppressive therapy. *Kidney Int* **50**:1089–1100.

Bennett WM, DeMattos A, Norman DJ et al (1996b) Which cyclosporin formulation? *Lancet* **348**:205.

Berg LC, Copenhaver CM, Morrison VA et al (1992) B-cell lymphoproliferative disorders in solid-organ transplant patients: detection of Epstein–Barr virus by in situ hybridization. *Hum Pathol* **23**:159–163.

Birkeland SA (1998) Steroid-free immunosuppression after kidney transplantation with antithymocyte globulin induction and cyclosporine and mycophenolate mofetil maintenance therapy. *Transplantation* **66**:1207–1210.

Birkeland SA, Andersen IIK, Hamilton-Dutoit SJ (1999) Preventing acute rejection, Epstein–Barr virus infection, and posttransplant lymphoproliferative disorders after kidney transplantation: use of acyclovir and mycophenolate mofetil in a steroid-free immunosuppressive protocol. *Transplantation* **67**:1209–1214.

Borel JF, Feurer C, Gubler HU, Stahelin H (1976) Biological effects of cyclosporin A: a new antilymphocytic agent. *Agents Actions* **6**:468–475.

Boubenider S, Hiesse C, Goupy C et al (1997) Incidence and consequences of post-transplantation lymphoproliferative disorders. *J Nephrol* **10**:136–145.

Bry W, Warvariv V, Bohannon L et al (1991) Cadaveric renal transplant without prophylactic prednisone therapy. *Transplant Proc* **23**:994–996.

Budde K, Smettan S, Fritsche L et al (1998) Long-term outcome of tacrolimus rescue therapy in late rejection after renal transplantation. *Transplant Proc* **30**:1780–1781.

Bullingham R, Monroe S, Nicholls A, Hale M (1996) Pharmacokinetics and bioavailability of mycophenolate mofetil in healthy subjects after single-dose oral and intravenous administration. *J Clin Pharmacol* **36**:315–324.

Calne RY (1960) The rejection of renal homograft inhibition in dogs by 6-mercaptopurine, *Lancet* **1**:417.

Calne RY, White DJ, Thiru S et al (1978) Cyclosporin A in patients receiving renal allografts from cadaver donors. *Lancet* **2**:1323–1327.

Calne RY, Collier DS, Lim S et al (1989) Rapamycin for immunosuppression in organ allografting. *Lancet* **ii**:227.

Carl S, Wiesel M, Daniel V et al (1997) Rescue therapy with interleukin-2 receptor antibody in high risk kidney transplant patients: a 3-year follow-up study. *Transplant Proc* **29**:320–322.

Ciancio G, Burke GW, Roth D, Miller J (1999) Tacrolimus and mycophenolate mofetil regimens in transplantation. *Bio Drugs* **11**:395–407.

Curtis JJ, Dubovsky E, Whelchel JD et al (1986) Cyclosporin in therapeutic doses increases renal allograft vascular resistance. *Lancet* **ii**:477–479.

DiJoseph JF, Sharma RN, Chang JY (1992) The effect of rapamycin on kidney function in the Sprague-Dawley rat. *Transplantation* **53**:507–513.

DiMartini AF, Trzepacz PT, Pajer KA et al (1997) Neuropsychiatric side effects of FK506 vs cyclosporine A. *Psychosomatics* **38**:565–569.

Drachenberg CB, Klassen DK, Weir MR et al (1999) Islet cell damage associated with tacrolimus and cyclosporine: morphological features in pancreas allograft biopsies and clinical correlation. *Transplantation* **68**:396–402.

Drath DB, Kahan BD (1983) Alterations in rat pulmonary macrophage function by the immuno-suppressive agents cyclosporine, azathioprine, and prednisolone. *Transplantation* **35**:588–592.

English J, Evan A, Houghton DC, Bennett WM (1987) Cyclosporine-induced acute renal dys-function in the rat. Evidence of arteriolar vasoconstriction with preservation of tubular function. *Transplantation* **44**:135–141.

European FK506 Multicentre Liver Study Group (1994) Randomized trial: comparing tacrolimus (FK506) and cyclosporine in prevention of liver allograft rejection. *Lancet* **344**:423–428.

European Mycophenolate Mofetil Cooperative Study Group (1995) Placebo-controlled study of mycophenolate mofetil combined with cyclosporin and corticosteroids for prevention of acute rejection. *Lancet* **345**:1321–1325.

Ferguson R (1994) Acute rejection episodes: best predictor of long-term primary cadaveric renal transplant survival. *Clin Transplant* **8**:328–331.

Feutren G, Mihatsch MJ (1992) Risk factors for cyclosporine-induced nephropathy in patients with autoimmune diseases. International Kidney Biopsy Registry of Cyclosporine in Autoimmune Diseases. *N Engl J Med* **326**:1654–1660.

First MR, Alloway R, Schroeder TJ (1998) Development of Sang-35: a cyclosporine formulation bioequivalent to Neoral. *Clin Transplant* **12**:518–524.

Flechner SM, Kerman RH, Van Buren CT, Kahan BD (1985) Mixed lymphocyte culture hyporesponsiveness as a marker for steroid withdrawal in cyclosporine-treated living related renal recipients. *Transplant Proc* **17**:1260–1264.

Friedman J, Barnes L, Sheahan M et al (1987) Orthoclone OKT3 treatment of acute renal allo-graft rejection. *Transplant Proc* **19**:46.

Fung JJ, Starzl TE (1995) FK506 in solid organ transplantation. *Ther Drug Monit* **17**:592–595.

Fung JJ, Todo S, Tsakis A et al (1991) Conversion of liver allograft recipients from cyclosporine to FK506-based immunosuppression: benefits and pitfalls. *Transplant Proc* **23**:14–21.

Fung JJ, Eliaziw M, Todo S et al (1996) The Pittsburgh randomized trial of tacrolimus compared to cyclosporine for hepatic transplantation. *J Am Coll Surg* **183**:117–125.

Gaber AO, First MR, Tesi RJ et al (1998) Results of the double-blind, randomized, multicenter, phase III clinical trial of thymoglobulin versus ATGAM in the treatment of acute graft rejection episodes after renal transplantation. *Transplantation* **66**:29–37.

Gallo R, Padurean A, Jayaraman T et al (1999) Inhibition of intimal thickening after balloon angioplasty in porcine coronary arteries by targeting regulators of the cell cycle. *Circulation* **99**:2164–2170.

Geerling RA, de Bruin RWF, Scheringa M et al (1994) Suppression of acute rejection prevents graft arteriosclerosis after allogenic aorta transplantation in the rat. *Transplantation* **58**:1258–1263.

Goodwin WE, Kaufman JJ, Mims MM et al (1963) Human renal transplantation. I. Clinical experiences with six cases of renal homotransplantation. *J Urol* **89**:13–24.

Goto T, Kino T, Hatanaka H et al (1987) Discovery of FK506, a novel immunosuppressant iso-lated from *Streptomyces tsukubaensis*. *Transplant Proc* **19**:4–8.

Graves LM, Bornfeldt KE, Argast GM et al (1995) cAMP- and rapamycin-sensitive regulation of the association of eukaryotic initiation factor 4E and the translational regulator PHAS-I in aortic smooth muscle cells. *Proc Natl Acad Sci USA* **92**:7222–7226.

Gregory CR, Huang X, Pratt RE et al (1995) Treatment with rapamycin and mycophenolic acid reduces arterial intimal thickening produced by mechanical injury and allows endothelial replacement. *Transplantation* **59**:655–661.

Grinyó JM, Gil-Vernet S, Seron D et al (1997) Steroid withdrawal in mycophenolate mofetil-treated renal allograft recipients. *Transplantation* **63**:1688–1690.

Grinyó JM, Gil-Vernet S, Seron D et al (1998) Primary immunosuppression with mycophenolate mofetil and antithymocyte globulin for kidney transplant recipients of a suboptimal graft. *Nephrol Dial Transplant* **13**:2601–2604.

Groth CG, Backman L, Morales JM et al (1999) Sirolimus (rapamycin)-based therapy in human renal transplantation. *Transplantation* **67**:1036–1042.

Gruessner RWG, Burke GW, Stratta R et al (1996) A multicenter analysis of the first experience with FK506 for induction and rescue therapy after pancreas transplantation. *Transplantation* **61**:261–273.

Halloran P, Mathew T, Tomlanovich MS et al (1997) Mycophenolate mofetil in renal allograft recipients. *Transplantation* **63**:39–47.

Hariharan S, Munda R, Demmy TJ et al (1995) Conversion from cyclosporine to tacrolimus after pancreas transplantation. *Transplant Proc* **27**:2981–2982.

Hariharan S, Peddi VR, Munda R et al (1997) Long-term renal and pancreas function with tacrolimus rescue therapy following pancreas transplantation. *Transplant Proc* **29**:652–653.

Hebert MF, Ascher NL, Lake JR et al (1999) Four-year follow-up of mycophenolate mofetil for graft rescue in liver allograft recipients. *Transplantation* **67**:707–712.

Hojo M, Morimoto T, Maluccio M et al (1999) Cyclosporine induces cancer progression by a cell-autonomous mechanism. *Nature* **397**:530–534.

Hollander AA, van Saase JL, Kootte AM et al (1995) Beneficial effects of conversion from cyclosporin to azathioprine after kidney transplantation. *Lancet* **345**:610–614.

Hong JC, Kahan BD (1999) Use of anti-CD25 monoclonal antibody in combination with rapamycin to eliminate cyclosporine treatment during the induction phase of immunosuppression. *Transplantation* **68**:701–704.

Hricik DE, Bartucci MR, Moir EJ et al (1991) Effects of steroid withdrawal on posttransplant diabetes mellitus in cyclosporine-treated renal transplant recipients. *Transplantation* **51**:374–377.

Hricik DE, Lautman J, Bartucci MR et al (1992a) Variable effects of steroid withdrawal on blood pressure reduction in cyclosporine-treated renal transplant recipients. *Transplantation* **53**:1232–1235.

Hricik DE, Whalen CC, Lautman J et al (1992b) Withdrawal of steroids after renal transplantation: clinical predictors of outcome. *Transplantation* **53**:41–45.

Hricik DE, O'Toole MA, Schulak JA, Herson J (1993) Steroid-free immunosuppression in cyclosporine-treated renal transplant recipients: a meta-analysis. *J Am Soc Nephrol* **4**:1300–1305.

Hricik DE, Seliga RM, Fleming-Brooks S et al (1995) Determinants of long-term allograft function following steroid withdrawal in renal transplant recipients. *Clin Transplant* **9**:419–423.

Hueso M, Bover J, Seron D et al (1998) Low-dose cyclosporine and mycophenolate mofetil in renal allograft recipients with suboptimal renal function. *Transplantation* **66**:1727–1731.

Isoniemi HM, Krogerus L, von Willebrand E et al (1992) Histopathological findings in well-functioning, long-term renal allografts. *Kidney Int* **41**:155–160.

Iwasaki Y, Porter KA, Amend JR et al (1967) The preparation and testing of horse antidog and antihuman antilymphoid plasma or serum and its protein fractions. *Surg Gynecol Obstet* **124**:1–24.

Jaffe HW, Pellett PE (1999) Human herpesvirus 8 and Kaposi's sarcoma: some answers, more questions. *N Engl J Med* **340**:1912–1913.

Jain A, Fung J, Todo S (1996) More than six years actual follow-up: conversion from cyclosporine to tacrolimus for chronic liver allograft rejection. *Hepatology* **24**:181.

Jonas S, Kling N, Bechstein WO et al (1995) Rejection episodes after liver transplantation during primary immunosuppression with FK506 or a cyclosporine-based regimen: a controlled, prospective, randomized trial. *Clin Transplant* 9:406–414.

Jordan ML, Naraghi R, Shapiro R et al (1997) Tacrolimus rescue therapy for renal allograft rejection: 5 years' experience. *Transplantation* 63:223–228.

Julian BA, Laskow DA, Dubovsky J et al (1991) Rapid loss of vertebral mineral density after renal transplantation. *N Engl J Med* 325:544–550.

Kahan BD (1985a) Individualization of cyclosporine therapy using pharmacokinetic and pharmacodynamic parameters. *Transplantation* 40:457–476.

Kahan BD (1985b) Overview: individualization of cyclosporine therapy using pharmacokinetic and pharmacodynamic parameters. *Transplantation* 40:457–476.

Kahan BD (1989) Cyclosporine. *N Engl J Med* 321:1725–1738.

Kahan BD (1998) The role of rapamycin in chronic rejection prophylaxis: a theoretical consideration. *Graft* 1(2 Suppl II):93–96.

Kahan BD (1999) Considerations concerning generic formulations of immunosuppressive drugs. *Transplant Proc* 31:1635–1641.

Kahan BD, Van Buren CT, Flechner SM et al (1985) Clinical and experimental studies with cyclosporine in renal transplantation. *Surgery* 97:125–140.

Kahan BD, Kramer WG, Wideman C et al (1986) Demographic factors affecting the pharmacokinetics of cyclosporine estimated by radioimmunoassay. *Transplantation* 41:459–464.

Kahan BD, Kerman RH, Van Buren CT et al (1989) Clinical outcome in 36 patients after at least 1 and up to 5 years of steroid withdrawal based upon specific mixed lymphocyte reaction hyporesponsiveness toward the living related donor. *Transplant Proc* 21:1579–1580.

Kahan BD, Dunn J, Fitts C et al (1995) Reduced inter- and intra-subject variability in cyclosporine pharmacokinetics in renal transplant recipients treated with a microemulsion formulation in conjunction with fasting, low fat or high fat meals. *Transplantation* 59:505–511.

Kahan BD, Welsh M, Schoenberg L et al (1996b) Variable oral absorption of cyclosporine: a biopharmaceutical risk factor for chronic renal allograft rejection. *Transplantation* 62:599–606.

Kahan BD, Podbielski J, Napoli KL et al (1998a) Immunosuppressive effects and safety of a sirolimus/cyclosporine combination regimen for renal transplantation. *Transplantation* 66:1040–1046.

Kahan BD, Podbielski J, Van Buren CT (1998b) Rapamycin for refractory renal allograft rejection (abst 711). *XVII Annual Meeting of the American Society of Transplant Physicians*, May 9–13, 1998, Chicago, IL.

Kahan BD, for the USA Rapamune Study Group (1999a) Pivotal phase III multicenter, randomized, blinded trial of sirolimus versus azathioprine in combination with cyclosporine and prednisone in primary renal transplants (abst 68), *25th Annual Meeting of the American Society of Transplant Surgeons*, May 19–21, Chicago, IL.

Kahan BD, Julian BA, Pescovitz MD et al for the Rapamune Study Group (1999b) Sirolimus reduces the incidence of acute rejection episodes despite lower cyclosporine doses in Caucasian recipients of mismatched primary renal allografts: a phase II trial. *Transplantation* 68:1526–1532.

Kahan BD, Rajagopalan PR, Hall M for the United States Simulect Renal Study Group (1999c) Reduction of the occurrence of acute cellular rejection among renal allograft recipients treated with basiliximab, a chimeric anti-interleukin-2-receptor monoclonal antibody. *Transplantation* 67:276–284.

Kahan BD, Wong RL, Carter C et al (1999d) A phase I study of a four-week course of the rapamycin analogue SDZ-RAD (RAD) in quiescent cyclosporine-prednisone-treated renal transplant recipients. *Transplantation* 68:1100–1106.

Kasiske BL, Heim-Duthoy K, Ma JZ (1993) Elective cyclosporine withdrawal after renal transplantation. *JAMA* 269:395–400.

Katari SR, Magnone M, Shapiro R et al (1997) Clinical features of acute reversible tacrolimus (FK506) nephrotoxicity in kidney transplant recipients. *Clin Transplant* 11:237–242.

Keane WF (1999) Lipids and progressive renal disease: the cardio-renal link. *Am J Kidney Dis* 34:xliii–xlvi.

Keenan RJ, Konishi H, Kawai A et al (1995) Clinical trial of tacrolimus versus cyclosporine in lung transplantation. *Ann Thorac Surg* 60:580–584.

Khajehdehi P, Yip D, Bastani B (1999) The impact of (1:1) cyclosporine A conversion to its microemulsion formulation on the kidney function of patients with cardiac allografts. *Clin Transplant* 13:176–180.

Klintmalm GB, Goldstein R, Gonwa T et al (1993) Use of Prograf (FK506) as rescue therapy for refractory rejection after liver transplantation, *Transplant Proc* 1:679–688.

Knoll GA, Bell RC (1999) Tacrolimus versus cyclosporin for immunosuppression in renal transplantation: meta-analysis of randomised trials. *BMJ* 318:1104–1107.

Kobashigawa J, Miller L, Renlund D et al (1998) A randomized active-controlled trial of mycophenolate mofetil in heart transplant recipients. Mycophenolate Mofetil Investigators. *Transplantation* 66:507–515.

Kovarik JM, Kahan BD, Rajagopalan PR et al (1999) Population pharmacokinetics and exposure–response relationships for basiliximab in kidney transplantation. The US Simulect Renal Transplant Study Group. *Transplantation* 68:1288–1294.

Kupin W, Venkat KK, Oh HK, Dienst S (1988) Complete replacement of methylprednisolone by azathioprine in cyclosporine-treated primary cadaveric renal transplant recipients. *Transplantation* 45:53–55.

Langrehr JM, Nussler NC, Neumann U et al (1997) A prospective randomized trial comparing interleukin-2 receptor antibody versus antithymocyte globulin as part of a quadruple immunosuppressive induction therapy following orthotopic liver transplantation. *Transplantation* 63:1772–1781.

Laskow DA, Vincenti F, Neylan JF et al (1996) An open-label, concentration-ranging trial of FK506 in primary kidney transplantation. *Transplantation* 62:900–905.

Lindholm A, Kahan BD (1993) Influence of cyclosporine pharmacokinetics, trough concentrations, and AUC monitoring on outcome after kidney transplantation. *Clin Pharmacol Ther* 54:205–218.

Lindholm A, Welsh M, Alton C, Kahan BD (1992) Demographic factors influencing cyclosporine pharmacokinetic parameters in uremic patients: racial differences in bioavailability. *Clin Pharmacol Ther* 52:359–371.

Lorber MI, Flechner SM, Van Buren CT et al (1987) Cyclosporine toxicity: the effect of combined therapy using cyclosporine, azathioprine, and prednisone. *Am J Kidney Dis* 9:476–484.

Lown KS, Mayo RR, Leichtman AB et al (1997) Role of intestinal P-glycoprotein (mdr1) in interpatient variation in the oral bioavailability of cyclosporine. *Clin Pharmacol Ther* 62:248–260.

MacDonald AS, for the Rapamune Global Study Group (1998) A randomized, placebo-controlled trial of Rapamune in primary renal allograft recipients (abst 426). *Abstracts of the Transplantation Society XVII World Congress* July 12–17, 1998, Montreal, Canada.

Marx SO, Jayaraman T, Go LO, Marks AR (1995) Rapamycin-FKBP inhibits cell cycle regulators of proliferation in vascular smooth muscle cells. *Circ Res* 76:412–417.

Mason J (1989) Pharmacology of cyclosporine (Sandimmune) VII. Pathology and toxicology of cyclosporine in humans and animals. *Pharmacol Rev* 42:423–434.

Mathew T, for the Tricontinental Mycophenolate Mofetil Renal Transplantation Study Group (1998) A blinded, long term, randomized multicenter study of mycophenolate mofetil in cadaveric renal transplantation. *Transplantation* 65:1450–1454.

Matsunami C, Hilton AF, Dyer JA et al (1994) Ocular complications in renal transplant patients. *Aust NZ J Ophthalmol* 22:53–57.

Mayer AD, Dmitrewski J, Squifflet JP et al (1997) Multicenter randomized trial comparing tacrolimus and cyclosporine in the prevention of renal allograft rejection. *Transplantation* 64:436–443.

Meiser BM, Billingham ME, Morris RE (1991) Effects of cyclosporin, FK506, and rapamycin on graft-vessel disease. *Lancet* 338:1297–1298.

Miller J for the FK506/MMF Dose Ranging Kidney Transplant Study Group (1999) Tacrolimus and mycophenolate mofetil in renal transplant recipients: 1 year results of a multicenter, randomized dose ranging trial. *Transplant Proc* 31:276–277.

Millis JM, McDiarmid SV, Hiatt JR et al (1989) Randomized prospective trial of OKT3 for early prophylaxis of rejection after liver transplantation. *Transplantation* 47:82–88.

Mohacsi PJ, Tuller D, Hullinger B, Wijngaard PL (1997) Different inhibitory effects of immunosuppressive drugs on human and rat aortic smooth muscle and endothelial cell proliferation stimulated by platelet-derived growth factor or endothelial cell growth factor. *J Heart Lung Transplant* 16:484–492.

Morris RE, Wang J, Blum JR et al (1991) Immunosuppressive effects of the morpholinoethyl ester of mycophenolate acid (RS-61443) in rat and nonhuman primate recipients of heart allografts. *Transplant Proc* 23:19–25.

Morris RE, Huang X, Gregory CR et al (1995) Studies in experimental models of chronic rejection: use of rapamycin (sirolimus) and isoxazole derivatives (leflunomide and its analogue) for the suppression of graft vascular disease and obliterative bronchiolitis. *Transplant Proc* 27:2068–2069.

Mourad G, Vela C, Ribstein J, Mimran A (1998) Long-term improvement in renal function after cyclosporine reduction in renal transplant recipients with histologically proven chronic cyclosporine nephropathy. *Transplantation* 65:661–667.

Murgia MG, Jordan S, Kahan BD (1996) The side effect profile of sirolimus: a phase I study in quiescent cyclosporine-prednisone-treated renal transplant patients. *Kidney Int* 49:209–216.

Murray JE, Merrill JP, Harrison JH (1963) Prolonged survival of human kidney homografts by immunosuppressive drug therapy. *N Engl J Med* 268:1315.

Musarò A, McCullagh KJA, Naya FJ et al (1999) IGF-1 induces skeletal myocyte hypertrophy through calcineurin in association with GATA-2 and NF-Atc1. *Nature* 400:581–585.

Mycophenolate Mofetil Acute Renal Rejection Study Group (1998) Mycophenolate mofetil for treatment of first acute renal rejection. *Transplantation* 65:235–241.

Myers BD, Ross J, Newton L et al (1984) Cyclosporine-associated chronic nephropathy. *New Engl J Med* 311:699–705.

Najarian JS, Simmons RL, Condie RM et al (1976) Seven years' experience with antilymphoblast globulin for renal transplantation from cadaver donors. *Ann Surg* 184:352–368.

Napoli KL, Kahan BD (1996) Routine clinical monitoring of sirolimus (rapamycin) whole-blood concentrations by HPLC with ultraviolet detection. *Clin Chem* 42:1943–1948.

Napoli KL, Wang M-E, Stepkowski SM, Kahan BD (1998) Relative tissue distributions of cyclosporine and sirolimus following concomitant peroral administration to the rat: evidence for pharmacokinetic interactions. *Ther Drug Monit* 20:123–133.

Nashan B, Schlitt HJ, Schwinzer R et al (1996) Immunoprophylaxis with a monoclonal anti-IL-2-receptor antibody in liver transplant patients. *Transplantation* 61:546–554.

Nashan B, Moore R, Amlot P et al (1997) Randomized trial of basiliximab versus placebo for control of acute cellular rejection in renal allograft recipients. CHIB 201 International Study Group. *Lancet* 350:1193–1198.

Nashan B, Light S, Hardie IR et al (1999) Reduction of acute renal allograft rejection by daclizumab. Daclizumab Double Therapy Study Group. *Transplantation* 67:110–115.

Neylan JF (1997) Immunosuppressive therapy in high-risk transplant patients. *Transplantation* 64:1277–1282.

Neylan JF (1998) Racial differences in renal transplantation after immunosuppression with tacrolimus versus cyclosporine. *Transplantation* **65**:515–523.

Niese D, Keown P (1998) Safety and efficacy of microemulsion versus conventional cyclosporine in de novo renal allograft recipients. *Kidney Int* **54**:938–944.

Novick AC, Ho-Hsiegh H, Steinmuller D et al (1986) Detrimental effect of cyclosporine on initial function of cadaver renal allografts following extended preservation. *Transplantation* **42**:154–158.

Obata T, Kashiwagi A, Maegawa H et al (1996) Insulin signaling and its regulation of system A amino acid uptake in cultured rat vascular smooth muscle cells. *Circ Res* **79**:1167–1176.

Odorico JS, Pirsch JD, Knechtle SJ et al (1998) A study comparing mycophenolate mofetil to azathioprine in simultaneous pancreas–kidney transplantation. *Transplantation* **66**:1751–1759.

Offermann G, Schwarz A, Krause PH (1993) Long-term effects of steroid withdrawal in kidney transplantation. *Transplant Int* **6**:290–292.

Oksenhendler E, Cazals-Hatem D, Schulz TF et al (1998) Transient angiolymphoid hyperplasia and Kaposi's sarcoma after primary infection with human herpesvirus 8 in a patient with human immunodeficiency virus infection. *N Engl J Med* **338**:1585–1590.

Ortho Multicenter Transplant Study Group (1985) A randomized clinical trial of OKT3 monoclonal antibody for acute rejection of cadaveric renal transplants. *N Engl J Med* **313**:337–342.

Pascual M, Saidman S, Tolkoff-Rubin N et al (1998) Plasma exchange and tacrolimus-mycophenolate rescue for acute humoral rejection in kidney transplantation. *Transplantation* **66**:1460–1464.

Pescovitz MD, Barone G, Choc MG Jr et al (1997) Safety and tolerability of cyclosporine microemulsion versus cyclosporine: 2-year data in primary renal allograft recipients. *Transplantation* **63**:778–780.

Pham SM, Kormos RL, Hatter BG et al (1996) A prospective trial of tacrolimus (FK506) in clinical heart transplantation: intermediate-term results. *J Thorac Cardiovasc Surg* **111**:764–772.

Pirsch JD, Miller J, Deierhoi MH et al (1997) A comparison of tacrolimus and cyclosporine for immunosuppression after cadaveric renal transplantation. *Transplantation* **63**:977–983.

Platz KP, Eckhoff DE, Hullett DA, Sollinger HW (1991) RS-61443 studies: review and proposal. *Transplant Proc* **23**:33–35.

Pollard SG, Lear PA, Ready AR et al (1999) Comparison of microemulsion and conventional formulations of cyclosporine A in preventing acute rejection in de novo kidney transplant patients. *Transplantation* **68**:1325–1331.

Quesniaux VFJ, Wehrli S, Steiner C et al (1994) The immunosuppressant rapamycin blocks in vitro responses to hematopoietic cytokines and inhibits recovering but not steady-state hematopoiesis in vivo. *Blood* **84**:1543–1552.

Radermacher J, Meiners M, Bramlage C, Henry JP (1998) Pronounced renal vasoconstriction and systemic in renal transplant patients treated with cyclosporine A versus FK 506. *Transplant Int* **11**:3–11.

Randhawa PS, Shapiro R, Jordan ML et al (1993) The histopathological changes associated with allograft rejection and drug toxicity in renal transplant recipients maintained on FK506. *Am J Surg Pathol* **17**:60–68.

Ratcliffe PJ, Dudley CR, Higgins RM et al (1996) Randomised controlled trial of steroid withdrawal in renal transplant recipients receiving triple immunosuppression. *Lancet* **348**:643–648.

Regamey N, Tamm M, Wernli M et al (1998) Transmission of human herpesvirus 8 infection from renal-transplant donors to recipients. *N Engl J Med* **339**:1358–1363.

Reichart B, Meiser B, Vigano M et al (1998) European Multicenter Tacrolimus (FK506) heart pilot study: 1-year results—European Tacrolimus Multicenter Heart Study Group. *J Heart Lung Transplant* **17**:775–781.

Rosenthal JT, Hakala TR, Iwatsuki S et al (1983) Cadaveric renal transplantation under cyclosporine-steroid therapy. *Surg Gynecol Obstet* **157**:309–315.

Ross DJ, Waters PF, Levine M et al (1998) Mycophenolate mofetil versus azathioprine immuno-suppressive regimens after lung transplantation: preliminary experience. *J Heart Lung Transplant* **17**:768–774.

Roth D, Colona J, Burke GW et al (1998) Primary immunosuppression with tacrolimus and mycophenolate mofetil for renal allograft recipients. *Transplantation* **65**:248–252.

Sanchez-Fructuoso AI, Naranjo P, Torrente J et al (1998) Effect of antithymocyte globulin induction treatment on renal transplant outcome. *Transplant Proc* **30**:1790–1792.

Schmid RA, Yamashita M, Boasquevisque CH et al (1997) Carbohydrate selectin inhibitor CY-1503 reduces neutrophil migration and reperfusion injury in canine pulmonary allografts. *J Heart Lung Transplant* **16**:1054–1061.

Schmouder R, Arns W, Merkel F (1999) Pharmacokinetics of ERL080A: a new enteric coated formulation of mycophenolic acid-sodium (abst 787). *18th Annual Meeting of the American Society of Transplantation*, May 15–19, 1999, Chicago, IL.

Schulak JA, Hricik DE (1994) Steroid withdrawal after renal transplantation. *Clin Transplant* **8**:211–216.

Schulak JA, Mayes JT, Moritz CE, Hricik DE (1990) A prospective randomized trial of prednisone versus no prednisone maintenance therapy in cyclosporine-treated and azathioprine-treated renal transplant patients. *Transplantation* **49**:327–332.

Schweitzer EJ, Yoon S, Fink J et al (1998) Mycophenolate mofetil reduces the risk of acute rejection less in African-American than in Caucasian kidney recipients. *Transplantation* **65**:242–248.

Scott PH, Belham CM, Al-Hafidh J et al (1996) A regulatory role for cAMP in phosphatidylinositol 3-kinase/p70 ribosomal S6 kinase-mediated DNA synthesis in platelet-derived-growth-factor-stimulated bovine airway smooth-muscle cells. *Biochem J* **318**:965–971.

Semsarian C, Wu M-J, Ju Y-K et al (1999) Skeletal muscle hypertrophy is mediated by a Ca^{2+}-dependent calcineurin signalling pathway. *Nature* **400**:576–581.

Shaffer D, Simpson MA, Conway P et al (1995) Normal pancreas allograft function following simultaneous pancreas kidney transplantation after rescue therapy with tacrolimus (FK506). *Transplantation* **59**:1063–1066.

Shapiro R, Jordan ML, Scantlebury VP et al (1998) Alopecia as a consequence of tacrolimus therapy. Letter. *Transplantation* **65**:1631.

Shapiro R, Jordan ML, Scantlebury VP et al (1999a) A prospective, randomized trial of tacrolimus/prednisone versus tacrolimus/prednisone/mycophenolate mofetil in renal transplant recipients. *Transplantation* **67**:411–415.

Shapiro R, Scantlebury VP, Jordan ML et al (1999b) Pediatric renal transplantation under tacrolimus-based immunosuppression. *Transplantation* **67**:299–303.

Sharma VK, Bologa RM, Xu G-P et al (1996) Intragraft TGF-β_1 mRNA: a correlate of interstitial fibrosis and chronic allograft nephropathy. *Kidney Int* **49**:1297–1303.

Sher LS, Cosenza CA, Michel J et al (1997) Efficacy of tacrolimus as rescue therapy for chronic rejection in orthotopic liver transplantation. *Transplantation* **64**:258–263.

Shield CF III, Jacobs RJ, Wyant S, Das A (1996) A cost-effectiveness analysis of OKT3 induction therapy in cadaveric kidney transplantation. *Am J Kidney Dis* **27**:855–864.

Shumway SJ, Kaye MP (1988) The International Society for Heart Transplantation Registry. In: Terasaki PI (ed.). *Clinical Transplants 1988*. Los Angeles: UCLA Tissue Typing Laboratory, pp. 1–4.

Simm A, Nestler M, Hoppe V (1997) PDGF-AA, a potent mitogen for cardiac fibroblasts from adult rats. *J Mol Cell Cardiol* **29**:357–368.

Simmons RL, Condie R, Najarian JS (1972) Antilymphoblast globulin for renal allograft prolongation. *Transplant Proc* **4**:487–490.

Sinclair NRSC for the Canadian Multicentre Transplant Study Group (1992) Low-dose steroid therapy in cyclosporine-treated renal transplant recipients with well-functioning grafts. *Can Med Assoc J* 147:645–657.

Slaton JW, Kahan BD (1996) Case report: sirolimus rescue therapy for refractory renal allograft rejection. Brief communication. *Transplantation* 61:977–979.

Sollinger HW, Belzer FO, Deierhoi MH et al (1992) RS-61443 (mycophenolate mofetil). A multicenter study for refractory kidney transplant rejection. *Ann Surg* 216:513–518.

Sollinger HW for the US Renal Transplant Mycophenolate Mofetil Study Group (1995) Mycophenolate mofetil for the prevention of acute rejection in primary cadaveric renal allograft recipients. *Transplantation* 60:225–232.

Solomon H, Gonwa TA, Mor E et al (1993) OKT3 rescue for steroid-resistant rejection in adult liver transplantation. *Transplantation* 55:87–91.

Starzl TE (1993) France and the early history of organ transplantation. *Perspect Biol Med* 37:35–47.

Starzl TE, Marchioro TL, Huntley RT et al (1964) Experimental and clinical homotransplantation of the liver. *Ann NY Acad Sci* 120:730–750.

Starzl TE, Iwatsuki S, Van Thiel DH et al (1982) Evolution of liver transplantation. *Hepatology* 2:614–636.

Starzl TE, Todo S, Fung J et al (1989) FK506 for liver, kidney, and pancreas transplantation. *Lancet* 2:1000–1004.

Stratta RJ, Armbrust MJ, Oh CS et al (1988) Withdrawal of steroid immunosuppression in renal transplant recipients. *Transplantation* 45:323–328.

Swinnen LJ, Costanzo-Nordin MR, Fisher SG et al (1990) Increased incidence of lymphoproliferative disorder after immunosuppression with the monoclonal antibody OKT3 in cardiac transplant recipients. *N Engl J Med* 323:1723–1728.

Tejani A, Butt KM, Rajpoot D et al (1989) Strategies for optimizing growth in children with kidney transplants. *Transplantation* 47:229–233.

Teraoka S, Babazono T, Koike T et al (1995) Effect of rescue therapy using FK506 on relapsing rejection after combined pancreas and kidney transplantation. *Transplant Proc* 27:1335–1339.

Timonen P, Friend P, Abeywickrama K et al (1990) Efficacy of low-dose cyclosporin A in psoriasis: results of dose-finding studies. *Br J Dermatol* 122(Suppl 36):33–39.

Tricontinental Mycophenolate Mofetil Renal Transplantation Study Group (1996) A blinded, randomized clinical trial of mycophenolate mofetil for the prevention of acute rejection in cadaveric renal transplantation. *Transplantation* 61:1029–1037.

Tsamandas AC, Pham SM, Seaberg EC et al (1997) Adult heart transplantation under tacrolimus (FK506) immunosuppression: histopathologic observations and comparison to a cyclosporine-based regimen with lympholytic (ATG) induction. *J Heart Lung Transplant* 16:723–734.

US Multicenter FK506 Liver Study Group (1994) A comparison of tacrolimus (FK506) and cyclosporine for immunosuppression in liver transplantation. *N Engl J Med* 331:1110–1115.

Van Gelder T, Mulder AH, Balk AHMM et al (1995a) Intragraft monitoring of rejection after prophylactic treatment with monoclonal anti-interleukin-2 receptor antibody (BT563) in heart transplant recipients. *J Heart Lung Transplant* 14:346–350.

Van Gelder T, Zietse R, Mulder AH et al (1995b) A double-blind, placebo-controlled study of monoclonal anti-interleukin-2 receptor antibody (BT563) administration to prevent acute rejection after kidney transplantation. *Transplantation* 60:248–252.

Vathsala A, Chou T-C, Kahan BD (1990) Analysis of the interactions of immunosuppressive drugs with cyclosporine in inhibiting DNA proliferation. *Transplantation* 49:463–472.

Vianello A, Mastrosimone S, Calconi G et al (1993) The role of hypertension as a damaging factor for kidney grafts under cyclosporine therapy. *Am J Kidney Dis* 21:79–83.

Vincenti F, Kirkman R, Light S et al (1998) Interleukin-2 receptor blockade with daclizumab to prevent acute rejection in renal transplantation. *N Engl J Med* **338**:161–165.

Vincenti F, Grinyó J, Ramos E et al (1999) Can antibody prophylaxis allow sparing of other immunosuppressives? *Transplant Proc* **31**:1246–1248.

Wacher VJ, Wu CY, Benet LZ (1995) Overlapping substrate specificities and tissue distribution of cytochrome P450 #A and P-glycoprotein: implications for drug delivery and activity in cancer chemotherapy. *Mol Carcinog* **13**:129–134.

Wechter WJ, Brodie JA, Morrell RM et al (1979) Antithymocyte globulin (ATGAM) in renal allograft recipients. Multicenter trials using a 14-dose regimen. *Transplantation* **28**:294–302.

Weir MR, Anderson L, Fink JC et al (1997) A novel approach to the treatment of chronic allograft nephropathy. *Transplantation* **64**:1706–1710.

Wenger R (1986) Cyclosporine and analogues: structural requirements for immunosuppressive activity. *Transplant Proc* **18**(Suppl 5):213–218.

Wiesel M, Carl S (1998) A placebo controlled study of mycophenolate mofetil used in combination with cyclosporine and corticosteroids for the prevention of acute rejection in renal allograft recipients: 1 year results. *J Urol* **159**:28–33.

Wiesel M, Carl S, Pomer S et al (1995) Effect of the anti-IL2 receptor monoclonal antibody inolimomab in treatment of acute interstitial renal rejection. *J Urol* **153**(Suppl):399.

Wiesner RH (1998) A long term comparison of tacrolimus (FK506) versus cyclosporine in liver transplantation: a report of the United States FK506 study group. *Transplantation* **66**:493–499.

Woodle ES, Thistlethwaite JR, Gordon JH et al (1996) A multicenter trial of FK506 (tacrolimus) therapy in refractory acute renal allograft rejection: a report of the Tacrolimus Kidney Transplantation Rescue Study Group. *Transplantation* **62**:594–599.

Woodruff MF, Anderson NA (1963) Effect of lymphocyte depletion by thoracic duct, fistula, and administration of anti-lymphocytic serum on the survival of skin homografts in rats. *Nature* **200**:702.

Yamamoto T, Noble NA, Miller DE, Border WA (1994) Sustained expression of TGF-β_1 underlies development of progressive kidney fibrosis. *Kidney Int* **45**:916–927.

Yang HC, Holman MJ, Langhoff E et al (1999) Tacrolimus/'low-dose' mycophenolate mofetil versus microemulsion cyclosporine/'low-dose' mycophenolate mofetil after kidney transplantation: 1-year follow-up of a prospective, randomized clinical trial. *Transplant Proc* **31**:1121–1124.

Zanker B, Schneeberger H, Rothenpieler U et al (1998) Mycophenolate mofetil-based, cyclosporine-free induction and maintenance immunosuppression: first-3-months, analysis of efficacy and safety in two cohorts of renal allograft recipients. *Transplantation* **66**:44–49.

Zimmerman J, Kahan BD (1997) Pharmacokinetics of sirolimus in stable renal transplant patients after multiple oral dose administration. *J Clin Pharmacol* **37**:405–415.

10 IMMUNOSUPPRESSIVE DRUGS: NEW STRATEGIES

INTRODUCTION

The last two decades have witnessed the development of selective T-cell inhibitors—cyclosporine (CsA), anti-CD3 and anti-CD25 monoclonal antibodies (MAbs), tacrolimus (TRL), and sirolimus (SRL)—each of which exerts a unique action to block signals generated by histocompatibility antigens or by cytokine mediators critical to the immune response. Owing to their selective properties, these agents have improved the levels of safety and potency beyond those previously obtained with immunosuppressive strategies utilizing steroids, antiproliferative drugs, such as azathioprine (AZA) and mycophenolate mofetil (MMF), and/or polyclonal antilymphocyte sera. On the horizon are a variety of strategies to further increase the therapeutic efficacy by blocking novel sites in the immune response, or by disrupting the ischemia–reperfusion cascades that enhance the antigenicity of the graft, as well as its vulnerability to antigen-dependent and -independent injuries.

The agents presently under development can be classified according to eight paradigms of their mechanisms of action (Table 10.1), which are presented in the order of their potential development. Among the drugs developed to address the proliferation paradigm, the nonselective agent AZA and the modestly selective agent MMF may be supplanted by the far more potent inhibitors of pyrimidine biosynthesis, brequinar and leflunomide. Within the framework of the cytokine paradigm, the archetypal agents CsA and TRL may yield to new strategies based either upon an improved selectivity for the immunophilin (indolyl ascomycin), or upon competition by specific peptide inhibitors for the calcineurin (CaN) site that binds nuclear factor of activated T cells (NF-AT), but not other substrates for dephosphorylation. In addition, refinement of existing antibodies, such as the production of humanized forms to succeed the purely murine form of anti-CD3 MAbs, may provide greater safety and tolerability of this therapy. Other agents in development to interrupt the cytokine paradigm include target intermediates that are relatively specific for the activation and/or transduction cascades of T-cells receptors (ZAP70), MAbs directed against the coreceptors that are critical for effective generation of signal one (CD2 or CD4), and drugs that inhibit the enzyme activity linked to Janus kinase 3 activity for T-cell-specific lymphokines (AG490, prodigiosin).

Generation	Paradigm	Agents	
		Established	New
First	Proliferation	Azathioprine (AZA)	Brequinar
		Mycophenolate mofetil (MMF)	Leflunomide
Second/third	Cytokine Generation	Cyclosporine (CsA), tacrolimus (TRL)	Indolyl ascomycin; peptide inhibitor NF-AT
	Reception	α-IL-2R monoclonal antibodies (MAbs)	None
	Transduction	Sirolimus (SRL), SDZ RAD	AG490, Prodigiosin
New strategies	Co-receptor	None	Anti-CD2, anti-CD4, anti-ICAM-1, or anti-LFA-1 MAbs
	Ischemia/reperfusion/migration	None	Anti-selectin MAbs; anti-ICAM-1 MAbs; FTY720
	Anti-inflammatory	None	Soluble tumor necrosis factor; cyclo-oxygenase (COX) inhibitors
Tolerance	T-cell depletion	None	Anti-T cell MAbs
	Costimulation	None	Anti-B7, anti-CD154 MAbs; CTLA-4Ig receptor conjugates
	Altered ligand	None	Peptides; allochimeric antigens

Table 10.1. Eight paradigms of immunosuppressive therapy

Increasingly, the ischemia/reperfusion/migration paradigm has been implicated in both early and late graft destruction. Injury to the graft provokes lymphocytes to adhere to its endothelium and to undergo diapedesis into its interstitium, resulting in direct antigen recognition. The rolling of leukocytes, the first step in the adhesion process, may be blocked by selectin inhibitors; the tethering, the second step, by antagonists of intercellular adhesion molecule-1 (ICAM-1) or its ligand, lymphocyte function antigen-1 (LFA-1; CD11a/CD18); and the migration response to chemokines, the third step, by the sphingosine analog FTY720. Furthermore, recent developments in the understanding of the mechanisms of action of cyclo-oxygenase (COX) inhibitors proffer the possibility of dampening tissue damage in newly engrafted and in rejecting allografts—the anti-inflammatory paradigm.

The final three paradigms are designed to achieve transplantation tolerance. First, profound T-cell depletion without or with reconstitution by donor-type bone marrow ('chimerism') has been amply documented in animal models to favor tolerance induction. Second, interruption of costimulatory events in T-cell activation by blockade of the B7-1/B7-2 markers on antigen-presenting cells (APC) prevents binding to CD28/CTLA-4 surface proteins on T cells. Initial encouraging experiments in animal models suggest that administration of either anti-B7 MAbs or CTLA-4 receptor conjugate without or with adjunctive treatment with anti-CD40 ligand (CD154) markedly prolongs graft survival. While at least the initial mechanism of unresponsiveness is the emergence of anergy, namely, a failure to mount a destructive response, in the longer term, alloreactive cells may undergo an apoptotic mechanism that leads to deletion. Third, administration of specific peptides or tailored histocompatibility antigens may represent the most powerful approach to induce tolerance, since these substances do not produce any adverse reactions. The next decade should witness the rapid introduction of a variety of strategies designed to interrupt the immune response with high degrees of selectivity and synergy, as well as the specificity required to achieve the goal of immunosuppressive therapy—transplant tolerance.

ISCHEMIA/REPERFUSION/MIGRATION PARADIGM

The ischemia–reperfusion injury begins during the preretrieval phase as the result of pathophysiologic insults to the donor that predispose the renal graft to damage. Even when removed under ideal circumstances, the kidney suffers at least a modest ischemic injury caused by the period of lack of blood perfusion. This injury is only modestly dampened by the use of special preservation solutions and by organ storage at cold temperatures. The inflammatory mechanisms triggered during the preretrieval process and the ischemic injuries incurred during the preservation period are exacerbated as warm host blood enters the graft and thus initiates the reperfusion cascade. Although the interventions to mitigate these events remain primarily within the realm of investigations in animal models, recent recognition of their seminal importance to the long-term outcome of transplants has sparked intense interest in the clinical application of new countermeasure strategies.

Pathophysiologic mechanisms of ischemia

Ion and water fluxes

During the nonoxygenated period after kidney removal, ongoing anaerobic metabolism in the graft depletes intracellular ATP, thus interrupting critical ion transport processes that are necessary to maintain transmembrane gradients, prevent intracellular accumulation of water, and preserve cell permselectivity (Figure 10.1, Table 10.2). Ischemia causes dysfunction of the junctional proteins, including occludin, the main functional component of the tight junction within the zonula occludens, and vascular endothelial (VE)-cadherin, the principle transmembrane protein for cell-to-cell adhesion within the zonula adherens. These alterations disturb both the barrier-to-intracellular penetration of water and the associations between membrane structures and cytoskeletal actin (Lampugnani et al 1992), thus interfering with cellular function and architecture. The ischemic effects may activate proteases (caspases and metalloproteinases) and predispose to internalization of surface proteins, particularly cadhedrin, resulting in the formation of endothelial gaps. Kevil et al (1998) hypothesized that the ATP depletion results in the generation of activated oxidative intermediates, which are responsible for these effects.

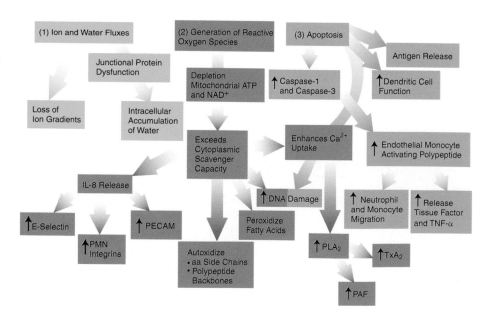

Figure 10.1. Schematic representation of mechanisms of the three major types of ischemic injuries: (1) ion and water fluxes, (2) generation of reactive oxygen species, and (3) apoptosis.

Type of injury	Potential therapeutic approach
Ischemic	
Free radicals of oxygen and hydroxyl	Allopurinol, Vitamin C, SOD
Antiapoptosis	
Mitochondrial protectants	TMZ, anti-TNF-α MAb
Caspase inhibitors	ZAD-fmk
Enhanced Bcl-2	Transfection Bcl-2 genes
Reperfusion	
Ligand inhibitors	
Selectins	MAbs, molecular antagonists, activators of receptor degradation
Endothelial surface markers	Anti-ICAM-1 antisense oligodeoxynucleotides MAbs, peptide antagonists, FTY720
Lymphocyte integrins	MAbs, peptide antagonists, FTY720
Inhibitors of humoral responses	
Vasoconstriction	
Prostacyclin	Beraprost, prostaglandin E
Endothelin (ET)	ET-A receptor antagonist
TNF-α	Soluble TNF receptor

Table 10.2. Potential therapies for allograft injuries

Reactive oxygen species

The lack of blood perfusion necessitates that ischemic tissues convert substrates to water to derive energy for ongoing metabolic processes. This anaerobic metabolism generates highly chemically reactive free radicals of oxygen, including superoxide anion (O_2^-), hydroxyl radical ($OH^{\bullet}$), its byproduct hydrogen peroxide (H_2O_2), and nitric oxide radical ($NO^{\bullet}$). During anaerobic metabolism, ATP is converted to ADP and AMP, and eventually to hypoxanthine, which is metabolized by xanthine oxidase to the potentially toxic metabolite uric acid, which in turn releases reactive oxygen species.

Owing to the presence of an odd number of electrons in their atoms, free radicals contain an open bond that renders them highly chemically reactive. Normally, these radicals are only produced in mitochondria, where they are promptly eliminated by electron transport systems, a process that depletes ATP and nicotinamide adenine dinucleotide (NAD^+) intermediates. When the content of these radicals, generated by the pathologic stimuli of ischemia, exceeds the metabolic capacities of mitochondrial mechanisms, they are released from these organelles into the cytoplasm of macrophages, leukocytes, and endothelial cells. If their intracellular content further exceeds the natural antioxidant scavenger capacity of the cell via glutathione and N-acetyl cysteine intermediates, as well as the catalytic activity of superoxide dismutase (SOD), catalase, and peroxidase, the free radicals auto-oxidize amino acid side chains (especially cysteine) as well as polypeptide backbones of endogenous and exogenous macromolecular substrates; peroxidize polyunsaturated fatty acids in intracellular membranes; damage and break the strands of DNA; and induce upregulated expression of adhesion markers, such as P-selectin, on endothelial cells. Accumulation of reactive oxygen metabolites also stimulates interleukin-8 (IL-8) release, resulting in enhanced expression of E-selectin, of polymorphonuclear leukocyte (PMN) integrins, and of PECAM-1, which guides transendothelial migration between intercellular junctions.

ATP depletion promotes Ca^{2+} uptake into anoxic endothelial cells, thereby activating the catalytic activity of phospholipase A_2 (PLA_2), which hydrolyzes arachidonic acid-containing phospholipids, thereby generating platelet activating factor (PAF) and thromboxane A_2 (TxA_2). This network of interactions disseminates the ischemic injury from the primary endothelial target to host leukocytes and then to the graft interstitium and tubular cells, the last of which show persistently elevated free radical activity for several days after injury. The vicious cycle caused by the increased levels of reactive oxygen species and by the consequent complement activation (Chávez-Cartaya et al 1995) is known as 'oxidative stress', a state that provokes a variety of homeostatic and pathologic modulations.

Apoptosis

Another component of the ischemic damage to endothelial, epithelial, and tubular cells is apoptosis, or programmed cell death. The characteristic morphologic features of DNA fragmentation result from increased activities of the death proteases caspase-1 and caspase-3. Caspase upregulation may activate endothelial monocyte-activating polypeptide II (Knies et al 1998), which not only serves as a potent chemokine to stimulate neutrophil and monocyte migration (Kao et al 1994), but also releases tissue factor from endothelial cells and tumor necrosis factor (TNF)-α from monocytes. Furthermore, Albert et al (1998) and Rovere et al (1998) found that release of antigen from apoptotic cells triggers the activation of dendritic APCs.

The apoptotic events may be triggered by enhanced release of ceramide from damaged plasma membranes (Zager et al 1997), and/or by upregulated expression of p53 (Raafat et al 1997), of TNF-α (Daemen et al 1999a), and/or of Fas (Nogae et al 1998). In addition, the mitochondrial damage produced by free radical generation causes cytochrome C to be released into the cytosol (White 1996, Kroemer 1997). This enzyme degrades Bcl-2, an intermediate critical not only to prevent mitochondrial dysfunction due to proapoptotic stimuli, but also to block the cytotoxic effects mediated by the perforin and granzyme products of cytotoxic lymphocytes. Cytochrome C cleaves the regulatory domain of Bcl-2, thereby destroying the antiapoptotic function of the molecule and releasing a proapoptotic activity (Uckan et al 1997). Downregulated Bcl-2 expression in bile duct epithelial cells has been observed in liver allografts undergoing acute rejection (Gapany et al 1997), possibly accounting for their increased rate of apoptosis (Krams et al 1995).

Therapeutic approaches to ischemia

Organ preservation solutions

Available organ preservation solutions seek to mitigate the increased permeability of ischemic graft cells. Most solutions contain an ionic composition similar to that of intracellular fluid, namely, a large amount of potassium and phosphate relative to sodium and chloride, as well as additional glucose and mannitol to provide an energy source for anaerobic metabolism and to reduce the osmotic differential between the aqueous medium and the tissue, thus contravening the water flux that causes cell swelling. However, these solutions are not entirely effective. Using dual well chambers, Trocha et al (1999) observed that diffusion of University of Wisconsin preservation solution (Viaspan, DuPont Pharma, Wilmington, DE, USA) from the lower chamber through human umbilical endothelial cell monolayers in the upper chamber produced a decreased content of both occludin and later of VE-cadherin, as well as an alteration in their functional organization with F-actin. Further understanding of the molecular events mediating these processes will be necessary to tailor more effective preservation solutions.

Antioxidants

Therapeutic interventions designed to dampen the release or to enhance the scavenger capacity of tissues for reactive oxygen species have not been effective to mitigate the ischemic injury in the clinical setting. Addition to the organ procurement solution of allopurinol, an inhibitor of xanthine oxidase catalytic activity during anaerobic ischemia, has been shown to produce beneficial effects on the ischemic injury in animal models (Williams 1990), but not in the clinical setting. Schneeberger et al (1989) observed a trend to a more rapid return of creatinine clearance among kidneys treated with SOD, compared to untreated organs, at the time of reperfusion. Using an in situ ischemia model in pigs, Hoshino et al (1988) observed that pretreatment with SOD ameliorated the reperfusion injury, and that intra-arterial delivery of SOD at the time of transplantation of renal allografts modulated the injury resulting from 18 hours of storage. Although treatment of renal transplant recipients with 200 mg doses of recombinant (rh) SOD produced little benefit on kidney function in the early period, Land and Messmer (1996) suggested that this treatment reduced the proclivity of the graft to chronic transplant failure.

A third use of antioxidants seeks to selectively block lipid peroxidation. For example, pretreatment of rat cardiac transplants with the antioxidant probucol (Hoechst-Marion-Roussel, Bridgewater, NJ, USA), which is designed to prevent peroxidation of low-density lipoproteins, mitigated the diastolic dysfunction engendered by a 2-hour period of ischemia (Rabkin et al 1999). Using malondialdehyde (MDA) as a surrogate of lipid peroxidation consequent to the generation of free radicals, Rabl et al (1992), Davenport et al (1995), and Hower et al (1996) reported that pretreatment with vitamin C (500 mg intravenously during surgery) dampened the MDA surge in renal venous blood in animal models. In contrast, Bonventre (1993) consistently failed to observe either increased lipid peroxidation or a benefit of antioxidant treatment in this model. Although none of the antioxidant approaches is presently under active investigation, the plethora of potential clinical applications beyond transplantation is bound to reawaken interest in this field.

Antiapoptotic strategies

Trimetazidine (TMZ; Servier Institute, Paris, France) is a trioxymethyl benzene compound that promotes Ca^{2+} efflux from cells, thereby counteracting the destructive effects of this ion on anoxic endothelium. This effect is particularly pronounced on the mitochondrial organelles of endothelial cells in kidneys contemporaneously exposed to CaN antagonists (CNAs) CsA or TRL. Upon addition to storage solutions, TMZ restored the cellular content of NAD^+ and ATP that had been depressed by an ischemic injury (Baumert et al 1999), and thereby promoted renal graft recovery (Salducci et al 1996). One possible mechanism of action of this agent is the inhibition of release of cytochrome C from the mitochondria to the cytosol. Thus, there is no enzyme available to activate caspases. Trimetazidine may act in a fashion complementary to Bcl-2, which also suppresses mitochondrial release of cytochrome C.

A gene engineering approach may also be useful to prevent apoptosis. In other settings, overexpression of Bcl-2 has been shown to mitigate a variety of vascular insults, particularly in the central nervous system (Garcia et al 1992; Shimazaki et al 1994; Lawrence et al 1996). To protect the liver against the ischemia–reperfusion cascade, Gapany et al (1997) treated hosts prior to injury by intravenous transfection with a hepatotropic adenovirus vector containing the gene encoding the Bcl-2 polypeptide. Transfected livers showed dampened ischemic effects: namely, a reduction in the content of transaminases, the number of apoptotic cells, and the host mortality rate. However, this strategy has limited clinical application, due both to the need to perform the gene transfer prior to the injury and to the rapid elimination of the adenoviral vector, which limits the period of transgene expression.

A third approach to avert apoptosis was reported by Daemen et al (1999b): treatment at the time of reperfusion either with the tripeptide caspase inhibitor ZAD-fmk (Z-Val-Ala-Asp [Ome]-CH_2F) or with insulin-like growth factor-1 (IGF-1) abrogated renal functional impairment, early apoptotic events, and inflammation in renal grafts, possibly by promoting the generation of the renal vasodilator nitric oxide. These investigators also observed that administration of anti-TNF-α antibodies dampened apoptotic events following in situ ischemic injuries of murine kidneys.

Pathophysiologic mechanisms of reperfusion

The reperfusion injury that occurs after implantation of the allograft includes enhanced triggering of a cascade of receptor–ligand interactions (Springer 1994; Butcher and Picker 1996) and the production of proinflammatory mediators. The stored kidney may be particularly vulnerable to injuries caused by premorbid humoral events in the donor, namely, excessive catecholamine release, which produces autonomic storm; increased serum levels of IL-6; as well as enhanced transcriptional upregulation of TNF-α and IL-6 synthesis (Pratschke et al 1999). These events cause the injured organ to alter the rheologic properties of host blood entering the kidney (Figure 10.2).

Vasoconstrictive effects

Reduced blood flow to the graft is caused by at least three ischemic processes that are exacerbated upon reperfusion: (1) augmented translocation of water from the intravascular to the inter- and intracellular spaces, producing local hemoconcentration and increased blood viscosity; (2) endothelial cell swelling, causing luminal narrowing; and (3) acidosis, reducing erythrocyte membrane elasticity.

Endothelial cells independently release the vasoconstrictor TxA$_2$, which is also a platelet activator (Zamora et al 1993). The consequent platelet accumulation on endothelium shows a high correlation with the degree of preservation–reperfusion injury (Cywes et al 1993). In addition, platelet aggregation and thrombosis are potentiated by

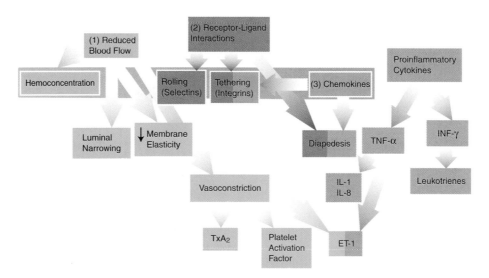

Figure 10.2. Schematic representation of the three major mechanisms of the reperfusion injury: (1) reduced blood flow, (2) receptor–ligand interaction, and (3) generation of chemokines and of proinflammatory cytokines.

423

a reduced production of prostacyclin and by a paralysis of natural anticoagulant pathways. Another potent vasoconstrictor is endothelin (ET), which is produced by endothelial cells and macrophages. ET-1, the strongest vasoconstrictor among the three isotypes, binds predominantly to ET-A as opposed to ET-B receptors (Yanagisawa and Masaki 1989). Augmented production of ET-1 during ischemia results from TNF-α stimulation of the de novo synthesis of prepro-ET and the activation of ET-converting enzyme (Lundblad and Giercksky 1995). A potential role of this mediator in the dysfunction of renal grafts is suggested by the observations that not only do mice transgenic for human ET-1 display renal changes akin to those of chronic rejection, but also organ transplant patients show elevated plasma ET-1 levels (Lerman et al 1992). Furthermore, the presence of ET-1 is often demonstrated by histologic staining of human cardiac allografts undergoing chronic rejection processes (Watschinger et al 1995).

Receptor–ligand interactions: rolling

Lymphocytes and granulocytes marginate, contact, and roll along the endothelium by forming transient, low-affinity interactions between selectin surface molecules both on circulating elements (L-selectin) and on endothelial cells (E- and P-selectins). Selectins are single-chain transmembrane glycoproteins of approximate molecular weight 120 kD. They consist of five domains: a membrane-distal, amino terminal, Ca^{2+}-dependent, lectin recognition unit; an epidermal growth factor-like region; a variable number of short sequences similar to complement-regulatory proteins; a transmembrane area; and a short carboxy-terminal intracellular portion (Figure 10.3). Each type of selectin molecule mediates rolling at a characteristic speed of blood flow, with L-selectin at the highest and E-selectin (CD62E) at the lowest velocity. Thus, L-selectin most efficiently captures leukocytes from the flow, whereas E-selectin promotes stable rolling; P-selectin (CD62P) displays both functions (Jung and Ley 1999). Local generation of the cytokine mediators IL-1 and TNF-α in response to tissue injury upregulates the expression of selectin molecules and triggers endothelial cell activation, which in turn leads to PAF generation, thereby enhancing PMN-mediated release of proteolytic enzymes and reactive oxygen species (Bulkley 1983). Upon cytokine stimulation, E-selectin is transiently synthesized at and expressed on the surface of endothelial cells at 4–6 hours, thereafter decaying by 24–48 hours. In contrast, within 5–10 min after exposure to thrombin, histamine, or hydrogen peroxide, P-selectin, which is produced constitutively and stored in the granules of platelets and the Weibel–Palade bodies of endothelial cells, is rapidly expressed on the cell surface; P-selectin returns to basal levels by 60 min. Cytokine release upon reperfusion may also upregulate new P-selectin synthesis by endothelial and kidney cells (Hughes et al 1995).

The mononuclear leukocyte ligands for selectins are sialylated and fucosylated lactosamine determinants (Figure 10.3a). Among the T-helper (Th) group, $CD4^+$ Th_1 (but not Th_2) cells express a functionally intact P-selectin glycoprotein ligand-1 (PSGL-1) that binds to P- and E-selectins (Austrup 1997). Thus, $CD4^+$ Th_1 cells are the predominant invaders at an inflammatory site (Borges et al 1997). In contrast, L-selectins

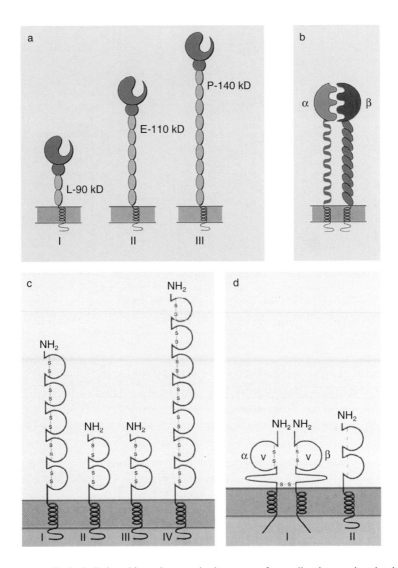

Figure 10.3. Endothelial and lymphocyte–leukocyte surface adhesion molecules in cell–cell adhesion. (a) Structures showing the complement regulatory repeat units (orange '0'), the epidermal growth factor region (red '0'), and the lectin binding domain (blue) of L-selectin (I, 90 kD), E-selectin (II, 110 kD), and P-selectin (III, 140 kD). (b) Integrins contain α and β chains in noncovalent complexes to produce different isoforms. (c) Cell-surface molecules of the immunoglobulin gene superfamily, including I. ICAM-1; II. ICAM-2; III. CD2; and IV. VCAM-1. (d) Coreceptor ligand pairs of the immunoglobulin gene superfamily: I. CD28; II. B7.

are predominantly expressed on CD8$^+$ lymphocytes. In addition to the binding of endothelial E- and P-selectins on the endothelium to the specific glycoprotein ligands— sialyl Lewis^x (sLe^x), sLe^a, and PSGL-1—P- and L-selectins also bind to sulfatide and sulfated glycosoaminoglycan markers on matrix components (Figure 10.4).

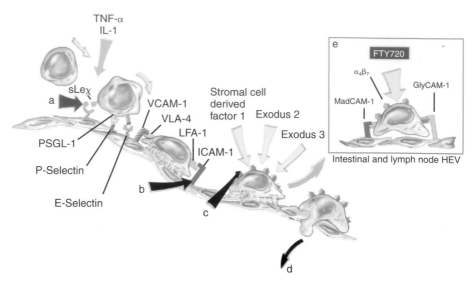

Figure 10.4. The ischemia–reperfusion–migration paradigm. (a) Rolling. (b) Tethering. (c) Integrin activation. (d) Diapedesis. (e) Unique phenotype of the cells generated by FTY720.

Ligation of L-selectin on lymphocytes triggers an increased intracellular content of calcium, which activates extracellular signal-regulated kinases (ERK, including Ras) to catalyze phosphorylation of tyrosine. This process enhances the ruffling of plasma membranes and promotes the cytoskeletal reorganization of actin assemblies, thereby altering cell deformability, an effect that is necessary for the formation of pseudopodia at the leading edge and uropods at the rear of the migrating cell (Simon et al 1999). Furthermore, ligation promotes clustering of L-selectin, as well as enhances the surface expression of and colocalizes with the β_2 integrin leukocyte function antigen-1 in the plasma membrane.

Receptor–ligand interactions: tethering

While L-selectin initiates leukocyte capture on endothelium, production of cytokines, such as IL-8 and/or PAF as well as chemokines, upregulates expression of cell surface integrin markers and induces distinctive patterns of lymphocyte adhesion. Integrins contain α and β subunits; each $\alpha\beta$ combination displays distinct binding and signaling properties (Figure 10.3b). The β_2-lymphocyte integrin LFA-1, which contains a unique α-chain (CD11a) and a β_2-integrin-common β-chain (CD18), binds to the endothelial cell marker ICAM-1. Upregulated expression of endothelial cell ICAM-1 is a common feature of grafts exposed to an ischemia–reperfusion cycle (Briscoe et al 1991; Taylor et al 1992). ICAM-1 provides an excellent coreceptor stimulus to CD8$^+$ CTL responses, particularly when combined with B7-1 (CD86) and with the generation of MIP-1β and 'the regulated on activation of normal T cells expressed and secreted factor'

(RANTES; Kim et al 1999). Alternatively, ICAM-1 can bind to LFA-3 (CD58; 50–70 kD), an interaction that specifically enhances activation, proliferation, and cytokine production by Th cells. The β_1-integrin vascular cell adhesion molecule (VCAM; CD106; 110 kD) binds to the PMN marker very late antigen-4 (VLA-4), producing arteriolar plugging and the no-reflow phenomenon upon reperfusion of the graft, but has no effect on T-cell responses (Ames et al 1968).

After binding to their ligands on the surface of endothelial cells, and following upregulation of the heterodimer CD98, an early marker of T-cell activation, integrins form clusters in the lymphocyte membrane. These high-density complexes display an increased avidity for their ligands. The heavy chain of CD98, which crosslinks integrins, induces an intracellular cascade, thus producing a conformation change in the ligand binding sites (Fenczik et al 1997). Because their cytoplasmic tails are short and devoid of enzymatic activities, integrins must associate with adapter proteins that connect them to the cytoskeleton, promoting the formation of actin filaments, and to cytoplasmic kinases and to transmembrane growth factor receptors (Giancotti and Ruoslahti 1999).

Among T lymphocytes, one can distinguish a subpopulation of $\alpha_4\beta_7$-negative cells, which embody memory for systemic (nonintestinal) responses (Santamaria Babi et al 1995; Salmi et al 1998; Butcher et al 1999) and bear a sLe^x-related carbohydrate epitope, denoted as cutaneous lymphocyte antigen and functioning as a 'homing' receptor for inflamed skin. In contrast, lymphocytes bearing the $\alpha_4\beta_7$-integrin pair are attracted to the mucosal addressin cell adhesion molecule (MadCAM-1) homing receptor and to intestinal antigen lymphoid structures (Mackay et al 1996; Williams and Butcher 1997; Butcher et al 1999). In addition to expression of unique integrin pairs, special ligands characteristic of the high endothelial venules (HEVs) of various tissues control the selective pattern of lymphocyte emigration. Lymph node HEVs display two forms of sialyl-glycoproteins: the addressins (PNAd) and vascular adhesion protein-1 (VAP-1). Both sialyl-glycoproteins exist in two isoforms: PNAd as the 50-kD mucin-type molecule glyCAM-1 or the 17-kD sulfated protein podocalyxin; VAP-1 as a 90- or 170-kD isoform. For example, sialyl residues on VAP-1 molecules selectively bind to an unknown ligand that is present on CD8$^+$, but not on CD4$^+$, lymphocytes, B cells, or monocytes.

Receptor–ligand interactions: diapedesis

Because the lymphocyte arrest on endothelial cells is transient, rapid signals are necessary to initiate diapedesis. The emigration of lymphocytes into tissues is an integral function of normal immune surveillance mechanisms. However, whereas the percolation of cells through tissues is normally rapid, the presence of an inflammatory postperfusion syndrome causes lymphocytes to remain in the tissues, wherein they contact donor interstitial dendritic cells, an interaction that strongly triggers T-cell alloactivation by direct recognition. This aberrant behavior is explained at least in part by the influence of cytokines (Pober and Cotran 1990), and by the upregulated expression of L-selectins, as well as of ICAM-1 (CD54; 90–114 kD) and VLA-4 (Oppenheimer-Marks and Lipsky

1993) ligands, which function as coreceptors in the immune response. Lymphocyte interactions with these ligands facilitate both the emigration and the activation of T cells (van Seventer et al 1990).

Humoral mediators: chemokines

Among the army of more than 30 chemotactic cytokines (including Exodus factors) that are produced by ischemic tissue, six important chemokines trigger rapid but transient integrin-mediated adhesion of rolling leukocytes: namely, (1) stromal cell-derived factor-1 (SDF-1); (2) 6-C-kine (Exodus 2), which attracts most circulating $CD4^+$ cells; (3) macrophage inflammation protein-3α (MIP-3α); (4) MIP-3β (Exodus 3) for memory but not naïve $CD4^+$ T cells (Campbell et al 1998); (5) interferon (IFN)-α inducible protein 10 (IP-10); and (6) RANTES. Other substances among the army of chemokines that have complex and overlapping functions to facilitate cell tethering to endothelium are PAF (as well as related substances) and leukotrienes (KT3) (Lehr et al 1991), all of which produce leakage of macromolecules, thus promoting the development of interstitial edema.

Chemokines trigger G protein-coupled receptors, which are trimeric αβγ-chains bound to seven-pass surface membrane structures. Upon ligand binding, the receptors dissociate from Gαβγ to Gβγ heterodimers and Gα subunits (Jordan and Devi 1999). The Gα units, which are sensitive to the action of pertussis toxin, associate with a GTPase activating protein Rap1, which in turn regulates ERKs. The chemokine receptors may also be linked to Gs proteins, which activate adenyl cyclase, and/or to Gq proteins, which activate phospholipidase C, and in turn generate second messengers, including diacylglycerol.

Chemokine reception increases the intralymphocyte calcium concentrations and promotes chemotaxis. The G receptor signal transduction pathways include three members of a family of small guanine nucleotide-binding proteins: Cdc42, Rac, and Rho (Keely et al 1997). The small GTPase, Rho, converts GTP to the inactive GDP-bound form in response to serum and cellular lysophosphatidic acid. In some cells, a Rho-associated kinase (ROCK) phosphorylates LIM-kinase, thus triggering the formation of actin stress fibers (Maekawa et al 1999). The Rho family of GTP-binding proteins, in concert with phosphoinositol triphosphate (PI-3) and PI-5 signal transduction molecules, are necessary for actin arrangement, namely, simultaneous attachment at the leading edge and detachment at the rear of the motile cell, events that are essential for the migration event. Thus, the participation of Rho is necessary to enable lymphocytes to extend filopodia, Cdc42 to form local adhesions, and Rac to spread across the extracellular matrix. In addition, Rac promotes cell cycle progression and integrin clustering.

RANTES augments pseudopod formation and promotes actin rearrangement via a pathway sensitive to the PI-3 kinase inhibitor Wortmannin, and to the Rho GTP-binding protein inhibitor, known as epidermal cell differentiation inhibitor (Kawai et al 1999). RANTES activates two T-cell signaling pathways: an initial, transient, G protein-dependent signal, and a second, long-lasting, protein tyrosine kinase signal. In conjunction with the cytoskeletal protein moesin, RANTES induces redistribution of ICAM-3 at the uropod.

IFN-γ induces production of the chemokine SDF-1, which binds to the CX chemokine receptor-4 (CXCR4) receptors present on all T-cell subsets and upregulates LFA-1-mediated lymphocyte adhesion to ICAM-1. IFN-γ stimulation of endothelial cells induces RANTES, which binds to CCR5, selectively enhancing diapedesis of CD4 Th$_1$ cells. These cells express CXCR3 preferentially, and also CXCR4. Both the intestinal- and the skin-affinity lymphocyte subsets respond to MIP-3β, a ligand for CCR7, and to SDF-1, a ligand for CXCR4. The chemokines TARC and MDC attract skin-homing cells that display CCR4 receptors and that express the cutaneous lymphocyte antigen (Campbell et al 1999). Although CXCR3 receptors are present on resting, naïve cells, their expression is markedly upregulated on recently activated, undifferentiated cells. In contrast, the CC chemokine receptors CCR2, CCR3, and CCR5 are not expressed on fresh naïve or activated, but only on fully differentiated, CD4$^+$ cells (Rabin et al 1999). For example, CCR5, which is present only on memory CD4 but not CD8 cells, serves as the receptor for three chemokines: MIP-1α, MIP-1β, and RANTES. In contrast, Th$_2$-type CD4$^+$ cells preferentially express CCR4 and CCR8, as well as CCR3 and CXCR3. CCR7 is distinctive for lymphocytes as opposed to PMNs, monocytes or erythrocytes.

Humoral mediators: proinflammatory cytokines

Ischemic tissues induce local release of cytokines that cause lymphocytes to adhere to endothelium, diapedese into the interstitium, and produce tissue inflammation. The extent and range of cytokines released from an organ upon reperfusion are markedly increased by prolonged periods of cold storage or by profound inflammatory events ('explosive brain death') in the donor prior to recovery (Takada et al 1998) (Figure 10.2).

An important cytokine vector of the acute postperfusion response to local injury is TNF-α, which is produced by activated monocytes and macrophages. This cytokine displays several critical effects: (1) it upregulates the expression of major histocompatibility complex (MHC) surface antigens and adhesion molecules on endothelial cells (Arai et al 1998); (2) it increases IL-1 production by monocytes and macrophages; and (3) it enhances the actions of IL-6 to recruit and integrate lymphocyte responses and of IL-8 to stimulate chemotactic migration. In addition, production of TNF-α may trigger renal cell apoptosis (Schulze-Osthoff et al 1992), reduce glomerular filtration rates, activate PMNs, induce expression of ICAM-1, P-, and E-selectins, as well as provoke the synthesis of MCP-1 and the release of IL-8. IL-10 may potentially counterregulate these effects of TNF-α, thereby mitigating tissue damage (Daemen et al 1999a).

A second critical cytokine in the early cascade of ischemia–reperfusion events is IFN-γ, which even more intensely upregulates the expression of MHC products: initially class I antigens on tubular cells, and subsequently class II antigens on tubular and interstitial cells. In aggregate, these events increase the immunogenicity of the graft, accounting for the increased incidence of acute rejection episodes among kidneys that have displayed delayed graft function, as well as their enhanced susceptibility to chronic attrition. Halloran et al (1995) and Goes et al (1995) observed that temporary occlusion of the pedicle of an in situ kidney induced upregulated production of IL-18 (at day 1) and IL-12 (at day 6), two potent IFN-γ producers. In addition to IFN-γ synthesis, these workers observed upregulated IL-2, IL-10, and TGF-β expression, findings that were confirmed in a syngeneic graft model for IL-10 and TGF-β, but not for IFN-γ and IL-2 (Connolly et al 1995). In the clinical setting, the concentration of IL-6, but neither TNF-α nor IFN-γ, was increased in renal venous blood at 30 and 60 min after revascularization of a renal graft (Hower et al 1996), and TNF-α and IL-6 were augmented at the same time intervals after liver reperfusion.

Therapeutic approaches to reperfusion

Pharmacologic interruption or modulation of the endothelial cell damage accompanying reperfusion and ischemic injuries seeks to promote early graft function, to reduce the strength of alloimmune responses, and to minimize the progression of vascular dysfunction and transplant senescence.

Disruption of vasoconstrictive mediators

Prostacyclin analogs such as beraprost sodium have been shown to disrupt preservation-induced injury, presumably because of their action to inhibit platelet adhesion (Okada et al 1998b). In the clinical arena, the vasodilator and antiplatelet effects of prostaglandin E seem to aid the functional recovery of cadaveric-donor liver grafts (Greig et al 1989; Himmelreich et al 1993). However, the risks of bleeding caused by the platelet dysfunction probably outweigh the potential benefits.

A second group of agents seeks to block the reception of endothelin (ET) humoral signals, which not only produce vasoconstriction, but also stimulate the mitogenesis and the activity of inflammatory cells. Anti-ET MAbs have been shown to mitigate the vasculopathic component of CsA-induced nephropathy. Using nonselective blockade of ET-A and ET-B receptors with TAK-044, a cyclic hexapeptide, Mitsuoka et al (1999) observed mitigation of the microcirculatory disturbances produced by ischemic changes. A selective ET-A receptor antagonist was shown by Braun et al (1999) to mitigate the development of chronic rejection in the Fisher-to-Lewis rat model. Compared to untreated controls, animals treated with the ET-A receptor antagonist exhibited better creatinine clearance rates and histopathologic appearances, but no differences in the hypertensive or proteinuric stigmata of chronic rejection. In another model, oral administration of the selective ET-A receptor antagonist LU135252 was reported to prevent the development of arteriosclerosis (Okada et al 1998a).

Selectin inhibitors

Three approaches to inhibit selectin function are presently undergoing evaluation: MAbs, ligand antagonists, and activators of receptor degradation. These strategies are likely to be relevant to transplantation, since sLe^x-L-selectin interactions are critical to lymphocyte extravasation into renal allografts (Turunen et al 1994).

The novel immunoglobulin G (IgG) MAb KPL1 targets the human leukocyte ligand PSGL-1, which interacts with endothelial cell P-selectin (McEver 1998; Snapp et al 1998). Pretreatment of murine liver allografts with KPL1 inhibited neutrophil infiltration, thereby mitigating both the cold and the warm ischemic injuries, as evidenced by dampened transaminase release and histologic damage (Dulkanchainun et al 1998). Across an H-2D to H-2K disparity, Yamazaki (1998) observed that a combination of anti-P plus anti-E selectin MAbs prolonged murine cardiac allograft survival to 30 days from 10 days. These observations are consistent with the findings in knockout mice: while E-selectin knockout mice show few or no abnormalities, and P-selectin-deficient mice display only partial inhibition of rolling and of delayed-type hypersensitivity responses, dual knockout mice suffer profound impairments, demonstrating a cooperative interaction between selectins.

A second therapeutic approach administers sLe^x analogs: CY-1503 (Schmid et al 1997), which blocks P-, E-, and L-selectin binding, has been shown in animal models to mitigate myocardial ischemia reperfusion injuries (Lefer et al 1994). Indeed, the effect on the reperfusion injury following myocardial ischemia is potentiated by the combination of infusion of sLe^x oligosaccharide molecular antagonist prior to ischemia, and administration of IgG$_1$ (κ) antibodies raised against a truncated form of rat P-selectin after the ischemic event (Tojo et al 1996). Another sLe^x analog, a novel, small, nonoligosaccharide molecule (TBC-1269; Texas Biotechnology Corporation, Houston, TX, USA), blocks selectins and dampens the ischemic injury displayed after temporary occlusion of in situ kidney or liver tissue (Palma-Vargas et al 1997). Similarly, rat hosts pretreated with either a soluble form of P-selectin glycoprotein ligand (sPSGL; Genetics Institute, Cambridge, MA, USA) or CTLA-4Ig (Bristol-Myers Squibb, Princeton, NJ, USA) prior to explosive brain injury caused by balloon-mediated increase in intracranial pressure displayed a reduced renal injury response (Takada et al 1998).

A third strategy uses neoglycopolymers that noncovalently associate with and thereby disrupt selectin binding to cognate surface ligands. The polymer, a 15-unit structure of disulfated trisaccharide 3,6-sulpho-sialyl hex4 monomers, mimics the structure of mucins, which are able to cluster L-selectin molecules into caps—an action similar to that of glyCAM-1, the natural glycosylation-dependent cell adhesion molecule. Once the agent has complexed with selectins, it promotes proteolytic cleavage of these adhesion molecules (Gordon et al 1998). Ex vivo treatment of PMNs with this agent causes a rapid shedding of selectins from the cell surface without augmenting the synthesis of these surface markers, suggesting that different proteases mediate the shedding versus the activation processes. Further preclinical refinement of all of these agents will be necessary prior to human testing. While it is likely that selectin inhibition per se will not provide full protection against leukocyte-induced tissue injury, this target may be useful in the development of a multimodality strategy.

Tethering inhibitors

The reperfusion injury has not been mitigated by any of the several strategies tested in experimental models, including leukocyte depletion using filters, administration of poly-clonal anti-Mac-1 or anti-LFA-1 antibodies to inhibit leukocyte adherence and macro-molecular leakage, or delivery of inhibitors of either LTB synthesis or PAF activity (Land and Messmer 1996). One study has claimed that upregulated ICAM-1 expression is blunted by the presence of an organ preservation solution (Viebahn et al 1995), and enhanced by human cytomegalovirus (CMV) infection via an effect on the ICAM-1 gene promoter in endothelial cells (Burns et al 1999). Three new approaches seem more likely to disrupt tethering mediated by LFA-1 adhesion to ICAM-1: namely, specific humanized MAbs, competitive molecular antagonists, and oligodeoxynucleotides (oligos) that interrupt ligand synthesis.

Tethering inhibitors: monoclonal antibodies

Treatment with MAbs directed toward cell adhesion molecules blunts macromolecular extravasation and mitigates ischemic injuries in experimental animal models (Harlan et al 1992). An anti-CD11b MAb was shown to blunt canine myocardial insults (Simpson et al 1988). In addition, a large number of studies support the activities of various forms of anti-CD18 MAbs to blunt feline intestinal injury (Hernandez et al 1987), myocardial ischemia (Ma et al 1991), reperfusion dysfunction (Vedder et al 1990), and neutrophil and lymphocyte extravasation as well as VCAM-1 expression (Akimoto et al 1996).

Nolte et al (1994) observed that an anti-ICAM-1 MAb prevented ischemic renal injuries to in situ kidneys in mice. In a nonhuman primate model, another anti-ICAM-1 MAb was shown to delay the onset of acute allograft rejection (Cosimi 1995). However, despite initially promising clinical trials (Haug et al 1993), the murine antihu-man ICAM-1 MAb failed to mitigate preservation injuries or to reduce the occurrence of acute rejection episodes in a subsequent multicenter trial. Similarly, preoperative administration and a 5-day postoperative course of the murine anti-LFA-1 IgG_{2a} MAb (Enlimomab, Boehringer Ingleheim, Germany) initially showed good tolerability and a reduced incidence of acute rejection episodes in one study (Hourmant et al 1996) and a protective effect on delayed graft function in another study (Troppman et al 1995). However, a subsequent randomized, blinded, placebo-controlled study failed to demon-strate a reduced risk of delayed graft function or of acute rejection episodes (Salmela et al 1999). The higher rate of infectious complications observed among the MAb- versus the placebo-treated patients suggested that the reagent did bear some immunosuppres-sive activity. While these results are not particularly encouraging, an humanized anti-LFA-1 MAb (Xoma/Genentech, San Francisco, CA, USA) has been shown in recent phase I trials to display a prolonged circulation time, an absence of prothrombotic activ-ity, and good tolerability in psoriasis patients. Binding of the humanized MAb to the LFA-1 ligand seems to trigger endocytosis of the antigen–antibody complexes; therefore, the peripheral blood leukocytes are denuded of LFA-1 ligand but not coated with anti-body Fc regions that would otherwise trigger prothrombotic events mediated by Fc receptors on platelets or leukocytes. This reagent will soon be tested in de novo renal transplant recipients.

Combined treatment with antibodies directed against LFA-1 and ICAM-1 induced transplant tolerance in mouse models (Isobe et al 1992). In contrast, the effect could only be obtained in rat models if these MAbs were combined with both sulfatide and TRL (Horimoto et al 1998). In addition, prolonged graft survival has been reported in a mouse model using a combination of MAbs directed against VCAM-1 and VLA-4 (Isobe et al 1994), and in the rat with MAbs against LFA-1 and VLA-4 (Paul et al 1996). Thus, demonstration of a clinical effect may demand the use not only of humanized forms of MAbs, but also combinations of MAbs without or with other therapeutic interventions to disrupt the ischemia–reperfusion injury.

Tethering inhibitors: molecular antagonists

Low-molecular-weight peptide antagonists have been designed to inhibit LFA-1 or ICAM-1 (Tibbetts et al 1999). Fewer than 25 amino acids in length, these peptides represent counterreceptor contact domains that mediate the adhesion and coreceptor functions of the LFA-1/ICAM-1 interaction. In addition, the peptides block the adhesion between, but not the viability of, homotypic cells, and interrupt proliferation in mixed lymphocyte cultures without inducing immune activation. Further analysis of the in vivo activities of these antagonists is likely to be of great import to the transplant community.

Tethering inhibitors: antisense ICAM-1 oligodeoxynucleotides

The rationale for the development of oligos is based on their three unique features: (1) the specificity of the genetic code, wherein a unique DNA sequence stipulates only a single mRNA; (2) a unique mechanism of action that disrupts mRNA protein translation; and (3) a distinctive side-effect profile, which does not overlap that of other immunosuppressive agents. Disruption of the synthesis of ICAM-1 in response to proinflammatory cytokines, such as TNF-α, that upregulate endothelial cell expression of this ligand eliminates binding by the constitutively expressed β_2-integrin LFA-1 and thereby prevents tethering of leukocytes (Figure 10.4b).

ISIS 2302 (ISIS Pharmaceuticals Inc., Carlsbad, CA, USA), a phosphorothioate oligo containing 20 bases ($C_{192},H_{225},N_{75},Na_{19},O_{98},P_{19},S_{79}$; GCCCAAGCTGGCATC-CGTCA), is produced by solid-phase phosphoramide synthesis. The oligo was designed to hybridize to the 3'-untranslated region of human ICAM-1 mRNA (Figure 10.5), thereby inhibiting protein translation (Figure 10.6b). The protein translation mechanism seems a more likely mode of drug action than an association of the oligo with the complementary DNA chains to form a triplex (Figure 10.6a), or a nonspecific binding of highly negatively charged oligo to protein products (Figure 10.6c). The disruption of protein synthesis probably results from the formation of a two-chain oligo-mRNA complex (Figure 10.6b), the presence of which in the cytoplasm provokes the action of

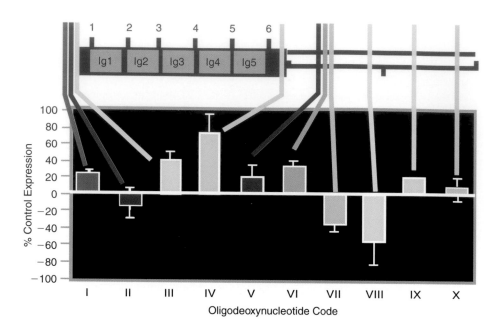

Figure 10.5. Effect of various oligo sequences to dampen upregulated ICAM-1 expression in vitro. Oligonucleotides (I-X) hybridize with specific mRNA sequences on either side of the protein coding region (shown in brown) based on the 5-Ig-like domains. Each oligo was tested by in vitro pre-exposure to endothelial cells to dampen the effect of TNF-α to upregulate ICAM-1. Oligo VIII (ISIS 3082) displayed the greatest inhibitory effect.

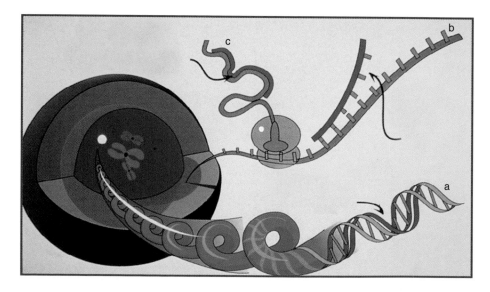

Figure 10.6. Potential mechanisms of oligo inhibition of protein synthesis. Mechanism (a) anti-ICAM-1 oligo forms a DNA triplex. Mechanism (b) anti-ICAM-1 oligo binds to mRNA. Mechanism (c) anti-ICAM-1 oligo complexes with protein. The oligo is indicated as the red band.

RNase H that cleaves the specific mRNA and selectively prevents protein translation of the ICAM-1 message.

Administration of anti-ICAM-1 oligos has been shown to produce beneficial effects in transplant models. Whether the anti-ICAM-1 oligo is delivered solely pretransplant to the donor (Figure 10.7a), directly into the allograft, or exclusively posttransplant to the recipient (Figure 10.7b), kidney allograft rejection is significantly delayed in rats (Stepkowski et al 1998b; Chen et al 1999). Another antisense ICAM-1 oligo has been shown to attenuate reperfusion injury and progression to renal failure after either in situ ischemia (Haller et al 1996) or isograft transplantation in rats (Dragun et al 1998).

ISIS 2302 is undergoing phase II clinical trials at The University of Texas at Houston to determine whether it promotes more rapid return of graft function and/or enhances acute rejection prophylaxis among cadaveric kidney transplant recipients. The study was initiated after a phase I trial in which ISIS 2302 was administered to stable transplant recipients revealed that the adverse effects of the oligo were mild, namely, prolongation of the partial thromboplastin time, modest activation of complement component C3a, and a trend toward a decrease in the platelet count (Lappin et al

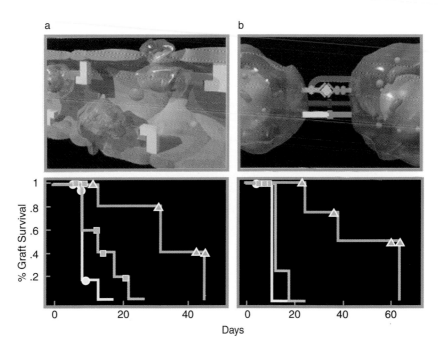

Figure 10.7. Potential therapeutic actions of anti-ICAM-1 antisense oligos. (a) Mitigation of the ischemic injury, shown diagrammatically as endothelial ICAM-1 (yellow) and lymphocyte LFA-1 (blue). (b) Disruption of alloactivation, shown diagrammatically as LFA-1 (blue) on lymphocytes linking ICAM-1 (yellow) on APCs. The bottom panels show the prolongation of graft survival with the antisense molecule (green line), compared to the sense molecule (same sequence as the native mRNA), and unable to hybridize (pink line), and no treatment (yellow line). In (a) treatment was given only to the donor; in (b) only to the recipient.

1998). Indeed, the phase I trial, in which oligo was added to a baseline regimen of CsA-Pred in renal transplant recipients, revealed an adverse event profile that was more modest than that previously observed in normal volunteers (Glover et al 1997).

Although clinical trials are under way, two major concerns may limit the use of ISIS 2302. First, anti-ICAM-1 oligos only block critical steps in the activation of lymphocytes. Thus, treatment with a VCAM-1 antisense oligo may be necessary to interrupt adhesion of granulocytes. Indeed, a combination of oligos might enhance the therapeutic effect by blocking the critical ligands of firm adhesion for both granulocytes and lymphocytes. Second, the high negative charge of oligos may restrict their penetration into cells. Strategies to address this shortcoming include novel delivery systems or the development of structural analogs with a lower negative charge. In experimental animals, the former approach has used liposomes bearing encapsulated oligos (Haller et al 1996); however, because of their lipid components, liposomes may be diverted from their endothelial target by a higher uptake in phagocytes. The latter shortcoming is being addressed with the less highly charged peptidic or methoxy-, rather than phosphorothioate, derivatives. Another alternate delivery system is ex vivo transfection. Cardiac allografts incubated with an anti-ICAM-1 antisense oligonucleotide under 3 atm pressure showed nuclear incorporation of the oligo, with consequent reduction in the expression of ICAM-1, as well as moderate immunosuppressive effects, when used in combination with anti-LFA-1 MAb, but not when administered alone or in combination with SRL (Poston et al 1999).

Indeed, it is likely that combination strategies will be necessary to obtain therapeutic benefits with anti-ICAM-1 oligos. Combinations with anti-LFA-1 MAbs and/or with L-selectin blockade are likely to be required, since double-deficient knockout mice for ICAM-1 and selectin markers showed a synergistic effect to vitiate leukocyte rolling and entry into tissues (Steeber et al 1999). Similarly, Räisänen-Sokolowski et al (1999) found that the combination of ICAM-1 and P-selectin knockouts of the donor organ (but not the recipient) prevented the development of acute rejection, but not of the long-term arteriosclerotic changes in transplants.

Integrin inhibitors

Therapeutic approach: FTY720

FTY720 (2-amino-2 [2-4-{-octylphenyl) ethyl}-1,3-propanediol hydrochloride, $C_{19}H_{33}NO_2 \times HCl$; MW 343.94; Yoshitomi, Osaka, Japan, now licensed to Novartis, Basle, Switzerland) is a synthetic analog of the sphingosine-like compound Myriocin (ISP-1), which is produced by the ascomycete *Isaria sinclairii* (Figure 10.8a). The mechanism of FTY720 drug action is not understood. Suzuki et al (1996b) initially observed that FTY720 treatment profoundly decreased the number of peripheral blood lymphocytes, but affected neither granulocytes nor monocytes (Figure 10.9). He proposed that lymphocyte depletion owed to an effect of FTY720 to induce lymphocyte apoptosis (Wang et al 1992; Shimizu et al 1998): in vitro addition of the drug to cell

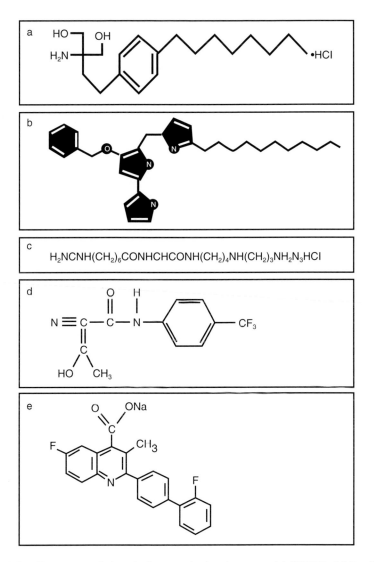

Figure 10.8. Structures of chemical agents in development. (a) FTY720. (b) Prodigiosin-156804. (c) 15-Deoxyspergualin. (d) Leflunomide active component A77 1726. (e) Brequinar.

cultures caused DNA fragmentation, as evidenced by a ladder pattern of nucleic acid fragments in agarose gel analyses of extracts from treated cells. In addition, Suzuki et al (1997) observed that in vivo administration of FTY720 (1 mg/kg per day) decreased the cellularity of the otherwise hyperplastic spleen and lymph nodes from, as well as reduced the content of the antiapoptotic factor Bcl-2 in lpr mice, which are bred to spontaneously develop autoimmune disease.

437

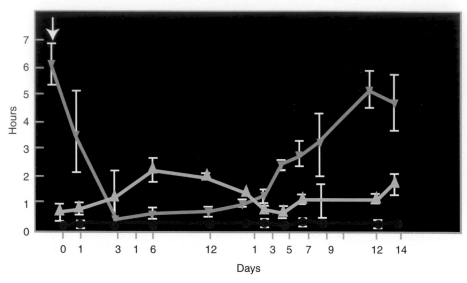

Figure 10.9. Effect of oral gavage of FTY720 (10 mg/kg) on numbers of circulating lymphocytes. After drug administration (as denoted by the arrow), numbers of cells at serial hours/days are counted, including lymphocytes (orange line), neutrophils (green line), and monocytes (red line). (Suzuki S, Enosawa S, Kakefuda T et al. A novel immunosuppressant, FTY720, with a unique mechanism of action, induces long-term graft acceptance in rat and dog allotransplantation. *Transplantation* 1996; **61**:200–205. © Lippincott Williams & Wilkins. All rights reserved.)

One possible mechanism of drug-induced apoptosis is inhibited conversion to sphingosine of ceramide, an antimitogenic, proapoptotic, intracellular lipid intermediate (Flores et al 1998). However, two pieces of evidence refute the role of ceramide in FTY720-induced apoptosis: first, ceramide tends to induce changes that occur well after exposure, whereas the drug produces immediate effects; second, FTY720-sensitive Jurkat cells do not undergo apoptosis upon treatment with the membrane permeable analog C2-ceramide. Another possible molecular target of FTY720 is phospholipase C, which mediates Ca^{2+} release, activates Ca^{2+}-dependent endonucleases and Ca^{2+}-activated proteinases, as well as causes damage to mitochondria. On the one hand, FTY720-induced apoptosis requires the activation of the ERK cascade (Matsuda et al 1999), but is independent of the Fas pathway. On the other hand, the apoptotic event was unaffected by pertussis toxin, leading Shinomiya et al (1997) to conclude that it was not dependent upon G-protein activation. To explain the apoptotic effect, one might postulate that FTY720 directly activates caspase 3, c-Jun NH_2 terminal kinase, and/or p38 CSAID-binding protein.

However, two pieces of evidence refute the hypothesis that the primary mechanism of FTY720 action is to induce apoptosis. First, drug treatment does not delete donor-specific lymphocyte clones. Limiting dilution analysis revealed a frequency of activated specific antidonor cytotoxic elements among the lymph node and spleen cells of FTY720-treated, transplanted hosts similar to that found in rejecting hosts. Second, FTY720 treatment at the time of a repeat transplant neither produces clonal stripping of donor-reactive cells nor disrupts the rapid progression of accelerated rejection (SM Stepkowski, unpublished work).

An alternate proposal to explain the mechanism of drug action is that FTY720 alters lymphocyte recirculation and homing, thereby diverting cells away from the graft, particularly into mesenteric lymph nodes and Peyer's patches (Chiba et al 1998). This hypothesis postulates that FTY720 alters the normal pattern of lymphocyte trafficking, possibly via blunted stimulation of chemokine release by the tissues or, more likely, by modifying chemokine reception that rapidly upregulates integrin expression or the reception of humoral signals necessary for the adhesion and arrest of lymphocytes on graft endothelium. For example, FTY720 seems to induce upregulated function of human $\alpha_4\beta_7$ glycoprotein homing receptors (Jalkanen et al 1987), which direct lymphocytes to adhere to the gastrointestinal MadCAM-1, as well as to glyCAM-1 addressins on endothelial cells, particularly in the lamina propria, Peyer's patches, and mesenteric lymph nodes (Berlin et al 1993, 1995). This hypothesis is consistent with the findings of Kantele et al (1999): adoptive transfer of lymphocytes from hosts immunized via the oral route into syngeneic hosts results in their preferential return to Peyer's patches. In contrast, upregulated L-selectin expression directs cells to peripheral lymph nodes (Steeber et al 1996), and cutaneous lymphocyte antigen, to the skin (Picker et al 1991). Thus, FTY720 may impose the chemokine receptor and integrin characteristics and/or responses of cells homing to lymphoid structures upon at least 80% of the peripheral blood lymphocyte population.

The possibility that FTY720 alters the generation of the T-cell chemokines is unlikely. Lymphocytes harvested from FTY720-treated donors and labeled with a fluorescent marker show homing patterns to Peyer's patches and mesenteric lymph nodes, whether they are transferred into untreated secondary hosts or treated primary hosts, suggesting that the drug acts primarily on the circulating cells (K Yuzawa and SM Stepkowski, unpublished work). Thus, FTY720 may either induce upregulated expression/activity of chemokine receptor 7 or of $\alpha_4\beta_7$ on, or, alternatively, inhibit the reception by/response to chemokines by lymphocytes. In contradistinction to the findings of Shinomiya et al (1997), Brinkmann et al (1999) observed that FTY720 blocked the function of G protein-coupled lymphocyte receptors that mediate integrin aggregation and cytoskeletal interactions.

A third possible mechanism of action is an effect of FTY720 to interrupt sphingolipid cascades necessary for early activation events in integrin signal transduction. For example, inhibited sphingosine generation may prevent Ca^{2+} release from intracellular stores independent of inositol 1,4,5-triphosphate production (Fatatis and Miller 1999); this effect would complement the immunosuppressive action of CsA. Further, FTY720-mediated inhibition of downstream integrin signaling, namely, activation of the mitogen-activated protein kinase (MAPK) c-Jun NH_2-terminal kinase (JNK) and regulation of the activities of cyclin-dependent kinases (cdk 4/6 and cdk 2), would be predicted to be enhanced by SRL, since the mammalian target of rapamycin (mTOR) is critical for cell cycle progression through G_1.

In animal transplant models, FTY720 prolongs renal allograft survival (Kawaguchi et al 1996; Suzuki et al 1996a, b) and reduces the numbers of animals undergoing acute

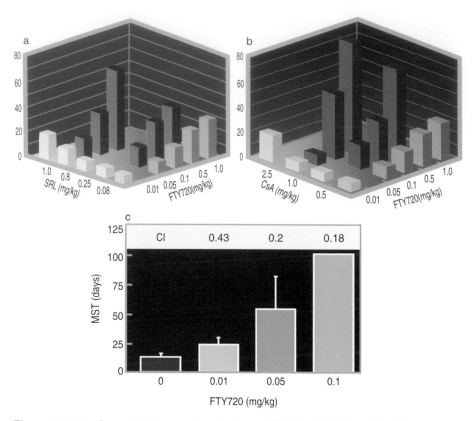

Figure 10.10. Synergistic interactions between FTY720 with CsA and/or SRL. (a) Interaction between SRL alone (yellow) and FTY720 alone (orange) versus the combination (red). (b) CsA (yellow) and FTY720 (pink) versus the combination (red). (c) Impact on mean survival time (MST, days) of addition of increasing amounts of FTY720 (x-axis) to a fixed dose combination of CsA (0.5 mg/kg per day) and SRL (0.08 mg/kg per day). CI = combination index; CI values <1.0 denote a synergistic interaction. (Modified from Wang ME, Tejpal N, Qy X et al. Immunosuppressive effects of FTY720 alone or in combination with cyclosporine or sirolimus. *Transplantation* 1998; **65**:899–905. © 1998 Lippincott Williams & Wilkins. All rights reserved.)

rejection episodes (Yuzawa et al 1998) with 10- to 100-fold greater potency than CsA (Suzuki et al 1996a; Yanagawa et al 1998). FTY720 acts synergistically with CsA and/or SRL in rodent models (Wang et al 1998), and displays at least an additive interaction with CsA in canine (Kawaguchi et al 1996; Suzuki et al 1997) and in subhuman primate transplant models (Troncoso et al 1999). Figure 10.10 shows that the interactions of FTY720 with CsA and/or SRL in the rat heterotopic cardiac model displayed combination index (CI) values less than 1.0, indicating synergism (Wang et al 1998).

In the first human study, 32 adult patients treated with CsA and Pred to maintain renal transplants in a quiescent state received a single dose (0.25–3.5 mg) of either placebo or FTY720 (Brunkhorst et al 1999). As in animal models, the drug caused a dose-dependent, rapidly reversible fall in the peripheral blood lymphocyte count: the nadir occurred at approximately 6–12 hours, recovering to the normal range by 48–72 hours. Lymphocyte counts decreased to a mean of 27% of the baseline value among patients in the 3.5 mg dose group. Although no serious adverse events were reported, bradycardia occurred in the seven patients whose heart rates were no more than 60 beats/min prior to FTY720 dosing, as well as in three other subjects. In addition to this potential side-effect, patients in the current multiple-dose phase I study are being carefully monitored for exercise-induced hypoxia, since subhuman primates showed evidence of pulmonary diffusion defects. To date, the 22 Houston patients who have been entered into a phase I multiple-dose, ascending-exposure study using a 1-month treatment schedule have not experienced serious adverse events. A multicenter trial incorporating FTY720 into de novo immunosuppressive regimens has already begun in the year 2000.

Disruption of cytokines: soluble tumor necrosis factor receptor

Soluble TNF receptor (Etanercept, Enbrel, Immunex, Seattle, WA, USA) is a conjugate of a dimer of the p75 TNF-α receptor and the Fc portion of IgG_1. The fusion peptide acts by antagonizing the effects of TNF-α, a cytokine produced by lymphocytes that augments the cytotoxic effects of macrophages and polymorphonuclear leukocytes, and regulates the production of other cytokines. TNF-α not only participates in the systemic inflammatory responses occurring during the effector phase of allograft rejection, but also in the cytokine release syndrome in response to OKT3 administration. The primary path of drug development and the US Food and Drug Administration (FDA)-approved indication for treatment with the soluble receptor is moderate-to-severe rheumatoid arthritis among patients unresponsive to other modalities (Moreland et al 1997). However, the agent also has been tested in renal allograft recipients undergoing treatment of a moderate-to-severe acute rejection episode. The trial sought to establish whether administration of the soluble receptor would modify the cytokine release syndrome induced by administration of OKT3. Unfortunately, none of the doses (0.05–0.75 mg/kg per day) significantly decreased TNF-α responses or mitigated the symptoms of the cytokine release syndrome (Wee et al 1997). However, the reagent has not been tested in the ischemia–reperfusion syndrome, in which TNF-α has been shown to adversely affect allografts by upregulating the expression of VCAM-1 and ICAM-1. Since the agent neither causes dose-limiting adverse events nor stimulates the production of neutralizing antibodies, it should be further explored in transplant settings. Although it works in a fashion that theoretically might complement the action of CsA, the combination of the dimeric TNF-αβ receptor and CsA showed little benefit to prolong renal graft survival beyond that achieved with CsA alone (Eason et al 1995). Interestingly, the soluble TNF-α receptor has been reported to dampen the development of intimal thickening in heterotopic hearts transplanted into rabbit hosts fed a high-cholesterol diet (Molossi et al 1994).

CYTOKINE PARADIGM

Pathophysiologic mechanisms

Strategies to intervene in the cytokine paradigm seek to disrupt events that trigger cytokine production, reception, and signal transduction processes necessary for T and B cell activation (Figure 10.11). These strategies are summarized in Figure 10.12 as the cytokine paradigm. Inhibited generation of the first antigen-driven signal might be obtained by utilizing MAb reagents directed toward common antigenic markers on class I (or class II) MHC antigens to block APC functions, or MAbs reactive with T-cell receptors (TCR). Although Smith et al (1997) reported that administration of recipient-specific anti-MHC class II antibody—the first strategy—did prolong the survival of murine vascularized heart grafts, this approach has not yet been developed for clinical trials.

Investigators have made considerably more progress toward the development of reagents that target the TCR. Isoimmunization of rodents by administration of T cells bearing specific anti-donor TCR yielded MAbs that, upon passive transfer to syngeneic hosts, produced indefinite graft survival. Since clinical application of this principle would demand an array of specific anti-TCR reagents from which the physician would select the one reactive toward the donor-type antigen binding site ('idiotype'), the only feasible approach in the clinic is to produce specific MAbs directed against antigenic determinants common to *all* human TCRs. The alternate approach to more effectively

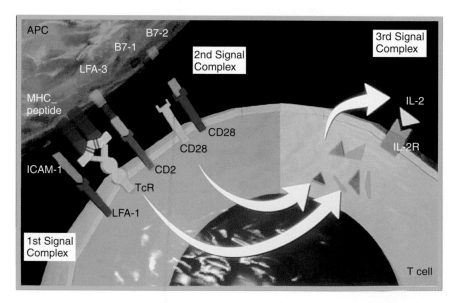

Figure 10.11. Three signals of the T cell response. Signal one (red) is delivered by the MHC–peptide–TCR complex with coreceptor pairs ICAM-1/LFA-1 and LFA-3/CD2; Signal two (orange), B7–1/B7–2 with CD28; Signal three (green), cytokine/cytokine receptor.

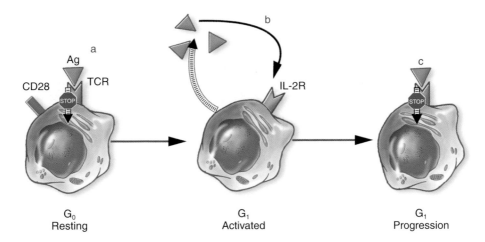

Figure 10.12. The cytokine paradigm showing potential sites of disruption of T-cell maturation events. (a) Signal one/two events; blockade of transcriptional activation of gene expression that leads to cytokine synthesis. (b) Blockade of cytokine receptors. (c) Interruption of signal transduction events after cytokine triggering.

disrupt the CD3 transduction of the TCR signal is to utilize humanized variants of the Orthoclone (OKT3; Ortho Pharmaceutical Corp., Raritan, NJ, USA) MAbs in an attempt to mitigate the cytokine release syndrome.

Both the immunosuppressive effects and the drug-induced toxicities of CsA and TRL seem to result from inhibition of the activity of the CaN target, rather than the formation of complexes with peptidyl prolyl isomerase immunophilins (Sigal et al 1991; Figure 10.13). The therapeutic challenge is to produce an inhibitor selective preferably for the CaN, or possibly for the peptidyl prolyl, isoforms characteristic of lymphocytes, as opposed to endothelial, neural, or other cell types.

The costimulatory signal that promotes cytokine synthesis frequently utilizes members of the NF-κB family, which are critical regulators of DNA transcription leading to the synthesis of the proinflammatory factors, including the cytokines TNF-α, IL-6, IL-8, MHC class II antigens, ICAM-1, inducible nitric oxide synthase, and cyclo-oxygenase-2 (COX-2). NF-κB transcriptional factors are homodimers or heterodimers of Rel proteins. In resting cells, these molecules interact with and are bound to the proteins of the IκB family. A 300-amino acid homology region on c-Rel proteins binds to multiple ankyrin repeat sequences on IκB molecules, thereby masking the NF-κB nuclear localization signal. The inhibited NF-κB/IκB dimers are sequestered in the cytoplasm. Delivery of costimulatory signals for example, via the p55 or p75 components of IL-1 or TNF-α surface receptors or via CD28, activates phospholipidases type A_2 and C (including the phosphatidyl-choline type), sphingomyelinase, protein kinase Cζ, ceramide-activated protein kinase, and MAPK. The downstream consequence of these events is to trigger activation of NIK (NF-κB, inducing kinase) and Akt/protein kinase β (Ozes et al 1999), which upregulate α and β IκB kinases (IKKs),

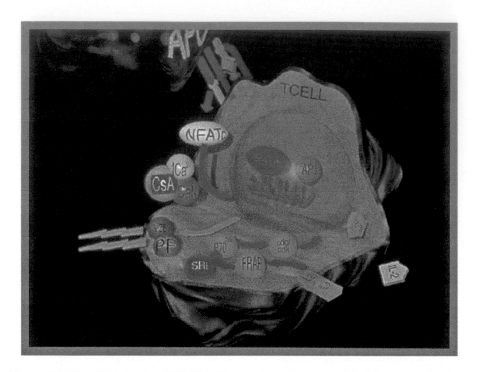

Figure 10.13. Critical role of NF-AT (yellow oval) as the target of CsA (orange sphere) inhibition in the signal one pathway to cytokine synthesis. In addition, the figure shows the action of sirolimus (SRL) to inhibit FK-rapamycin-associated protein (FRAP), also known as mammalian target of rapamycin (mTOR).

possibly by promoting linkage of a third peptide, IKKγ. The kinases phosphorylate two specific serine residues in the N-terminal region of IκB, permitting the heterodimerization necessary for ubiquination and proteolysis of the substrate in the 26S proteasome, thereby releasing NF-κB for translocation to the nucleus.

An alternate strategy to the use of MAbs to disrupt binding of IL-2 (Figure 10.12) is to target early receptor-linked events. In contrast to the CD25 target, which is exclusive for IL-2Rα, one approach targets the γ-chain, which is common to all cytokine receptors of the IL-2 family: namely, IL-2, IL-4, IL-7, IL-9, and IL-15. In humans, mutations of the γ-chain result in severe, combined immunodeficiency (Leonard 1996), particularly impeding the development of CD8$^+$ T cells. The selective targeting of upstream events differs from the inhibition by SRL of downstream cascades common to lymphoid and hematologic/vascular growth factor receptors (Figure 10.14), an effect that may be responsible for the toxic side-effects of SRL. T-cell activation via the IL-2Rγ chain depends upon phosphorylation of JAK3, a tyrosine kinase that is predominantly expressed in leukocytes, including monocytes as well as T, B, and natural killer (NK) cells. JAK3 activity is required for cell development and function (Thomis and Berg 1997); mutations that interrupt JAK3 functions cause a severe combined immunodefi-

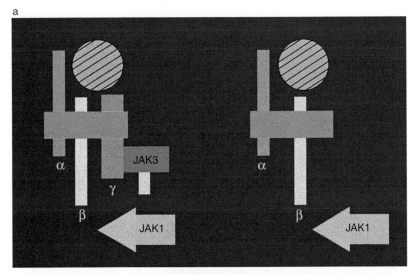

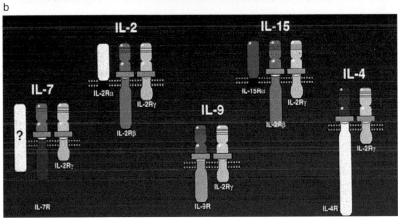

Figure 10.14. (a) Two families of receptors for cytokines. On the left is the lymphoid IL-2 type; on the right, the vascular-hematologic cytokines, namely, IL-6, IL-11, granulocyte-monocyte colony stimulating factor, erythropoietin, basic fibroblast growth factor, and vascular endothelial growth factor. The latter group do not contain the receptor γ-chain or the linkage to JAK3 as does the IL-2 family (left). (b) IL-2 family of receptors, namely, for IL-2, -4, -7, -9, and -15, all of which share the γ-chain and the transduction element JAK3. (Sugamura K, Asao H, Kondo M et al. The interleukin-2 receptor gamma chain: its role in the multiple cytokine receptor complexes and T cell development in XSCID. *Annu Rev Immunol* 1996; **14**:179–205. © 1996 Annual Reviews. Reprinted with permission.)

ciency (Macchi et al 1995). A major action of JAK3 is to phosphorylate specific tyrosine residues in the β-chain of the IL-2R, and in Stat5a and Stat5b (Figure 10.15); the latter effects (in conjunction with serine phosphorylation by MAPK) are necessary for nuclear localization of the Stat transcription factors.

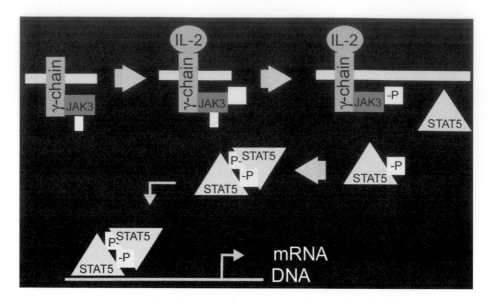

Figure 10.15. The γ-chain transduction pathway. Upon activation, JAK3 is phosphorylated, leading to association and phosphorylation of Stat5, which then dimerizes and enters the nucleus as a regulatory protein for gene transcription.

Therapeutic approaches: antigen signal reception (Figure 10.12)

Anti-T cell receptor MAbs: T10B9

T10B9, a murine IgM antihuman α/β T-cell receptor MAb directed against a common determinant, was developed by John Thompson and licensed by MedImmune (Gaithersburg, MD, USA). Thompson reported five mechanisms of T10B9 action: modulation of the expression of the α/β TCR/CD3 complex, induction of apoptosis; stimulation of IL-10 release; inhibition of IL-2 generation; and synergy with CNAs. Two 4-year, blinded phase II clinical trials demonstrated that administration of T10B9 (6 mg twice daily) did not elicit the cytokine release syndrome. However, T10B9 was as effective as OKT3 both to prevent and to reverse acute allograft rejection episodes in both renal (Waid et al 1997a) and cardiac (Waid et al 1997b) transplant recipients. Despite these promising results, MedImmune is not proceeding with the clinical development of T10B9.

Anti-T cell receptor MAbs: BMA 031

BMA 031 is an IgG$_{2b}$ mouse antihuman α/β TCR MAb (Behring, Marburg, Germany) that was initially shown in anecdotal reports to inhibit alloactivation processes in patients at high risk for allograft rejection (Hillebrand et al 1989; Chatenoud et al 1990; Dendorfer et al 1990; Smely et al 1990). A randomized, blinded phase II study conducted at The University of Texas at Houston (Knight et al 1994) utilized peripheral intravenous injections of 50 mg BMA 031 MAb before as well as on days 2 and 4 after transplantation. Owing to its IgG_{2b} isotype, administration of BMA 031 was not associated with the cytokine release syndrome. The antibody reduced peripheral T cell numbers to less than 10% of baseline at 7–14 days and delayed the onset (but did not reduce the incidence) of acute rejection episodes. However, administration was not-infrequently accompanied by production of human antimouse antibodies (HAMA), which limited therapeutic efficacy. Behring is not currently exploring the use of this reagent in transplantation.

Humanized anti-CD3 MAbs

To overcome the cytokine release syndrome—the major limitation of Orthoclone (OKT3, Ortho, Raritan, NJ, USA)—a genetically engineered human IgG_1 MAb was engrafted with the six complementarity-determining regions from the mouse OKT3 MAb molecule. In a phase I pilot study using 5 or 10 mg doses, Woodle et al (1999) reported reversal of first acute rejection episodes among five out of seven kidney or simultaneous kidney–pancreas transplant recipients. The reagent elicited neither the cytokine release syndrome nor xenoantibody production. In contradistinction to the modulation mechanism of OKT3 action, the humanized form may act as an altered ligand, which fails to deliver a full TCR signal and thus induces only low levels of ZAP70 phosphorylation (Smith et al 1998).

Another humanized anti-CD3 MAb utilizes an IgG_2 antibody backbone, bearing mutations in the upper CH_2 region of the Fc domain (Hsu et al 1999). These manipulations reduced the affinity of the molecule for Fc receptors, as well as mitigated its capacity to trigger cytokine release or to stimulate lymphocyte proliferation in chimpanzee hosts. After the last of three 10-mg injections, the antibody depleted $CD2^+$ and $CD3^+$ T cells for 10 days. A phase I trial confirmed that the MAb did not evoke the cytokine release syndrome. Although these modifications are undoubtedly useful to improve their tolerability, future commercial development of anti-CD3 MAbs may be imperiled due to the markedly reduced rate of acute allograft rejection episodes presently observed under immunosuppressive drug maintenance regimens including CsA, TRL, MMF, and/or SRL.

Therapeutic approaches: inhibitors of T cell activation/cytokine synthesis

In two companion papers, Peterson et al (1998) and Dumont et al (1998) reported the properties of a TRL analog, indolyl-ascomycin (IAC), bearing a hydroxyethyl indole moiety at the C32 position of the macrocyclic lactone structure. On the one hand, IAC displayed a 10-fold-lower rate of association with FK-binding proteins (FKBPs); on the other hand, the FKBP-IAC heterodimers displayed a greater stability of their pentameric complexes with CaN, owing to the additional contact point on IAC. The authors suggested that the reduced binding to FKBP-12 might selectively mitigate drug-induced toxicity in tissues with a low ratio of FKBP-12 to CaN, such as brain and kidney. Although the authors observed a two-fold-reduced nephrotoxicity of IAC compared with TRL, human trials will be necessary to assess the clinical applicability of this analog.

A second strategy to enhance the tissue specificity of CNAs might utilize molecular modeling based upon possible structural differences between isoforms of either the immunophilin or CaN expressed in nonimmune versus T or B cells. Thus, molecules are being designed to associate with a specific CaN target isoform, based upon rational synthesis using crystallographic measurements.

A third and potentially exciting strategy was reported by Aramburu et al (1999), who designed a peptide inhibitor (MAGPHPVIVITGPHEE) that competes 25-fold more avidly than the natural NF-AT for association with the CaN site (Figure 10.13). Because CsA inhibits the dephosphorylation of the model peptide in the same fashion that it blocks the dephosphorylation of NF-AT, both processes are likely to reflect inhibition at close if not identical sites on CaN. Furthermore, in vitro experiments documented that the model peptide selectively inhibited the NF-AT-dependent, inducible expression of IL-2, IL-3, IL-13, TNF-α, GM-CSF, and MIP-1α. In contrast, the model peptide had no effects on CaN-mediated events that were independent of the participation of NF-AT, namely, generation of NF-κB, TNF-β, or lymphotoxin-β. The availability of this peptide, which has not yet been tested in vivo, may proffer the opportunity not only to determine whether CaN substrates other than NF-AT mediate CsA- and TRL-induced drug toxicities, but also to develop a new battery of selective agents.

Therapeutic approaches: inhibitors of NF-κB

A variety of compounds inhibit TNF-α upregulation of NF-κB and of ICAM-1 expression. The binding of cytosolic phospholipidase A_2 (PLA$_2$) to arachidonic acid is prevented by two substances: the trifluoromethyl ketone analog of arachidonic acid, and the methyl-arachidonyl fluorophosphate. The release of arachidonic acid—an action that is necessary but not sufficient to produce the response to TGF-α—is prevented by two other drugs: the lysine-modified 12-epi-scalaradial, and the active site inhibitor LY311727r, an analog of indomethacin that does not inhibit COX (Thommesen et al 1998). Curcumin, a spice that is the major constituent of tumeric powder, a traditional medicine for inflammatory disorders, may block NF-κB by inhibiting the signal leading to IKK activation, without interfering with IKK or NIK activities in intestinal epithelial cell cultures (Jobin et al 1999).

Of considerable interest is the report by Lai et al (1999) that a bisbenzylin/quinolone alkaloid tetrandrine, purified from a tuberous root, and particularly its analog, dauricine, inhibit the CD3 or PMA plus anti-CD28-stimulated lymphoproliferation and cytokine generation, a CsA-resistant pathway utilized by both CD4$^+$ and CD8$^+$ cells. The authors suggest that the agent acts to inhibit the protein kinase (Ho et al 1999), but not the calcium-dependent, pathway. They observed that the immunosuppressive effect of tetrandrine was synergistic with that of CsA.

Deoxyspergualin (15-DSG, Gusperimus, Behring, Marburg, Germany; Figure 10.8c) is a derivative of spergualin that blocks T- and B-cell maturation. This action is attributed at least in part to inhibition of IL-1 synthesis and consequent disruption of costimulation (Yuh and Morris 1993). The agent not only prevents acute rejection (Yuh and Morris 1993), but also prolongs the survival of xenografts (Marchman et al 1992). In clinical trials, 15-DSG reversed both early (Okubo et al 1993) and late (Amada et al 1998) acute rejection episodes, particularly when used in combination with high doses of corticosteroids. However, because it must be administered parenterally and because of its severe myelosuppressive properties, 15-DSG is unlikely to become a major component of immunosuppressive regimens. Although intraperitoneal administration of Tresperimus (Group Fournier, Paris, France), an analog of 15-DSG, was shown to prolong rat cardiac allograft survival (Dutartre et al 1995), the drug is primarily under development to attenuate graft-versus-host disease (Annat et al 1996).

Therapeutic approaches: enhanced production of natural immunosuppressive cytokines

Adenoviral gene transfer of viral IL-10, a 35-kD homodimeric product of Th_2 cells, B cells, and macrophages, produces anti-inflammatory, immunosuppressive, or immunostimulatory effects, depending upon the target cell. The immunosuppressive effects are due primarily to dampened APC functions, including downregulated expression of MHC class II molecules, as well as of B7–1 and B7–2 (Willems et al 1994). Although IL-10 enhances humoral immunity, an action that may contravene its use as an immunosuppressant in humans, retroviral-mediated transfer of IL-10 in a murine model prolonged cardiac graft survival (Qin et al 1996). Clinical trials utilizing transfected cells have not yet been initiated in transplantation.

Therapeutic approaches: inhibitors of cytokine reception—IL-2 antagonists

Compared with the natural IL-2 ligand, the two available anti-IL-2R MAbs—daclizumab and basiliximab—display relatively low affinity and are therefore relatively weak competitors for binding to IL-2R. Two new chimeric reagents bind to IL-2R with similar affinities as the IL-2 ligand: an IL-2-diphtheria toxin-related fusion protein (Penkewycz et al 1989), and an IL-2/Fc fusion protein (Zheng et al 1999). The latter fusion protein bears an amino acid sequence of the CH_1 portion of the human Fc region that has been mutated to render it unable to mediate either antibody-dependent cell-mediated or complement-dependent cytotoxicity. Furthermore, the IL-2/Fc fusion protein overcomes the limitations of the toxin conjugate: namely, the high immunogenicity, short half-life, and lower relative affinity to IL-2R of the toxin. These reagents await further testing in primates prior to clinical study.

Therapeutic approaches: inhibitors of lymphokine signal transduction

Anti-γ-chain strategies: MAbs

Dai et al (1999) observed that blockade of the γ-chain by MAbs increased the proportion of apoptotic cells, a finding consistent with the decreased content of Bcl-2 previously observed in γ-chain knockout mice. Although anti-γ-chain MAbs tend to display a low potency, administration to mice was shown to prolong the survival of pancreatic islet grafts, one of the most vulnerable immunologic targets.

Anti-γ-chain strategies: JAK3 inhibitors

The JAK3 inhibitor AG490 (Calbiochem, San Diego, CA, USA) blocks both Stat5 phosphorylation and the Shc/Ras/Raf MAPK cascade, without inhibiting the other tyrosine kinases, Lck, Lyn, Btk, Syk, Src, JAK1, or Tyk2 (Wang et al 1999a). AG490 has been shown to inhibit the growth of mycosis fungoides cells (Nielsen et al 1997) and to prevent experimental allergic encephalomyelitis (Bright et al 1999). In transplant models, AG490 prolongs allograft survival in a fashion that is synergistic with CsA (Kirken et al 1999).

A structural analog of a natural product of *Serratia marcescens,* the JAK3 inhibitor Prodigiosin 156804 (4-benzyloxy-5-[(5-undecyl-2H-pyrrol-2-ylidene)methyl]-2,2′-bi-1H pyrrole, hydrochloride; Pharmacia-Upjohn; Madison, NJ, USA; Figure 10.8b) is five times more potent than AG490. Prodigiosin 156804 selectively inhibits the kinase activity of JAK3, more selectively than JAK1 or JAK2. This blockade of JAK3 interrupts lymphocyte development in the mid-G_1 phase, and may also dampen NF-κB and AP-1 generation, both of which are required for cell proliferation in response to IL-2 (Mortellaro et al 1999). The drug may also inhibit CD40 crosslinking in B cells, thereby preventing the degradation of IκB-α and -β that is required for NF-κB generation. However, Prodigiosin 156804 does not inhibit c-myc or Bcl-2 mRNA induction (Mortellaro et al 1999). When administered intravenously on an alternate-day schedule, the agent produces modest prolongation of allograft survival; when used in conjunction with CsA, it shows a synergistic interaction (Wang et al 1999b).

CORECEPTOR PARADIGM

Pathophysiologic mechanisms

Because the affinity of TCRs for the peptide/MHC-APC unit is relatively low, effective TCR recognition depends upon the formation of an immunologic synapse—the signal one complex—including also the interactions of multiple coreceptors, adhesion, and/or costimulatory molecules (Grakoui et al 1999; Malissen 1999). These coreceptor interactions determine whether the TCR peptide encounter triggers an aggression versus an acceptance alloimmune response. For example, blockade of the CD28/B7 costimulation pair seems to promote and, contrariwise of the ICAM-1/LFA-1 coreceptor complexes, to inhibit Th_2 cell development (Salomon and Bluestone 1998).

In addition to their role as adhesion molecules (as discussed above in 'Ischemia–reperfusion–migration paradigm'), the ICAM-1/LFA-1 coreceptor pair provides a costimulatory signal that activates T cells. T cell reception of the antigen signal produces conformational changes in LFA-1, resulting in its signal-dependent release from other noncovalent attractions and association thereafter with the cytoskeleton, two events that increase the avidity of LFA-1 for ICAM-1 (Van Seventer et al 1992; Lollo et al 1993). The amplified engagement of this ligand pair augments the TCR signal, thus facilitating the generation of T cell killing, particularly by $CD8^+$ cells; the induction of some Th, B, and NK cell responses; and the mediation of antibody-dependent, cell-mediated cytotoxicity. In addition, LFA-1 generates transmembrane signals (Kanner et al 1993; Arroyo et al 1994) that increase the cytosolic content of Ca^{2+}, prolong the phosphorylation of phospholipase $C\gamma_1$, and upregulate the activities of acidic sphingomyelinase and JNK, thereby generating NF-κB, phosphoinositol-3-kinase, as well as a possibly unique pattern of tyrosine phosphorylations (albeit with a decreased activity of Fyn). Although ligation of LFA-1 transiently upregulates IL-2 synthesis, it cannot replace the durable CD28 signal nor support clonal proliferation in the fashion that B7-1 ligation of CD28 promotes T-cell activation (Ni et al 1999). Indeed, in the absence of the CD28 signal, LFA-1 ligation does not upregulate Bcl expression, and lymphocytes undergo apoptosis (Zuckerman et al 1998). Thus, stimulation of $CD4^+$ cells by APC ICAM-1 alone (without B7 and/or CD40) is incomplete, resulting in tolerance induction rather than in clonal expansion (Zuckerman et al 1998).

Therapeutic approaches

Anti-CD4

Based upon the results of rodent transplantation experiments (Yin et al 1998a), anti-CD4 MAbs seem to proffer more potent immunosuppressive reagents than anti-CD8 MAbs. Prixilimab (Centara; Centocor; Malvern, PA, USA) is a chimeric anti-CD4 MAb constructed from the antigen-binding variable region of the murine antibody M-T412 and the constant region of human IgG_1 κ immunoglobulin. Priliximab (at doses of 50 or 100 mg/day but not 10 mg/day) almost completely coats CD4 sites on helper T cells (Van der Lubbe et al 1994). Although chills and fever were not-infrequently encountered, heart transplant patients receiving the anti-CD4 MAb experienced a lower incidence of acute rejection episodes and better tolerability than those treated with antithymocyte globulin (Meiser et al 1994). Another murine anti-CD4 MAb (Ortho) was employed by Norman et al (1993) for induction treatment of renal transplant patients; the more severe clinical side-effect profile observed in this cohort compared with recipients treated with OKT3 led to its recent modification as a humanized MAb, which should be suitable for clinical trials. An alternate approach to block the CD4 marker might utilize a synthetic CD4 antagonist that blocks the homologous epitope from binding to the α_3 receptor region of class II MHC molecules, thus interfering with full immune activation.

Anti-CD2

The pan T-cell marker CD2, which is also present on NK cells, binds to APC markers (Boussiotis et al 1994). Transplantation tolerance has been induced in mice treated with a combination of MAbs directed toward CD2 and MAbs directed against CD3 (Punch et al 1999). The original anti-CD2 agent developed for use in humans, BTI 322, a rat IgG_{2b} κ MAb, was administered at daily doses of 5 mg for the initial 10 days posttransplant in combination with CsA, AZA, and steroids. Squifflet et al (1997) reported not only good tolerability, but also a reduced incidence of acute rejection episodes. Similarly, MEDI-507 (Biotransplant Inc., Charlestown, MA, USA), the humanized form of BTI 322, is well tolerated. A phase I/II clinical trial suggested a benefit of MEDI-507 in 55% of patients whose graft-versus-host disease after bone marrow transplantation was unresponsive to steroids, and a 58% reduction in the occurrence of acute renal allograft rejection episodes compared with patients receiving only CsA-AZA-Pred. Based on the hypothesis that, after immunodepletion, the foreign bone marrow can educate the host thymus to accept donor tissues as 'self', MEDI-507 is planned to be used in a tolerance induction protocol: renal transplant patients are first treated with MEDI-507, followed by radiation therapy, bone marrow transplantation from the organ donor, and, finally, implantation of the organ.

Anti-ICAM-1/anti-LFA-1

MAbs directed against LFA-1 or its ligands have been shown to inhibit T-cell activation in vitro (Springer et al 1987). In vivo administration of anti-LFA-1 (CD11a) antibodies to mice induces tolerance to protein antigens (Benjamin et al 1998) and prolongs the survival of tissue and organ allografts (van Dijken et al 1990; Isobe et al 1992; Nakakura et al 1993; Talento et al 1993; He et al 1994; Nishihara et al 1995; Kato et al 1996). Murine anti-CD11a MAbs were demonstrated to reduce the incidence of acute rejection episodes among recipients of human renal allografts (Hourmant et al 1994; Le Mauff 1995, 1996), but the therapeutic effects were beclouded by a high incidence of HAMA. A recently developed humanized IgG_1 κ version of the murine antihuman CD11a MAb (Werther et al 1996) has been shown to block LFA-1 functions in vitro (Champe et al 1995) and to display excellent tolerability in phase I trials in psoriatic patients. This reagent is being prepared for phase I/II trials in renal transplantation (Xoma/Genentech, San Francisco, CA, USA). An alternate strategy, treatment of allograft recipients with an anti-ICAM-1 antisense oligo, has been shown to disrupt ICAM-1 expression on APCs, preventing this coreceptor function and thus providing a novel mechanism of immuno-suppression (Stepkowski et al 1998a).

PROLIFERATION PARADIGM

Pathophysiologic mechanisms

The proliferation paradigm is based on the critical role of cell division to increase the number of donor-specific immunoreactive cells—clonal amplification—upon reception of a foreign antigenic challenge (Figure 10.16). Two types of agents have been used to interrupt cell proliferation: those that interfere with the de novo synthesis (or recycling) of nucleotide bases, and those that prevent the separation of DNA chains. The model compound for the latter action is cyclophosphamide, an alkylating agent that crosslinks DNA chains. Owing to the frequent occurrence and severe degree of bone marrow toxicity and to the high incidence of leukemia (as well as hemorrhagic cystitis) induced by cyclophosphamide, the drug is infrequently utilized for immunosuppression. The only currently recognized (but generally not accepted) indication for its use is as a selective antiproliferative agent against activated B cells.

The group of immunosuppressive drugs that display a more acceptable safety profile includes agents that disrupt the synthesis of purines, namely, AZA and MMF. However, pyrimidines may represent a better target to inhibit nucleotide synthesis, because their cytosolic content is much lower than that of purines. Two new drugs, leflunomide and brequinar, share a common site of action, namely, inhibition of dihydro-orotic acid dehydrogenase, the third step in the biosynthesis of pyrimidines.

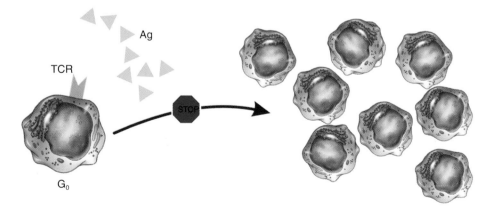

Figure 10.16. Proliferation paradigm. Introduction of antigen (Ag) triggers resting T cell (G_0) bearing the corresponding T cell receptor (TCR) to undergo proliferation, unless inhibited (stop sign) by an antiproliferative agent.

Therapeutic approaches

Leflunomide

The heterocyclic derivative leflunomide ($C_{12}H_9F^3N_2O_2$, Arava; Hoechst-Marion-Roussel; now licensed to Fujisawa) is an oral prodrug of the active major circulating metabolite A77 1726 (Figure 10.8d), which is produced by opening of the isoxazole ring. This antiproliferative agent interrupts a variety of stimulatory signals (Chong et al 1996). Leflunomide appears to be a bifunctional inhibitor: at high ($5-10~\mu M$) concentrations, it blocks the protein tyrosine kinase $p56^{lck}$ and MEK, dampening the generation of NF-κB (Manna and Aggarwal 1999). At low concentrations, it more potently ($179~nM-2.7~\mu M$) suppresses the activity of dihydro-orotate dehydrogenase (Davis et al 1996). It has been suggested that the two inhibitory activities can be studied separately, because the latter action is counteracted by addition of uridine.

In animal models, leflunomide modestly prolongs rat cardiac allograft survival (D'Silva et al 1995) and displays an additive interaction with CsA (Williams et al 1994). When coadministered with uridine, the activity of leflunomide to prolong xenograft survival is antagonized, leaving only a modest effect on allograft survival (Chong et al 1999). Although it extends the survival of renal allografts, leflunomide is toxic to dogs (Yuh et al 1995). When used in combination with CsA and MMF, the drug has been reported to prolong the survival of islet transplants—both allografts (Guo et al 1997a) and xenografts (Guo et al 1997b; Wennberg et al 1997)—rather than solid organ transplants. However, the utility of leflunomide is likely to be limited by its toxicities of anemia, diarrhea, and pathologic changes in the small bowel and liver.

Brequinar

Brequinar (DuPont-Merck, Wilmington, DE, USA, now licensed to Novartis, Basle, Switzerland), a substituted 4-quinoline carboxylic acid, is a potent inhibitor of dihydro-orotate dehydrogenase, the third enzyme in the de novo synthesis of pyrimidines (Chen et al 1989; Figure 10.8e). The drug prolongs allograft survival in rats and mice (Cramer et al 1992; Stepkowski et al 1994). An initial phase I dose-escalation study revealed that brequinar displays a lower oral clearance in quiescent transplant recipients than that previously observed in cancer patients. In both settings, the drug displays a long elimination half-life, allowing alternate-day dosing (Joshi et al 1997). A phase I/II dose-finding study revealed that the potency of the therapeutic effects correlated better with the peak than with the trough concentration of the drug (BD Kahan, unpublished work). The phase II multicenter trial to assess efficacy was inconclusive, owing to the large proportion of patients who experienced a single episode of thrombocytopenia and were thereafter discontinued from the study, as mandated by the protocol.

INFLAMMATION PARADIGM

Pathophysiologic mechanisms

The rejection of allografts includes not only the responses of specific elements of the adaptive T- and B-cell armies, but also inflammatory responses by macrophage, mono-cyte, granulocyte, and NK cell elements of nonspecific host resistance (Table 10.3). In addition to the T cell lymphokine and cytotoxic products, activated macrophages release cytokines, eicosanoids, PAFs, enzymes, and free radicals. Furthermore, immunoglobulin fixation on target cells may activate the complement cascade, as well as trigger adhesion of polymorphonuclear leukocytes and Fc receptor positive (K) lymphocytes and mono-cytes, events that activate the coagulation cascade.

T-cell products
Lymphokines (TNF-α, TNF-β, IFN-γ)
Cytotoxic molecules (perforins, serine esterases, endonucleases, others)

Activated macrophage products
TNF-α, IFN-α, IFN-β, IL-6, IL-1
Eicosanoids
Platelet aggregating factors
Enzymes
O-free radicals

Immunoglobulin and related mechanisms
Complement, polymorphs
Fc receptor-bearing cytotoxic cells (natural killer cells, monocytes)

Secondary effectors
Coagulation cascade

Table 10.3. Humoral effectors of rejection

Therapeutic approaches

Cyclo-oxygenase (COX) inhibitors

Aspirin (ASA) and nonsteroidal anti-inflammatory drugs (NSAIDs) inhibit prostaglandin synthesis by blocking the action of COX, which occurs in two isoforms, COX-1 and COX-2. COX-1 is constitutively expressed in many tissues, where it serves several 'housekeeping' functions. COX-2 is inducible and activated in response to cytokines.

While ASA inhibits COX-2 10–100 times more potently than COX-1 activities (Kalgutkar et al 1998), NSAIDs display a nonselective action (Dubois et al 1998).

Celebrex (Monsanto, St. Louis, MO, USA) was developed as a selective COX-2 inhibitor. However, the drug is likely to have limited application in renal transplantation, owing to its adverse reaction to produce interstitial nephritis—a property that Celebrex shares with NSAIDs. However, recent findings suggest that ASA might be an excellent structure for therapeutic drug modeling. In addition to its inhibitory activity on COX, high concentrations of ASA (IC_{50} = 50 μM) blocked IKKβ catalysis, namely, the transfer of phosphate groups from ATP to IκB, the event that triggers degradation of IκB with release of NF-κB (Yin et al 1998b). Furthermore, these authors observed that high ASA concentrations inhibited activation of the JNKs that mediate the phosphorylation of c-Jun, a step that is necessary for activation of this transcriptional regulator. Interestingly, these concentrations of ASA have been observed among patients treated chronically for inflammatory disorders. Thus, synthetic modification to produce a structural analog of ASA may be predicted to yield an agent that is selectively active on enzymes of interest to the transplant clinician, without engendering the toxicities of headaches, tinnitus, or dizziness associated with the high ASA concentrations that are presently necessary to inhibit these enzymes.

TOLERANCE PARADIGMS

T-cell depletion: pathophysiologic mechanisms

The seminal observation of the critical role of T cells in the development of both T and B cell-mediated resistance to transplants suggested that their depletion might facilitate alloacceptance. The application of extreme depletion methods, radiation and thoracic duct drainage, engendered a high degree of vulnerability to infectious complications. MAbs with or without toxic conjugates have been designed to bind at high avidity to elements of host resistance and thereby to deplete T-cell elements. Recognizing the potential danger of this approach—the annihilation of all T cells—a strategy of single-dose treatment has been used to only briefly interrupt host recognition and, it is hoped, result in a situation akin to neonatal animals that more readily react to a foreign antigen by alloacceptance rather than alloaggression.

Another approach that is more gentle than the physical process of thoracic duct drainage of lymphocytes from the body is the use of photopheresis. Patient peripheral blood lymphocytes separated by leukapheresis are exposed ex vivo to a photoactive compound (Methoxsalen), which is then activated by ultraviolet A radiation. Thereafter, the cells are reinfused into the patient. The proposed mechanisms of the effect of photopheresis include modulation of cytokine responses, induction of regulatory programs, deviation to apoptosis pathways, or alteration of TCR function.

A third approach to produce T-cell depletion is the induction of apoptosis. The expression of Fas ligand (FasL) in the testis and eye may explain the 'privileged' status of transplants in these sites (Suda et al 1993), that is, their ability to be engrafted without producing allorejection, as occurs with virtually every other organ. Binding of FasL, which is constitutively expressed on a wide variety of cells, including the testis, to Fas on T cells induces apoptosis of the immune elements.

T-cell depletion: therapeutic approaches

The original T-cell depletion procedures using either total body or total lymphoid irradiation were not only toxic to the bone marrow, but also cumbersome to implement in clinical practice. The strategy of thoracic duct drainage (Franksson 1968) was technically challenging, and patients frequently showed only partial depletion of T cells. Recently, a physical depletion strategy based on ex vivo irradiation of blood lymphocytes has been subjected to clinical trials. However, a more feasible strategy utilizes MAbs either with or without conjugation to diptheria toxin to potentiate cell killing.

Photopheresis

In an international multicenter trial, cardiac transplant recipients who underwent prophylactic photopheresis treatments—24 during the first 6 months—displayed a reduced number of rejection episodes, namely, 1.44 ± 1.0 versus 0.91 ± 1.0 ($P = 0.04$; Barr et al 1998), without an evident increase in infectious episodes. Photopheresis has also been used for treatment of refractory bronchiolitis obliterans after lung transplantation (Salerno et al 1999).

Diphtheria toxin immunoconjugates

Pretransplant administration to monkeys of the holoimmunotoxin FN18-CRM9, which bears a murine antirhesus-CD3 MAb linked to a diphthcria toxin binding site mutant (Neville et al 1985), produces T-cell depletion and prolongs renal allograft survival (Knechtle et al 1997). However, when given at the time of transplantation, the agent is associated with the development of interstitial nephritis and chronic rejection (Knechtle et al 1998). In attempting to understand these effects, Hamawy et al (1999) observed that the MAb portion activates T cells for adhesion and cytokine (INF-γ and TNF-α) expression, effects that can be deleterious to a transplant, while the toxin portion inhibits protein synthesis and cell proliferation, probably by inhibition of tyrosine phosphorylation.

Campath-1-IgG antibody

Campath-1-IgG, a rat antihuman IgG$_{2b}$ MAb developed by Hale and Waldmann (1994) and licensed to Glaxo Wellcome (UK), binds CD52, a surface antigen common to B and T lymphocytes. Ex vivo exposure of bone marrow transplant inocula to 20 mg doses of the reagent depletes donor lymphocytes, reduces the incidence of acute rejection episodes, and eliminates chronic graft-versus-host disease (Arnold et al 1993). However, patients treated with the combination of Campath-1-IgG, CsA, and methotrexate display both lymphoproliferative and infectious complications, particularly due to CMV (Hertenstein et al 1995).

Campath-1-IgG has recently been administered in a 20 mg dose intravenously on day 1 postrenal transplant to induce depletion of peripheral blood lymphocytes. During the second day, a 'window for opportunity', all immunosuppressive therapy is withheld in an attempt to permit a period of interaction between the immune-impaired host and his graft, and, it is hoped, to achieve 'prope' (almost) tolerance. Thereafter, on day 3, CsA treatment is administered at reduced doses, targeting the amounts needed to achieve trough concentrations of 100 ± 25 ng/ml (Calne et al 1998). No concomitant corticosteroid is given. Following antibody administration, the peripheral blood lymphocyte count falls to zero and recovers at about 1 month. Among 31 patients treated with the regimen, the acute rejection rate was 16%. The three graft losses owed to death from congestive heart failure, recurrent kidney disease, and poor renal function (Calne et al 1999). The remainder of the patients continue to be steroid-free. Recently, to permit the possibility of multiple courses of antibody therapy, Galliland et al (1999) designed a monomeric non-cell-binding variant that tolerized hosts to prevent them from forming antibody against the wild-type, cell-binding form of the MAb. The efficacy of this strategy was confirmed in humans; patients treated with the monomeric form did not generate antibody responses (Rebello et al 1999).

Anti-CD7 antibody

Another therapeutic approach is the development of chimeric mouse/human MAb directed toward the CD7, since this epitope is upregulated upon activation of T cells. Lazarovits et al (1993) reported a randomized but open-label study of 20 CsA-Pred-treated patients, demonstrating approximately equal efficacy of six doses of anti-CD7 MAb versus 10 doses of OKT3. In contrast to OKT3, the anti-CD7 MAb did not produce the cytokine release syndrome. Indeed, the anti-CD7 elicited only mild side-effects (Kirkham et al 1992): three of 10 patients experienced minor tremor and diarrhea, and one patient, fever. Only one recipient of anti-CD7 experienced a serious infection, compared with four patients treated with anti-CD3. Formal reports of subsequent trials are not yet published.

Anti-TIRC7

Upregulated expression of a variety of T-cell proteins occurs during T-cell activation. Using a strategy of differential display of mRNA transcripts, a new product, TIRC7, was identified to be expressed within 24 hours; this event is inhibited by CsA. Antibodies directed against this epitope prolonged renal allograft survival in rats without causing T-cell depletion (Utku et al 1998).

Induction of Fas ligand (FasL)

Another strategy seeks to transfect expression of FasL into transplanted organs to protect them against the ravages of T cells. Initial attempts to apply this strategy in pancreatic islet transplantation produced inconsistent results, but, in general, the transfected tissue appeared to be destroyed more quickly compared to nontransfected islets (Muruve et al 1997). However, Li et al (1998) suggest that tight control of the degree of FasL expression on hepatic allografts and the use of a nonviral vector may overcome the proapoptotic effects of FasL, leading to prolonged transplant survival. In view of these uncertainties, it is unlikely that this strategy will be employed clinically in the near future.

Costimulation blockade: pathophysiologic mechanisms

The second major therapeutic approach has been to prevent the costimulatory signal necessary for full activation of T cells. Lafferty and Cunningham (1975) suggested that two signals are necessary to trigger T-cell activation: one signal provided by antigen presented in the context of MHC, and a second signal of an uncertain nature. It now appears that one of the major components of the second signal is the reciprocal binding of surface markers on professional APCs and T cells, namely, B7 (B7-1 (CD80) and B7-2 (CD86)) and CD28, as well as CD40 and CD40 ligand (CD40L, CD154), respectively (Figure 10.17). An alternate approach to disrupt signal two is to deliver an antigen in the absence of a costimulatory signal, thus producing anergy. Reception of the costimulatory signal via CD28 is followed by sustained downregulation of IκBα protein and enhanced nuclear translocation of Rel/NF-κB transcription factors from the cytosol (Bryan et al 1994), a step that is inhibited by SRL (Lai and Tan 1994). The presence of Rel/NF-κB produces transcriptional activation of the CD28 response element within the IL-2 promoter enhancer region (Lai et al 1995). In addition, CD28 signaling events activate JNK (Su et al 1994) and induce the expression of the antiapoptotic factor Bcl-xL (Boise et al 1995), increase cytokine mRNA stability (Lindstein et al 1989), and activate important transcription factors, including NF-AT (Ghosh et al 1996), as well as an AMP-responsive element (Hsueh et al 1997).

CD40 is a 50-kD molecule constitutively expressed on APCs, whereas CD154 is a 30–33-kD transmembrane protein that is structurally related to the cytokine TNF-α. CD154 is transiently expressed on CD4[+] T cells, mast cells, basophils, and platelets (Henn et al 1998). In addition to its expression on macrophages, monocytes, dendritic cells, and B cells, CD40 is present on endothelial cells, platelets, fibroblasts, and keratinocytes. Following ligation of CD40 markers by CD154, cells undergo activation, resulting in induction of B7, ICAM-1 (CD54), and VCAM-1 (Yellin et al 1995), as well as production of proinflammatory cytokines such as IL-1β, TNF-α, and IL-12. The critical role these ligands play in T- (and B-) cell activation has raised increased interest in their blockade.

One line of evidence supporting this paradigm is the observation that hepatic APCs

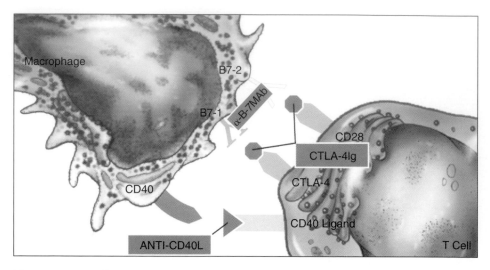

Figure 10.17. The costimulatory paradigm. Cell–cell interactions across the immunologic synapse include not only MHC-TCR, but also B7–1/B7–2 with CD28 and CD40 with CD40 ligand (CD154). Shown are strategies using receptor conjugates or MAbs.

do not deliver costimulatory signals (Gorczynski et al 1996). Thus, in animal models, delivery of allogeneic cells (Kenick et al 1987; Yoshimura et al 1990; Nakano et al 1992; Morita et al 1999) or of soluble antigen (Wang et al 1997) by the portal venous route, frequently in combination with a brief course of CsA, tends to produce donor-specific anergy and operational tolerance (Figure 10.18).

Costimulation blockade: therapeutic approaches

CTLA-4Ig-receptor conjugate

Developed by Linsley et al (1991), a conjugate of the extracellular domain of the CTLA-4 marker was fused to the heavy chain of IgG_1. This reagent blocks B7 with greater avidity than the natural ligand CD28. Not only does CTLA-4Ig act as an efficient competitive inhibitor of B7 binding to CD28, but also it prevents binding of B7 to CTLA-4 (CD152), which is subsequently expressed and serves as a negative regulatory molecule. Because the CTLA-4 marker shows a 10–20-fold-greater affinity for B7 than CD28 (Judge et al 1999), it is able to terminate the immune response. While this negative regulation clearly owes in part to antagonism of ligand binding to CD28 (Blazar et al 1999), it may also be caused by an effect of CTLA-4 ligation to reduce the cytoplasmic generation of NF-AT and of the nuclear regulatory factor of the IL-2-independent molecule CdR6, as well as to persistence of the cell cycle control molecule p27 (Brunner et al 1999). Administration of the CTLA-4Ig conjugate prolongs graft survival in a variety of rodent heart, kidney, lung, and islet transplant models (Sayegh and Turka 1998).

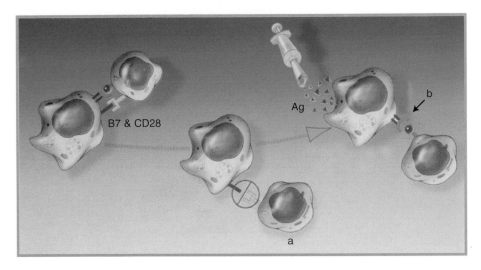

Figure 10.18. Two methods of tolerance induction. (a) Blockade of second signal generated by professional (P) APC. (b) Antigen (Ag) fed to nonprofessional APC delivers only partial signal since these APCs are incapable of delivering the costimulatory signal.

However, permanent allograft survival has only been achieved when the receptor conjugate was administered concomitantly with donor-antigen, in the form either of splenocytes or of blood transfusions (Lin et al 1993). An alternate strategy to deliver conjugate treatment ex vivo utilizes transduction of the allograft with a recombinant adenovirus encoding the CTLA-4Ig gene (Yang et al 1999).

CTLA-4Ig has been examined in two types of clinical trials. Administration of 25 or 50 mg/kg CTLA-4Ig to patients afflicted with *Psoriasis vulgaris* resulted in significant improvement in nine of 11 patients; the response rates were substantially lower at reduced doses. Although the immunomodulation persisted for up to 5 months, it did not eventuate in tolerance induction (Abrams et al 1999). In the second type of clinical trial, in vitro incubation of CTLA-4Ig with alloreactive bone marrow T cells from HLA-haploidentical donors mitigated their capacity to cause graft-versus-host disease after bone marrow transplantation (Guinan et al 1999).

Anti-B7 MAb

An alternate tool to therapeutically manipulate the B7/CD28 costimulation cascade is the use of anti-B7 MAb (Genetics Institute, Cambridge, MA, USA). Knockout animals showing defective expression of both B7–1 (CD80) and B7–2 (CD86) display indefinite survival of allografts (Mandelbrot et al 1999), suggesting that antibodies against both determinants provide greater benefit than those directed against a single determinant. Blockade of B7 costimulation (Sayegh et al 1995) promotes but is not essential for long-term transplant survival (Lakkis et al 1997). Indeed, the effect of blockade of both B7 markers seems to be greater than that observed either with CTLA-4Ig (Woodward et al

461

1998) or with dual blockade of the CD40/CD154 costimulatory pair. Infusion of a combination of anti-B7-1 and anti-B7-2 MAbs eliminated graft-versus-host disease lethality by reducing (but not completely vitiating) $CD4^+$ and $CD8^+$ mediated resistance (Blazar et al 1996).

Anti-CD154 MAb

Administration of anti-CD154 MAbs in combination with CTLA-4Ig to nonhuman primates was reported to prevent acute rejection, producing long-term graft survival or even tolerance (Kirk et al 1997). As in the case with CTLA-4Ig, ex vivo treatment of donor bone marrow inocula with anti-CD154 MAb mitigated graft-versus-host disease in a murine model (Blazar et al 1998). When used as a single agent, anti-CD154 was more potent than CTLA-4Ig to prevent organ transplant rejection. However, despite the prolonged survival of grafts engendered by anti-CD154, host antidonor alloantibodies were present in the circulation, and infiltrating activated lymphocytes, in the transplant. The failure of anti-CD154 MAbs to block alloantibody responses was unexpected, since it would have been predicted that the MAb would interrupt the function of B-cell CD154, a limiting factor in the humoral response to T cell-dependent antigens (Pérez-Melgosa et al 1999). One of the primary obstacles to clinical applications of this reagent was the finding that the immunosuppressive effects of humanized anti-CD154 MAbs were antagonized by steroids, MMF, or TRL (Kirk et al 1999), as well as CsA (Larsen et al 1996), presumably owing to the effects of these drugs to prevent full expression/function of CD154 on T cells.

An initial clinical trial using a humanized anti-CD154 MAb (20 mg/kg), administered on alternate weeks to de novo renal transplant patients treated with a baseline regimen of MMF and steroids, failed to protect patients from acute rejection episodes. Unfortunately, clinical trials of patients afflicted with *Psoriasis vulgaris* and of de novo posttransplant recipients, particularly with the 40 mg/kg dose, revealed that the reagent was associated with an increased rate of thrombotic events. While the toxicity may owe in part to the expression of CD40 on vascular endothelial cells, it is more likely that the binding of antibody to CD154 on platelets enhances their agglutination (Rosenberg and Aird 1999), as well as potentiates tissue factor-dependent procoagulant activity, resulting in thrombogeneration and fibrin deposition (Zhou et al 1998). Additionally, one cannot exclude the possibility that anti-CD154 MAb affects the intrinsic or extrinsic coagulation cascade; endothelial cell expression of CD40; the activation, generation or regulation of plasminogen activator or thrombin receptors; and/or the expression of selectins, ICAM-1, or VCAM. A reasonable alternate strategy to mitigate these negative effects would be to combine low doses of anti-CD154 MAb with other maintenance immunosuppressive agents, such as SRL.

Altered ligand stimulation: pathophysiologic mechanisms

A third potential approach to tolerance induction is the delivery of peptides that trigger alloacceptance rather than alloaggression. In contrast to antagonists, which prevent T-cell recognition and probably have to be administered chronically, partial agonists induce an altered pattern of T-cell development, with the predominant emergence of cells bearing features of the Th_2 subset and mediating immune unresponsiveness (Figure 10.19). However, growing evidence indicates that Th_2 cells also participate in transplant resistance, suggesting that the concept of disparate responses by T helper subpopulations is probably an oversimplification.

Using a hemoglobin model peptide system to stimulate cloned T cells, Sloan-Lancaster et al (1994) showed that treatment with an altered peptide ligand (partial agonist) induces incomplete $CD3\zeta$ phosphorylation of all T cells, resulting in a failure of this transduction molecule to associate with ZAP70. In contrast, immunogenic peptides cause $CD3\zeta$ phosphorylation, leading to association with ZAP70 and intense reciprocal phosphorylation (Figure 10.20). Daniel et al (1998) observed that a partial agonist peptide was able to antagonize alloactivation via a specific TCR in vitro.

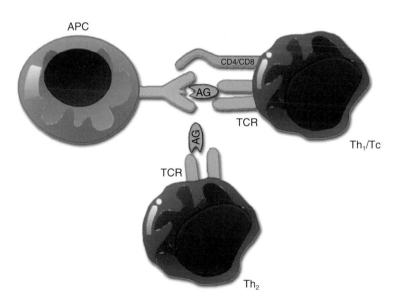

Figure 10.19. Antigen presentation by APC to helper (or cytotoxic) T cell (Th_1/Tc) producing alloaggression versus effect on regulatory T cell (thought to be T helper subset 2). An antagonist prevents Th_1/Tc activation, whereas a partial agonist triggers regulatory Th_2 cells.

463

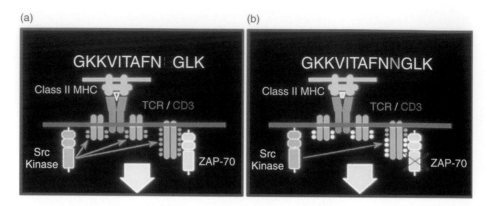

Figure 10.20. Comparison of partial with full T cell activation. (a) Full T cell activation by an immunogenic peptide of murine hemoglobin produces phosphorylation of CD3ζ (shown by blue circles), as well as association with and full phosphorylation of ZAP70. (b) Partial T cell activation by altered peptide ligand bearing a single amino acid substitution, leading to only partial phosphorylation of CD3ζ (white circles), as well as lack of association with and minimal phosphorylation of ZAP70. (Sloan-Lancaster J, Shaw AS, Rothbard JB, Allen PM. Partial T cell signaling: altered phospho-zeta and lack of zap70 recruitment in APL-induced T cell anergy. *Cell* 1994; **79**(5):913–922. © 1994 Cell Press. Reprinted with permission.)

Altered ligand stimulation: therapeutic approaches

The recognition of alloantigen by Th, Tc, or B cells, which triggers the host response, may be disrupted by antagonists or partial agonists of T-cell receptor function. Krensky and Clayberger (1994) observed that peptides derived from conserved domains of MHC class I or class II molecules inhibit T-cell activation in vitro and, in combination with CsA, graft rejection in vivo. However, the effect was limited to relatively weak donor–recipient incompatibilities.

An altered peptide signal delivered in the form of a modified or incomplete histocompatibility antigen may provide a tolerogen. For example, Brouard et al (1999) used concepts of rational synthesis of a peptide analogous to the amino acid sequence in the α_1 helical region of the class I MHC molecule. This peptide was immunosuppressive; it inhibited heme oxygenase, an intermediate in the development of upregulated immune effector functions. A recent finding by Hin et al (1999) proffers hope for more effective therapy: N-hydroxylation of an antigenic epitope generated an antagonist (mimotope) peptide that was 100-fold more potent than, and thus overcame the presence of, the cognate epitope agonist. The amino acid that was changed is not one expressed toward or even accessible to the TCR, but rather one that is buried inside the peptide binding groove. Thus, the effect must owe to indirect conformational changes that alter TCR binding. In contrast to strategies that seek to modify the side chains of the peptide (Jameson et al 1993; Preckel et al 1997), this technique leaves the side chains intact and thus should improve the antigenic specificity of the antagonist. Another approach that has been shown to induce specific tolerance is the production of allochimeric molecules that bear foreign donor-type antigenic epitopes substituted onto host-type class I MHC molecules (Wang et al 1997). However, because this strategy is specific for the donor–recipient combination, it is difficult to envision how it would be readily applied to the clinical setting.

A major issue in clinical therapy using peptides is the difficulty of their delivery into cells. One strategy harnesses gene therapy, which introduces DNA that encodes the synthesis of the desired product (Anderson 1998). An alternate epigenetic strategy is protein transport, linking the desired amino acid sequence to an NH_2-terminal 111-amino acid domain from the human immunodeficiency virus (HIV) transactivation transcription (TAT) regulatory factor, a 'Trojan protein'. This protein contains domains of highly basic amino acids that readily penetrate the cell, carrying other proteins of molecular sizes greater than 100 kD. For example, Schwarze et al (1999) used this strategy to demonstrate cellular uptake of the 110 kD protein galactosidase into virtually every organ following intraperitoneal injection of conjugate in mice.

CONCLUSION

The field of immunosuppression is developing rapidly, driven by the clinical demands of physicians engaged in the treatment of patients either bearing organ transplants or afflicted with autoimmune disease. Because of their relatively nonselective mechanisms of action, the first-generation antiproliferative agents are likely to play a diminishing role in the therapeutic armamentarium of the next millennium. The second-generation CNAs occupy a solid role in current therapy, owing to their greater selectivity of inhibition of T and B cells rather than polymorphonuclear or monocyte/macrophage activities. However, in the coming decade, CsA and TRL are likely to be displaced by the introduction of CNAs that are specifically designed as structural analogs or cognate peptides. Similarly, the remarkable progress engendered by the discovery of the synergistic effects of combining CNAs with the third-generation agents SRL (or SDZ RAD), as represented by the cytokine paradigm, is likely to be succeeded by more selective agents that overcome the pleiotropic toxicities of SRL, unless it can be documented that the broad spectrum of action of SRL on a wide variety of cytokine effects actually mitigates the vasculopathy associated with rejection. Drugs that disrupt more specific targets, such as the lymphokine-specific γ-chain transduction events of JAK3 catalysis and Stat5 generation, seem to be more likely candidates for development.

A new pathway for therapeutic intervention is the adhesion/migration/homing paradigm, since the ischemia–reperfusion injuries upregulate expression of foreign histocompatibility antigens, which increases the risk of rejection, and of adhesion molecules, which predisposes to vascular dysfunction.

While new MAbs that block coreceptor functions or novel anti-inflammatory drugs may provide other therapeutic alternatives, the major target of transplantation research in the new millennium is the induction of specific tolerance. T-cell depletion paradigms have been widely recognized to strip the immune system back to a primordial state, where its elements can interact in a fashion more likely to eventuate in alloacceptance; however, this state may be hazardous, particularly in the presence of concomitant infection. Interruption of the costimulatory pathway of lymphocyte activation has been proffered as an immunologically attractive approach; however, the initial clinical data suggest that these agents may be toxic. Possibly, the most desirable approach is antigen-specific immunosuppression using modified peptides or proteins. It is hoped that this last group of strategies will yield a specific state of immunosuppression, since induction of immunologic tolerance will achieve permanent graft survival without the need for ongoing treatment and with only a modest defect in the host T-cell repertoire.

REFERENCES

Abrams JR, Lebwohl MG, Guzzo CA et al (1999) CTLA4Ig-mediated blockade of T-cell costimulation in patients with psoriasis vulgaris. *J Clin Invest* **103**:1243–1252.

Akimoto H, McDonald TO, Weyhrich JT et al (1996) Antibody to CD18 reduces neutrophil and T lymphocyte infiltration and vascular cell adhesion molecule-1 expression in cardiac rejection. *Transplantation* **61**:1610–1617.

Albert ML, Sauter B, Bhardwaj N (1998) Dendritic cells acquire antigen from apoptotic cells and induce class I-restricted CTLs. *Nature* **392**:86–89.

Amada N, Okazaki H, Sato T et al (1998) Beneficial effects of 15-deoxyspergualin on late acute rejection occurring more than three months after renal transplantation. *Transplant Proc* **30**:2246–2247.

Ames A, Wright RL, Kowada M et al (1968) Cerebral ischemia. II. The no-reflow phenomenon. *Am J Pathol* **52**:437–453.

Anderson WF (1998) Human gene therapy. *Nature* **392**(6679 Suppl):25–30.

Annat J, Churaqui E, Dutartre P, Bruley-Rosset M (1996) Prevention of lethal graft-versus-host disease following allogeneic bone marrow transplantation in mice by short course administration of LF 08-0299. *Transplantation* **62**:721–729.

Arai T, Kelly SA, Brengman ML et al (1998) Ambient but not incremental oxidant generation effects intercellular adhesion molecule 1 induction by tumour necrosis factor alpha in endothelium. *Biochem J* **331**:853–861.

Aramburu J, Yaffe MB, López-Rodríguez C et al (1999) Affinity-driven peptide selection of an NFAT inhibitor more selective than cyclosporin A. *Science* **285**:2129–2133.

Arnold R, Bunjes D, Wiesneth M et al (1993) In vitro and in vivo depletion of T cells. *Bone Marrow Transplant* **12**(Suppl 3):S11–12.

Arroyo AG, Campanero MR, Sanchez-Mateos P et al (1994) Induction of tyrosine phosphorylation during ICAM-3 and LFA-1-mediated intercellular adhesion, and its regulation by the CD45 tyrosine phosphatase. *J Cell Biol* **126**:1277–1286.

Austrup F, Vestweber D, Borges E et al (1997) P- and E-selectin mediate recruitment of T-helper-1 but not T-helper-2 cells into inflamed tissues. *Nature* **385**:81–83.

Barr ML, Meiser BM, Eisen HJ et al (1998) Photopheresis for the prevention of rejection in cardiac transplantation. *N Engl J Med* **339**:1744–1751.

Baumert H, Goujon J-M, Richer J-P et al (1999) Renoprotective effects of trimetazidine against ischemia–reperfusion injury and cold storage preservation: a preliminary study. *Transplantation* **68**:300–303.

Benjamin RJ, Qin SX, Wqise MP et al (1988) Mechanisms of monoclonal antibody-facilitated tolerance induction: a possible role for the CD4 (L3T4) and CD11a (LFA-1) molecules in self–non-self discrimination. *Eur J Immunol* **18**:1079–1088.

Berlin C, Berg EL, Briskin MJ et al (1993) $\alpha_4\beta_7$ integrin mediates lymphocyte binding to the mucosal vascular addressin MAdCAM-1. *Cell* **74**:185–195.

Berlin C, Bargatze RF, Campbell JJ et al (1995) α_4 integrins mediate lymphocyte attachment and rolling under physiologic flow. *Cell* **80**:413–422.

Blazar BR, Sharpe AH, Taylor PA et al (1996) Infusion of anti-B7.1 (CD80) and anti-B7.2 (CD86) monoclonal antibodies inhibits murine graft-versus-host disease lethality in part via direct effects on CD4$^+$ and CD8$^+$ T cells. *J Immunol* **157**:3250–3259.

Blazar BR, Taylor PA, Noelle RJ, Vallera DA (1998) CD4(+) T cells tolerized ex vivo to host alloantigen by anti-CD40 ligand (CD40L:CD154) antibody lose their graft-versus-host disease lethality capacity but retain nominal antigen responses. *J Clin Invest* **102**:473–482.

Blazar BR, Taylor PA, Panoskaltsis-Mortari A et al (1999) Opposing roles of CD28:B7 and CTLA-4:B7 pathways in regulating in vivo alloresponses in murine receipients of MHC disparate T cells. *J Immunol* **162**:6368–6377.

Boise LH, Minn AJ, Noel PJ et al (1995) CD28 costimulation can promote T cell survival by enhancing the expression of Bcl-XL. *Immunity* **3**:87–98.

Bonventre JV (1993) Mechanisms of ischemic acute renal failure. *Kidney Int* **43**:1160–1178.

Borges E, Tietz W, Steegmaier M et al (1997) P-selectin glycoprotein ligand-1 (PSGL-1) on T helper 1 but not on T helper 2 cells binds to P-selectin and supports migration into inflamed skin. *J Exp Med* **185**:573–578.

Boussiotis V, Freeman G, Griffin J et al (1994) CD2 is involved in maintenance and reversal of human alloantigen-specific clonal anergy. *J Exp Med* **180**:1665–1673.

Braun C, Conzelmann T, Vetter S et al (1999) Prevention of chronic renal allograft rejection in rats with an oral endothelin A receptor antagonist. *Transplantation* **68**:739–746.

Bright JJ, Du C, Sriram S (1999) Tyrphostin B42 inhibits IL-12-induced tyrosine phosphorylation and activation of Janus kinase-2 and prevents experimental allergic encephalomyelitis. *J Immunol* **162**:6255–6262.

Brinkmann V, Pinschewer D, Feng L (1999) FTY 720 suppresses immune responses by modulating G-protein coupled receptors on lymphocytes resulting in altered lymphocyte homing. *18th Annual Meeting of the American Society of Transplantation*, May 15–19, Chicago, IL.

Briscoe DM, Schoen FJ, Rice GE et al (1991) Induced expression of endothelial-leukocyte adhesion molecules in human cardiac allografts. *Transplantation* **51**:537–539.

Brouard S, Cuturi MC, Pignon P et al (1999) Prolongation of heart xenograft survival in a hamster-to-rat model after therapy with a rationally designed immunosuppressive peptide. *Transplantation* **67**:1614–1618.

Brunkhorst R, Neumayer H-H, Hiss M et al (1999) Human safety and pharmacology of FTY720 (abst 585). *18th Annual Meeting of the American Society of Transplantation*, May 15–19, Chicago, IL.

Brunner MC, Chambers CA, Chan FK-M et al (1999) CTLA-4-mediated inhibition of early events of T cell proliferation. *J Immunol* **162**:5813–5820.

Bryan RG, Li Y, Lai JH et al (1994) Effect of CD28 signal transduction on c-Rel in human peripheral blood T cells. *Mol Cell Biol* **14**:7933–7942.

Bulkley GB (1983) The role of oxygen free radicals in human disease processes. *Surgery* **94**:407–411.

Burns LJ, Pooley JC, Walsh DJ et al (1999) Intercellular adhesion molecule-1 expression in endothelial cells is activated by cytomegalovirus immediate early proteins. *Transplantation* **67**:137–144.

Butcher EC, Picker LJ (1996) Lymphocyte homing and homeostasis. *Science* **272**:60–66.

Butcher EC, Williams M, Youngman K et al (1999) Lymphocyte trafficking and regional immunity. *Adv Immunol* 72:209–253.

Calne R, Friend P, Moffatt S et al (1998) Prope tolerance, perioperative campath 1H, and low-dose cyclosporin monotherapy in renal allograft recipients. *Lancet* 351:1701–1702.

Calne R, Moffatt SD, Friend PJ et al (1999) Campath IH allows low-dose cyclosporine monotherapy in 31 cadaveric renal allograft recipients. *Transplantation* 68:1613–1616.

Campbell JJ, Hedrick J, Zlotnik A et al (1998) Chemokines and arrest of lymphocytes rolling under flow conditions. *Nature* 279:381–384.

Campbell JJ, Haraldsen G, Pan J et al (1999) The chemokine receptor CCR4 in vascular recognition by cutaneous but not intestinal memory T cells. *Nature* 400:776–780.

Champe M, McIntyre BW, Berman PW (1995) Monoclonal antibodies that block the activity of leukocyte function-associated antigen 1 recognize three discrete epitopes in the inserted domain of CD11a. *J Biol Chem* 270:1388–1394.

Chatenoud L, Ferran C, Legendre C et al (1990) Immunological follow-up of renal allograft recipients treated with the BMA 031 (anti-TCR) monoclonal antibody. *Transplant Proc* 22:1787–1788.

Chávez-Cartaya R, Cozzi E, Pino-DeSola G et al (1995) Regulation of complement activation in rat liver ischemia and reperfusion: expression of endothelial CD59 (RIP). *Transplant Proc* 27:2852–2854.

Chen S-F, Ruben RL, Dexter DL (1989) Mechanism of action of the novel anticancer agent DuP 785 [6-fluoro-2-(2'-fluoro-1,1'-biphenyl-4-yl)-3-methyl-4-quinolinecarboxylic acid sodium salt]: inhibition of de novo pyrimidine nucleotide biosynthesis. *Cancer Res* 46:5014–5019.

Chen W, Bennett CF, Wang ME et al (1999) Perfusion of kidneys with unformulated 'naked' intercellular adhesion molecule-1 antisense oligodeoxynucleotides prevents ischemic/reperfusion injury. *Transplantation* 68:880–887.

Chiba K, Yanagawa Y, Masubuchi Y et al (1998) FTY720, a novel immunosuppressant, induces sequestration of circulating mature lymphocytes by acceleration of lymphocyte homing in rats. I. FTY720 selectively decreases the number of circulating mature lymphocytes by acceleration of lymphocyte homing. *J Immunol* 160:5037–5044.

Chong AS, Rezai K, Gebel HM et al (1996) Effects of leflunomide and other immunosuppressive agents on T cell proliferation in vitro. *Transplantation* 61:140–145.

Chong AS, Huang W, Liu W et al (1999) In vivo activity of leflunomide: pharmacokinetic analyses and mechanism of immunosuppression. *Transplantation* 68:100–109.

Connolly JK, Guy SP, Parrot NR (1995) Cytokine gene expression and eicosanoid production in renal reperfusion injury. *Transplant Proc* 27:2816–2818.

Cosimi AB (1995) Current and future application of monoclonal antibodies in clinical immunosuppressive protocols. *Clin Transplant* 9:219–226.

Cramer DV, Chapman FA, Jaffee BD et al (1992) The effect of a new immunosuppressive drug, brequinar sodium, on cardiac, hepatic, and renal allograft rejection in the rat. *Transplantation* 53:303–308.

Cywes R, Mullen JB, Stratis MA et al (1993) Prediction of the outcome of transplantation in man by platelet adherence in donor liver allografts. Evidence of the importance of prepreservation injury. *Transplantation* 56:316–323.

Daemen MARC, Van de Ven MWCM, Heineman E, Buurman WA (1999a) Involvement of endogenous interleukin-10 and tumor necrosis factor-α in renal ischemia–reperfusion injury. *Transplantation* 67:792–800.

Daemen MARC, van 't Veer C, Denecker G et al (1999b) Inhibition of apoptosis induced by ischemia–reperfusion prevents inflammation. *J Clin Invest* 104:541–549.

Dai Z, Arakelov A, Wagener M et al (1999) The role of common cytokine receptor γ-chain in regulating IL-2-dependent, activation-induced CD8$^+$ T cell death. *J Immunol* 163:3131–3137.

Daniel C, Grakoui A, Allen PM (1998) Inhibition of an in vitro CD4$^+$ T cell alloresponse using altered peptide ligands. *J Immunol* **160**:3244–3250.

Davenport A, Hopton M, Bolton C (1995) Measurement of malondialdehyde as a marker of oxygen free radical production during renal allograft transplantation and the effect on early graft function. *Clin Transplant* **9**:171–175.

Davis JP, Cain GA, Pitts WJ et al (1996) The immunosuppressive metabolite of leflunomide is a potent inhibitor of human dihydroorotate dehydrogenase. *Biochemistry* **35**:1270–1273.

Dendorfer U, Hillebrand G, Kasper C et al (1990) Effective prevention of interstitial rejection crises in immunological high risk patients following renal transplantation: use of high doses of the new monoclonal antibody BMA 031. *Transplant Proc* **22**:1789–1790.

Dragun D, Lukitsch I, Tullius SG et al (1998) Inhibition of intercellular adhesion molecule-1 with antisense deoxynucleotides prolongs renal allograft survival in the rat. *Kidney Int* **54**:2113–2122.

D'Silva M, Candinas D, Achilleos O et al (1995) The immunomodulatory effect of leflunomide in rat cardiac allotransplantation. *Transplantation* **60**:430–437.

Dubois RN, Abramson SB, Crofford L et al (1998) Cyclooxygenase in biology and disease. *FASEB J* **12**:1063–1073.

Dulkanchainun TS, Goss JA, Imagawa DK et al (1998) Reduction of hepatic ischemia/reperfusion injury by a soluble P-selectin glycoprotein ligand-1. *Ann Surg* **227**:832.

Dumont FJ, Koprak S, Staruch MJ et al (1998) A tacrolimus-related immunosuppressant with reduced toxicity. *Transplantation* **65**:18–26.

Dutartre P, Annat J, Derrepas P (1995) LF 08-0299 induces tolerance after short-term treatment in a fully major histocompatibility mismatched rat cardiac allograft model. *Transplant Proc* **27**:440–442.

Eason JD, Wee S, Kawai T et al (1995) Inhibition of the effects of TNF in renal allograft recipients using recombinant human dimeric tumor necrosis factor receptors. *Transplantation* **59**:300–305.

Fatatis A, Miller RJ (1999) Cell cycle control of PDGF-induced Ca^{2+} signaling through modulation of sphingolipid metabolism. *FASEB J* **13**:1291–1301.

Fenczik CA, Sethi T, Ramos JW et al (1997) Complementation of dominant suppression implicates CD98 in integrin activation. *Nature* **390**:81–85.

Flores I, Martinez-A C, Hannun YA, Merida I (1998) Dual role of ceramide in the control of apoptosis following IL-2 withdrawal. *J Immunol* **160**:3528–3533.

Franksson C (1968) Cannulating of the thoracic duct. A diagnostic and therapeutic method [in Swedish]. *Lakartidningen* **65**:2658–2660.

Galliland LK, Walsh LA, Frewin MR et al (1999) Elimination of immunogenicity of therapeutic antibodies. *J Immunol* **162**:3663–3671.

Gapany C, Zhao M, Zimmerman A (1997) The apoptosis protector, bcl-2 protein, is downregulated in bile duct epithelial cells in human liver allografts. *J Hepatol* **26**:535–542.

Garcia I, Martinou I, Tsujimoto Y, Martinou JC (1992) Prevention of programmed cell death of sympathetic neurons by the bcl-2 proto-oncogene. *Science* **258**:302–304.

Ghosh P, Sica A, Cippitelli M et al (1996) Activation of nuclear factor of activated T cells in a cyclosporin A-resistant pathway. *J Biol Chem* **271**:7700–7704.

Giancotti FG, Ruoslahti E (1999) Integrin signaling. *Science* **285**:1028–1032.

Glover JM, Leeds JM, Mant TG et al (1997) Phase I safety and pharmacokinetic profile of an intercellular adhesion molecule-1 antisense oligodeoxynucleotide (ISIS 2302). *J Pharmacol Exp Ther* **282**:1173–1180.

Goes N, Urmson J, Ramassar V, Halloran PF (1995) Ischemic acute tubular necrosis induces an extensive local cytokine response. Evidence for induction of interferon-gamma, transforming growth factor-β_1, granulocyte-macrophage colony-stimulating factor, interleukin-2, and interleukin-10. *Transplantation* **59**:565–572.

Gorczynski RM, Chen Z, Hoang Y, Rossi-Bergman B (1996) A subset of T-cell receptor-positive cells produce T-helper type-2 cytokines and regulate mouse skin graft rejection following portal venous pretransplant preimmunization. *Immunology* 87:381–389.

Gordon EJ, Sanders WJ, Kiessling LL (1998) Synthetic ligands point to cell surface strategies. *Nature* 392:30–31.

Grakoui A, Bromley SK, Sumen C et al (1999) The immunological synapse: a molecular machine controlling T cell activation. *Science* 285:221–226.

Greig PD, Woolf GM, Sinclair SB et al (1989) Treatment of primary liver graft nonfunction with prostaglandin E1. *Transplantation* 48:447–453.

Guinan EC, Boussiotis VA, Neuberg D et al (1999) Transplantation of anergic histoincompatible bone marrow allografts. *N Engl J Med* 340:1704–1714.

Guo Z, Chong AS, Shen J et al (1997a) Prolongation of rat islet allograft survival by the immuno-suppressive agent leflunomide. *Transplantation* 63:711–716.

Guo Z, Chong AS, Tian Y et al (1997b) Effect of leflunomide and cyclosporine on concordant xenogeneic islet transplantation in streptozotocin-induced and autoimmune diabetic mice. *Transplant Proc* 29:2155.

Hale G, Waldmann H (1994) Control of graft-versus-host disease and graft rejection by T cell depletion of donor and recipient with Campath-1 antibodies. Results of matched sibling transplants for malignant diseases. *Bone Marrow Transplant* 13:597–611.

Haller H, Dragun D, Miethke A et al (1996) Antisense oligonucleotides for ICAM-1 attenuate reperfusion injury and renal failure in the rat. *Kidney Int* 50:473–480.

Halloran PF, Batiuk TD, Goes NB, Campbell P (1995) Strategies to improve the immunologic management of organ transplants. *Clin Transplant* 9:227–236.

Hamawy MM, Tsuchida M, Manthei ER et al (1999) Activation of T lymphocytes for adhesion and cytokine expression by toxin-conjugated anti-CD3 monoclonal antibodies. *Transplantation* 68:693–698.

Harlan JM, Winn RK, Doerschuk CM et al (1992) In vivo models of leukocyte adherence to endothelium. In: Harlan JM, Liu D (eds). *Adhesion: Its Role in Inflammatory Disease*. New York: WH Freeman, p. 117.

Haug CE, Colvin RB, Delmonico FL et al (1993) A phase I trial of immunosuppression with anti-ICAM-1 (CD54) mAb in renal allograft recipients. *Transplantation* 55:766–772.

He Y, Mellon J, Apte R, Niederkorn JY (1994) Effect of LFA-1 and ICAM-1 antibody treatment on murine corneal allograft survival. *Invest Ophthalmol Vis Sci* 35:3218–3225.

Henn V, Slupsky JR, Grafe M et al (1998) CD40 ligand on activated platelets triggers an inflammatory reaction of endothelial cells. *Nature* 391:591–594.

Hernandez LA, Grisham MB, Twohig B et al (1987) Role of neutrophils in ischemia–reperfusion-induced microvascular injury. *Am J Physiol* 253:H699–H703.

Hertenstein B, Hampl W, Bunjes D et al (1995) In vivo/ex vivo T cell depletion for GVHD prophylaxis influences onset and course of active cytomegalovirus infection and disease after BMT. *Bone Marrow Transplant* 15:387–393.

Hillebrand G, Rothaug E, Hammer C et al (1989) Experience with a new monoclonal antibody in clinical kidney transplantation. *Transplant Proc* 21:1776–1777.

Himmelreich G, Hundt K, Neuhaus P et al (1993) Evidence that intraoperative prostaglandin E1 infusion reduces impaired platelet aggregation after reperfusion in orthotopic liver transplantation. *Transplantation* 55:819–826.

Hin S, Zabel C, Bianco A et al (1999) Cutting edge: N-hydroxy peptides: a new class of TCR antagonists. *J Immunol* 163:2363–2367.

Ho LJ, Chang DM, Lee TC et al (1999) Plant alkaloid tetrandrine downregulates protein kinase C-dependent signaling pathway in T cells. *Eur J Pharmacol* 367:389–398.

Horimoto H, Ito T, Hayashi T et al (1998) Transplantation tolerance by a combined therapy with sulfatide, anti-LFA-1/ICAM-1 monoclonal antibodies and FK506 in rat cardiac transplantation. *Transplant Int* 11(Suppl 1):S310–S312.

Hoshino T, Maley WR, Bulkley GB, Williams GM (1988) Ablation of free radical-mediated reperfusion injury for the salvage of kidneys taken from non-heartbeating donors. A quantitative evaluation of the proportion of injury caused by reperfusion following periods of warm, cold, and combined warm and cold ischemia. *Transplantation* 45:284–289.

Hourmant M, Le Mauff B, Le Meur Y et al (1994) Administration of an anti-CD11a monoclonal antibody in recipients of kidney transplantation: a pilot study. *Transplantation* 58:377–380.

Hourmant M, Bedrossian J, Durand D et al (1996) A randomized multicenter trial comparing leukocyte function-associated antigen-1 monoclonal antibody with rabbit antithymocyte globulin as induction treatment in first kidney transplantations. *Transplantation* 62:1565–1570.

Hower R, Minor T, Schneeberger H et al (1996) Assessment of oxygen radicals during kidney transplantation–effect of radical scavenger. *Transplant Int* 9(Suppl 1):S479–S482.

Hsu D-H, Shi JD, Homola M et al (1999) A humanized, anti-CD3 antibody, HuM291, with low mitogenic activity, mediates complete and reversible T-cell depletion in chimpanzees. *Transplantation* 68:545–554.

Hsueh YP, Liang HE, Ng SY, Lai MZ (1997) CD28-costimulation activates cyclic AMP-responsive element-binding protein in T lymphocytes. *J Immunol* 158:85–93.

Hughes DA, McLean A, Roake JA et al (1995) Free oxygen species (FOS), FOS-scavenging enzyme P-selectin and monocyte activity in cell populations aspirated from early human renal allografts. *Transplant Proc* 28:2879.

Isobe M, Yagita H, Okumura K, Ihara A (1992) Specific acceptance of cardiac allograft after treatment with anti-ICAM-1 and anti-LFA-1. *Science* 255:1125–1127.

Isobe M, Suzuki J, Yagita H et al (1994) Immunosuppression to cardiac allografts and soluble antigens by anti-vascular cellular adhesion molecule-1 and anti-very late antigen-4 monoclonal antibodies. *J Immunol* 153:5810–5818.

Jalkanen S, Bargatze RF, de los Toyos J, Butcher EC (1987) Lymphocyte recognition of high endothelium: antibodies to distinct epitopes of an 85–95-kD glycoprotein antigen differentially inhibit lymphocyte binding to lymph node, mucosal, or synovial endothelial cells. *J Cell Biol* 105:983–990.

Jameson SC, Carbone FR, Bevan MJ (1993) Clone-specific T cell receptor antagonists of major histocompatibility complex class I-restricted cytotoxic T cells. *J Exp Med* 177:1541–1550.

Jobin C, Bradham CA, Russo MP et al (1999) Curcumin blocks cytokine-mediated NF-κB activation and proinflammatory gene expression by inhibiting inhibitory factor I-κB kinase activity. *J Immunol* 163:3474–3483.

Jordan BA, Devi LA (1999) G-protein-coupled receptor hetermodimerization modulates receptor function. *Nature* 399:697–700.

Joshi AS, King SYP, Zajac BA et al (1997) Phase I safety and pharmacokinetic studies of brequinar sodium after single ascending oral doses in stable renal, hepatic and cardiac allograft recipients. *J Clin Pharmacol* 37:1121–1128.

Judge TA, Wu Z, Zheng XG et al (1999) The role of CD80, CD86, and CTLA4 in alloimmune responses and the induction of long-term allograft survival. *J Immunol* 162:1947–1951.

Jung U, Ley K (1999) Mice lacking two or all three selectins demonstrate overlapping and distinct functions for each selectin. *J Immunol* 162:6755–6762.

Kalgutkar AS, Crews BC, Rowlinson SW et al (1998) Aspirin-like molecules that covalently inactivate cyclooxygenase-2. *Science* 280:1268–1270.

Kanner SB, Grosmaire LS, Ledbetter JA, Damle NK (1993) β_2-integrin LFA-1 signaling through phospholipase C-gamma 1 activation. *Proc Natl Acad Sci USA* 90:7099–7103.

Kantele A, Zivny J, Hakkinen M et al (1999) Differential homing commitments of antigen-specific T cells after oral or parenteral immunization in humans. *J Immunol* 162:5173–5177.

Kao J, Fan YG, Haehnel I et al (1994) A peptide derived from the amino terminus of endothelial-monocyte-activating polypeptide II modulates mononuclear and polymorphonuclear leukocyte functions, defines an apparently novel cellular interaction site, and induces an acute inflammatory response. *J Biol Chem* **269**:9774–9782.

Kato Y, Yamataka A, Yagita H et al (1996) Specific acceptance of fetal bowel allograft in mice after combined treatment with anti-intercellular adhesion molecule-1 and leukocyte function-associated antigen-1 antibodies. *Ann Surg* **223**:94–100.

Kawaguchi T, Hoshino Y, Rahman F et al (1996) FTY720, a novel immunosuppressant possessing unique mechanisms. III. Synergistic prolongation of canine renal allograft survival in combination with cyclosporine A. *Transplant Proc* **28**:1062.

Kawai T, Seki M, Horimatsu K et al (1999) Selective diapedesis of Th1 cells induced by endothelial RANTES. *J Immunol* **163**:3269–3278.

Keely PJ, Westwick JK, Whitehead IP et al (1997) Cdc42 and Rac1 induce integrin-mediated cell motility and invasiveness through PI(3)K. *Nature* **390**:632–636.

Kenick S, Lowry RP, Forbes RD, Lisbona R (1987) Prolonged cardiac allograft survival following portal venous inoculation of allogeneic cells: what is 'hepatic tolerance'? *Transplant Proc* **19**:478–480.

Kevil CG, Ohno N, Gute DC et al (1998) Role of cadherin internalization in hydrogen peroxide-mediated endothelial permeability. *Free Radic Biol Med* **24**:1015–1022.

Kim JJ, Tsai A, Nottingham LK et al (1999) Intracellular adhesion molecule-1 modulates β-chemokines and directly costimulates T cells in vivo. *J Clin Invest* **103**:869–877.

Kirk AD, Harlan DM, Armstrong NN et al (1997) CTLA4-Ig and anti-CD40 ligand prevent renal allograft rejection in primates. *Proc Natl Acad Sci USA* **94**:8789–8794.

Kirk AD, Burkly LC, Batty DS et al (1999) Treatment with humanized monoclonal antibody against CD154 prevents acute renal allograft rejection in nonhuman primates. *Nat Med* **5**:686–693.

Kirken R, Erwin-Cohen R, Behbod F et al (1999) Tyrphostin AG490 blocks activation of JAK3 and rejection of heart allografts in rats (abstr 110). *25th Annual Meeting American Society of Transplant Surgeons*, May 19–21, Chicago, IL.

Kirkham BW, Thien F, Pelton BK et al (1992) Chimeric CD7 monoclonal antibody therapy in rheumatoid arthritis. *J Rheumatol* **19**:1348–1352.

Knechtle SJ, Vargo D, Fechner J et al (1997) FN-18-CRM9 immunotoxin promotes tolerance in primate renal allografts. *Transplantation* **63**:1–6.

Knechtle SJ, Fechner JH Jr, Dong Y, Stavrou S, Neville DM Jr et al (1998) Primate renal transplants using immunotoxin. *Surgery* **124**:438–447.

Knies UE, Behrensdorf HA, Mitchell CA et al (1998) Regulation of endothelial monocyte-activating polypeptide II release by apoptosis. *Proc Natl Acad Sci USA* **95**:12322–12327.

Knight RJ, Kurrle R, McClain J et al (1994) Clinical evaluation of induction immunosuppression with a murine IgG2b monoclonal antibody (BMA 031) directed toward the human α/β-T cell receptor. *Transplantation* **57**:1581–1588.

Krams SM, Egawa H, Quinn MB et al (1995) Apoptosis as a mechanism of cell death in liver allograft rejection. *Transplantation* **59**:621–625.

Krensky AM, Clayberger C (1994) The induction of tolerance to alloantigens using HLA-based synthetic peptides. *Curr Opin Immunol* **6**:791–796.

Kroemer G (1997) The proto-oncogene Bcl-2 and its role in regulating apoptosis. *Nat Med* **3**:614–20. (Erratum, *Nat Med* 1997, **3**:934.)

Lafferty KJ, Cunningham AJ (1975) A new analysis of allogeneic interactions. *Aust J Exp Biol Med Sci* **53**:27–42.

Lai J-H, Tan TH (1994) CD28 signaling causes a sustained down-regulation of IκBα which can be prevented by the immunosuppressant rapamycin. *J Biol Chem* **269**:30077–30080.

Lai J-H, Horvath G, Subleski J et al (1995) RelA is a potent transcriptional activator of the CD28 response element within the interleukin 2 promoter. *Mol Cell Biol* 15:4260–4271.

Lai J-H, Ho L-J, Kwan C-Y et al (1999) Plant alkaloid tetrandrine and its analog block CD8-stimulated activities of human peripheral blood T cells. *Transplantation* 68:1383–1392.

Lakkis FG, Konieczny BT, Saleem S et al (1997) Blocking the CD28-B7 T cell costimulation pathway induces long term cardiac allograft acceptance in the absence of IL-4. *J Immunol* 158:2443–2448.

Lampugnani MG, Resnati M, Raiteri M et al (1992) A novel endothelial-specific membrane protein is a marker of cell–cell contacts. *J Cell Biol* 118:1511–1522.

Land W, Messmer K (1996) The impact of ischemia/reperfusion injury on specific and non-specific early and late chronic events after organ transplantation. *Transplant Rev* 10:108–127.

Lappin J, Podbielski J, Welsh M et al (1998) A phase I study: the side-effect profile of an intercellular adhesion molecule-1-antisense phosphorothiote oligodeoxynucleotide, ISIS 2302 (abst). *Transplantation* 65:S63.

Larsen CP, Elwood ET, Alexander DZ et al (1996) Long-term acceptance of skin and cardiac allografts after blocking CD40 and CD28 pathways. *Nature* 381:434–438.

Lawrence MS, Ho DY, Sun GH et al (1996) Overexpression of Bcl-2 with herpes simplex virus vectors protects CNS neurons against neurological insults in vitro and in vivo. *J Neurosci* 16:486–496.

Lazarovits AI, Rochon J, Banks L et al (1993) Human mouse chimeric CD7 monoclonal antibody (SDZCHH380) for the prophylaxis of kidney transplant rejection. *J Immunol* 150:5163–5174.

Lefer DJ, Flynn DM, Phillips ML et al (1994) A novel sialyl Lewis X analog attenuates neutrophil accumulation and myocardial necrosis after ischemia and reperfusion. *Circulation* 90:2390–2401.

Lehr HA, Guhlmann A, Nolte D et al (1991) Leukotrienes as mediators in ischemia–reperfusion injury in a microcirculation model in the hamster. *J Clin Invest* 87:2036–2041.

Le Mauff B, Hourmant M, Le Meur Y et al (1995) Anti-LFA-1 adhesion molecule monoclonal antibody in prophylaxis of human kidney allograft rejection. *Transplant Proc* 27:865–866.

Le Mauff B, Le Meur Y, Hourmant M et al (1996) A dose-searching trial of an anti-LFA1 monoclonal antibody in first kidney transplant recipients. *Kidney Int* 53:S44–S50.

Leonard WJ (1996) The molecular basis of X-linked severe combined immunodeficiency: defective cytokine receptor signaling. *Ann Rev Med* 47:229–239.

Lerman A, Kubo SH, Tschumperlin LK, Burnett JC Jr (1992) Plasma endothelin concentrations in humans with end-stage heart failure and after heart transplantation. *J Am Coll Cardiol* 20:849–853.

Li XK, Okuyama T, Tamura A et al (1998) Prolonged survival of rat liver allografts transfected with Fas ligand-expressing plasmid. *Transplantation* 66:1416–1423.

Lin H, Bolling SF, Linsley PS et al (1993) Long-term acceptance of major histocompatibility complex mismatched cardiac allografts induced by CTLA4Ig plus donor-specific transfusion. *J Exp Med* 178:1801–1806.

Lindstein T, June CH, Ledbetter JA et al (1989) Regulation of lymphokine messenger RNA stability by a surface-mediated T cell activation pathway. *Science* 244:339–343.

Linsley PS, Brady W, Urnes M et al (1991) CTLA-4 is a second receptor for the B cell activation antigen B7. *J Exp Med* 174:561–569.

Lollo BA, Chan KW, Hanson EM et al (1993) Direct evidence for two affinity states for lymphocyte function-associated antigen 1 on activated T cells. *J Biol Chem* 268:21693–21700. (Erratum, *J Biol Chem* 1994, 269:10184).

Lundblad R, Giercksky KE (1995) Endothelin concentrations in experimental sepsis: profiles of big endothelin and endothelin 1-21 in lethal peritonitis in rats. *Eur J Surg* 161:9–16.

Ma XL, Tsao PS, Lefer AM (1991) Antibody to CD18 exerts endothelial and cardiac protective effects of myocardial ischemia and reperfusion. *J Clin Invest* 88:1237–1243.

Macchi P, Villa A, Giliani S et al (1995) Mutations of Jak-3 gene in patients with autosomal severe combined immune deficiency (SCID). *Nature* 377:65–68.

Mackay CR, Andrew DP, Briskin M et al (1996) Phenotype, and migration properties of three major subsets of tissue homing T cells in sheep. *Eur J Immunol* 26:2433–2439.

Maekawa M, Ishizaki T, Boku S et al (1999) Signaling from Rho to the actin cytoskeleton through protein kinases ROCK and LIM-kinase. *Science* 285:895–898.

Malissen B (1999) Dancing the immunological two-step. *Science* 285:207–208.

Mandelbrot DA, Furukawa Y, McAdam AJ et al (1999) Expression of B7 molecules in recipient, not donor, mice determines the survival of cardiac allografts. *J Immunol* 163:3753–3757.

Manna SK, Aggarwal BB (1999) Immunosuppressive leflunomide metabolite (A77 1726) blocks TNF-dependent nuclear factor-κB activation and gene expression. *J Immunol* 162:2095–2102.

Marchman W, Araneda D, DeMasi R et al (1992) Prolongation of xenograft survival after combination therapy with 15-deoxyspergualin and total-lymphoid irradiation in the hamster-to-rat cardiac xenograft model. *Transplantation* 53:30–34.

Matsuda S, Minowa A, Suzuki S, Koyasu S (1999) Differential activation of c-Jun NH2-terminal kinase and p38 pathways during FTY720-induced apoptosis of T lymphocytes that is suppressed by the extracellular signal-regulated kinase pathway. *J Immunol* 162:3321–3326.

McEver RP (1998) Leukocyte adhesion through selectins under flow. *Immunologist* 6:61.

Meiser BM, Reiter C, Reichenspurner H et al (1994) Chimeric monoclonal CD4 antibody: a novel immunosuppressant for clinical heart transplantation. *Transplantation* 58:419–423.

Mitsuoka H, Suzuki S, Sakaguchi T et al (1999) Contribution of endothelin-1 to microcirculatory impairment in total hepatic ischemia and reperfusion injury. *Transplantation* 67:514–520.

Molossi S, Clausell N, Sett S et al (1994) Effects of the TNF-α blockade and CsA in the expression of VCAM-1, ICAM-1 and fibronectin in rabbit cardiac allograft vasculopathy. *J Heart Lung Transplant* 13:84.

Moreland LW, Baumgartner SW, Schiff MH et al (1997) Treatment of rheumatoid arthritis with a recombinant human tumor necrosis factor receptor (p75)-Fc fusion protein. *N Engl J Med* 337:141–147.

Morita H, Nakamura N, Sugiura K et al (1999) Acceptance of skin allografts in pigs by portal venous injection of donor bone marrow cells. *Ann Surg* 230:114–119.

Mortellaro A, Songia S, Gnocchi P et al (1999) New immunosuppressive drug PNU156804 blocks IL-2-dependent proliferation and NK-κB and AP-1 activation. *J Immunol* 162:7102–7109

Muruve DA, Nicolson AG, Manfro RC et al (1997) Adenovirus-mediated expression of Fas ligand induces hepatic apoptosis after systemic administration and apoptosis of ex vivo-infected pancreatic islet allografts and isografts. *Hum Gene Ther* 8:955–963.

Nakakura EK, McCabe SM, Zheng B et al (1993) Potent and effective prolongation by anti-LFA-1 monoclonal antibody monotherapy of non-primary vascularized heart allograft survival in mice without T cell depletion. *Transplantation* 55:412–417.

Nakano Y, Monden M, Valdivia LA et al (1992) Permanent acceptance of liver allografts by intra-portal injection of donor spleen cells in rats. *Surgery* 111:668–676.

Neville DM Jr, Scharff J, Hu HZ et al (1985) A new reagent for the induction of T-cell depletion, anti-CD3-CRM9. *J Immunother* 2:85–92.

Ni HT, Deeths MJ, Li W et al (1999) Signaling pathways activated by leukocyte function-associated Ag-1-dependent costimulation. *J Immunol* 162:5183–5189.

Nielsen M, Kaltoft K, Nordahl M et al (1997) Constitutive activation of a slowly migrating isoform of Stat3 in mycosis fungoides: tyrphostin AG490 inhibits Stat3 activation and growth of mycosis fungoides tumor cell lines. *Proc Natl Acad Sci USA* 94:6764–6769.

Nishihara M, Gotoh M, Fukuzaki T et al (1995) Potent immunosuppressive effect of anti-LFA-1 monoclonal antibody on islet allograft rejection. *Transplant Proc* 27:372.

Nogae S, Miyazaki M, Kobayashi N et al (1998) Induction of apoptosis in ischemia–reperfusion model of mouse kidney: possible involvement of Fas. *J Am Soc Nephrol* 9:620–631.

Nolte D, Hecht R, Schmid P et al (1994) Role of Mac-1 and ICAM-1 in ischemia–reperfusion injury in a microcirculation model of BALB/C mice. *Am J Physiol* 267:H1320–H1328.

Norman DJ, Bennett WM, Cobanoglu A et al (1993) Use of OKT4A (a murine monoclonal anti-CD4 antibody) in human organ transplantation: initial clinical experience. *Transplant Proc* 25:802–803.

Okada K, Nishida Y, Murakami H et al (1998a) Role of endogenous endothelin in the development of graft arteriosclerosis in rat cardiac allografts: antiproliferative effects of bosentan, a nonselective endothelin receptor antagonist. *Circulation* 97:2346–2351.

Okada Y, Marchevsky AM, Kass RM, Matloff JM, Jordan SC (1998b) A stable prostacyclin analog, beraprost sodium, attenuates platelet accumulation and preservation-reperfusion injury of isografts in a rat model of lung transplantation. *Transplantation* 66:1132–1136.

Okubo M, Tamura K, Kamata K et al (1993) 15-Deoxyspergualin 'rescue therapy' for methylprednisolone-resistant rejection of renal transplants as compared with anti-T cell monoclonal antibody (OKT3). *Transplantation* 55:505–508.

Oppenheimer-Marks N, Lipsky PE (1993) The adhesion and trans-endothelial migration of human T-lymphocytes subsets. *Behring Inst Mitt* 92:44.

Ozes ON, Mayo LD, Gustin JA et al (1999) NF-κB activation by tumour necrosis factor requires the Akt serine-threonine kinase. *Nature* 401:82–85.

Palma-Vargas JM, Toledo-Pereya L, Dean RE et al (1997) Small-molecule selectin inhibitor protects against liver inflammatory response after ischemia and reperfusion. *J Am Coll Surg* 185:365.

Paul LC, Davidoff A, Benediktsson H, Issekutz T (1996) Anti-integrin (LFA-1, VLA-4, and Mac-1) antibody treatment and acute cardiac graft rejection in the rat. *Transpl Int* 9:420–425.

Penkewycz O, Mackie J, Hassarjian R et al (1989) Interleukin-2-diptheria toxin fusion protein prolongs murine islet cell engraftment. *Transplantation* 47:318–322.

Pérez-Melgosa M, Hollenbaugh D, Wilson CB (1999) Cutting edge: CD40 ligand is a limiting factor in the humoral response to T cell-dependent antigens. *J Immunol* 163:1123–1127.

Peterson LB, Cryan JG, Rosa R et al (1998) A tacrolimus-related immunosuppressant with biochemical properties distinct from those of tacrolimus. *Transplantation* 65:10–18.

Picker LJ, Kishimoto TK, Smith CW et al (1991) ELAM-1 is an adhesion molecule for skin-homing T cells. *Nature* 349:796–799.

Pober JS, Cotran RS (1990) Cytokines and endothelial cell biology. *Physiol Rev* 70:427–451.

Poston RS, Mann MJ, Hoyt EG et al (1999) Antisense oligodeoxynucleotides prevent acute cardiac allograft rejection via a novel, nontoxic, highly efficient transfection method. *Transplantation* 68:825–832.

Pratschke J, Wilhelm MJ, Kusaka M et al (1999) Brain death and its influence on donor organ quality and outcome after transplantation. *Transplantation* 67:343–348.

Preckel T, Grimm R, Martin S, Weltzien HU (1997) Altered hapten ligands antagonize trinitrophenyl-specific cytotoxic T cells and block internalization of hapten-specific receptors. *J Exp Med* 185:1803–1813.

Punch JD, Lin J, Bluestone J, Bromberg JS (1999) CD2 and CD3 receptor-mediated tolerance. *Transplantation* 67:741–748.

Qin L, Chavin KD, Ding Y et al (1996) Retrovirus-mediated transfer of viral IL-10 gene prolongs murine cardiac allograft survival. *J Immunol* 156:2316–2323.

Raafat AM, Murray MT, McGuire T et al (1997) Calcium blockade reduces renal apoptosis during ischemia reperfusion. *Shock* 8:186–192.

Rabin RL, Park MK, Liao F et al (1999) Chemokine receptor responses on T cells are achieved through regulation of both receptor expression and signaling. *J Immunol* 162:3840–3850.

Rabkin DG, Jia C-X, Spotnitz HM (1999) Attenuation of reperfusion injury with probucol in the heterotopic rat cardiac isograft. *J Heart Lung Transplant* **18**:775–780.

Rabl H, Khoschsorur G, Colombo T et al (1992) Human plasma lipid peroxide levels show a strong transient increase after successful revascularization operations. *Free Radic Biol Med* **13**:281–288.

Räisänen-Sokolowski A, Glysing-Jensen T, Russell ME (1999) Donor and recipient contributions of ICAM-1 and P-selectin in parenchymal rejection and graft arteriosclerosis: insights from double knockout mice. *J Heart Lung Transplant* **18**:735–743.

Rebello PR, Hale G, Friend PJ et al (1999) Anti-globulin responses to rat and humanized campath-1 monoclonal antibody used to treat transplant rejection. *Transplantation* **68**:1417–1420.

Rosenberg RD, Aird WC (1999) Vascular-bed-specific hemostasis and hypercoagulable states. *N Engl J Med* **350**:1555–1564.

Rovere P, Vallinoto C, Bondanza A et al (1998) Bystander apoptosis triggers dendritic cell maturation and antigen-presenting function. *J Immunol* **161**:4467–4471.

Sugamura K, Asao H, Kondo M et al (1996) The interleukin-2 receptor gamma chain: its role in the multiple cytokine receptor complexes and T cell development in XSCID. *Annu Rev Immunol* **14**:179–205.

Salducci MD, Chauvet-Monges AM, Tillement JP et al (1996) Trimetazidine reverses calcium accumulation and impairment of phosphorylation induced by cyclosporine A in isolated rat liver mitochondria. *J Pharmacol Exp Ther* **277**:417–422.

Salerno CT, Park SJ, Kreykes NS et al (1999) Adjuvant treatment of refractory lung transplant rejection with extracorporeal photopheresis. *J Thorac Cardiovasc Surg* **117**:1063–1069.

Salmela K, Wramner L, Ekberg H et al (1999) A randomized multicenter trial of the anti-ICAM-1 monoclonal antibody (enlimomab) for the prevention of acute rejection and delayed onset of graft function in cadaveric renal transplantation. *Transplantation* **67**:729–736.

Salmi M, Hellman J, Jalkanen S (1998) The role of two distinct endothelial molecules, vascular adhesion protein-1 and peripheral lymph node addressin, in the binding of lymphocyte subsets to human lymph nodes. *J Immunol* **160**:5629–5636.

Salomon B, Bluestone JA (1998) Cutting edge: LFA-1 interaction with ICAM-1 and ICAM-2 regulates Th2 cytokine production. *J Immunol* **161**:5138–5142.

Santamaria Babi LF, Picker LJ, Perez Soler MT et al (1995) Circulating allergen-reactive T cells from patients with atopic dermatitis and allergic contact dermatitis express the skin-selective homing receptor, the cutaneous lymphocyte-associated antigen. *J Exp Med* **181**:1935–1940.

Sayegh MH, Turka LA (1998) The role of T-cell costimulatory activation pathways in transplant rejection. *N Engl J Med* **338**:1813–1821.

Sayegh MH, Akalin E, Hancock WW et al (1995) CD28-B7 blockade after alloantigenic challenge in vivo inhibits Th1 cytokines but spares Th2. *J Exp Med* **181**:1869–1874.

Schmid C, Heemann U, Tilney NL (1997) Factors contributing to the development of chronic rejection in heterotopic rat heart transplantation. *Transplantation* **64**:222–228.

Schneeberger H, Illner WD, Abendroth D et al (1989) First clinical experiences with superoxide dismutase in kidney transplantation: results of a double-blind randomized study. *Transplant Proc* **21**:1245–1246.

Schulze-Osthoff K, Bakker AC, Vanhaesenbroeck B et al (1992) Cytotoxic activity of tumor necrosis factor is mediated by early damage of mitochondrial functions: evidence for the involvement of mitochondrial radical generation. *J Biol Chem* **267**:5713–5723.

Schwarze SR, Ho A, Vocero-Akbani A, Dowdy SF (1999) In vivo protein transduction: delivery of a biologically active protein into the mouse. *Science* **285**:1569–1572.

Shimazaki K, Ishida A, Kawai N (1994) Increase in bcl-2 oncoprotein and the tolerance to ischemia-induced neuronal death in the gerbil hippocampus. *Neurosci Res* **20**:95–99.

Shimizu C, Li X, Kimura M et al (1998) A novel immunosuppressant, FTY720, increases the efficiency of a superantigen-induced peripheral T-cell deletion whilst inhibiting negative selection in the thymus. *Immunology* 94:503–512.

Shinomiya T, Li X-K, Amemiya H, Suzuki S (1997) An immunosuppressive agent, FTY720, increases intracellular concentration of calcium ion and induces apoptosis of HL-60. *Immunology* 91:594–600.

Sigal NH, Dumont F, Durette P et al (1991) Is cyclophilin involved in the immunosuppressive and nephrotoxic mechanism of action of cyclosporin A? *J Exp Med* 173:619–628.

Simon SI, Cherapanov V, Nadra I et al (1999) Signaling functions of L-selectin in neutrophils: alterations in the cytoskeleton and colocalization with CD18. *J Immunol* 63:2891–2901.

Simpson PJ, Todd RF III, Fantone JC et al (1988) Reduction of experimental canine myocardial reperfusion injury by a monoclonal antibody (anti-Mo1, anti-CD11b) that inhibits leukocyte adhesion. *J Clin Invest* 81:624–629.

Sloan-Lancaster J, Shaw AS, Rothbard JB, Allen PM (1994) Partial T cell signaling: altered phospho-zeta and lack of Zap70 recruitment in APL-induced T cell anergy. *Cell* 79:913–922.

Smely S, Weschka M, Hillebrand G et al (1990) Prophylactic use of the new monoclonal antibody BMA 031 in clinical kidney transplantation. *Transplant Proc* 22:1785–1786.

Smith JA, Tong Q, Bluestone JA (1998) Partial TCR signals delivered by FcR-nonbinding anti-CD3 monoclonal antibodies differentially regulate individual Th subsets. *J Immunol* 160:4841–4849.

Smith RM, Chen ZK, Foulkes R et al (1997) Prolongation of murine vascularized heart allografts survival by recipient-specific anti-major histocompatibility complex class II antibody. *Transplantation* 64:525–528.

Snapp KR, Ding II, Atkins K et al (1998) A novel P-selectin glycoprotein ligand-1 monoclonal antibody recognizes an epitope within the tyrosine sulfate motif of human PSGL-1 and blocks recognition of both P- and L- selectin. *Blood* 91:154.

Springer TA (1994) Traffic signals for lymphocyte recirculation and leukocyte emigration: the multistep paradigm. *Cell* 76:301–314.

Springer TA, Dustin ML, Kishimoto TK, Marlin SD (1987) The lymphocyte function-associated LFA-1, CD2, and LFA-3 molecules: cell adhesion receptors of the immune system. *Ann Rev Immunol* 5:223–252.

Squifflet J-P, Besse T, Malaise J et al (1997) BTI-322 for induction therapy after renal transplantation: a randomized study. *Transplant Proc* 29:317–319.

Steeber DA, Green NE, Sato S, Tedder TF (1996) Lymphocyte migration in L-selectin-deficient mice. Altered subset migration and aging of the immune system. *J Immunol* 157:1096–1106.

Steeber DA, Tang MLK, Green NE et al (1999) Leukocyte entry into sites of inflammation requires overlapping interactions between the L-selectin and ICAM-1 pathways. *J Immunol* 163:2176–2186.

Stepkowski SM, Yu T, Chou T-C, Kahan BD (1994) Synergistic interaction of cyclosporine, rapamycin, and brequinar on cardiac allograft survival in mice. *Transplant Proc* 26:3025–3027.

Stepkowski SM, Wang ME, Amante A et al (1998a) ICAM-1 antisense oligodeoxynucleotide blocks kidney allograft rejection in cynomolgus monkeys (abst). *XVII Annual Meeting of the American Society of Transplant Physicians*, May 9–13, 1998, Chicago, IL.

Stepkowski SM, Wang ME, Condon TP et al (1998b) Protection against allograft rejection with ICAM-1 antisense oligodeoxynucleotides. *Transplantation* 66:699–707.

Su B, Jacinto E, Hibi M et al (1994) JNK is involved in signal integration during costimulation of T lymphocytes. *Cell* 77:727–736.

Suda T, Takahashi T, Golstein P, Nagata S (1993) Molecular cloning and expression of the Fas ligand, a novel member of the tumor necrosis factor family. *Cell* 75:1169–1178.

Suzuki S, Enosawa S, Kakefuda T et al (1996a) Long-term graft acceptance in allografted rats and dogs by treatment with a novel immunosuppressant, FTY720. *Transplant Proc* 28:1375.

Suzuki S, Enosawa S, Kakefuda T et al (1996b) A novel immunosuppressant, FTY720, with a unique mechanism of action, induces long-term graft acceptance in rat and dog allotransplantation. *Transplantation* **61**:200–205.

Suzuki S, Li X-K, Shinomiya T et al (1997) The in vivo induction of lymphocyte apoptosis in MRL-lpr/lpr mice treated with FTY720. *Clin Exp Immunol* **107**:103–111.

Takada M, Nadeau KC, Hancock WW et al (1998) Effects of explosive brain death on cytokine activation of peripheral organs in the rat. *Transplantation* **65**:1533–1542.

Talento A, Nguyen M, Blake T et al (1993) A single administration of LFA-1 antibody confers prolonged allograft survival. *Transplantation* **55**:418–422.

Taylor PM, Rose ML, Yacoub MH, Pigott R (1992) Induction of vascular adhesion molecules during rejection of human cardiac allografts. *Transplantation* **54**:451–457.

Thomis DC, Berg LJ (1997) The role of Jak3 in lymphoid development, activation, and signaling. *Curr Opin Immunol* **9**:541–547.

Thommesen L, Sjursen W, Gasvik K et al (1998) Selective inhibitors of cytosolic or secretory phospholipase A$_2$ block TNF-induced activation of transcription factor nuclear factor-κB and expression of ICAM-1. *J Immunol* **161**:3421–3430.

Tibbetts SA, Chirathaworn C, Nakashima M et al (1999) Peptides derived from ICAM-1 and LFA-1 modulate T cell adhesion and immune function in a mixed lymphocyte culture. *Transplantation* **68**:685–692.

Tojo SJ, Yokota S, Koike H et al (1996) Reduction of rat myocardial ischemia and reperfusion injury by sialyl Lewis X oligosaccharide and anti-rat P-selectin antibodies. *Glycobiology* **6**:463–469.

Trocha SD, Kevil CG, Mancini MC, Alexander JS (1999) Organ preservation solutions increase endothelial permeability and promote loss of junctional proteins. *Ann Surg* **230**:105–113.

Troncoso P, Stepkowski SM, Wang ME et al (1999) Prophylaxis of acute renal allograft rejection using FTY720 in combination with subtherapeutic doses of cyclosporine. *Transplantation* **67**:145–151.

Troppmann C, Gillingham KJ, Benedetti E et al (1995) Delayed graft function, acute rejection, and outcome after cadaver renal transplantation. The multivariate analysis. *Transplantation* **59**:962–968.

Turunen JP, Paavonen T, Majuri ML et al (1994) Sialyl Lewis(x)- and L-selectin-dependent site-specific lymphocyte extravasation into renal transplants during acute rejection. *Eur J Immunol* **24**:1130–1136.

Uckan D, Steele A, Cherry et al (1997) Trophoblasts express Fas ligand: a proposed mechanism for immune privilege in placenta and maternal invasion. *Mol Hum Reprod* **3**:655–662.

Utku N, Heinemann T, Tullius SG et al (1998) Prevention of acute allograft rejection by antibody targeting of TIRC7, a novel T cell membrane protein. *Immunity* **9**:509–518.

van der Lubbe PA, Reiter C, Miltenburg AM et al (1994) Treatment of rheumatoid arthritis with a chimeric CD4 monoclonal antibody (cM-T412): immunopharmacological aspects and mechanisms of action. *Scand J Immunol* **39**:286–294.

van Dijken PJ, Ghayur T, Mauch P et al (1990) Evidence that anti-LFA-1 in vivo improves engraftment and survival after allogeneic bone marrow transplantation. *Transplantation* **49**:882–886.

Van Seventer GA, Shimizu Y, Horgan KJ, Shaw S (1990) The LFA-1 ligand ICAM-1 provides an important costimulatory signal for T cell receptor-mediated activation of resting T cells. *J Immunol* **144**:4579–4586.

Van Seventer GA, Bonvini E, Yamada H et al (1992) Costimulation of T cell receptor/CD3-mediated activation of resting human CD4$^+$ T cells by leukocyte function-associated antigen-1 ligand intercellular cell adhesion molecule-1 involves prolonged inositol phospholipid hydrolysis and sustained increase of intracellular Ca^{2+} levels. *J Immunol* **149**:3872–3880.

Vedder NB, Winn RK, Rice CL et al (1990) Inhibition of leukocyte adherence by anti-CD18 monoclonal antibody attenuates reperfusion injury in the rabbit ear. *Proc Natl Acad Sci USA* 87:2643–2646.

Viebahn R, Schmidt M, Prolap R et al (1995) ICAM and MHC are upregulated after reperfusion injury: immunohistological study in 20 human liver transplants (abst). *VII Congress ESOT.* October 1995, Vienna, Austria.

Waid TH, Lucas BA, Thompson JS et al (1997a) Treatment of renal allograft rejection with T10B9.1A31 or OKT3: final analysis of a phase II clinical trial. *Transplantation* 64:274–281.

Waid TH, Thompson JS, McKeown JW et al (1997b) Induction immunotherapy in heart transplantation with T10B9.1A-31: a phase I study. *J Heart Lung Transplant* 16:913–916.

Wang LH, Kirken RA, Erwin RA et al (1999a) JAK3, STAT, and MAPK signaling pathways as novel molecular targets for the tyrphostin AG-490 regulation of IL-2-mediated T cell response. *J Immunol* 162:3897–3904.

Wang ME, Stepkowski SM, Ferraresso M, Kahan BD (1992) Evidence that rapamycin rescue therapy delays rejection of major (MHC) plus minor (non-MHC) histoincompatible heart allografts in rats. *Transplantation* 54:704–709.

Wang M, Stepkowski SM, Yu J et al (1997) Localization of cryptic tolerogenic epitopes in the α_1 helical region of the RT1.A^u alloantigen. *Transplantation* 63:1373–1379.

Wang ME, Tejpal N, Qu X et al (1998) Immunosuppressive effects of FTY720 alone or in combination with cyclosporine or sirolimus. *Transplantation* 65:899–905.

Wang ME, Kirken R, Behbod F et al (1999b) Inhibition of JAK3 tyrosine kinase by PNU 15804 blocks heart allograft rejection (abst 465). *American Society of Transplantation 18th Annual Scientific Meeting*, May 15–19, Chicago, Il.

Watschinger B, Sayegh MH, Hancock WW, Russell ME (1995) Upregulation of endothelin-1 mRNA and peptide expression in rat cardiac allografts with rejection and arteriosclerosis. *Am J Pathol* 146:1065–1072.

Wee S, Pascual M, Eason JD et al (1997) Biological effects and fate of a soluble, dimeric, 80-kDa tumor necrosis factor receptor in renal transplant recipients who receive OKT3 therapy. *Transplantation* 63:570–577.

Wennberg L, Karlsson-Parra A, Sundberg B et al (1997) Efficacy of immunosuppressive drugs in islet xenotransplantation: leflunomide in combination with cyclosporine and mycophenolate mofetil prevents islet xenograft rejection in the pig-to-rat model. *Transplantation* 63:1234–1242.

Werther WA, Gonzalez TN, O'Connor SJ et al (1996) Humanization of an anti-lymphocyte function-associated antigen (LFA)-1 monoclonal antibody and reengineering of the humanized antibody for binding to rhesus LFA-1. *J Immunol* 157:4986–4995.

White E (1996) Life, death, and the pursuit of apoptosis. *Genes Dev* 10:1–15.

Willems F, Marchant A, Delville JP et al (1994) Interleukin-10 inhibits B7 and intercellular adhesion molecule-1 expression on human monocytes. *Eur J Immunol* 24:1007–1009.

Williams GM (1990) Quantitation of free radical-mediated reperfusion injury in renal transplantation. *Methods Enzymol* 186:748–751.

Williams JW, Xiao F, Foster P et al (1994) Leflunomide in experimental transplantation. Control of rejection and alloantibody production, reversal of acute rejection, and interaction with cyclosporine. *Transplantation* 57:1223–1231.

Williams MB, Butcher EC (1997) Homing of naive and memory T lymphocyte subsets to Peyer's patches, lymph nodes, and spleen. *J Immunol* 159:1746–1752.

Woodle ES, Xu D, Zivin RA et al (1999) Phase I trial of a humanized, Fc receptor nonbinding OKT3 antibody, huOKT3γ1(Ala-Ala) in the treatment of acute renal allograft rejection. *Transplantation* 68:608–616.

Woodward JE, Bayer AL, Chavin KD et al (1998) T-cell alterations in cardiac allograft recipients after B7 (CD80 and CD86) blockade. *Transplantation* 66:14–20.

Yamazaki S, Isobe M, Suzuki J-I et al (1998) Role of selectin-dependent adhesion in cardiac allograft rejection. *J Heart Lung Transplant* 17:1007–1016.

Yanagawa Y, Sugahara K, Kataoka H et al (1998) FTY720, a novel immunosuppressant, induces sequestration of circulating mature lymphocytes by acceleration of lymphocyte homing in rats: II. FTY720 prolongs skin allograft survival by decreasing T cell infiltration into grafts but not cytokine production in vivo. *J Immunol* 160:5493.

Yanagisawa M, Masaki T (1989) Molecular biology and biochemistry of the endothelins. *Trends Pharmacol Sci* 10:374–378.

Yang Z, Rostami S, Koeberlein B et al (1999) Cardiac allograft tolerance induced by intra-arterial infusion of recombinant adenoviral CTLA4Ig. *Transplantation* 67:1517–1523.

Yellin MJ, Brett J, Baum D et al (1995) Functional interactions of T cells with endothelial cells: the role of CD40L-CD40 mediated signals. *J Exp Med* 182:1857–1864.

Yin D-P, Sankary HN, Tailor-Edwards C et al (1998a) Anti-CD4 therapy in combined heart–kidney, heart–liver, and heart–small bowel allotransplants in high-responder rats. *Transplantation* 66:1–5.

Yin MJ, Yamamoto Y, Gaynor RB (1998b) The anti-inflammatory agents aspirin and salicylate inhibit the activity of I(κ)B kinase-β. *Nature* 396:77–80.

Yoshimura N, Matsui S, Hamashima T et al (1990) The effects of perioperative portal venous inoculation with donor lymphocytes on renal allograft survival in the rat. I. Specific prolongation of donor grafts and suppressor factor in the serum. *Transplantation* 49:167–171.

Yuh DD, Morris RE (1993) The immunopharmacology of immunosuppression by 15-deoxyspergualin. *Transplantation* 55:578–591.

Yuh DD, Gandy KL, Morris RE et al (1995) Leflunomide prolongs pulmonary allograft and xenograft survival. *J Heart Lung Transplant* 14:1136–1144.

Yuzawa K, Otsuka M, Taniguchi H et al (1998) An effect of FTY720 on acute rejection in canine renal transplantation. *Transplant Proc* 30:1046.

Zager RA, Iwata M, Conrad DS et al (1997) Altered ceramide and sphingosine expression during the induction phase of ischemic acute renal failure. *Kidney Int* 52:60–70.

Zamora CA, Baron DA, Heffner JE (1993) Thromboxane contributes to pulmonary hypertension in ischemia–reperfusion lung injury. *J Appl Physiol* 74:224–229.

Zheng XX, Steele AW, Hancock WW et al (1999) IL-2 receptor-targeted cytolytic IL-2/Fc fusion protein treatment blocks diabetogenic autoimmunity in nonobese diabetic mice. *J Immunol* 163:4041–4048.

Zhou L, Stordeur P, de Lavareille A et al (1998) CD40 engagement on endothelial cells promotes tissue factor-dependent procoagulant activity. *Thromb Haemost* 79:1025–1028.

Zuckerman LA, Pullen L, Miller J (1998) Functional consequences of costimulation by ICAM-1 on IL-2 gene expression and T cell activation. *J Immunol* 160:3259–3268.

11 REJECTION AND OTHER RENAL COMPLICATIONS

In collaboration with A Tarantino[*]

REJECTION

The nature of alloantigen disparity between recipient and donor is considered a barrier to engraftment. The recipient responds to this challenge by mounting an immune response involving both the cellular (T cell) and humoral (B cell) arms of the immune response (see Chapter 2). There are three main patterns of rejection diagnosed on the basis of time of onset, pathogenetic mechanisms (humoral or cellular immunity), clinical and histologic features: hyperacute, acute, and chronic.

Hyperacute rejection

Hyperacute rejection is the term used to describe an irreversible antibody-mediated rejection that generally occurs within minutes or hours after transplantation. It is initiated by alloantibodies present in the serum of the recipient at the time of transplantation and produced by previous pregnancies, blood transfusions or renal allografts. Graft is damaged by the binding of these alloantibodies to donor endothelium and by complement activation.

Hyperacute rejection is very rare nowadays because a crossmatch between the serum of the recipient and the lymphocytes of the donors is regularly performed before transplantation. The modern crossmatching techniques, such as flow-cytometry crossmatch, are capable of revealing even a low grade of immunization.

In its typical form, hyperacute rejection may be recognized by the surgeon in the operating theatre. Immediately following the completion of vascular anastomoses or a few minutes later, the graft appears flaccid and blue, instead of having the normal firm pink appearance. There is no urine formation. At histology, the most striking features are seen in the small vessels (Figure 11.1). At an early stage there is intense engorgement affecting both glomerular and peritubular capillaries with clumping of red blood cells. These changes rapidly involve the small arteries, in particular the afferent glomerular arterioles. Somewhat later, interstitial hemorrhages are seen most markedly at the corticomedullary junction, while there is infiltration of neutrophils. After 24 hours or more, tubular necrosis, thrombosis and fibrinoid necrosis of small vessels with complete cortical necrosis can be seen.

*Division of Nephrology, Ospedale Maggiore, Milan

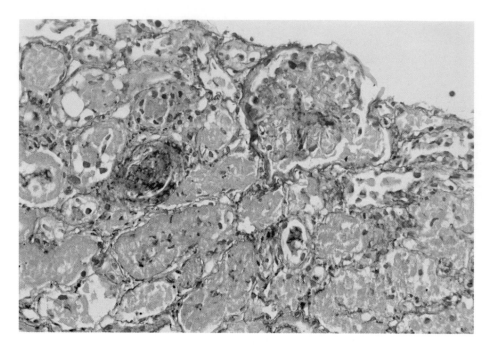

Figure 11.1. Complete necrosis and thrombosis of a small preglomerular arteriole and glomerular thrombosis characterize severe vascular ('accelerated') rejection. (AFOG ×160)

Differential diagnosis

Hyperacute rejection must be distinguished from acute tubular necrosis (ATN), thrombosis of renal artery or vein, ureteric obstruction or disruption. Investigations should include a perfusion scan, an echo-color Doppler and an angiogram if necessary. A decrease in the platelet count or an increase in fibrinogen degradation products may support the diagnosis of hyperacute rejection, but these findings may also be seen in cyclosporine (CsA) or tacrolimus-induced hemolytic uremic sindrome. Graft biopsy can confirm the diagnosis of hyperacute rejection. A repeat crossmatch may be performed after graft nephrectomy to confirm the diagnosis.

Therapy

There is no effective therapy for hyperacute rejection. Graft nephrectomy may be mandatory when severe systemic toxicity from necrotic renal tissue and consumption coagulopathy develop. Some trials have been conducted in order to prevent hyperacute rejection in highly sensitized patients. Plasma exchange or immunoadsorption can reduce the concentration of panel-reactive antibodies so that there is a window of time (weeks or months) during which a kidney with negative crossmatch might be found

(Taube et al 1984; Ross et al 1993; Reisaeter et al 1995; Higgins et al 1996). Another approach consists of the removal of antiHLA antibodies by one-shot immunoadsorption immediately before transplantation after identification of a suitable cadaver kidney. The potential advantage of this approach is the reduction of infection when compared to prolonged plasma exchanges or immunoadsorption.

Acute rejection

Despite improved immunosuppression acute rejection still remains a major obstacle for the success of renal transplantation. Acute rejection is particularly frequent in the early posttransplant period but it can occur at any time, even after years of immunological quiescence. The immunobiology of acute rejection is described in detail in Chapter 2.

Clinical diagnosis

The typical presentation of acute rejection is characterized by fever, graft tenderness, oliguria and proteinuria. However, these findings are not specific at all and are becoming more and more rare after the advent of cyclosporine (CsA) and other new powerful immunosuppressants. In clinical practice, an acute rejection is suspected whenever there is an acute graft dysfunction, which is usually detected by a rapid increase in plasma creatinine. How much plasma creatinine should increase to diagnose rejection is still controversial, however. Some clinicians consider diagnostic an absolute increase in plasma creatinine of 0.3 mg/dl or more. Such an approach exposes the patient to the risk of an overdiagnosis in the case of elevated basal levels of plasma creatinine. Looking at a percentage increase in plasma creatinine is probably more correct. However, a mild increase can give a good sensitivity but a poor specificity while a large increase may offer a good specificity but a poor sensitivity. Considering the elevated coefficient of variability of plasma creatinine, which may also expose the patient to the risk of an incorrect diagnosis, a percentage increase of 30% over the baseline may be considered as a reasonable compromise (Ponticelli and Campise 1997). It has to be pointed out, however, that many rejections may not show relevant clinical or biochemical abnormalities and may be difficult to recognize by renal biopsy (Rush et al 1999).

Another major problem is that a number of causes other than rejection can produce an increase in plasma creatinine (Table 11.1).

A number of immunological tests have been proposed for early confirmation of acute rejection. But these tests are either expensive or time-consuming or have low sensitivity or specificity. Enzymuria, lymphocyturia, dosage of coagulation proteins, amyloid A, β2 microglobulins, neopterin, thromboxane α2 and C-reactive protein have also been proposed but have not been adopted in clinical practice, because of the possibility of false results. As there is no specific noninvasive test confirmatory of acute rejection, the clinical diagnosis mainly rests on the exclusion of other causes of graft dysfunction.

Noninvasive imaging is helpful in this setting. Ultrasonography, echo-color Doppler,

Laboratory errors (double check!)
Drugs (trimethoprim, flucytosine, vitamin C)
Acute rejection
Volume depletion
Tubular necrosis
Lymphocele
Urine tract obstruction
Urine extravasation
Vascular occlusion
Infection
Cyclosporine/tacrolimus
Other nephrotoxic drugs
Chronic rejection
Recurrent primary disease

Table 11.1.   Causes of increases in plasma creatinine

and/or radionuclide imaging can detect the presence of lymphocele or urological complications and can give information on the vascularization and viability of the allograft. In spite of initial enthusiasm, the value of noninvasive imaging for a confirmatory diagnosis of acute rejection is questionable (Perrella et al 1990; Tublin and Dodd 1995), as the sensitivity and the specificity of findings suggesting acute rejection are relatively poor (Table 11.2). A number of clinicians feel that while imaging techniques are very important for assessing whether the allograft is viable and for diagnosing urological and/or vascular complications, they provide information little better than that obtained by careful clinical observation for the diagnosis of acute rejection.

The differential diagnosis between acute rejection and toxicity caused by calcineurin inhibitors may be difficult. Some clinical data may orientate the diagnosis, but in the more difficult cases a renal biopsy may be needed. Even more difficult can be the clinical diagnosis when an increase in plasma creatinine occurs months or years after transplantation. In late acute rejection the increase in plasma creatinine is usually slow and is not associated with other clinical findings with the possible exception of proteinuria and hypertension. Late acute rejection should be suspected if a patient is poorly compliant or if immunosuppression was reduced days or weeks before the increase in plasma creatinine. In the other cases the differential diagnosis between chronic rejection, toxicity of CsA or tacrolimus, and, recurrence of glomerulonephritis is very difficult. Finally, a clinical diagnosis of acute rejection is almost impossible in the case of posttransplant anuria. In these instances and whenever there is an unexpected response to the adopted therapeutic measures, invasive procedures, fine needle aspiration or renal biopsy are required.

Fine needle aspiration biopsy (FNAB) is performed by the introduction of a

Ultrasonography
   Renal enlargement
   Increased cortical thickness
   Hyper–hypoechogenicity of renal cortex
   Loss of corticomedullary differentiation
   Prominent pyramids
   Collecting system thickening
   Effacement of the central sinus echocomplex
   Gray scale

Duplex Doppler sonography
   Elevated pulsatily index (high resistance) ($\geq$0.72? $\geq$0.90?)
   Grade of renal vascularization

Renal scintigraphy
   Delayed or decreased DTPA perfusion and o-iodohippurate excretion

Table 11.2. Findings that might support the diagnosis of acute rejection with imaging techniques. The sensitivity and specificity as well as the predictive value of these findings are usually low

Lymphoblasts	1.0
Monoblasts	1.0
Macrophages	1.0
Plasmablasts	1.0
Activated lymphocytes	0.5
Large granular lymphocytes	0.2
Other lymphocytes	0.1
Polymorphonuclear cells	0.1

Table 11.3. The corrected increment with FNBA is obtained by summing the scores of white blood cells found in graft aspiration after subtraction of WBC from blood. The higher the corrected increment the higher the immunological activation (Häyry 1989)

25-gauge lumbar-puncture needle with stylet and a transparent hub into the renal cortex. After removal of the stylet and its replacement with a syringe renal tissue is aspirated. A sample of blood is obtained from the fingertip. Fine needle aspiration biopsy allows recognition of both parenchymal cells and white blood cells (WBC) infiltrating the kidney. The study of tubular cells may show necrosis (acute tubular necrosis) or vacuolization (CsA toxicity). The number of WBC remaining after subtraction from blood WBC would express the degree of immunological activity (Table 11.3). While FNAB is reliable in the case of cellular acute rejection (Manfro et al 1995), the technique is of little help in the case of vascular acute rejection (Häyry 1989). Moreover it has little sensitivity and specificity in the cases of tubular necrosis and CsA toxicity (Delaney et al 1993).

Renal biopsy remains the cornerstone for a correct diagnosis of intragraft events.

Pathology of acute rejection

Renal biopsy is helpful not only for a correct diagnosis but also for assessing the prognosis and for establishing the treatment of acute rejection. Obviously the sample of kidney tissue should be adequate. One artery with endothelialitis is sufficient for the diagnosis of acute rejection, but a portion of cortex with minimal infiltrate does not exclude acute rejection even if many glomeruli are present. Medulla alone is insufficient for a correct diagnosis. Finally, subcapsular specimens, which usually show inflammation and fibrosis, are not useful (Colvin 1996).

The typical histological features in acute rejection are a pleiomorphic interstitial infiltrate of mononuclear cells, associated with interstitial edema and a variable amount of hemorrhage (Figures 11.2 and 11.3). The infiltrating cells are mainly represented by T cells. CD8$^+$ cells are predominant in the renal cortex, while CD4$^+$ are more numerous in perivascular aggregates (Tuazon et al 1987). Macrophages are often present, sometimes predominant. Mononuclear cells invade tubules and insinuate between tubular epithelial cells. This 'tubulitis' (Figure 11.4) has been regarded as a reliable marker of

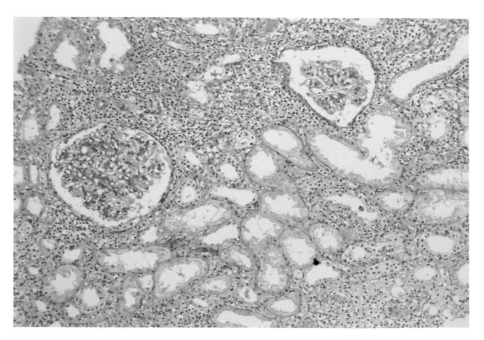

Figure 11.2. Acute cellular rejection. A dense and diffuse infiltrate of mononuclear cells occupies the interstitial space and focally invades tubular structures. (PAS ×160).

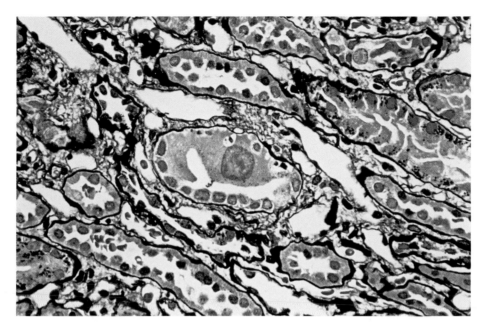

Figure 11.3. Peritubular capillary congestion and focal erythrocyte extravasation into the interstitium may accompany severe cellular rejection. (AFOG ×250)

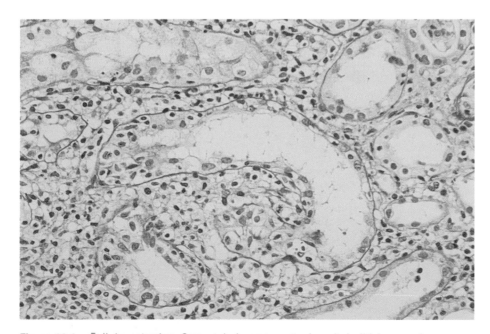

Figure 11.4. Cellular rejection. Some tubular segments show 'tubulitis'; several inflammatory mononuclear cells have crossed the tubular basement membrane and lie beneath epithelial cells (arrows). (PAS ×400)

acute rejection (Solez et al 1993), although it can be seen even in other forms of acute interstitial nephritis (Colvin 1996).

Endarteritis is another characteristic feature of acute rejection (Figures 11.5 and 11.6). Infiltration of mononuclear cells under arteriolar endothelium (endothelialitis) is considered to be pathognomonic. More uncertain is the significance of lymphocytes on the surface of endothelium (Colvin 1996). However, endothelialitis is seen in only about half the cases of acute rejection. The media of the artery usually shows few changes but in severe cases the cellular infiltration may cause medial necrosis and thrombosis. With the exception of the latter cases, the presence of endothelialitis per se does not have a bad prognostic significance. In fact graft survival is similar for grafts with cellular arteritis and for those with tubulointerstitial lesions (Matas et al 1983).

A more severe vascular lesion is necrotizing arteritis (Figure 11.7), which unlike cellular arteritis does not show a mononuclear infiltrate within and around the artery. Thrombotic vasculopathy may also occur. The prognosis of necrotizing arteritis and of arterial thrombi is severe although some cases may be reversible.

While the intensity of interstitial infiltrate has no correlation with the outcome of acute rejection (Banfi et al 1981), the presence and the intensity of interstitial hemorrhage and interstitial fibrosis correlate with a poor long-term graft outcome (Banfi et al 1981; Matas et al 1983; Visscher et al 1991).

Glomeruli are usually spared or show only mild changes in acute rejection. Rarely, an

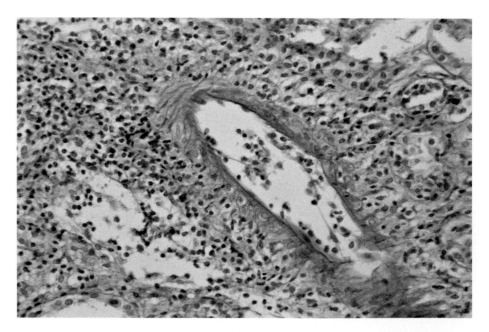

Figure 11.5. Mild endoarteritis ('endothelialitis'). Inflammatory mononuclear cells not only stick to the endothelium but also have penetrated underneath, lifting it up. (PAS ×250)

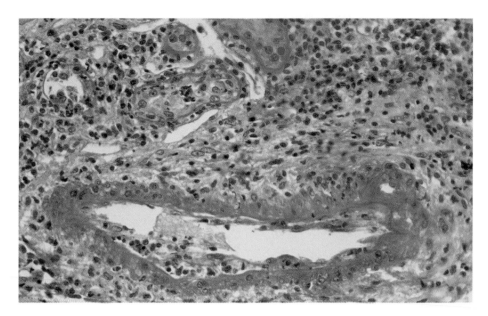

Figure 11.6. Moderate endoarteritis of an interlobular artery. Inflammatory cells infiltrate the subendothelial space and the intima which irregularly proliferates with partial luminal narrowing. Some inflammatory cells are also present in the deeper muscular layer and in the adventitia. (PAS ×250)

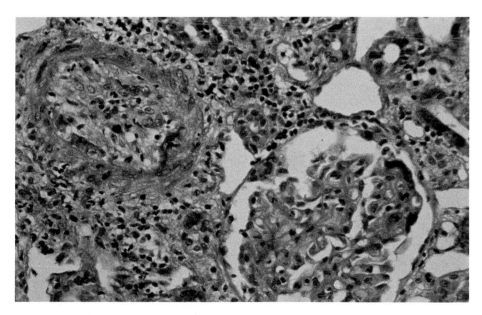

Figure 11.7. Severe endoarteritis. The lumen of an interlobular artery is completely obliterated by a messy myointimal proliferation and by infiltrating inflammatory cells. Lumpy fibrinoid insudates lean upon the lamina elastica which appears focally disrupted (arrow). (PAS ×250)

489

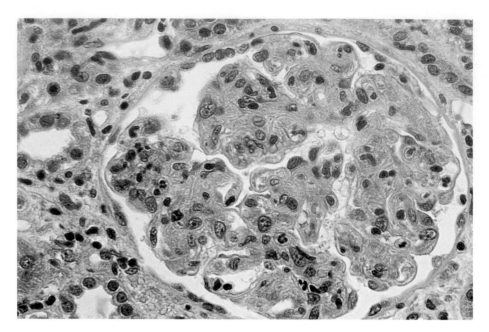

Figure 11.8. Acute transplant glomerulitis. Capillary lumina are severely narrowed by endothelial swelling and infiltrating inflammatory mononuclear cells. Capillary walls appear markedly thickened showing 'double contour' appearance. (Masson trichrome ×400)

acute glomerulopathy may develop, characterized by hypercellularity, injury and enlargement of endothelial cells, and glomerular infiltration of mononuclear cells (Figure 11.8). The prognosis of this form of acute rejection, which in the past was thought to be associated with cytomegalovirus infection, is severe (Richardson et al 1981). The presence of thrombi in glomeruli has also a bad prognosis.

Two types of classification and categorization of acute rejection have been proposed, the Banff classification (Solez et al 1993, 1996), which was recently modified and that of the National Institutes of Health (Colvin et al 1997). Although similar in many aspects the two classifications have some relevant differences (Table 11.4). If renal biopsy remains the more valid tool for a correct diagnosis and for therapeutic decision it must be pointed out that there are also limits with this technique, depending on the time of the biopsy (too early a renal biopsy may fail to assess the severity of rejection), the poor specificity of some lesions, and the difficulty of classifying some acute rejections (a biopsy section may contain hundreds of tubular cross-sections with different severities of infiltration). Moreover, the grading of acute rejection leans heavily on the presence of arterial vessels. This implies that graft biopsies without representative arteries should be considered inadequate. Finally the differential diagnosis between clinical and subclinical acute rejection is not always easy (Rush et al 1999) and rejection recurrence is independent of the histologic score of the first rejection (Gaber et al 1996).

Banff

Grade I   Interstitial inflammation >25% of parenchyma

A Tubulitis (>4 mononuclear cells/tubular cross section)

B Tubulitis (>10 mononuclear cells/tubular cross section)

Grade II   A Significant interstitial inflammation and/or mild to moderate arteritis

B Moderate to severe intimal arteritis comprising >25% of the luminal area

Grade III Transmural arteritis or fibrinoid necrosis of medial smooth muscle cells

Cooperative Clinical Trials in Transplantation

Mononuclear infiltrate in >5% of cortex

At least three tubules with tubulitis in 10 consecutive high-power fields. At least two of three features: edema, activated lymphocytes or tubular injury

Arterial or arteriolar endothelialitis with or without the preceding features

Arterial fibrinoid necrosis or transmural inflammation with or without thrombosis, parenchymal necrosis or hemorrhage

Table 11.4. Categorization of acute rejection according to Banff classification (1998) or CCTT classification (Colvin et al 1997)

In summary, the clinical diagnosis of acute rejection is mainly a diagnosis of exclusion. Renal biopsy can confirm the diagnosis, however the histology may be misleading in some few cases.

Consequences of acute rejection

The occurrence of acute rejection may have several consequences both in the short and in the long term. At onset, the severity of acute rejection may be difficult to assess on clinical grounds. It may be regarded as severe if the peak plasma creatinine level reaches 5 mg/dl or more. It may also be considered severe if it does not reverse after five consecutive intravenous steroid pulses. Renal biopsy may help in assessing severity. The presence of severe intimal arteritis or transmural arteritis, fibrinoid necrosis and/or interstitial hemorrhage carries a more severe prognosis. Some cases of acute rejection can be irreversible. In other cases the nadir of plasma creatinine after reversal of acute rejection remains more elevated than the prerejection values. In other patients the heavy immunosuppression used for handling acute rejection may result in infections or other

491

life-threatening complications; to overcome these complications, immunosuppression has often to be reduced or stopped with consequent loss of the allograft.

Acute rejection can also influence the long-term outcome. Acute rejection has been found to be correlated with the risk of chronic rejection (Flechner et al 1996); the graft half-life has been found to be longer in patients who never experienced acute rejection (Lindholm et al 1993; Ferguson 1994; Massy et al 1996, Cecka 1999) and long-term graft survival has been reported to be better in patients who had a single episode than in patients with two or more episodes of acute rejection (Montagnino et al 1997). It seems, however, that fully reversible acute rejection does not have a deleterious impact on long-term graft function. A recent analysis of the Collaborative Transplant Study showed that the 6-year graft survival was significantly lower in patients who needed anti-rejection treatment (60 versus 75%), but patients with acute rejection whose graft function returned to normal after treatment (serum creatinine lower than 1.5 mg/dl) had a 6-year graft survival only 2% lower than patients without acute rejection (Opelz 1997).

Treatment of acute rejection

The three most used approaches for treating acute rejection are high-dose steroids, ATG and OKT3. High-dose steroids prevent release of IL-1 by macrophages, block IL-2-mediated synthesis by T helper cells and inhibit tumor necrosis factor-alpha (TNF-α) and eicosanoids. These agents may be given by mouth (100–200 mg/24 hours prednisone gradually tapered over 1–3 weeks) or intravenously (0.25–2 g/24 hours methyl-prednisolone (MP) for 3–5 days). Most centers use intravenous MP pulses at a dose of 0.5 g every 24 hours for 3–5 days. About 75% of primary acute rejection episodes are reversible after treatment with MP; histological features may require as long as 10 days to disappear (Mazzucchi et al 1999).

Intravenous ATG lyses circulating T cells and perhaps favors the production of T suppressor cells. ATG has been claimed to be more effective than MP in reversing rejection and in preventing a second episode of acute rejection. The efficacy of ATG depends on the animal source. Rabbit ATG proved to be superior to horse ATG in reversing acute rejection and in preventing recurrent rejection (Gaber et al 1998). Treatment with ATG is expensive, may require hospitalization (ATG should be administered in a central vein) and may expose the patient to viral infection. The use of ATG is generally limited to acute rejection episodes that do not respond to steroids or to episodes with vascular involvement.

The monoclonal antibody OKT3 blocks the antigen receptor complex CD3 and prevents antigen recognition. It is administered intravenously, usually at a dose of 5 mg/day for 7–14 days. OKT3 is significantly more effective than steroids in reversing the first acute rejection episode, and can also reverse a number of steroid-resistant acute rejection episodes. The efficacy of OKT3 in reversing rejection seems to be similar to that of rabbit ATG (Waiser et al 1988; Mariat et al 1998), but the use of OKT3 is associated with more side effects. The first injection exposes the patient to the so-called cytokine release syndrome (chills, hyperpyrexia, tremor, sudden rise in plasma creatinine), to pulmonary edema in overhydrated patients, and rarely to aseptic meningitis or vascular

- Before the first dose:
  correct hydrosaline excess (<3% bodyweight)
  intravenous high-dose MP (0.25 g 6 hours and 1 hour before OKT3)
- Infusion of the first dose:
  infuse the first dose of OKT3 slowly (2 hours)
  infuse half-dose of OKT3
- During treatment:
  reduce or stop cyclosporine, or tacrolimus, or MMF
  administer ganciclovir
  limit the duration of treatment to 7–10 days

Table 11.5. Precautions with the use of OKT3

thrombosis. Before administration of OKT3 several precautions should be taken. Patients with overhydration should be treated with high-dose furosemide or with dialysis in order to avoid the bronchospasm and pulmonary edema that can follow the first injection. Premedication with intravenous MP may be useful in order to reduce the effects of the massive release of cytokines. The dose of MP should not exceed 8 mg/kg as higher doses could concur with OKT3 in producing a procoagulant effect with risk of arterial thrombosis (Abramowicz et al 1996). A slow infusion of OKT3, over 2 hours, has been found to reduce the intensity of cytokine release syndrome (Ten Berge et al 1996). A controlled trial did not however confirm the beneficial effect of pentoxyfillin (Vincenti et al 1996) in preventing the side-effects of OKT3. It has also been demonstrated that the use of a half-dose of OKT3 is as effective as the full dose and may also reduce side-effects (Midtvedt et al 1996). Similarly to ATG, OKT3 can also expose the patient to viral infection and to an increased risk of lymphoproliferative disorders. Thus, whenever antilymphocyte antibodies are used, the duration of treatment should be limited to 7–10 days, basic immunosuppression should be reduced, and antiviral agents, such as ganciclovir or acyclovir, should be administered (Table 11.5).

Good results have been reported with the use of FK506 (Woodle et al 1996) for rescue treatment of acute rejection. However, in other experiences this drug had only a mild benefit in reversing steroid-resistant rejections (Felldin et al 1997). High-dose mycophenolate mofetil also proved to be effective in some cases of acute rejection refractory to previous treatments (Mycophenolate Mofetil Study Group 1996).

Chronic rejection

One of the main problems with renal transplantation is represented by chronic rejection, which is the leading cause of late failure of kidney transplants.

Clinical diagnosis.

Clinically, chronic rejection is characterized by a slowly progressive decline of glomerular filtration rate, appearing months or years after transplantation. Chronic rejection is usually associated with proteinuria and arterial hypertension.

Chronic rejection is responsible of graft loss in around 5% of renal transplants per year. The cadaveric kidney grafts are more exposed to chronic rejection than kidneys from living donors, but when chronic rejection develops the outcome is the same. Chronic rejection may be diagnosed only in the absence of other complications responsible for late and progressive allograft dysfunction such as renal artery stenosis, ureteral obstruction, late acute rejection, de novo or recurrent glomerulonephritis, and drug-related nephrotoxicity. Progressively deteriorating renal function may show a linear relationship between the reciprocal of the serum creatinine level versus time (Modena et al 1991) but in many cases there is a large variability in the rate of progression (Kasiske et al 1991). Proteinuria commonly, ranges from 0.4 to 2 g/day, but nephrotic proteinuria can be observed in the presence of a transplant glomerulopathy. The concomitant development or worsening of proteinuria and hypertension has been considered as a poor prognostic indicator for graft failure (Kasiske et al 1991).

Pathology of chronic rejection

Histologically, chronic allograft rejection is characterized by arterial intimal fibrosis, glomerular mesangial expansion, glomerular basement membrane (GBM) thickening, tubular atrophy and interstitial fibrosis, in varied degrees and combinations. The vascular and glomerular lesions are the most distinctive and are the prime morphologic criteria of chronic rejection.

Specific chronic vascular changes are disruptions of the elastica, and inflammatory cells (foamy macrophages) in fibrotic intima. Proliferation of myofibroblasts in the expanded intima, formation of a second neointima and fibrointimal thickening of vessels are also significant findings, although not pathognomonic. The vascular lesions may be graded on the basis of their extent and degree of vascular lumen occlusion (Figures 11.9 and 11.10). Gouldsbrough and Axelsen (1994) identified four patterns of arterial pathology: (1) subendothelial inflammation (endothelialitis) with little intimal thickening; (2) endothelialitis with intimal thickening; (3) intimal thickening without endothelialitis, and (4) intimal thickening with calcification and cholesterol clefts (natural atherosclerosis). The authors suggested that the lesions of chronic vascular rejection evolve, at varying rates, from an early 'endothelialitis' to a later stage with pronounced intimal thickening but without subendothelial inflammation. However, while most patients with chronic rejection show arteriopathy with fibrointimal hyperplasia, in about a quarter of cases it is impossible to classify the nature of a chronic allograft nephropathy because of the absence of adequate vessels in the biopsy sample (Cosio et al 1999).

Glomerular changes in long-standing allografts, different from either recurrent or de novo glomerulonephritis, have been recognized for many years (Hamburger et al 1964).

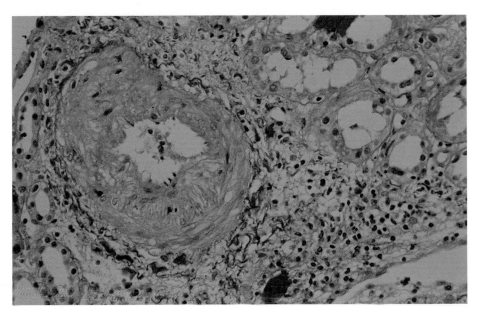

Figure 11.9. Transplant endoarteritis (chronic phase). Messy myointimal proliferation leads to a severe concentric although irregular thickening of the intimal layer. The muscular layer appears partially atrophic and, in a segment, replaced by fibrous material (scar of previous necrotic event) (arrow). (AFOG ×400)

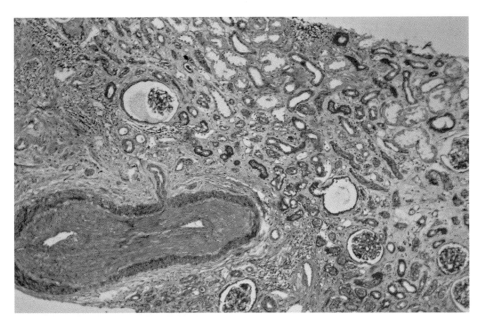

Figure 11.10. A sample of a graft removed for 'chronic rejection' shows arcuate artery almost occluded by a severe concentric proliferative endoarteritis in advanced fibrous transformation. (PAS ×100)

The more usual term for these lesions is 'allograft glomerulopathy' (AGP) which refers to the specific pattern of glomerular involvement (Figures 11.11–11.13). AGP is characterized by: widespread reduplication of the GBM due to a widening of the subendothelial space; moderate increase in mesangial matrix; and interposition of mesangial matrix and cells. The early lesions of AGP show prominent swelling of endothelial and mesangial cells, which together with the presence of monocyte-macrophages in the mesangial areas result in a diminished patency of the capillary lumens. The progression of this hypercellular type of involvement of glomeruli to the classic form of AGP with reduplication of GBM has been observed by some authors (Richardson et al 1981; Maryniak et al 1985), but others were not able to demonstrate this transition (Habib and Broyer 1993). Generally, AGP is found in association with vascular lesions of chronic rejection (Axelsen et al 1985), however, it can also be the unique lesion in long-functioning grafts. Allograft glomerulopathy is considered an ominous feature for the graft, but the delay between the finding of AGP and graft loss is extremely variable ranging from a few months to 2–3 years. The vascular changes in chronic rejection, which are invariably associated with AGP, are most likely responsible for the graft loss rather than the progression of the glomerular disease itself. In a few cases, remission of proteinuria and of histological alterations has been reported.

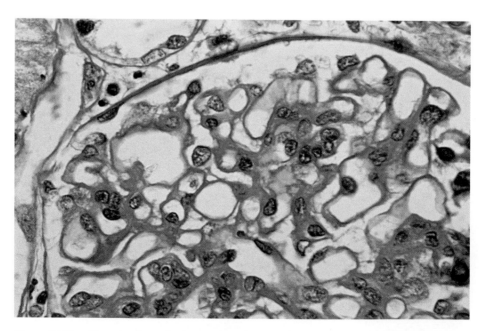

Figure 11.11. Chronic allograft glomerulopathy (initial phase). A slight but diffuse thickening of the capillary walls gives to the glomerulus a 'membranous nephropathy-like' appearance. (PAS ×400)

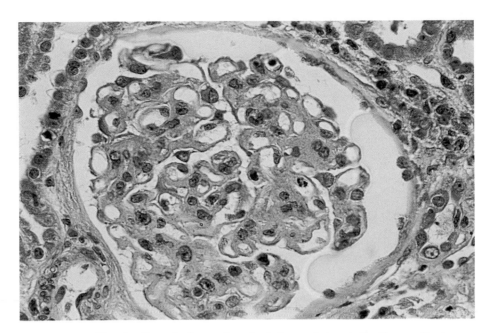

Figure 11.12. Chronic allograft glomerulopathy (advanced phase). Capillary walls show severe thickening and 'double contour' appearance. Cellular component is preserved while mesangial matrix is irregularly and moderately expanded. (Masson trichrome ×400)

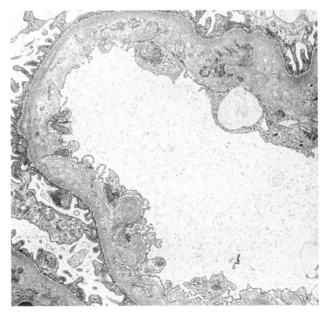

Figure 11.13. At electron microscopy chronic allograft glomerulopathy is characterized by a progressive widening of the lamina rara interna without cellular interposition and/or protein deposits. (×6800)

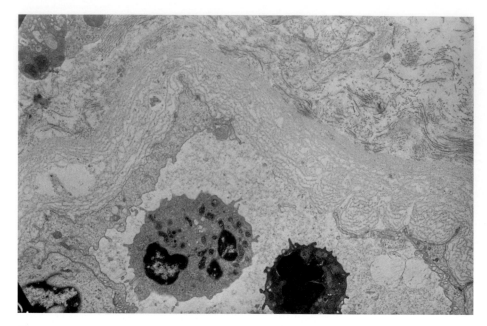

Figure 11.14.   A peritubular capillary wall shows splitting of the basement membrane in multiple layers. (×14 000. By courtesy of Professor G Mazzucco, University of Turin, Italy).

On electron microscopy, peritubular capillaries may show features consisting of the splitting and multilayered duplication of the basement membranes (Figure 11.14). These changes, analogous to those seen in the glomerular capillaries of transplant glomerulopathy, have been considered typical of chronic rejection by some investigators (Monga et al 1992; Drachenberg et al 1997). Diffuse interstitial fibrosis and tubular atrophy are seen in the advanced stages of chronic rejection.

Risk factors

There is evidence today that both alloantigen-dependent and alloantigen-independent mechanisms may be involved in the progressive allograft dysfunction (Table 11.6).

Immune-mediated factors might favor a continuous low-level host immune response to alloantigens expressed by the allograft. The importance of alloantigen-dependent factors is supported by several pieces of evidence. There is a stepwise decrease in graft survival rate and in graft half-life as the number of HLA mismatches increase (Feucht and Opelz 1996; Cecka 1999). The association between good histocompatibility and long-term graft function is a strong argument in favor of the immunological origin of chronic rejection. The deleterious long-term impact of cytotoxic anti-HLA antibodies developed after transplantation is another point supporting the immunological involve-

Immune-mediated mechanisms
HLA matching
Preformed humoral antibodies
Acute rejection
Immunosuppressive therapy
Compliance
CMV infections

Nonimmunological mechanisms
Donor source
Reduced renal mass
Ischemic-reperfusion injury
Renal toxicity of drugs
Hyperlipidemia
Hypertension

Table 11.6. Immunological and nonimmunological mechanisms involved in the pathogenesis of chronic rejection

ment in chronic rejection (Davenport et al 1994; Abe et al 1997; Costa et al 1997). Acute rejection has been recognized as one of the most important risk factors for chronic rejection, as already discussed above. The role of immunosuppressive therapy has also been investigated. Isoniemi et al (1992) found a lower incidence of histologically proven chronic rejection in patients given more powerful immunosuppressive regimens. Two randomized trials showed a significantly higher 10-year graft survival in patients assigned to receive CsA than in those assigned to receive azathioprine (Beveridge and Calne 1995; Ponticelli et al 1996). Many patients develop chronic rejection because of poor compliance to immunosuppressive drugs (Didlake et al 1988) or because of the use or inadequate doses of CsA (Almond et al 1993). Variable bioavailability of oral CsA also correlates with chronic rejection (Kahan et al 1996). Recent studies showed that cytomegalovirus infection may increase neointima formation of allografts when HLA incompatibility between recipient and donor is present (Li et al 1998) and may enhance the detrimental effects of rejection (Kosisken et al 1999). All these data support a major role for immune-mediated mechanisms in the development of chronic rejection.

The possibility that alloantigen-independent factors may increase the risk of late renal allograft failure has been recently pointed out. The better results observed with living-unrelated donors than with cadaveric HLA matched donors (Terasaki et al 1995) have been explained by the fact that the living donor kidneys are healthy without reduced nephron mass and/or pre-existing diseases. It has also been shown, however, that ischemic lesions in cadaver kidneys may upregulate the expression of HLA-DR antigens and cell adhesion molecules on tubular cells (Koo et al 1999) so favoring the development of rejection. It has been claimed that nephron underdosing could play an important role in the development of late graft dysfunction (Brenner et al 1992), although good results have also been obtained with elderly (Roodnat et al 1999) and/or size mismatched donors (Miles et al 1996). Delayed graft function caused by ischemic/reperfusion injury may be associated with graft dysfunction in the long term, particularly when it is combined with acute rejection (see later). Finally, several studies showed an association between chronic rejection and proteinuria (Hostetter 1994), hyperlipidemia (Dimeny et al 1993; Isoniemi et al 1994), oxidative stress (Cristol et al 1998) and hypertension (Opelz et al 1998). However, it is still unclear whether these abnormalities represent a cause or an effect of late graft failure.

Alloantigen-dependent and -independent factors are often intertwined and may have a common pathway eventually leading to graft failure (Ponticelli 1998). The demonstration that intrarenal TGF-β_1 mRNA expression is a molecular correlate of interstitial fibrosis and of chronic rejection (Sharma et al 1995) has raised a fibrogenic hypothesis for the pathogenesis of chronic rejection. The allograft injury caused by ischemia, rejection, nephrotoxic drugs, or other factors can result in TGF-β_1 expression (Ayanlar-Batuman et al 1991; Li et al 1991). In turn TGF-β_1 is able to stimulate its own production via specific response elements located in the TGF-β promoter region (Von Obberghen-Schilling et al 1985). Transforming growth factor-β_1 enhances the expression of some cytokines like platelet-derived growth factor (PDGF) and fibroblast growth factor, and of vasoactive protein like endothelin (Kiruhara et al 1989), which can lead to cellular proliferation, hypertension and chronic allograft dysfunction. Moreover, TGFβ_1 may block matrix degradation by stimulating protease inhibitors such as PAI-1 (Border and Noble 1995). It has been pointed out that tacrolimus may have a lower impact than CsA on the production of TGFβ_1 (El-Gamel et al 1998). A retrospective analysis found a better long-term graft survival in 544 cadaveric renal transplant recipients given tacrolimus than in 35 000 grafts treated with CsA (Gjertson et al 1995). However, there was a large disproportion between the numbers in the two groups, and most tacrolimus-treated patients participated in trials at excellent transplant centers whereas patients treated with CsA received the old formulation of the drug. However TGF-β quantitation can be tricky. The measurement may be limited by the analytical technique used or the possibility of artefacts. As a matter of fact, in liver transplantation neither cyclosporine nor tacrolimus induced active TGF-β_1 blood levels (Hughes et al 1999).

More recently, a possible role for accelerated senescence has been postulated (Halloran et al 1999). Research on the cell biology of aging and senescence demonstrated that somatic cells in culture have a limited cycling capacity (Hayflick and Moorhead 1961). At the end of its cycle, the cell irreversibility shuts down many processess and usually dies. In chronic rejection, the endothelial cells injured by several risk factors, cytokine release, and ischemia/reperfusion may lose their ability to control remodeling of the arterial wall, resulting in fibrosis. Since no specific lesions can separate chronic rejection from age-related disease, Halloran et al (1999) hypothesized that chronic rejection might be regarded as a senescence process accelerated by immunological and nonim-munological mechanisms. In order to attenuate the impact of this accelerated senescence the authors recommended measures to minimize the acute input stress, including the allocation of older kidneys to older recipients, in whom the immune and inflammatory response are blunted.

In summary, even if immunological factors probably play a major role in initiating chronic rejection, there is evidence that both alloantigen-dependent and -independent factors may contribute to the development and progression of chronic graft nephropa-thy. On the basis of the available knowledge, good HLA compatibility, prevention of viral infections, prevention of ischemia/reperfusion injury and, most importantly, ade-quate immunosuppression appear to be critical to prevent chronic rejection. Treatment of hyperlipidemia and hypertension is also warranted to prevent both progressive graft dysfunction and cardiovascular disease.

Therapeutic approaches

There is no effective treatment for established chronic rejection. While adequate immunosuppression is important to prevent either immunological activation or nephro-toxicity caused by excessive doses of calcineurin inhibitors, there is no evidence that a reinforcement of immunosuppressive therapy may be helpful in modifying the course of an already established chronic rejection (Kirkman et al 1992; Paul and Fellström 1992). Mycophenolate mofetil (MMF), which inhibits lymphocyte proliferation, adhesion mol-ecule glycosylation, and smooth muscle proliferation proved to be effective in preventing chronic vascular rejection in experimental models (Allison et al 1993; Raisanen-Sokolowski et al 1995). These results encouraged the use of MMF in patients with established chronic rejection in kidney transplantation. In one study (Glicklich et al 1998), the replacement of azathioprine with MMF showed no advantage. In contrast, another study (Weir et al 1997) reported a beneficial effect of MMF in 28 transplant recipients with progressive deterioration of renal function. In all patients CsA dose was reduced by 50% and azathioprine was discontinued, while MMF (1 g/day) was added. Renal function improved in 21 of 28 patients. Only one patient had continued deterio-ration of renal function. There was no acute rejection after the immunosuppression change. It is not clear, however, whether the benefit of this change in immunosuppres-sion was related to the reduced doses of CsA or to a specific effect of MMF.

Experimental studies showed that the administration of angiopeptin, a somatostatin lanreotide analog peptide, can reduce the growth factor expression and the replication rate of intimal and medial smooth muscle cells (Häyry et al 1993). These data indicate that the regulation of growth factor expression is a potential therapeutic approach but clinical data are lacking.

Some small studies investigated the role of a dietary protein restriction. Feehally et al (1986) reported that in five patients with advanced chronic renal rejection subjected to dietary protein restriction with no change in immunosuppression therapy the slope of the reciprocal serum creatinine significantly decreased. In another study (Kootte and

Paul 1988), patients assigned to a low protein diet tended to have better preservation of renal function although the number of patients who returned to dialysis was similar in the group with low protein intake. Rosenberg et al (1995) randomly assigned 14 patients with biopsy-proven chronic rejection to two 11-day periods, on low protein diet (0.55 g/kg per day) or on a high-protein diet (2 g/kg per day). The low protein diet was associated with a significant improvement in glomerular permselectivity without any change in blood pressure, glomerular filtration rate or renal plasma flow. The low protein diet was also associated with a significant reduction in plasma renin activity.

Another therapeutic approach was based on the assumption that the vascular lesions of chronic rejection could be favored by platelets, clotting factors, and complement. Teraoka et al (1987) randomly assigned 20 kidney transplant recipients with chronic rejection to be treated or not with anticoagulant, anticomplement (mafamstat mesilate and camstat mesilate), and antiplatelet agents (OP-41483, an analog of prostacyclin I_2 and ticlopidine). In 61% of the treated patients grafts remained functioning, whereas only 28% of untreated patients had functioning grafts. Fellström and Larsson (1993) obtained stabilization or improvement of graft function in 18/22 patients followed for 1 year by giving continuous intravenous infusion of epoprostenole for 1 week followed by oral salicylate (100–150 mg daily) and dipyridamole (225 mg daily). A significant reduction in the rate of graft function deterioration has also been reported with the use of fish oil (Sweny et al 1989).

Angiotensin-converting enzyme (ACE) inhibition has been shown to lower blood pressure and to reduce proteinuria in a variety of native kidney diseases and might oppose the production of $TGF\beta_1$ stimulated by angiotensin II (Campistol et al 1999). The beneficial effects of ACE inhibition on blood pressure and proteinuria were also found in patients with renal allografts (Traindl et al 1993; Oppenheimer et al 1995; Sennesael et al 1995). Little information is available on the role of ACE inhibition in altering the progressive course of chronic rejection. In a noncontrolled study on 40 patients with progressive transplant failure, the addition of lisinopril significantly reduced blood pressure and proteinuria, but the decline of creatinine clearance was lowered in only 19/40 patients (Barnas et al 1996).

The impact of these measures in lowering renal graft deterioration is difficult to establish, as in the above-mentioned studies the number of patients was very small, the follow-up was too short and the serum creatinine levels at entry were extremely variable. Hence, well-designed, well-sized, randomized, double-blind studies should be conducted in the future. Clinical and histologic criteria at entry and primary (graft loss) or surrogate endpoints (histologic parameters, percent of plasma creatinine variation) should be precisely identified.

DELAYED GRAFT FUNCTION

Delayed graft function (DGF) is a frequent complication in the early posttransplant period. Several different causes may account for DGF (Table 11.7). After excluding a bladder obstruction, either by urethral catheterization or by ultrasonography, the nature of DGF should be established as early as possible. In fact, an early diagnosis of the irreversible nature of DGF can avoid useless immunosuppression, which may be dangerous in an anuric patient. Irreversible cases can be easily recognized by isotopic scan and/or echocolor Doppler. Renal biopsy may confirm the existence of irreversible lesions and may help in identifying the causes of DGF (Figure 11.15).

Ultrasonography can demonstrate the presence of pyelectasia and calycectasia and may identify the causes of ureteric obstruction in the case of lymphocele, perirenal and periureteral hematoma or stone. Renal biopsy may show the presence of rejection, interstitial nephritis, acute nephrotoxicity or acute tubular necrosis (ATN), although the typical histological findings may also be absent in several cases.

Acute tubular necrosis

Acute tubular necrosis (ATN) is by far the most frequent cause of DGF. It may need dialysis within the first week after surgery in 20–50% of patients requiring a first cadaver graft (Troppman et al 1995; Feldman et al 1996). It is usually caused by the ischemic damage to the graft before or during harvesting and may be aggravated by the so-called reperfusion syndrome, in which polymorphonuclear cells probably play a major role (Land and Messmer 1996).

Irreversible
Nonviable kidney
Vascular thrombosis
Hyperacute rejection

Reversible
Acute tubular necrosis
Acute rejection
Ureteric obstruction (clotting, lymphocele, stenosis, etc.)
Acute drug toxicity (calcineurin-inhibitors, aminoglycosides, amphotericin, etc.)

Table 11.7. Main causes of posttransplant acute renal failure

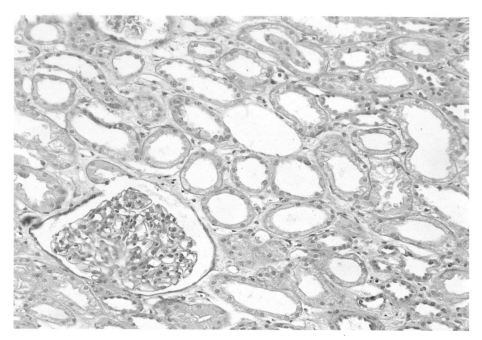

Figure 11.15. 'Acute tubular necrosis'. Tubuli show diffuse flattening of the epithelial cells. Some lumina are filled with clumps of necrotic epithelial cells. Scanty inflammatory infiltrates are present in the interstitium. (PAS ×160)

Risk factors

Several factors may contribute to the development of ATN. The preparation of the recipient may be important as hypovolemic recipients are more exposed to ATN. The dialysis modality before transplantation may also influence the development of ATN. The incidence of DGF is higher in patients treated with hemodialysis than in those treated with peritoneal dialysis (Bleyer et al 1999). The difference could be related to the different biocompatibility between the two modalities or to the overhydration status of patients on peritoneal dialysis when compared with those on hemodialysis (Maiorca et al 1992).

The use of high-dose CsA or tacrolimus may expose the patient to ATN (De Mattos et al 1996), particularly when these agents are combined with other nephrotoxic drugs such as aminoglycosides, nonsteroidal anti-inflammatory drugs or sulphonamides.

The source of donors is particularly important. Acute tubular necrosis is very rare in living kidney recipients while it may occur in 20–80% of cadaveric kidney transplants (Leichtman and Strom 1988). The difference is mainly accounted for by cytokine release and by hemodymanic instability associated with brain death. A massive release of cytokines and growth factors can cause injury, ischemia, and inflammation (Takada et al 1998), which can concur with the consequences of hemodynamic instability in producing ATN.

in tubular and glomerular cells. The use of monoclonal antibodies against CMV should be employed for a correct diagnosis. The presence of viruria may facilitate the diagnosis.

After diagnosis a course of treatment with ganciclovir is usually effective in eradicating viruses from kidney tissue. Whether or not immunosuppression should be reduced is uncertain, in view of the potential promotion of rejection by CMV (Grattan et al 1989). In the past, there have been contrasting opinions about the effect of CMV infection on graft function. It now seems that the outcome is determined by coexisting acute rejection or chronic allograft nephropathy rather than by viral infection or interstitial nephritis. In a recent series of 10 cases with CMV inclusions in the allograft and florid interstitial nephritis in seven, no graft loss primarily attributable to CMV was observed (Kashyap et al 1999).

Herpesvirus 1 and 2

Herpesvirus 1 or 2 rarely causes interstitial nephritis. Usually this occurs in the first weeks after transplantation and may be concomitant with mucocutaneous lesions. At renal biopsy, nuclear clearing, necrosis and inclusions in tubular cells may be seen. Acyclovir and reduction of immunosuppressive therapy may be helpful in reversing this type of interstitial nephritis, although there is little information about the clinical outcome of these cases.

Adenovirus

These viruses may cause necrotizing hemorrhagic interstitial nephritis with acute renal failure. At biopsy, tubular cells may show intranuclear inclusions with a halo surrounded by a ring of marginated chromatin and smudged nuclei. Glassy-appearing nuclear smudging and extensive tubular necrosis with moderate interstitial nephritis may allow a differential diagnosis with rejection (Colvin 1996). Immunoperoxidase stains for viral antigen can establish the etiology. The renal impairment is severe. Hemorrhagic cystitis may also occur.

Polyomavirus

The human polyomavirus family contains two viruses, the JC virus and the BK virus. These viruses are usually acquired in childhood probably through the oral route and remain latent in the kidney. Immunosuppression can favor the reactivation of polyomavirus in transplanted kidneys with development of an interstitial nephritis and significant risk of graft loss (Mathur et al 1997). Diabetes and potent immunosuppressive therapy predispose to infection and there is the clinical impression that the incidence of interstitial nephritis caused by polyomavirus is becoming more frequent after the introduction of newer immunosuppressive agents. An association with ureteral stenosis has been reported by some investigators (Hogan et al 1980) but not by others (Randhawa et al 1999). The presentation may be similar to that of acute rejection with

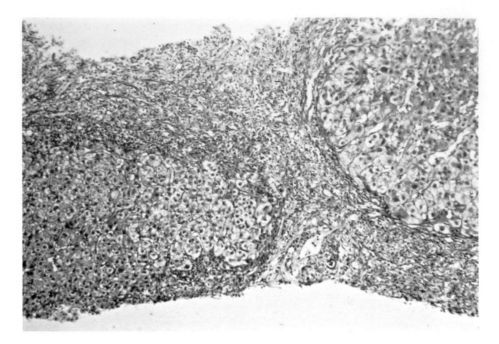

Figure 11.16. Giant nuclear transformation of a tubular cell in a case of polyoma infection (arrow). (Jones ×400. By courtesy of Dr F Egidi, Univeristy of Tenessee, Memphis.)

deterioration of renal function. Rarely, there is a hemorrhagic cystitis but the disease may also be asymptomatic. The differential diagnosis with acute rejection may be difficult (Binet et al 1999) but in some cases cytopathic changes can suggest diagnosis (Figure 11.16). In situ hybridization or electron microscopy may be required to identify the viral etiology. Reduction of immunosuppression may stabilize graft function in some few cases (Randhawa et al 1999), but in many patients there is progressive deterioration of renal function with ultimate graft loss (Mathur et al 1997).

Drug-induced interstitial nephritis

A number of drugs may be responsible for interstitial nephritis. These include antibiotics, sulphonamides, allopurinol, diuretics, nonsteroidal anti-inflammatory drugs, etc. The clinical diagnosis may be difficult. Fever, skin rash, and eosinophilia may be lacking or mild because the basic immunosuppression may mask the typical signs and symptoms of interstitial nephritis. A superimposed interstitial nephritis may be suspected when a sudden increase in plasma creatinine occurs in a transplant patient who took even a single dose of a potentially allergic drug.

As drug-associated interstitial nephritis may show histologic features identical to those of acute rejection, namely tubulitis, mononuclear interstitial infiltrate and eosinophilia, the differential diagnosis can also be difficult with renal biopsy. However, endothelialitis is typical of acute rejection and, when present, allows a correct diagnosis.

While in some cases the removal of the offending drug may be sufficient to reverse renal dysfunction, in other instances a course of high-dose corticosteroids may be necessary.

PYELONEPHRITIS

Infection of the urinary tract is frequent in renal transplant recipients. Most infections are localized in the lower urinary tract and are often asymptomatic. More rare are the infections of the upper urinary tract that may be responsible for acute or chronic pyelonephritis. Urological complications, vesicoureteral reflux and diabetes mellitus may predispose to the development of pyelonephritis.

Acute pyelonephritis

Although acute pyelonephritis may occur at any time, it occurs more frequently in the early posttransplant period because of catheterization, stenting, and/or antirejection treatment. This form of acute interstitial nephritis, due to bacterial invasion of the kidney, usually produces a septic picture. Symptoms develop rapidly and include high fever, shaking chills, tachycardia, muscular tenderness, nausea, vomiting and diarrhea. Cystitis and/or macroscopic hematuria may or may not be present. Severe hypotension and oliguria may develop in the most severe cases.

Laboratory investigations show leukocytosis in most patients, however, transplant recipients under treatment with azathioprine, MMF or ATG may show neutropenia. Leukocytes, erythrocytes and leukocyte casts are usually seen in the urine sediment. However, if the infective focus does not communicate with urine both the urinary sediment and the urine culture may be negative. In case of severe sepsis, bacteria can be isolated from the blood culture. An increase in plasma creatinine is frequent, often favored by profuse sweating, vomiting and/or diarrhea. This may raise some problems of differential diagnosis with acute rejection particularly in the early posttransplant period. Prior complications and/or instrumentation of the urinary tract orientate towards acute pyelonephritis. Ultrasonography may be helpful if urinary obstruction, fistula or stones are present. Renal biopsy may show a massive interstitial infiltrate rich in polymorphonuclear cells, with focal disruption of the tubular structure (Figure 11.17). However, if the infiltrates are striped (or patchy), not uniform, the renal biopsy can also be unrepresentative.

Most cases of acute pyelonephritis are due to Gram-negative bacteria such as *E. coli*, *Proteus* species, and *Pseudomonas* species. *Enterobacter* is the predominant Gram-positive

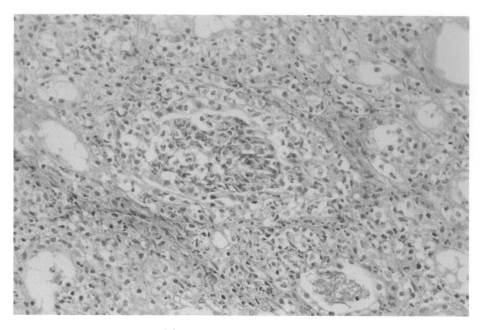

Figure 11.17. Acute pyelonephritis: tubuli display severe disruption by inflammatory cells constituted mainly by neutrophils which fill, together with necrotic tubular cells, the lumina. (AFOG ×250)

bacterium. Opportunistic microorganisms and fungi may also be responsible for acute pyelonephritis.

Usually, acute pyelonephritis responds favorably to antibiotics but those cases caused by acute urinary obstruction or urine fistula require urine diversion or surgery. Pending urine culture and sensitivity, parenteral antimicrobial therapy should be promptly instituted together with electrolyte and fluid replacement. Immunosuppressive treatment should be reduced if signs of sepsis are present. Third-generation cephalosporins, ampicillin sulbactam, imipenem, aztreonam and fluoroquinolones are active against the bacteria most frequently involved. Aminoglycosides are very useful, but should be handled with caution because of their potential nephrotoxicity. Intravenous therapy should be continued for at least 48 hours after fever disappears. Then, oral antimicrobial agents should be given for at least 4 weeks in order to prevent relapses.

Chronic pyelonephritis

Chronic pyelonephritis due to bacterial infection of the allograft is a rare cause of progressive chronic allograft dysfunction. The few cases are usually caused by recurrent stones, ureteral stenosis or massive vesicoureteral reflux (Debruyne et al 1978). However, some studies reported that vesicoureteral reflux in the transplanted kidney neither influences the long-term graft function and survival (Mastrosimone et al 1993) nor is associated with an increased risk of urinary infection (Grünberger et al 1993).

Clinically, chronic pyelonephritis may be asymptomatic. Some patients with stones may have renal colic, others may complain of cystitis. Usually the diagnosis is established because a patient with a persistently positive urine culture and/or progressive increase in plasma creatinine is submitted to ultrasonography. This reveals changes of decreased renal size and segmental cortical scarring. Intravenous pyelography confirms these findings and also shows blunting and dilatation of the calyces, and ureteral dilatation in case of vesicoureteral reflux. Urinary tuberculosis can give similar changes, but ureteral strictures and a contracted bladder can also be frequently found.

Surgical treatment is indicated in patients with urinary obstruction or stones resistant to lithotripsy. Continuous prophylaxis with low-dose sulphamethoxazole–trimethoprim, nitrofurantoin or other antimicrobial agents may be indicated to reduce the risk of acute infections.

Cyclosporine and tacrolimus nephrotoxicity

Owing to the similar mechanisms of action, it is not surprising that CsA and tacrolimus may exert a similar nephrotoxicity, including reversible acute renal function deterioration, hemolytic-uremic syndrome and chronic renal insufficiency. Most of the available data come, however, from the longer and larger experience with CsA.

Acute renal toxicity

Acute nephrotoxicity of calcineurin-inhibitors may manifest with variable severity, which is usually, but not always, dose-dependent. In the milder forms of toxicity, there is a slight reduction of glomerular filtration rate and renal blood flow associated with sodium retention, hypomagnesemia, hyperuricemia, hyperkalemia, and hyperchloremic acidosis. Interestingly, no signs of proxymal tubular dysfunction are seen. These functional changes are caused by afferent arteriolar vasoconstriction, which has been attributed to activation of the renin–angiotensin system, increased sympathetic activity, altered prostaglandin metabolism, and/or to enhanced endothelin secretion (De Mattos et al 1996; Kliem and Brunkhorst 1998). In several cases there are no morphologic abnormalities, but more often tubular lesions can be seen, such as isometric vacuolization, giant mitochondria and microcalcification (Figures 11.18 and 11.19). These lesions are not pathognomonic although they are particularly frequent in patients treated with CsA or tacrolimus. Although these abnormalities are not particularly severe, they may be a sign of general cytotoxicity that can also occur in endothelial cells. Both the functional and morphologic changes may be reversible if the doses of calcineurin-inhibitor are reduced (Mihatsch et al 1995).

More severe nephrotoxicity may lead to an important increase in plasma creatinine. This condition is often associated with an arteriolopathy, characterized by focal myocyte necrosis in the media of small arteries (Figures 11.20 and 11.21), in the absence of intimal changes (Mihatsch et al 1988, 1995). The differential diagnosis with

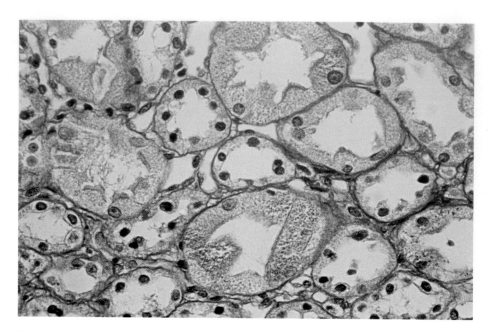

Figure 11.18. Cyclosporine tubular toxicity. Tubular cells show fine isometric vacuolization of the cytoplasm. (AFOG ×400)

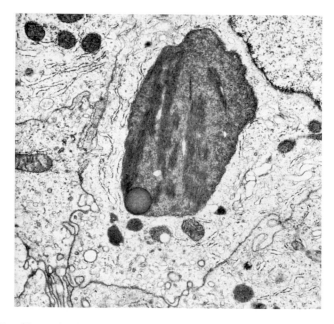

Figure 11.19. Giant mitochondria in a case of cyclosporine toxicity. (EM ×25 000)

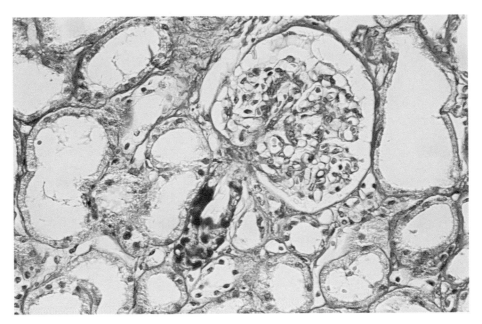

Figure 11.20. Cyclosporine arteriolopathy. A preglomerular arteriole shows severe nodular hyalinosis of the wall. (AFOG ×250)

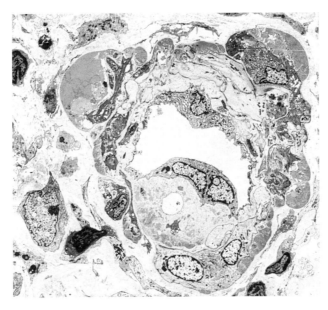

Figure 11.21. Cyclosporine arteriolopathy. At electron microscopy myocytes of a small arteriole show necrosis and cytoplasma filled with lumpy amorphous material. (×4800)

	Calcineurin-inhibitor toxicity	Acute rejection
Tubules	Isometric vacuolization	Tubulitis
	Giant mitochondria	
	Microcalcification	
Interstitium	Little or no change	Mononuclear cell infiltration
Arterioles	Focal myocyte necrosis in the media	Cellular arteritis (no involvement of the media)

Table 11.8. The typical morphological changes that may allow a differential diagnosis between acute rejection and acute nephrotoxicity caused by cyclosporine or tacrolimus. In a number of cases, however, arteriolar abnormalities are absent. In these cases, the differential diagnosis may be difficult as tubular and interstitial changes are not typical

acute rejection may be difficult. Usually acute rejection occurs earlier, the increase in plasma creatinine is higher and more rapid in acute rejection, fever and proteinuria are absent in the case of nephrotoxicity. Renal biopsy shows the typical interstitial infiltrate, tubulitis and cellular arteritis in the case of acute rejection. These findings are usually absent in the case of CsA or tacrolimus nephrotoxicity (Table 11.8). Decreasing the doses of calcineurin inhibitors can reverse renal dysfunction and morphological changes.

The most severe form of acute toxicity is represented by the hemolytic-uremic syndrome which has been described both in CsA-treated (Neild et al 1985) and in tacrolimus-treated (Randhawa et al 1993) renal transplant patients. Clinically, these cases may show a typical picture of hemolytic-uremic syndrome with acute renal failure, hypertension, microangiopathic hemolytic anemia, hyperbilirubinemia and thrombocytopenia. In other cases the diagnosis may be more difficult, as some signs and symptoms may be absent. Histologically, the characteristic features of thrombotic microangiopathy can be seen. The small arteries and arterioles show mucinoid intimal thickening, necrosis, and glomerular thrombi (Figure 11.22). While in the past most patients with thrombotic microangiopathy lost their grafts even with discontinuance of calcineurin inhibitors (Sommer et al 1985), more recent papers reported a total salvage of 92% of kidney allografts after discontinuance of the offending drug and later rechallenge (Young et al 1996).

Chronic renal toxicity

The main problem with the use of calcineurin inhibitors is the possible development of a progressive nephrotoxicity. The mechanisms responsible for this chronic nephropathy have not been completely elucidated. Mihatsch et al (1995) suggested that the arteriolopathy may eventually lead to vascular occlusion with consequent striped interstitial fibrosis (Figure 11.23) and tubular atrophy. Alternatively, CsA might alter the renal cytokine profiles (Ghiggeri et al 1994) and increase the production of the fibrogenic

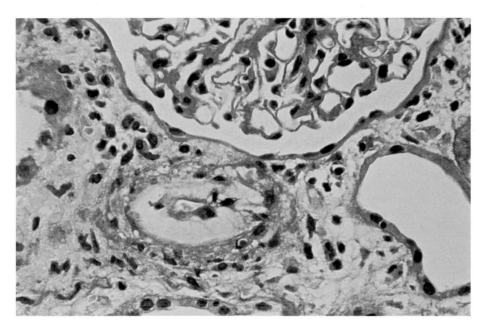

Figure 11.22. Hemolytic-uremic syndrome-like cyclosporine arteriolopathy. A preglomerular arteriole shows mucinoid intimal thickening with severe luminal restriction. (AFOG ×400)

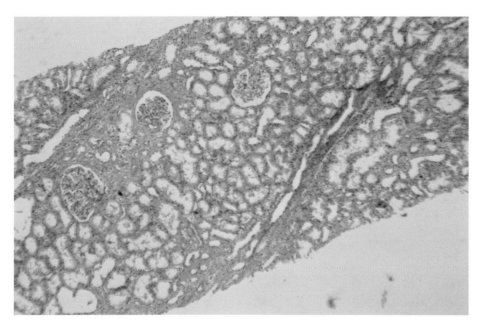

Figure 11.23. 'Stripe-fibrosis' of the interstium suggesting chronic cyclosporine toxicity. (AFOG ×80).

cytokine $TGF\beta_1$ (Ketteler et al 1995). In turn, the activation of the renin–angiotensin system stimulates osteopontin, a chemotactic agent which activates macrophage/mono-cyte/T cells with further production of $TGF\beta_1$ (Bennett et al 1996). It has also been hypothesized that CsA and tacrolimus might favor the accumulation of endogenous toxins or toxin metabolites by inhibiting P-glycoprotein, the multidrug resistance trans-porter, which is expressed in proximal tubular epithelia (Bennett et al 1996).

Clinically the chronic nephropathy caused by calcineurin inhibitors is indistinguish-able from chronic rejection, being characterized by a slowly progressive graft dysfunc-tion, hypertension and mild to moderate proteinuria. At renal biopsy, the chronic toxic nephropathy is heralded by arteriolar lesions characterized by either a mucinoid intimal thickening similar to that seen in hemolytic-uremic syndrome or by nodular hyaline deposits replacing myocytes as seen in malignant hypertension (Mihatsch et al 1995). At a later stage, scarring of arterioles, glomerular obsolescence and striped interstitial fibro-sis may develop, eventually leading to diffuse interstitial fibrosis and glomerular sclerosis. The dimensions of the involved vessels may allow differentiation of toxic nephropathy from chronic rejection. While only small vessels are affected in the case of renal toxicity, the vascular lesions in chronic rejection can affect not only arterioles but also arcuated and interlobular arteries (Mihatsch et al 1995). However, in many biopsies large vessels are not present, in other instances chronic toxicity and chronic rejection may coexist so that a firm diagnosis of chronic toxicity caused by CsA or tacrolimus may often be very difficult or even impossible.

The chronic nephropathy, which is generally comparable for CsA and tacrolimus, has been considered as a major limit for prolonged renal allograft survival. The retrospective data of UNOS seem to support this concern. The half-life of cadaver renal transplants was reported to range around 7 years both in the period 1975–1979 when no cal-cineurin inhibitor was available and between 1985–1990 when most transplant centers were using CsA (Gjertson 1992). On the other hand, more recent studies reported a kidney graft half-life of around 20 years in CsA-treated renal transplant patients (Van-renterghem and Peeters 1994; Montagnino et al 1997; Opelz et al 1999), and two ran-domized trials reported a significantly better cadaver renal transplant survival in CsA-than in azathioprine-treated patients not only in the short term but also after 10 years (Beveridge and Calne, 1995; Ponticelli et al 1996). Moreover, although most CsA-treated patients show suboptimal renal function, plasma creatinine levels may remain stable even in the long term (Burke et al 1994; Matas et al 1995; Ponticelli et al 1999). In several cases plasma creatinine may improve years after transplantation if CsA is stopped or reduced (Pascual et al 1991; Mourad et al 1998), showing that even in the long term CsA-induced nephropathy may be functional, dose-related, and potentially reversible. Finally, repeat renal biopsies demonstrated the histological reversibility of arteriolopathy after reduction or discontinuance of CsA (Morozumi et al 1992; Mihatsch et al 1995).

In summary, although nephrotoxicity caused by calcineurin inhibitors remains a major concern for long-term kidney allograft function, there is evidence that the risk of progressive chronic nephropathy may be minimized if these agents are handled appropriately. In this regard it must be pointed out that there is a good correlation between trough levels and the area-under-the-curve both for tacrolimus (Mekki et al 1993) and for the new microemulsion of CsA, Neoral (Kovarik et al 1994). This facilitates correct monitoring, individualization of the dose and reduction of intrapatient variability, which may protect against chronic toxicity and rejection (Kahan et al 1996). Periodic determinations of peak levels and areas-under-the-curve may also be helpful for assessing the drug bioavailability. If there is a progressive increase in plasma creatinine, reduction of the dosage of calcineurin inhibitors may obtain a reversal or a stabilization of renal dysfunction (Mourad et al 1998). A more striking reduction or even discontinuance of cyclosporine after introduction of mycophenolate mofetil have been successfully tried (Ducloux et al 1998: Hueso et al 1998). Unfortunately the follow-up of these studies was relatively short. As it is likely that the same mechanisms may be responsible for both efficacy and toxicity of calcineurin inhibitors, the patient should be carefully monitored after any modification of the immunosuppressive regimen in order to catch the signs of late, subclinical rejection which, when untreated, may cause irreversible lesions.

REFERENCES

Abe M, Kawai T, Fatatsuyama K et al (1997) Postoperative production of anti-donor antibody and chronic rejection in renal transplantation. *Transplantation* **63**:1616–1619.

Abramowicz D, De Pauw L, Le Moine A et al (1996) Prevention of OKT3 nephrotoxicity after kidney transplantation. *Kidney Int* **49**(Suppl 53): S39–S43.

Allison AC, Eugui EM, Sollinger HW (1993) Micophenolate mofetil: mechanism of action and effects in transplantation. *Transplant Rev* **7**:129–139.

Almond PS, Matas A, Gillingham K et al (1993) Risk factors for chronic rejection in renal allograft recipients. *Transplantation* **55**:752–757.

Axelsen RA, Seymour AE, Mathew TH et al (1985) Glomerular transplant rejection: a distinctive pattern of early graft damage. *Clin Nephrol* **23**:1–11.

Ayanlar-Batuman O, Ferrero AD, Diaz A, Jimenez SA (1991) Regulation of transforming growth factor β_1 gene expression by glucocorticoids in normal human T lymphocytes. *J Clin Invest* **88**:1574–1580.

Banfi G, Imbasciati E, Tarantino A, Ponticelli C (1981) Prognostic value of renal biopsy in acute rejection of kidney transplantation. *Nephron* **28**:222–226.

Barnas U, Schmidt A, Haas M et al (1996) The effects of prolonged angiotensin-converting enzyme inhibition on excretory kidney function and proteinuria in renal allograft recipients with chronic progressive transplant failure. *Nephrol Dial Transplant* **11**:1822–1824.

Bennett WM, De Mattos A, Meyer MM et al (1996) Chronic cyclosporine nephropathy: the Achille's heel of immunosuppressive therapy. *Kidney Int* **50**:1089–1100.

Beveridge T, Calne RY, for the European Multicentre Trial Group (1995) Cyclosporine (Sandimmun) in cadaveric renal transplantation: ten-year follow-up of a multicentre trial. *Transplantation* **59**:1568–1569.

Binet L, Nickeleit V, Hirsch HH et al (1999) Polyomavirus disease under immunosuppressive drugs. *Transplantation* **67**:918–922.

Bleyer AJ, Burkart JM, Russel GB, Adams PL (1999) Dialysis modality and delayed graft function after cadaveric renal transplantation. *J Am Soc Nephrol* **10**:154–159.

Border WA, Noble NA (1994) Transforming growth factor-β in tissue fibrosis. *N Engl J Med* **331**:1286–1292.

Brenner BM, Cohen RA, Milford EL (1992) In renal transplantation, one size may not fit all. *J Am Soc Nephrol* **3**:162–169.

Burke JF, Pirsch JD, Ramos E et al (1994) Long term efficacy and safety of cyclosporine in renal transplant recipients. *N Engl J Med* **331**:358–363.

Büyükgebiz O, Aktan AÖ, Haklar G et al (1996) BQ-123, a specific endothelin (ET$_A$) receptor antagonist, prevents ischemia-reperfusion injury in kidney transplantation. *Transplant Int* **9**:201–207.

Campistol JM, Iñigo P, Jimenez W et al (1999) Losartan decreases plasma levels of TGF-β1 in transplant patients with chronic allograft nephropathy. *Kidney Int* **56**:714–719.

Cecka JM (1999) The UNOS Scientific Renal Transplant Registry. In: Cecka JM, Terasaki PI (eds). *Clinical Transplants 1998*. Los Angeles CA: UCLA Tissue Typing Laboratory, pp. 1–16.

Cecka JM, Terasaki PI (eds). *Clinical Transplants 1991*. Los Angeles CA: UCLA Tissue Typing Laboratory, pp. 225–235.

Colvin RB (1996) The renal allograft biopsy. *Kidney Int* **50**:1069–1082.

Colvin RB, Cohen AH, Saiontz C et al (1997) Evaluation of pathologic criteria for acute renal allograft rejection: reproducibility sensitivity and clinical correlation. *J Am Soc Nephrol* **8**:1930–1941.

Cosio FG, Pelletier PR, Falkenhain ME et al (1997) Impact of acute rejection and early allograft function on renal allograft survival. *Transplantation* **63**:1611–1615.

Cosio FG, Pelletier PR, Sedmak DD et al (1999) Pathologic classification of chronic allograft nephropathy: pathogenic and prognostic implications. *Transplantation* **67**:690–697.

Costa A, Scolari M, Iannelli M et al (1997) The presence of posttransplant HLA specific IgG antibodies detected by enzyme-linked immunosorbent assay correlates with specific rejection pathologies. *Transplantation* **63**:167–169.

Cristol J, Vela C, Maggi M et al (1998) Oxidative stress and lipid abnormalities in renal transplant recipients with or without chronic rejection. *Transplantation* **65**:1322–1328.

Davenport A, Youmie ME, Parson JEM, Klouda PT (1994) Development of cytotoxic antibodies following renal allograft transplantation is associated with reduced graft survival due to chronic vascular rejection. *Nephrol Dial Transplant* **9**:1315–1319.

De Mattos AM, Olyaei AJ, Bennett WM (1996) Pharmacology of immunosuppressive medications used in renal diseases and transplantation. *Am J Kidney Dis* **28**:631–667.

Debruyne FMJ, Wijoleveld PG, Koene RAP et al (1978) Uretero-neo-cystostomy in renal transplantation. Is an anti-reflux mechanism mandatory? *Br J Urol* **50**:378–382.

Delaney V, Ling BN, Campbell WG et al (1993) Comparison of fine-needle aspiration biopsy, doppler ultrasound and radionuclide scintigraphy in the diagnosis of acute allograft dysfunction in renal transplant recipients: sensitivity, specifity and cost analysis. *Nephron* **63**:263–272.

Didlake RH, Dreyfus K, Kerman RH et al (1988) Patient noncompliance: a major cause of late graft failure in cyclosporine treated renal transplants. *Transplant Proc* **20**:63–69.

Dimeny E, Fellstrom B, Larsson E et al (1993) Chronic vascular rejection and hyperlipoproteinemia in renal transplant recipients. *Clin Transplant* **7**:482–490.

Drachenberg CB, Steinberger E, Hoehn-Saric E et al (1997) Specificity of intertubular capillary changes: comparative ultrastructural studies in renal allografts and native kidneys. *Ultrastruct Pathol* **21**:227–233.

Dragun D, Tullius GS, Park KJ et al (1998) ICAM-1 antisense oligodesoxynucleotides prevent perfusion injury and enhance immediate graft function in renal transplantation. *Kidney Int* **54**:590–602.

Ducloux D, Fournier V, Bresson-Vautrin C et al (1998) Mycophenolate mofetil in renal transplant recipients with cyclosporine-associated nephrotoxicity. *Transplantation* **65**:1504–1506.

Edagawa M, Yoshida E, Matsuzaki Y et al (1999) Reduction of post-ischemic lung reperfusion injury by fibrinolytic activity suppression. *Transplantation* 67:944–949.

El-Gamel A, Awad M, Yonan B et al (1998) Does cyclosporin promote the secretion of transforming growth factor-beta 1 following pulmunary transplantation? *Transplant Proc* 30:1525–1527.

Feehally J, Harris KPG, Bennet SE, Walls J (1987) Is chronic renal transplant rejection a non-immunological phenomenon? *Lancet* ii:486–488.

Feldman HI, Berlin A, Roth D et al (1996) Delayed graft function reduces renal allograft survival independent of acute rejection. *Nephrol Dial Transplant* 11:1306–1313.

Felldin M, Bäckman L, Brattström C (1997) Rescue therapy with tacrolimus (FK506) in renal transplant recipients: a Scandinavian multicenter analysis. *Transplant Int* 10:13–18.

Fellström B, Larsson E (1993) Pathogenesis and treatment perspectives in chronic graft rejection. *Immunol Rev* 134:83–98.

Ferguson R (1994) Acute rejection episodes-best predictor of long-term primary cadaveric renal transplantation survival. *Clin Transplant* 8:328–331.

Feucht HE, Opelz G (1996) The humoral immune response towards HLA class II determinants in renal transplantation. *Kidney Int* 50:1464–1475.

Flechner SM, Modlin CS, Serrano DP et al (1996) Determinants of chronic renal allograft rejection in cyclosporine-treated recipients. *Transplantation* 62:1235–1241.

Gaber AO, First MR, Tesi R et al (1998) Results of the double-blind, randomized, multicenter, phase III clinical trial of thymoglobulin versus ATGAM in the treatment of acute graft rejection episodes after renal transplantation. *Transplantation* 66:29–37.

Gaber LW, Schroeder TJ, Moore LW et al (1996) The correlation of Banff scoring with reversibility of first and recurrent rejection episodes. *Transplantation* 61:1711–1715.

Ghiggeri GM, Altieri P, Oleggini R et al (1994) Selective enhancement by cyclosporin A of collagen expression by mesangial cells 'in culture'. *Eur J Pharmacol* 270:195–201.

Giral-Classe M, Hourmant M, Cantavorich D et al (1998) Delayed graft function of more than six days strongly decreases long-term survival of transplanted kidneys. *Kidney Int* 54:972–978.

Gjertson DW (1992) Survival trends in long-term first cadaver donor kidney transplants. In: **Gjertson DW**, Cecka JM, Terasaki PI (1995) The relative effects of FK506 on cyclosporine on short-term and long-term kidney graft survival. *Transplantation* 60:1384–1388.

Glicklich D, Gupta B, Schurter-Frey G et al (1998) Chronic renal allograft rejection. No response to mycophenolate mofetil. *Transplantation* 66:398–399.

Gnann JW, Ahlmen J, Svalander C et al (1988) Inflammatory cells in transplanted kidneys are infected by human cytomegalovirus. *Am J Pathol* 132:239–248.

Gouldsbrough DR, Axelsen RA (1994) Arterial endothelialitis in chronic renal allograft rejection: a histopathological and immunecytochemical study. *Nephrol Dial Transplant* 9:35–40.

Grattan MT, Moreno Cabral CE, Starnes VA et al (1989) Cytomegalovirus infection is associated with cardiac rejection and atherosclerosis. *JAMA* 261:3561–3566.

Grünberger T, Gnant M, Sautner T et al (1993) Impact of vesicoureteral reflux on graft survival in renal transplantation. *Transplant Proc* 25:1058–1059.

Habib R, Broyer M (1993) Clinical significance of allograft glomerulopathy. *Kidney Int* 44(Suppl 43):595–598.

Halloran PF, Melk A, Barth C (1999) Rethinking chronic allograft nephropathy: the concept of accelerated senescence. *J Am Soc Nephrol* 10:167–181.

Hamburger J, Crosnier J, Dormont JA (1964) Observations in patients with a well tolerated transplanted kidney. *Ann NY Acad Sci* 120:558–577.

Harris KR, Digard NJ, Lee HA (1996) Serum C-reactive protein. *Transplantation* 61:1593–1600.

Haug CE, Colvin RB, Delmonico FL et al (1993) A phase I trial of immunosuppression with anti-ICAM-1 (CD54) mAb in renal allograft recipients. *Transplantation* 55:766–773.

Hayflick L, Moorhead PS (1961) The serial cultivation of human diploid cell strains. *Exp Cell Res* 25:585–621.

Häyry P (1989) Fine needle aspiration in renal transplantation. *Kidney Int* 36:130–141.

Häyry P, Isoniemi E, Yilmaz S et al (1993) Chronic allograft rejection. *Immunol Rev* 134:33–81.

Hernandez A, Light AJ, Barhyte YD et al (1999) Ablating the ischemia-reperfusion injury in non-heart-beating donor kidneys. *Transplantation* 67:200–206.

Higgins RM, Bevan DJ, Carey BS et al (1996) Prevention of hyperacute rejection by removal of antibodies to HLA immediately before renal transplantation. *Lancet* ii:1208–1211.

Hogan TF, Border EC, Mc Bain JA et al (1980) Human polyomavirus infection with JC virus and BK virus in renal transplant patients. *Ann Intern Med* 92:373–378.

Hostetter TH (1994) Chronic transplant rejection. *Kidney Int* 46:266–279.

Hourmant M, Bedrossian J, Durand D et al (1996) A randomized multicenter trial comparing leukocyte function-associated antigen-1 monoclonal antibody with rabbit antithymocyte globulin as induction treatment in first kidney transplantation. *Transplantation* 62:1565–1570.

Hueso M, Bover J, Serón D et al (1998) Low-dose cyclosporine and mycophenolate mofetil in renal allograft recipients with suboptimal renal function. *Transplantation* 66:1727–1731.

Hughes JR, Hughes VF, Trull AK, Metcalfe SM (1999) Blood levels of TGβ1 in liver transplant recipients receiving either tacrolimus or micro-emulsified cyclosporine. *Transplantation* 68:583–586.

Isoniemi HM, Krogerus L, von Willebrand E et al (1992) Histopathological findings in well-functioning, long-term renal allografts. *Kidney Int* 41:155–160.

Isoniemi H, Nurminen M, Tikkanen M et al (1994) Risk factors predicting chronic rejection of renal allografts. *Transplantation* 57:68–72.

Kahan BD, Welsh M, Shoenberg L et al (1996) Variable oral absorption of cyclosporine: a bio-pharmaceutical risk factor for chronic renal allograft rejection. *Transplantation* 62:599–606.

Kashyap R, Shapiro R, Jordan M, Randhawa PS (1999) The clinical significance of cytomegaloviral inclusions in the allograft kidney. *Transplantation* 67:98–103.

Kasiske BL, Kalil RSN, Lee HS, Rao KV (1991) Histologic findings associated with a chronic progressive decline in renal allograft function. *Kidney Int* 40:514–522.

Kelley KJ, Williams WW Jr, Colvin RB, Bonventre JV (1995) Antibodies to intercellular adhesion molecule 1 protect the kidney against ischemic injury. *Proc Natl Acad Sci USA* 91:812–816.

Ketteler M, Noble NA, Border WA (1995) Transforming growth factor-β and the kidney. *J Nephrol* 8:143–147.

Kirkman RL, Strom TB, Weir MR, Tilney NL (1992) Late mortality and morbidity in recipients of long-term allografts. *Transplantation* 34:347–351.

Kiruhara H, Yoshizumi M, Sugiyama T et al (1989) Transforming growth factor β stimulates the expression of endothelin mRNA by vascular endothelial cells. *Biochem Biophys Res Commun* 159:1435–1440.

Kliem V, Brunkhorst R (1998) Tacrolimus in kidney transplantation. *Nephron* 79:8–20.

Koo DDH, Welsh KI, McLaren J et al (1999) Cadaver versus living donor kidneys: impact of donor factors on antigen induction before transplantation. *Kidney Int* 56:1551–1559.

Kootte AMM, Paul LC (1988) Cyclosporin therapy or dietary protein manipulation in chronic allograft rejection. *Transplant Proc* 20:821–826.

Kosisken PK, Kallio EA, Tikkanen JM et al (1999) Cytomegalovirus infection and cardiac allograft vasculopathy. *Transpl Infect Dis* 1:115–126.

Kovarik JM, Mueller EA, Van Bree JB et al (1994) Cyclosporine pharmacokinetics and variability from a microemulsion formulation: a multicenter investigation in kidney transplant patients. *Transplantation* 58:658–663.

Land W, Messmer K (1996) The impact of ischemia/reperfusion injury on specific and non-specific early late chronic events after organ transplantation. *Transplant Rev* 10:108–127.

Land W, Schneebeberger H, Schleibner ST et al (1994) Beneficial effect of human recombinant superoxide dismutase on both acute and chronic rejection events in recipients of cadaveric renal transplants. *Transplantation* **57**:211–217.

Lehtonen SRK, Isoniemi HM, Salmela KT et al (1997) Long-term graft outcome is not necessarily affected by delayed onset of graft function and early rejection. *Transplantation* **64**:103–107.

Leichtman AB, Strom TB (1988) Therapeutic approach to renal transplantation: triple therapy and beyond. *Transplant Proc* **20** (suppl 8): 1–6.

Li B, Sehajpal PK, Vlassara H et al (1991) Differential regulation of transforming growth factor β and interleukin-2 genes in human T cells: demonstration by usage of novel competitor DNA constructs in the quantitative polymerase chain reaction. *J Exp Med* **174**:1259–1262.

Li F, Yin M, Van Dam JG et al (1998) Cytomegalovirus enhances the neointima formation in rat aortic allografts. *Transplantation* **65**:1298–1304.

Lindholm A, Ohlman S, Albrechtsen D et al (1993) The impact of acute rejection episodes on long-term graft function and outcome in 1347 primary renal transplants treated by cyclosporine regimen. *Transplantation* **56**:307–315.

Lu C, Penfield IG, Kielar M et al (1999) Does the injury of transplantation initiate acute rejection? *Graft* **2**(Suppl II): S36–S41.

Manfro RC, Gonçalves LFS, Ribeiro de Moura LA (1995) Reproducibility of fine needle aspiration biopsy in the diagnosis of acute rejection of renal allografts. *Nephrol Dial Transplant* **10**:2306–2309.

Maorca R, Sardrini S, Cancarini GC et al (1992) Kidney transplantation in peritoneal dialysis patients. *Perit Dial Internat* **14** (suppl 3):S162–S168.

Marcén R, Orofino L, Pascual J et al (1998) Delayed graft function does not reduce the survival of renal transplant allografts. *Transplantation* **66**:461–466.

Mariat C, Alamartine E, Dial N et al (1988) A randomised prospective study comparing low-dose OKT3 to low-dose ATG for the treatment of acute steroid-resistant episodes in kidney transplant recipients. *Transplant Int* **11**:231–236.

Maryniak RK, First MR, Weiss MA (1985) Transplant glomerulopathy: evolution of morphologically distinct changes. *Kidney Int* **27**:799–806.

Massy ZA, Guijarro C, Wiederkehr MR et al (1996) Chronic renal allograft rejection: immunologic and nonimmunologic risk factors. *Kidney Int* **49**:518–524.

Mastrosimone S, Pignata G, Maresca MC et al (1993) Clinical significance of vesicoureteral reflux after kidney transplantation. *Clin Nephrol* **40**:38–42.

Matas AJ, Sibley R, Mauer M et al (1983) The value of needle renal allograft biopsy. I. A retrospective study of biopsies performed during rejection episodes. *Ann Surg* **197**:226–237.

Matas AJ, Almond PS, Moss A et al (1995) Effect of cyclosporine on renal transplant recipients: a 12 year follow-up. *Clin Transplant* **9**:450–455.

Mathur VS, Olson JL, Darragh TM, Yen TS (1997) Polyomavirus-induced interstitial nephritis in two renal transplant recipients: case reports and review of the literature. *Am J Kidney Dis* **29**:754–758.

Matzinger P (1994) Tolerance, danger, and the extended family. *Ann Rev Immunol* **12**:991–1045.

Mazzucchi E, Lucon AM, Nahas WC et al (1999) Histological outcome of acute cellular rejection in kidney transplantation after treatment with methylprednisolone. *Transplantation* **67**:430–434.

Mekki Q, Lee C, Aweeka F et al (1993) Pharmacokinetics of tacrolimus (FK506) in kidney transplant patients (abstract). *Clin Pharm Ther* **53**:238.

Menger MD (1995). Microcirculatory disturbances secondary to ischemia/reperfusion. *Transplant Proc* **27**:2863.

Midtevedt K, Tafjord AB, Hartmann A et al (1996) Half dose of OKT3 is efficient in treatment of steroid-resistant renal allograft rejection *Transplantation* **62**:38–42.

Mihatsch MJ, Thiel G, Ryffel B (1988) Morphologic diagnosis of cyclosporine nephrotoxicity. *Semin Diagn Pathol* **5**:104–121.

Mihatsch MJ, Ryffel B, Gudat F (1995) The differential diagnosis between rejection and cyclosporine toxicity. *Kidney Int* **48**(Suppl 52): S63–S69.

Miles AMV, Sumrani N, John S et al (1996) The effect of kidney size on cadaveric renal allograft outcome. *Transplantation* **61**:894–897.

Modena FM, Hostetter TH, Salahudeen AK et al (1991) Progression of kidney disease in chronic renal transplant rejection. *Transplantation* **52**:239–244.

Monga G, Mazzucco G. Messina M et al (1992) Intertubular capillary changes in kidney allografts: a morphologic investigation on 61 renal specimens. *Mod Pathol* **5**:125–130.

Montagnino G, Tarantino A, Cesana B et al (1997) Prognostic factors of long-term allograft survival in 632 CyA-treated recipients of a primary renal transplant. *Transplant Int* **10**:268–275.

Morozumi K, Thiel G, Albert FW et al (1992) Studies on morphological outcome of cyclosporine associated arteriopathy after discontinuation of cyclosporine in renal allografts. *Clin Nephrol* **38**:1–6.

Mourad G, Vela C, Ribstein J, Mimran A (1998) Long-term improvement in renal function after cyclosporine reduction in renal transplant recipients with histologically proven chronic cyclosporine nephropathy. *Transplantation* **65**:661–666.

Mycophenolate Mofetil Renal Refractory Rejection Study Group (1996) Mycophenolate mofetil for the treatment of refractory, acute, cellular renal transplant rejection. *Transplantation* **61**:722–729.

Neild Gh, Rueben R, Hartley RB, Cameron JS (1985) Glomerular thrombi in renal allograft associated with cyclosporine treatment. *J Clin Pathol* **38**:253–258.

Novitzky D (1997) Detrimental effects of brain death on the potential organ donor. *Transplant Proc* **29**:3770.

Opelz G, for the Collaborative Transplant Study (1997) Critical evaluation of the association of acute with chronic graft rejection in kidney and heart transplant recipients. *Transplant Proc* **29**:73–76.

Opelz G, Wujciak T, Ritz E (1998) Association of chronic kidney graft failure with recipient blood pressure. *Kidney Int* **53**:217–222.

Opelz G, Döler B, Wujciak T (1999) Current results as references for future improvements in immunosuppression under trial. In: Cochat P (ed.). *Proceedings of the 31st International Conference on Transplantation and Clinical Immunology.* Dordrecht: Kluwer Academic, pp. 3–9.

Oppenheimer F, Flores R, Cofan F et al (1995) Treatment with angiotensin converting enzyme inhibitors in renal transplantation with proteinuria. *Transplant Proc* **27**:2235–2236.

Pascual J, Marcen R, Orofino L et al (1991) Evidence that addition of azathioprine improves renal function in cyclosporine-treated patients with allograft dysfunction. *Transplantation* **52**:276–280.

Paul LC (1999) Chronic allograft nephropathy. *Kidney Int* **56**:783–793.

Paul LC, Fellström B (1992) Chronic vascular rejection of the heart and the kidney. Have rational treatment options emerged? *Transplantation* **53**:1169–1179.

Perrella RR, Duerincky AJ, Tessler FN et al (1990) Evaluation of renal transplant dysfunction by duplex Doppler sonography: a prospective study and review of literature. *Am J Kidney Dis* **15**:544–550.

Pfaff WW, Howard RJ, Pattorn PR et al (1998) Delayed graft function after transplantation. *Transplantation* **65**:219–223.

Pollak R, Andrisevic JH, Maddux MS et al (1999) A randomized double blind trial of the use of human recombinant superoxide dismutase in renal transplantation. *Transplantation* **55**:57–60.

Ponticelli C (1998) Chronic kidney allograft dysfunction in the cyclosporine era. *Curr Opin Organ Transplant* **3**:169–174.

Ponticelli C, Campise M (1997) Appropriate endpoints for renal transplantation. *Drug Inform J* **31**:207–212.

Ponticelli C, Civati G, Tarantino A et al (1996) Randomized study with cyclosporine in kidney transplantation: 10-year follow-up. *J Am Soc Nephrol* 7:792–797.

Ponticelli C, Aroldi A, Elli A et al (1999) The clinical status of cadaveric renal transplant patients treated for 10 years with cyclosporine therapy. *Clin Transplant* 13:324–329.

Raisanen-Sokolowski A, Vuoristo P, Myllarnierni M et al (1995) Mycophenolate mofetil inhibits inflammation and smooth muscle cell proliferation in rat aortic allografts. *Transplant Immunol* 3:342.

Randhawa PS, Shapiro R, Jordan ML et al (1993) The histopathological changes associated with allograft rejection and drug toxicity in renal transplant recipients maintained on FK 506. Clinical significance and comparison with cyclosporine. *Am J Surg Pathol* 17:60–68.

Randhawa PS, Finkelstein S, Scantlebury V et al (1999) Human polyoma virus-associated interstitial nephritis in the allograft kidney. *Transplantation* 67:103–109.

Reisaeter AV, Leivestad T, Albrechtsen D et al (1995) Pretransplant plasma exchange facilitates renal transplantation in immunized patients. *Transplantation* 60:242–248.

Richardson WP, Colvin RB, Cheeseman SH et al (1981) Glomerulopathy associated with cytomegalovirus viremia in renal allografts. *N Engl J Med* 305:57–62.

Roodnat JI, Zietse R, Mulder PGH et al (1999) The vanishing importance of age in renal transplantation. *Transplantation* 67:576–580.

Rosenberg EM, Salahudeen KA, Hostetter HT (1995) Dietary protein and the renin, angiotensin system in chronic renal allograft rejection. *Kidney Int* 48(Suppl 52):S102–S106.

Ross CN, Gaskin G, Macgregor S et al (1993) Renal transplantation following immunoadsorption in highly sensitised recipients. *Transplantation* 55:785–789.

Rush D, Grimm P, Jeffrey J et al (1999) Predicting rejection. *Graft* 2(Suppl 2):S31–S35.

Sennesael J, Lamote J, Violet I et al (1995) Comparison of perindopril and amlodipine in cyclosporine-treated renal allograft recipients. *Hypertension* 26:436–444.

Sharma VK, Bologa RM, Xu GP et al (1996) Intragraft TGFβ_1 mRNA: a correlate of interstitial fibrosis and chronic allograft nephropathy. *Kidney Int* 49:1297–1303.

Shokes D, Cecka IM (1998) Deleterious effects of delayed graft function in cadaveric renal transplant recipients independent of acute rejection. *Transplantation* 66:1697–1701.

Solez K, Axelsen RA, Benediktsson H et al (1993) International standardization of nomenclature and criteria for the histologic diagnosis of renal allograft rejection: the Banff working classification of kidney transplant pathology. *Kidney Int* 44:411–422.

Solez K, Benediktsson H, Cavallo T et al (1996) Report of the third Banff conference on allograft pathology (July 20–24, 1995) on classification and lesion scoring in renal allograft pathology. *Transplant Proc* 28:441–444.

Sommer BG, Innes JT, Whitehurst RM et al (1985) Cyclosporine-associated renal arteriopathy resulting in loss of allograft function. *Am J Surg* 149:756–764.

Sweny P, Wheeler DC, Lui SF (1989) Dietary fish oil supplements preserve renal function in renal transplant recipients with chronic vascular rejection. *Nephrol Dial Transplant* 4:1070–1075.

Takada M, Nadeau CK, Shaw DG, Tilney LN (1997) Prevention of late renal changes after initial ischemia/reperfusion injury by blocking early selectin binding. *Transplantation* 64:1520–1525.

Takada M, Nadeau KC, Hancock WW et al (1998) Effects of explosive brain death on cytokine activation of peripheral organs in the rat. *Transplantation* 61:1533–1542.

Taube DH, Williams DG, Cameron JS et al (1984) Renal transplantation after removal and prevention of resynthesis of HLA antibodies. *Lancet* i:824–826.

Ten Berge RJM, Buysmann S, van Diepen FNJ et al (1996) Consequence of OKT3 administration via continuous infusion as compared to bolus infusion. *Transplant Proc* 28:3217–3220.

Teraoka S, Takahashi K, Toma H et al (1987) New approach to management of chronic vascular rejection with prostacyclin analogue after kidney transplantation. *Transplant Proc* 19:2115–2119.

Terasaki PI, Cecka JM, Gjertson DW et al (1995) High survival rates of kidney transplants from spousal and living unrelated donors. *N Engl J Med* **333**:333–336.

Traindl O, Falger S, Reading S et al (1993) The effects of lisinopril on renal function in protein-uric renal transplant recipients. *Transplantation* **55**:1309–1313.

Troppmann C, Benedetti E, Almond S et al (1995) Delayed graft function, acute rejection and outcome after cadaver renal transplantation. *Transplantation* **59**:962–968.

Troppmann C, Gillingham KJ, Guessner RW et al (1996) Delayed graft function in the absence of rejection has no long-term impact. A study of cadaver kidney recipients with good graft function at 1 year after transplantation. *Transplantation* **61**:1331–1337.

Tuazon TV, Schneeberger EE, Bhan AK et al (1987) Mononuclear cells in acute allograft glomerulopathy. *Am J Pathol* **29**:119–132.

Tublin ME, Dodd GD III (1995) Sonography of renal transplantation. *Radiol Clin North Am* **33**:447–459.

Van der Hoevon JAB, Postema F, Van Suylichem PTR et al (1998) Effects of brain death on donor organ quality: endothelial cell activation and predisposition for ischemia/reperfusion damage in transplantation. *Transplantation* **65**:95–99.

Vanrenterghem Y, Peeters J (1994) The impact of cyclosporine on graft vasculopathy. *Transplant Proc* **26**:2560–2563.

Vincenti F, Danovich GM, Neylan JF et al (1996) Pentoxyfilline does not prevent cytokine induced first dose reaction following OKT3: a randomized double-blind placebo-controlled study. *Transplantation* **61**:573–577.

Visscher D, Carey I, Oh H et al (1991) Histologic and immunophenotypic evaluation of pre-treatment renal biopsies in OKT3-treated allograft rejections. *Transplantation* **51**:1023–1028.

Von Obberghen-Schilling E, Roche NS, Flanders KC et al (1985) Transforming growth factor-β positively regulates its own expression in normal and transformed cells. *J Biol Chem* **262**:7741–7746.

Waiser J, Budde K, Schreiber M et al (1998) Antibody therapy in steroid-resistant rejection. *Transplant Proc* **30**:1778–1779.

Weir RM, Anderson L, Fink CJ et al (1977) A novel approach to the treatment of chronic allograft nephropathy. *Transplantation* **64**:1706–1710.

Woodle ES, Thistlethwaite JR, Gordon JH, for the Tacrolimus Kidney Transplantation Rescue Study Group (1996) Tacrolimus therapy for refractory acute renal allograft rejection: a prospective multicenter trial. *Transplant Proc* **28**:3163–3164.

Young BA, Barsh CL, Alpers CE, Davis CL (1996) Cyclosporine-associated thrombotic microangiopathy/hemolytic uremic syndrome following kidney and kidney–pancreas transplantation. *Am J Kidney Dis* **28**:561–571

12 RECURRENT PRIMARY DISEASE AND DE NOVO NEPHRITIS

In collaboration with G Banfi*

Recurrence of the original disease following renal transplantation is a relatively frequent complication, which may contribute to the dysfunction and even to the loss of kidney allograft. The incidence and the severity of recurrence depend on the nature of primary disease. The length of graft survival is also important. The risk of recurrence was 2.8% at 2 years but 18.5% at 8 years in an analysis of 1577 transplants (Hariharan et al 1998). In other instances a de novo renal disease may develop in the allografted kidney. The recognition of recurrent or de novo renal disease is important not only to avoid wrong diagnosis and incorrect treatment but also to institute adequate therapeutic measures promptly, whenever possible. In this regard, renal biopsy and its thorough investigation, encompassing immunofluorescence and electron microscopy studies, have an irreplaceable role in most cases.

RECURRENCE OF PRIMARY DISEASE

Primary glomerulonephritis (GN)

All forms of GN may recur on the kidney allograft but the risk of recurrence is different for the various subtypes of GN (Table 3.4). However even for a single subtype of GN it is difficult to assess the risk of recurrence for several reasons. (1) In many renal transplant recipients the diagnosis of the primary disease is unknown, so that it is difficult to establish whether the glomerulonephritis of the kidney allograft represents a recurrence of GN, a de novo GN or a GN of the donor. (2) Because of the different indications for graft biopsy adopted by various transplant units it is impossible to assess the exact incidence of a recurrence of GN even in a recipient with a well-known diagnosis of the original disease. (3) In some cases the recurrence of histological lesions in the allograft is not heralded by signs and symptoms. (4) Sometimes the recurrent GN may show a morphology only partially reproducing that of the primary disease, probably as a consequence of the immunosuppressive therapy and of the different duration of the disease.

*Division of Nephrology and Dialysis, Ospedale Maggiore, Milan

For any type of GN the risk of recurrence seems particularly high when the original nephropathy had a rapid course.

Focal and segmental glomerulosclerosis (FSGS)

Patients with FSGS are at high risk of recurrence after renal transplantation. Approximately 15–50% of patients develop recurrence of FSGS in the first allograft (Ponticelli and Banfi 1997). At present, it is almost impossible to predict which patient will have a recurrence after transplantation and which will not. It seems, however, that in recipients with better HLA matching (Hariharan and Savin 1999), patients with collapsing variant of FSGS and in those who had a rapid progression uremia the risk of recurrence is higher (Tejani and Stablein 1992). Second grafts in those who have had recurrence in their first graft are accompanied in 85% by a further recurrence (Senguttuvan et al 1990).

In patients with recurrence, proteinuria and the early lesions of FSGS usually develop early (Figure 12.1), in median 10–18 days after transplantation (Cochat et al 1996), but the modalities of recurrence may vary from patient to patient, from immediate massive proteinuria to milder forms that develop after years. Spontaneous remission of proteinuria is exceptional. Patients with recurrence of FSGS have reduced graft survival. In a European pediatric survey the median survival of the graft from the appearance of nephrotic syndrome was 5 months (Ehrich et al 1992). A retrospective analysis of the literature found that 50–85% of patients with recurrence lost their allograft within 2 years (Ponticelli and Banfi 1997). It is possible that the high rate of acute renal failure and acute rejection observed in patients with recurrence may have contributed to this poor survival (Kim et al 1994).

The frequent occurrence of a rapid or even immediate relapse of proteinuria after transplantation suggests that at least some patients with FSGS have circulating factor(s) capable of altering glomerular permeability in normal grafts. Savin et al (1996) have isolated a circulating factor with an apparent molecular mass of about 50 daltons in patients with recurrent FSGS after transplantation, which might be responsible for initiating renal injury. Recently, Dantal et al (1998) reported that the albuminuric factors(s) are part of a complex with immunoglobulins. However, no firm evidence could be provided against a direct role of immunoglobulins.

The management of patients with recurrence of FSGS and nephrotic syndrome is difficult. Three large series have examined the frequency of recurrence in recipients treated with azathioprine or with cyclosporine. In none of the three series nor in the pooled data was there any difference in incidence (Habib et al 1987; Banfi et al 1990; Senguttuvan et al 1990). An amelioration of proteinuria has been reported in a few children given very high doses of cyclosporine (Ingulli and Tejani 1991). The aim of such an approach is to compensate the lipid binding of cyclosporine by elevated low density lipoprotein (LDL) concentrations. It is now recommended to give high-dose cyclosporine intravenously (target blood level 250–350 ng/ml) to children in order to keep a steady state blood level (Cochat et al 1996). However the long-term efficacy and

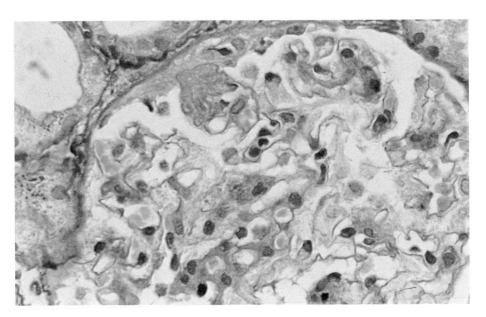

Figure 12.1. Recurrence of FSGS in a 16 year old boy 15 days after transplantation, profuse proteinuria developed immediately. Graft biopsy showed the typical early features of FSGS: initial collapse of a small peripheral loop, adhering to the capsule through a crown of hypertrophic epithelial cells. (AFOG ×600)

tolerance of such a therapy remains to be established. Artero et al (1992) treated nine patients with angiotensin-converting enzyme (ACE) inhibitors. Of them, five had lasting remission of proteinuria and stable renal function during treatment.

An alternative approach is represented by the use of early plasmapheresis. A review of the literature reported that of 17 adults treated with plasmapheresis because of a relapse of a nephrotic syndrome, five (29%) attained complete disappearance of proteinuria and another five patients showed a reduction of daily urine protein excretion to less than 3 g per day (Ponticelli and Banfi 1997). The response was better in patients treated earlier and more intensively. After stopping plasma exchange almost half of the responders relapsed. Some patients, however, responded to a new course of treatment. Even better are the results in children. The same review reported 17 cases of complete remission and four partial remissions in 23 children given plasmapheresis and concomitant intensified immunosuppression. A more specific apheresis, namely immunoadsorption with protein A, followed by intravenous infusion of human immunoglobulins has been proposed by Dantal et al (1994). However, among eight patients treated with such a technique only one attained a sustained remission while another patient had only a transient improvement in proteinuria. On the basis of the available results, we suggest that patients with

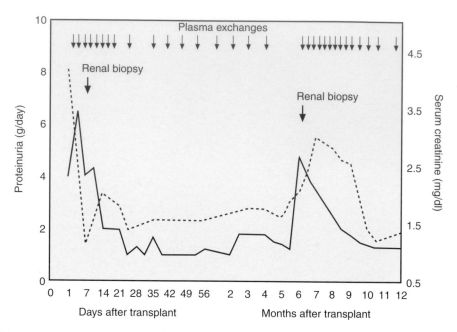

Figure 12.2. Effect of plasmapheresis on daily proteinuria (––) and serum creatinine (– – –) in a 26-year-old man with an early recurrence of focal and segmental glomerulosclerosis after renal transplantation and a relapse after stopping plasma exchanges.

recurrent FSGS and severe nephrotic syndrome should be treated as soon as possible with an intensive course of plasmapheresis (three exchanges per week for the first 2 weeks, then two per week for another 2 weeks, then one per week). If a complete disappearance of proteinuria is obtained we stop plasmapheresis. If proteinuria improves but remains over 2–3 g per day we continue plasma exchanges at longer intervals. A further course of plasmapheresis may be attempted in the case of relapse of nephrotic proteinuria (Figure 12.2). We also recommend the administration of high-dose ACE inhibitors in order to exploit the antiproteinuric effect of these agents. Whether reinforcement of immunosuppressive therapy might allow a more stable remission is still uncertain. Owing to the risk of overimmunosuppression the use of a more aggressive immunosuppressive therapy should be determined on an individual basis.

Membranous nephropathy (MN)

Membranous nephropathy can develop in a transplanted kidney either as recurrence of the original disease or as a de novo form. About one-third of allograft MN are caused by recurrence and two-thirds by a de novo glomerulonephritis.

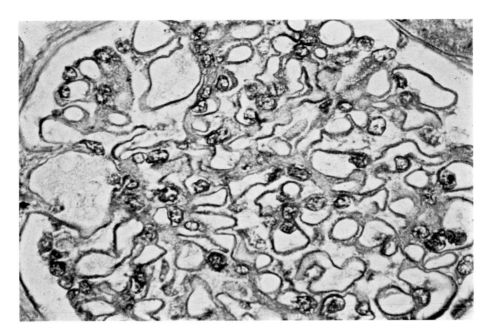

Figure 12.3. De novo membranous nephropathy in a patient transplanted because of polycystic kidney disease. Diffuse and regular thickening of capillary walls similar to that seen in idiopathic membranous nephropathy. (Jones silver ×480)

The proportion of recurrence of MN is difficult to assess (Ponticelli and Passerini 1997) as a de novo form may develop even in transplant recipients with an idiopathic MN as original disease with an indistinguishable histological pattern (Figures 12.3–12.5). The recurrence is exceptional in children. In adults the rate of recurrence averages 20–30% in the largest series (Odorico et al 1996; Cosyns et al 1998). The risk of recurrence seems to be higher in patients receiving a transplant from a living related donor than in those receiving a cadaveric kidney. The time of recurrence was earlier in recipients of a living-donor allograft (9.3 ± 3 months after transplantation) than in cadaveric transplant recipients (18.2 ± 7.5 months; Josephson et al 1994). Recurrence is not inhibited by cyclosporine (Montagnino et al 1989, Schwarz et al 1991). Obermiller et al (1985) suggested that more aggressive disease is more likely to recur after transplantation but others did not find any relationship between the duration of original disease and the rate of recurrence (Cosyns et al 1998).

Clinically, the recurrence is heralded by the appearance of proteinuria, which is often in a nephrotic range (more than 3.5 g per day). Rarely, proteinuria may spontaneously improve or even disappear (Marcen et al 1996). With the exception of these cases, the nephrotic syndrome is usually resistant to any treatment and about two-thirds of patients progress to end-stage renal failure in mean 4.1 ± 2.6 years after diagnosis of

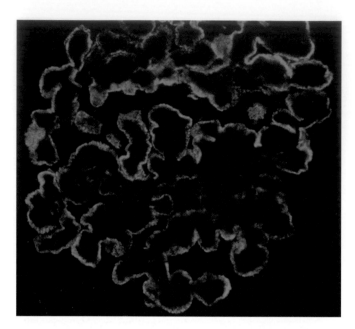

Figure 12.4. Immunofluorescence of the same case. Partial, fine granular deposits of IgG pathognomonic of membranous nephropathy. (×400)

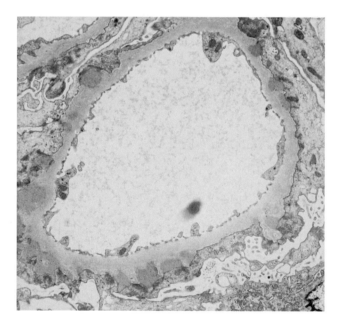

Figure 12.5. Membranous nephropathy, stage I–II: electron-dense globular deposits lay on the outer side of the glomerular basement membrane, separated by initial spikes. (×16 000)

recurrence (Josephson et al 1994). Renal vein thrombosis may also complicate the course of recurrent MN (First et al 1984). The bad prognosis is not always attributable to MN as many patients also showed histological evidence of rejection.

Membranoproliferative glomerulonephritis (MPGN)

Type I MPGN accounts for approximately 80% of cases of idiopathic MPGN. It is characterized by electron-dense subendothelial deposits that contain immunoglobulins and complement by immunofluorescence. Clinically the disease is characterized by hematuria, heavy proteinuria, hypertension and impairment of renal function. The recurrence rate is quite difficult to estimate because the feature lesions of type I MPGN on light microscopy (Figure 12.6) may mimic those seen in allograft glomerulopathy (Gallay et al 1995). However, at immunofluorescence patients with recurrent type I MPGN show greater intensity of C3 (Figure 12.7) while there is greater intensity for IgM in allograft glomerulopathy. On electron microscopy, type I MPGN shows subendothelial electron-dense deposits while transplant glomerulopathy shows an electron-lucent zone in the subendothelial space (Andresdottir et al 1998; Figure 12.8). In children, a French series reported recurrence in seven of 11 renal allograft recipients with graft loss in two patients (Habib et al 1987) while an American series found graft loss in only one child of 13 (Alexander et al 1990). A recent survey of the EDTA registry (Briggs and Jones 1999a) showed 6% of graft failure due to recurrence with a survival at 2 years of 86%. In adults the recurrence rate reached 48% at 4 years in a series

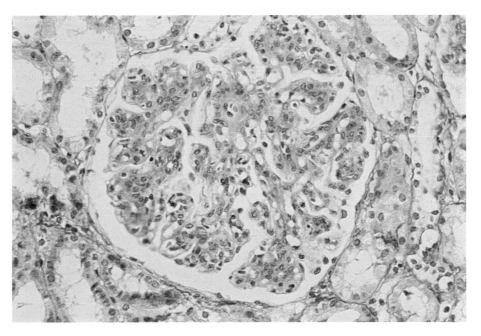

Figure 12.6. Recurrence of membranoproliferative glomerulonephritis type I. Diffuse hypercellularity, mainly due to mesangial cell proliferation, accompanied by mesangial matrix increase and diffuse, though irregular, thickening of the capillary walls. (AFOG ×300)

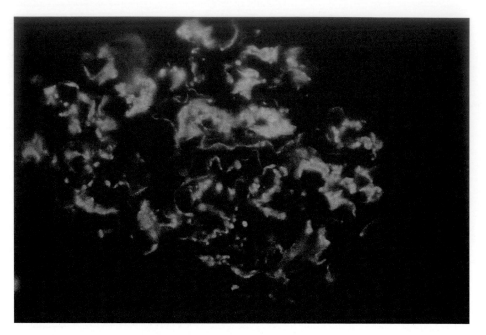

Figure 12.7. Immunostaining with C3 in coarse granular deposits in the mesangium and parietal position, corroborates the diagnosis of MPGN type I

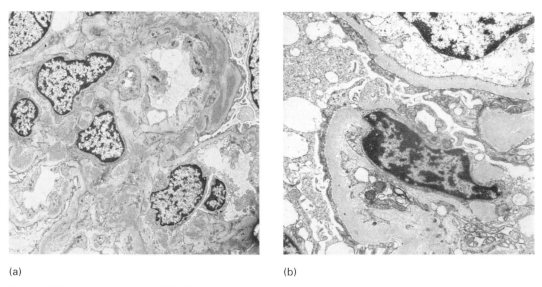

(a)   (b)

Figure 12.8. (a) Recurrence of MPGN type I. Together with the immunofluorescence pattern, electron microscopical investigation is mandatory to confirm the diagnosis of a recurrence of MPGN type I, disclosing the presence of deposits in the subendothelial and mesangial position ($\times$16 000). (b) For diagnostic purposes the ultrastructural features of a case of 'chronic transplant glomerulopathy' are shown. There is a fairly homogeneous thickening of the 'lamina rara interna', in the absence of electron-dense deposits and cellular interposition. ($\times$25 000)

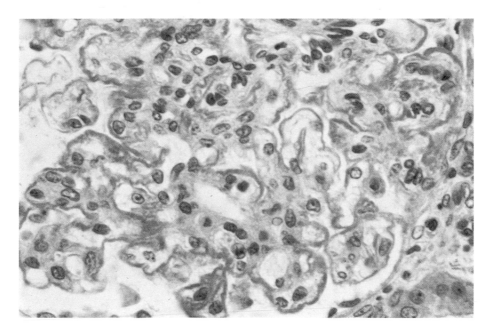

Figure 12.9. Recurrence of MPGN type II. Bright, continuous, ribbon-like deposits underline the capillary walls in this case of dense deposit disease (–), recurring 2 years after transplantation. (AFOG ×650)

(Andresdottir et al 1997). The risk of recurrence is considerably lower in Japan, around 3%, suggesting a role for racial predisposition (Shimizu et al 1998). There are no clinical features prior to transplantation that can predict the risk of recurrence. Cyclosporine does not seem to be able to prevent recurrence (Schwarz et al 1991) but may be protective against crescentic transformation (Ahsan et al 1997). The major clinical feature of recurrence is proteinuria, leading to the nephrotic syndrome and progression to renal insufficiency. Graft survival is poorer in patients with recurrence, being on average 40 months after the diagnosis of recurrence (Andresdottir et al 1997).

Type II MPGN, also called dense deposit disease, is characterized by intramembranous electron-dense deposits and is sometimes associated with partial lipodystrophy. C3 deposits can be found by immunofluorescence in the basal lamina surrounding the deposits and in the mesangium. The clinical expression of dense deposit disease is similar to that of MPGN type I. The histologic and ultrastructural features of recurrent type II MPGN are similar to those seen in the original disease (Figures 12.9 and 12.10). The histologic recurrence of dense deposits after renal transplantation ranges between 85 and 100% (Habib et al 1987; Cameron 1991; Mathew 1991) while clinical recurrence is much less common. Graft failure due to recurrent disease is 10–13% in adults (Cameron 1982; Mathew 1991) and around 28% in children (Habib et al 1987) but

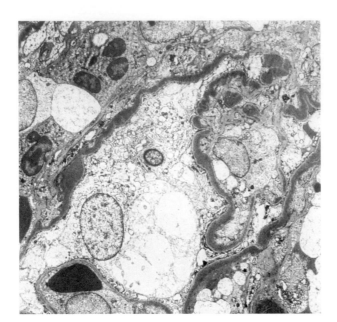

Figure 12.10. Recurrence of MPGN type II. Electron microscopy shows the characteristic dense transformation of the GBM.

these data are approximate as the number of reported cases is small and the follow-ups are variable.

A case of recurrence of type III MPGN, with electron-dense deposits in the mesangium, as well as in subepithelial and subendothelial positions, has been reported. The patient progressed to dialysis within 3 months after diagnosis. A second transplant was lost after 7 years because of recurrence (Morales et al 1997). There is no effective therapy for recurrent MPGN.

IgA nephropathy (IgAGN)

Histologic recurrence of mesangial IgAGN (Figures 12.11 and 12.12) is seen in about 60% of renal allografts in patients with a primary IgAGN (Odum et al 1994; Berger et al 1995; Kessler et al 1996). These figures may be underestimated as not all recipients are biopsied and in others IgA is not sought in the biopsy (Cameron 1991). Moreover, the prevalence of recurrent deposits largely depends on the timing of renal biopsy, being around 50% at 2–5 years but approaching 100% at 10–20 years after renal transplantation (Lee and Glassock 1997). The risk of recurrence is similar for recipients of living-related and cadaveric renal allografts. No pretransplant characteristics are predictive for recurrence (Coppo et al 1995; Ohmacht et al 1997).

Hematuria and low-grade proteinuria represent the clinical expression of recurrence. Rarely, a rapidly progressive renal failure caused by an underlying crescentic glomerulonephritis may occur (Diaz-Tejeiro et al 1990).

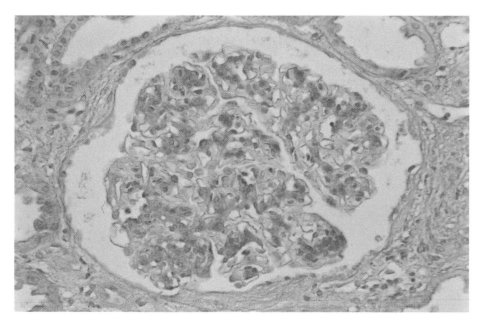

Figure 12.11. Recurrent IgAGN. Moderate mesangial enlargement due to mesangial cells proliferation and matrix increase. (PAS ×480)

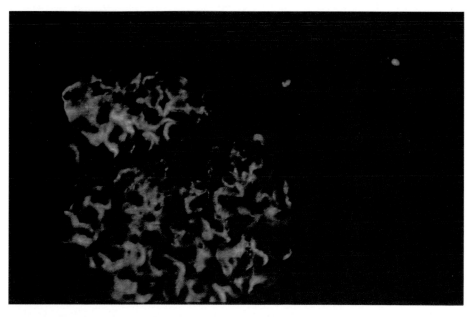

Figure 12.12. Recurrent IgAGN. The immunofluorescence shows the characteristic bright immunostaining for IgA, with parietal and mesangial pattern. (×400)

Previous reports have reported more favorable outcomes of the renal allograft in patients with IgAGN (Lim et al 1991; Alamartine et al 1994) but others found that graft survival in an IgA group was similar to that of non-IgA renal transplant recipients (Kim et al 1996; Bumgardner et al 1998). It now seems clear that the risk of graft loss caused by recurrence depends on the length of the follow-up. Hartung et al (1995) found a 15% lower cumulative graft survival rate at 5 years after transplantation in patients showing a recurrence when compared to those without recurrence. Odum et al (1994) followed 17 patients with recurrent IgAGN for 72 months. Graft loss occurred in five of them (29%). Bumgardner et al (1998) followed 18 renal transplant recipients with clinical and histologic signs of recurrence of IgAGN. At a mean follow-up of 61 months six patients (33%) lost their allograft and another four showed deteriorating renal function. Kimata et al (1996) reported that patients with recurrent disease who had proteinuria of more than 1 g per day and more than 30% glomerulosclerosis at renal biopsy, almost uniformly developed graft loss by 6 years after transplant. Thus, despite early reports that recurrent IgAGN is a benign process and despite the indolent course of the disease, it is now clear that in the long term IgAGN may be associated with deteriorating renal function and graft in a substantial proportion of patients. Living-related transplantation and HLA-matching do not appear to confer an advantage for graft survival (Bumgardner et al 1998).

There is no specific therapy for recurrent IgAGN. ACE inhibitors may be prescribed if hypertension and/or proteinuria are present, as these agents proved to be protective in primary IgAGN (Maschio et al 1994). If recurrent crescentic IgAGN develops, a trial with high-dose corticosteroids, cyclophosphamide and plasmapheresis may be attempted. Bumgardner et al (1998) reported the outcome of five patients retransplanted because of recurrence of IgAGN and graft loss. In spite of re-recurrence of IgAGN in three patients, all patients have a good graft function at an average follow-up of 54 months after their second transplant.

Antiglomerular basement membrane glomerulonephritis (antiGBM GN)

The recurrence of this disease is defined by linear deposits of IgG on glomerular capillary walls (Figure 12.13). AntiGBM GN recurs in 10–30% of allografts particularly if circulating antiGBM antibodies are present at the time of transplantation (Glassock 1997). Conversely, in patients in whom antibodies can not be detected, recurrent disease does not recur (Senguttuvan et al 1990).

Clinical disease consequent to the glomerular deposits of antiGBM antibodies occurs in less than 10% of cases and only rarely leads to graft loss. In the past, bilateral nephrectomy of the native kidneys was performed in order to allow disappearance of antibodies. This intervention is not recommended today. Most clinicians prefer to check the titer of circulating antiGBM antibodies periodically and wait for 6–12 months before transplantation until antiGBM antibodies disappear. With such a policy the recurrence of antiGBM GN has virtually disappeared.

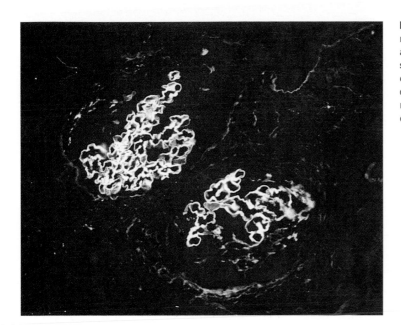

Figure 12.13. Early recurrence of antiGBM-GN in a patient with Goodpasture syndrome. Linear deposition of IgG along the GBM characterizes the reappearance of antiGBM disease in the graft. (×250)

Lupus nephritis

Recurrence of lupus nephritis is very rare (Figure 12.14). A review of the literature reported only eight cases of recurrence out of 823 patients transplanted for lupus nephritis (Stone et al 1997). A higher number of histologic recurrence at iterative renal allograft biopsy has been reported by Nyberg et al (1992) even if morphologic lesions were usually mild. At any rate, even if it is possible that recurrence of lupus nephritis may be more frequent than the 1% reported in the literature, this event occurs in a small minority of cases. Several hypotheses have been advanced to explain this low rate of recurrence even in patients with signs of clinical and serologic activity at the time of transplantation. (1) The immunosuppressive state induced by uremia might quench the lupus activity. (2) The natural course of the disease may gradually subside in the long term (Swaak et al 1989). (3) The kidney of patients with lupus nephritis may have some component that allows the appearance of nephritis and which is missing from the allografted kidney (Cameron 1991). It is possible, however, that the rate of recurrence has been underestimated because of underreporting, insufficient follow-up and/or failure to diagnose recurrence (Stone 1998).

From a clinical point of view, after transplantation many patients who were previously unresponsive to immunosuppression show little or no sign of active disease (Nossent et al 1991). Even in patients in whom recurrence has been clearly identified it is usually of little clinical relevance and does not justify a reinforcement of immunosuppression, which should be reserved for exceptional cases showing a severe lupus flare-up.

537

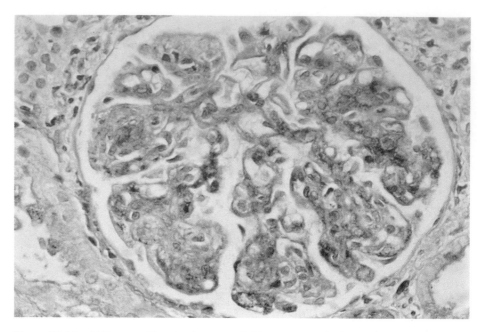

Figure 12.14. Diffuse proliferative lupus nephritis may recur in the graft with the same pattern, although sometimes with focal distribution. In this glomerulus hypercellularity is moderate; mesangial expansion with protein deposits, irregular but there is severe thickening of the capillary loops due to mesangial interposition and proteinaceous deposits. (AFOG ×400)

Henoch–Schönlein purpura

A review of the literature reported a recurrence of IgA mesangial deposits in 53% of renal allografts performed in patients with Henoch–Schönlein purpura. Clinical recurrence with microscopic hematuria and proteinuria occurred in 18% of cases; graft loss from recurrence occurred in 11% of cases at 5 years (Meulders et al 1994).

Recurrence is frequent in children, while it is quite rare in adults (Crown et al 1994). Some papers reported a higher risk of recurrence in living-related donor grafts than in cadaver kidney recipients (Nast et al 1987) but this was not confirmed by Meulders et al (1994). Recurrence can occur despite a delay of more than 1 year between disappearance of proteinuria and transplantation.

Clinical signs and symptoms may be absent. Hematuria, sometimes macroscopic, moderate proteinuria and hypertension are common in patients with clinical evidence of recurrence. Histologic recurrence is characterized by focal and segmental necrotizing GN (Figure 12.15) with mesangial IgA deposits. The prognosis is more severe in adults than in children (Hasegawa et al 1989; Meulders et al 1994). Graft survival in patients with recurrence is 57% at 2 years (Briggs and Jones 1999a).

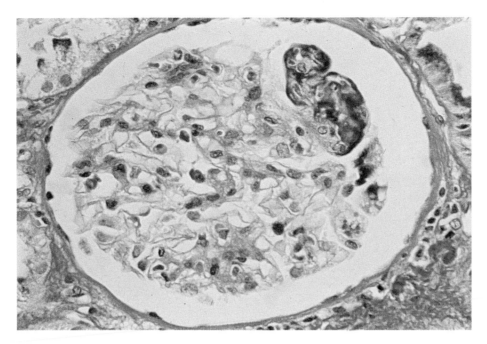

Figure 12.15. Recurrence of Henoch–Schönlein nephritis. Gross hematuria heralded the recurrence of focal and segmental necrotizing glomerulonephritis in this 35-year-old woman with Henoch–Schönlein purpura, 18 months after transplantation. (AFOG ×400)

Fibrillary/immunotactoid glomerulopathy (FG)

This rare disease is characterized by extracellular deposition of nonbranching micro-fibrils or microtubules within the mesangium and capillary walls of renal glomeruli. Proteinuria, generally in a nephrotic range, hematuria, hypertension and progressive course to renal failure are the main clinical features.

There is also limited information on the results of renal transplantation in FG because the diagnosis is difficult without electron microscopy (Figures 12.16 and 12.17). Fibril deposition recurred in 50% of cases, but the allografts functioned satisfactorily for over 5 years in the majority of cases. Interestingly, the rate of decline in renal function in allografts was slower than in native kidneys, suggesting some benefit of immunosuppressive therapy (Pronovost et al 1996).

Amyloidosis

Both primary and secondary amyloidosis may recur on the kidney allograft in 10–40% of cases (Heering et al 1989; Hartmann et al 1992).

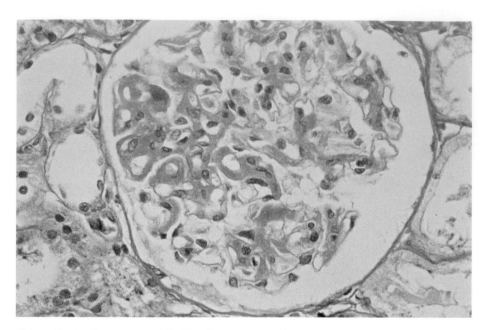

Figure 12.16. Recurrence of fibrillary/immunotactoid glomerulopathy. In the presence of an irregular 'membranoproliferative' pattern, as shown in this picture, one should also keep in mind the possibility of a recurrence of immunotactoid or fibrillary glomerulonephritis. (AFOG ×400)

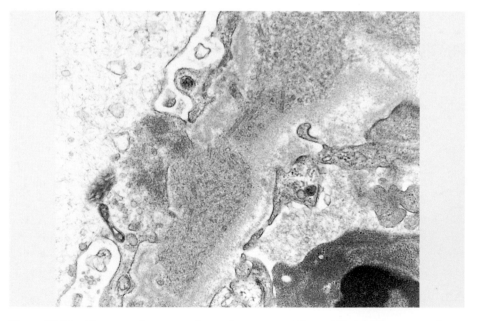

Figure 12.17. Electron microscopy shows the structured ('tactoid') deposits permeating the GBM.

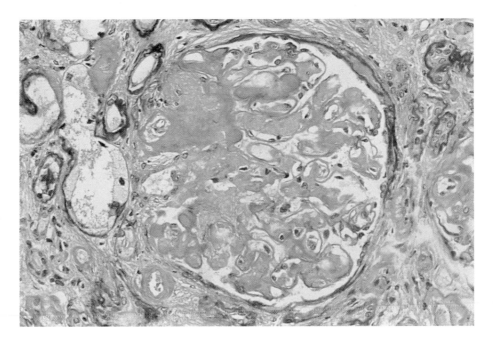

Figure 12.18. Recurrence of amyloidosis. The mesangial space is severely and irregularly dilated by the presence of a fluffy, cotton-like, slightly PAS-positive material in this patient with rheumatoid arthritis and recurrence of amyloidosis, 3.5 years after transplantation. (PAS ×300)

Recurrence develops within 3 years. In the secondary form, the risk of recurrence is correlated with the activity of the underlying primary disease, usually rheumatoid arthritis (Figure 12.18). Not all the patients with recurrence of amyloid deposits show signs of renal disease. Proteinuria, usually causing a nephrotic syndrome, is the cardinal clinical sign. It often heralds a progressive renal dysfunction. Unfortunately many patients die from infections or cardiovascular complications even if allograft function maintains stable.

Recurrence of amyloidosis may also occur in patients with familial Mediterranean fever. The early administration of colchicine, 1 mg/day indefinitely, can prevent the deposit of amyloid substance on the transplanted kidney (Livneh et al 1992).

Light-chain deposition disease (LCDD)

Light-chain deposition disease is characterized by the deposition of kappa- or lambda-immunoglobulin light chains in the kidneys and in other organs. About one-third of patients have no associated systemic illness, while in two-thirds LCDD is associated with multiple myeloma or other lymphoplasmacytic disease (Figures 12.19 and 12.20).

Recurrence of multiple myeloma and LCDD after renal transplantation is frequent

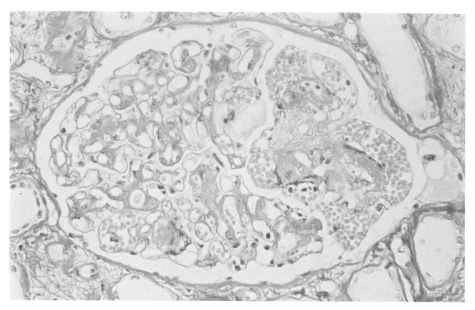

Figure 12.19. Recurrence of light-chain deposition disease. In this case, mesangial areas and capillary walls are markedly, although irregularly, widened by the presence of a homogeneous material that can mimic amyloid or glycosylated material of diabetes. (AFOG ×300)

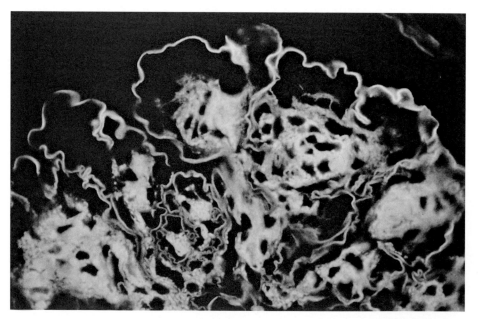

Figure 12.20. Recurrence of light-chain deposition disease. The immunofluorescence clarifies the nature of the disease showing linear parietal and homogeneous mesangial deposits of κ-chain (also present along TBM).

and involves an ominous prognosis. However, a few cases of prolonged allograft survival have been reported in patients who attained remission with melphalan and prednisone before transplantation (Gerlag et al 1986).

Hemolytic–uremic syndrome (HUS)

The possibility of recurrence of HUS after renal transplantation is well established but the risk is poorly defined. It has been estimated to range between 10 and 45% (Cameron 1991; Hebert et al 1991), the recurrence being more frequent in children.

At biopsy, thrombotic microangiopathy can be seen early following transplantation (Figure 12.21) but sometimes occurs later, after some months. Clinically, the recurrence of HUS may be associated with hemolytic microangiopathy anemia, thrombocytopenia, hypertension and progression to renal failure. In some cases, clinical signs and symptoms may be missing and the outcome may be benign. However, in most cases the recurrence of HUS leads to the loss of the allograft (Müller et al 1998). The differential diagnosis between recurrence and a de novo HUS, caused by cyclosporine or by malignant hypertension, can be difficult.

Whether the use of tacrolimus may or may not prevent the recurrence of HUS after

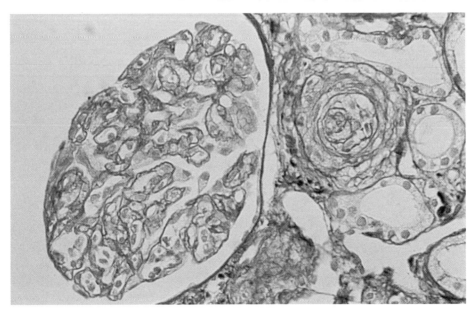

Figure 12.21. Recurrence of hemolytic–uremic syndrome. Acute graft deterioration developed 1 month after surgery in this woman who lost her native kidneys because of HUS. Graft biopsy revealed the recurrence of severe microangiopathy. The typical 'onion skin' aspect of a preglomerular arteriola is adjacent to the tributary glomerulus showing a moderate retraction of the tuft. (AFOG ×200)

transplantation is controversial. Some authors found a benefit by replacing cyclosporine with tacrolimus (Franz et al 1998) but others reported cases of HUS in patients treated with tacrolimus (Trimarchi et al 1999). There is no definite treatment for recurrent HUS. Withdrawal of cyclosporine may resolve the disease in a few cases (Van Buren et al 1985). Plasma infusions may be helpful for alleviating severe thrombocytopenia (Grinyó et al 1988).

VASCULITIS

Wegener granulomatosis (WG)

Although recurrence can occur after transplantation it is rare and many patients with WG have been transplanted successfully (Wrenger at al 1997). The optimal timing for transplantation is not clear. A successful outcome was obtained even in patients with a short interval between clinical onset and transplantation as well as in anti-neutrophil-cytoplasm antibodies (ANCA) positive patients with symptoms of active disease (Schmitt et al 1993). Cyclophosphamide and corticosteroids may stabilize renal function in most patients with recurrence (Ramos and Tisher 1994). The survival rate and graft function are similar in patients with WG to those of other kidney transplant recipients (Briggs and Jones 1999b). It must be pointed out, however, that many of these patients were older and most deaths were caused by cardiovascular death and extrarenal

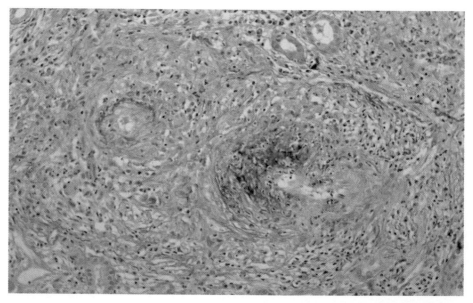

Figure 12.22. Recurrence of microscopic polyarteritis 8 years after renal transplantation. Segmental but complete necrosis of a branch of interlobular artery, with severe parietal inflammation is pathognomonic of ANCA-associated micropolyarteritis. (AFOG ×250)

complications. The risk of recurrence is low but a few patients may have recurrence even years after transplantation.

Microscopic polyarteritis

In a series, one of five patients showed a clinical recurrence with multiple relapses. However, reinforcement of immunosuppression could maintain stable graft function (Le Mao et al 1996). Frascà et al (1996) did not observe any recurrence in two patients with high titers of circulating ANCA at the time of transplantation (Figure 12.22).

Mixed cryoglobulinemic nephritis (MCN)

Mixed cryoglobidinemic nephritis is a rare disease characterized by vasculitis and by glomerular changes resembling a membranoproliferative glomerulonephritis usually associated with hepatitis C virus. Only few patients with MCN have been submitted to renal transplantation. By reviewing the literature Tarantino et al (1994) found a recurrence of MCN in 70% of cases. However, it is still unclear whether the recurrence of MCN may interfere with the evolution of the transplanted kidney. In our own experience of two patients with MCN submitted to transplantation, one lost his kidney because of acute rejection and the other still has his kidney allograft functioning 8 years after transplantation in spite of histological recurrence (Figure 12.23).

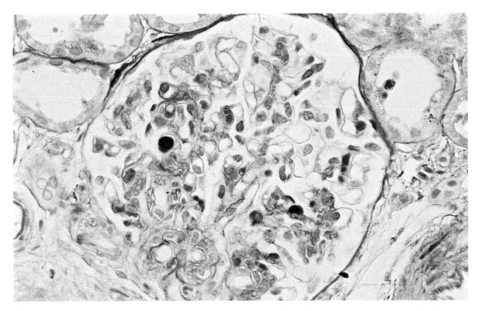

Figure 12.23. Recurrence of cryoglobulinemic nephritis. This case shows some highly characteristic features of cryoglobulinemic nephritis, which are irregularly and segmentally distributed. Pseudothrombi in some loops are associated with a segmental membranoproliferative pattern, without signs of monocyte inflammation. (AFOG ×400)

RECURRENCE OF METABOLIC DISEASE

Diabetic nephropathy

Recurrence of diabetic arteriolar lesions, mesangial expansion and glomerular basement thickening occur in 100% of diabetic patients within 4 years of transplantation (Najarian et al 1979). In patients with proteinuria and renal insufficiency the typical nodular intercapillary glomerulosclerosis (Figure 12.24) is seen infrequently, while vascular changes are predominant (Hariharan et al 1996).

The progression of histological lesions in the transplanted kidney is usually slow, but more rapid than in the original disease, perhaps because of the lower nephron mass, the use of nephrotoxic agents such as cyclosporine or tacrolimus, and the frequent hypertension. Microalbuminuria heralds the presence of renal morphological abnormalities. Overt proteinuria and nephrotic syndrome develop later preceding the onset of progressive renal failure. Frequent recurrence accounted for only 1.8% of graft losses in the largest series of renal transplants in diabetic recipients (Basadonna et al 1992). This is probably due to the fact that the mean interval between the onset of insulin-dependent diabetes and the development of overt nephropathy in renal transplant recipients is at least 7–8 years (Hariharan et al 1996).

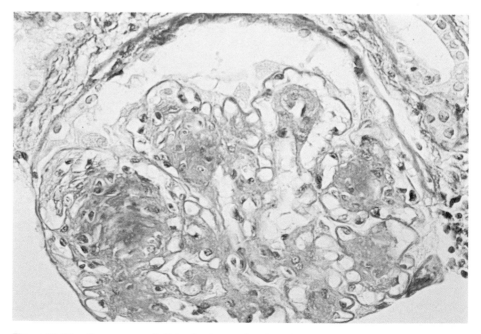

Figure 12.24. Recurrence of diabetic glomerulosclerosis. In its full pattern, as in this case, diabetic glomerulosclerosis usually recurs in the graft only after years of ill-controlled disease. (AFOG ×480)

Successful transplantation of both pancreas and kidney can prevent the development of diabetic nephropathy (Bohman et al 1985). In the case of kidney transplantation alone, strict glycemic control should be recommended. ACE inhibitors and/or angiotensin receptor antagonists may be helpful to slow the progression of renal disease and should be started as early as possible.

Oxalosis (type 1 primary hyperoxaluria)

This rare inborn error of metabolism is due to the deficiency of the hepatic enzyme glyoxylate aminotransferase. In infancy the disease is characterized by nephrocalcinosis and widespread oxalate deposition, particularly in blood vessel walls and in bone. Most commonly the disease is characterized by severely recurrent nephrolithiasis. After renal transplantation, patients may show a rapid recurrence with deposition of oxalate in the allograft that results in allograft loss (Figure 12.25). Measures to prevent progressive

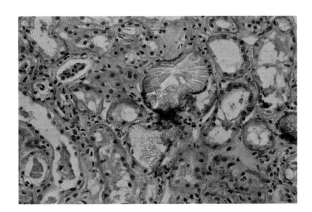

(a)

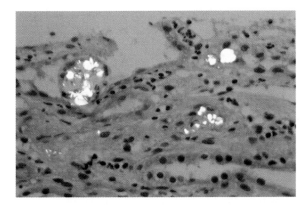

(b)

Figure 12.25. (a) Diffuse tubular damage with focal epithelial necrosis and diffuse interstitial inflammation. Some dilated tubular segments are filled with cellular debris and protein cast, but the central and largest segment is filled by needles of crystals, laying circumferentially on the luminal side of the tubular basement membrane, which shows partial disruption. (b) At polarized light the intraluminal crystals show birifringence. Such morphologic features are characteristic of crystals made of oxalic acid which, in this woman affected by primary oxaluria, massively precipitated destroying the graft 6 months after transplantation.

oxalate deposition include: early transplantation in patients with a glomerular filtration rate around 20 ml/min to minimize oxalate retention; preoperative dialysis to deplete the oxalate pool; forced diuresis; administration of pyridoxine, which may decrease the oxalate pool by converting glyoxylate to glycine; and avoidance of cyclosporine in the early posttransplant period (Scheinman 1991). Good results with isolated kidney allograft may be obtained in pyridoxine-responsive patients (Allen et al 1996; Saborio and Scheinman 1999).

In pyridoxine-resistant patients with prolonged renal failure the preferred treatment is combined liver and kidney transplantation (Marangella 1999). The transplanted liver can restore the missing enzyme and prevent cardiovascular disease, which is the major cause of death. Radiological and histological improvement of osteopathy has also been reported (Toussaint et al 1993).

Cystinosis

This is a rare metabolic disease inherited as an autosomal recessive trait and characterized by intracellular accumulation of free cystine in many organs including the kidney. Renal transplantation in children with cystinosis gives results comparable to those in children with other renal diseases (Ehrich et al 1991). Cystinosis does not recur, even if some accumulation of cystine may be seen in the renal interstitium. These cystine deposits are thought to derive from macrophage invasion of host origin and have no clinical consequences on the graft. Despite successful transplantation, accumulation of cystine in other organs continues and can lead to invalidating consequences. The early and continuous administration of cysteamine, however, may lower the content of cysteamine in leukocytes, and improve the annual growth rate. Cysteamine by eye-drop may prevent corneal accumulation.

Fabry's disease

This disease is caused by a deficiency of the enzyme alpha-galactosidase with consequent accumulation of glycosphyngolipids in most tissues including kidney. Angiokeratomata, corneal dystrophy, acroparesthesias, mitral valve defect and cardiovascular disease are frequent clinical features. Renal failure is the most common cause of death.

Poor results with renal transplantation were reported in the 1970s, but more recent data showed a good graft survival (Donati et al 1987; Nissenson and Port 1989). Recurrence of the disease on kidney allograft may occur (Figure 12.26), but this did not impede graft survival for 11 years in one patient (Mosnier et al 1991).

Lipoprotein glomerulopathy (LG)

This rare disease is characterized by intracapillary lipoprotein deposits associated with proteinuria often in a nephrotic range and qualitative changes in plasma apolipoprotein

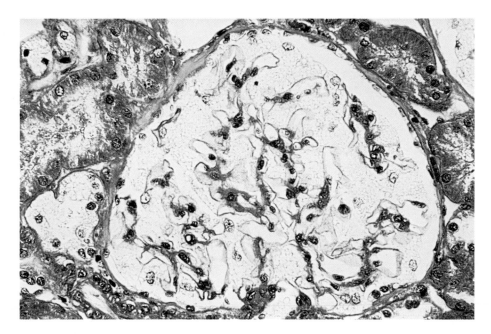

Figure 12.26. Recurrence of Fabry's disease. The glomerulus shows the characteristic fine web of foamy, enlarged visceral podocytes, wrapping up the loops, which appear well preserved. (AFOG ×250)

E. Cases of recurrence have been reported both in living kidney and cadaveric kidney recipients (Saito et al 1994; Mourad et al 1998). Although the majority of patients lost their graft after recurrence, one case with stable graft function 4 years after recurrence has been described (Mourad et al 1998).

DE NOVO RENAL DISEASES

Membranous nephropathy

De novo MN is the second cause of nephrotic syndrome after renal transplantation (Davison and Johnston 1992). A clinically overt disease may be seen in about 1.4% of renal allograft recipients (Schwarz et al 1994). However, a pediatric series, in which control allograft biopsy was performed even in the absence of signs of nephropathy, reported a de novo MN in 9% of cases. Of them, a quarter showed no sign of renal disease and another a quarter had only a mild proteinuria (Antignac et al 1988). A large number of cases of de novo MN was reported in retransplanted patients (Heidet et al 1994).

The pathogenesis is unclear. The disease has been considered an expression of chronic rejection, as lesions of rejection may be associated with MN or may even antedate it (Truong et al 1989). However, this hypothesis is challenged by the observation that de novo MN may also occur following transplantation between identical twins (Bansal et al 1986). It is possible that MN is caused by an autoimmune response to unknown antigens of glomerular or tubular origin, with consequent in situ deposition of immune complexes in a subepithelial position.

The prognosis in patients with proteinuria may be severe. Truong et al (1989) found that 42% of adults lost their allograft on average 3 years after the diagnosis. In children, 60% lost their graft on average 6 years after the diagnosis (Heidet et al 1994). On the other hand, Antignac et al (1988) did not observe a progressive course in patients with mild or absent proteinuria, and Schwarz et al (1994) reported that the 5-year graft survival rate was similar in 21 patients with de novo MN and in 851 other renal transplant recipients. In a few patients, remission of the nephrotic syndrome and stabilization of renal function were obtained by reinforcing the doses of oral prednisone.

Hepatitis C-associated glomerulonephritis

De novo cryoglobulinemic nephritis may develop after transplantation in patients infected with hepatitis C virus (HCV). Cruzado et al (1996) described six cases. All patients showed proteinuria of more than 1.5 g/day and microhematuria. Activation of classical serum complement pathway was constant. Cryoglobulins were detected in all cases but in very low plasma concentration. Renal biopsy showed a pattern of membranoproliferative glomerulonephritis with mesangial and sometimes endocapillary IgM and subendothelial cryoglobulin-like deposits.

Roth et al (1995) reported five cases of de novo membranoproliferative glomerulonephritis in HCV-infected renal allograft recipients. They failed to find evidence for cryoglobulinemia and circulating immune complexes, suggesting that a HCV-associated glomerulonephritis may develop even without cryoglobulinemia, although rarely. The prognosis is severe as most patients with HCV-associated type I MPGN progress to terminal renal failure (Hammoud et al 1996).

Cases of de novo MN have also been described in HCV-positive patients. In two Japanese patients the HCV core protein was found in the glomeruli, suggesting that HCV infection may cause MN through immune complex deposition (Okada et al 1996). It is now evident that the presence of antiHCV antibodies is a major risk factor for posttreatment proteinuria (Hastin et al 1998) and glomerular diseases (Cosio et al 1996). Cases of thrombotic microangiopathy associated with anticardiolipin antibodies have also been described in HCV-positive renal transplant patients (Baid et al 1999).

Hepatitis B-associated glomerulonephritis

While membranoproliferative glomerulonephritis is the commonest form of HCV-associated glomerulonephritis, membranous nephropathy seems to be the prevalent glomerular disease associated with hepatitis B infection. It is difficult to assess the prognosis from the few cases described but it is likely that glomerulonephritis may be progressive as it is in nontransplanted patients (Lai et al 1991).

Diabetic nephropathy

Some transplant recipients may develop diabetes mellitus, which may be caused by corticosteroids, cyclosporine or tacrolimus. However, the frequency of nephropathy due to de novo diabetes is unknown as there are no studies in which allograft biopsies were routinely performed. Posttransplantation diabetes is associated with an impaired long-term allograft survival. In the long term, the development of a diabetic nephropathy may contribute to the decline of renal function (Miles et al 1998; Dogu et al 1999).

Antiglomerular basement membrane (GBM) nephritis in Alport's syndrome

Approximately 15% of Alport patients who have undergone kidney transplantation develop transient IgG linear deposition along GBM without antiGBM antibodies.

The immunization of Alport patients is caused by the presence in the transplanted kidney of antigenic epitopes that are lacking in the native kidneys. Most of these antibodies are directed against the Goodpasture antigen located in the MC1 domain of the alpha-3 chain (Kalluri et al 1995).

The IgG deposition along GBM usually does not have any relevant effect on allograft function. However, some 3–5% of Alport patients, mainly those with a juvenile type, develop immunization against graft GBM, leading to severe crescentic glomerulonephritis. This complication manifests within the first year. The diagnosis is based on the detection of circulating antiGBM antibodies and renal biopsy. The prognosis is poor as three-quarters of patients lose their allograft (Grünfeld and Knebelmann 1988). Treatment consists of intensive plasma-exchange therapy in order to remove the antiGBM antibodies.

Nephrotic syndrome in congenital nephrosis

A massive steroid-resistant proteinuria has been reported to occur in about a quarter of children who received a kidney allograft for congenital nephrosis of the Finnish type (Laine et al 1993). The nephrotic syndrome developed 1–33 months after transplantation, and was often preceded by cytomegalovirus or Epstein–Barr virus infection. Histologic features consisted of endothelial swelling of glomerular capillaries with normal

GBM. This picture resembled that of transplant glomerulopathy. The nephrotic syndrome responds poorly to steroids and cyclophosphamide and heralds progression to graft failure in more than half of patients.

Hemolytic–uremic syndrome

In kidney graft recipients, HUS may occur not only as a recurrence of the disease but also as de novo HUS. Etiopathogenetic roles for cyclosporine (Franz et al 1998), tacrolimus (Trimarchi et al 1999) and OKT3 (Doutrelepont et al 1992) have been hypothesized. The clinicopathological findings are similar for the recurrent and de novo forms of posttransplant HUS. The prognosis is usually poor.

De novo immunotactoid glomerulopathy

The association of immunotactoid glomerulopathy with cytomegalovirus infection in a renal transplant recipient has been reported (Rao et al 1994). In the patient described, the morphologic lesions of immunotactoid glomerulopathy and clinical renal disease reversed after recovery from the viral infection.

Acute transplant glomerulopathy

Richardson et al (1981) reported that cytomegalovirus (CMV) infection could be associated with a peculiar glomerulopathy characterized by enlargement and necrosis of endothelial cells and subendothelial accumulation of amorphous material with IgM and C3 deposits at immunofluorescence. However, further studies concluded that there is no direct evidence for a specific CMV nephropathy. This acute transplant glomerulopathy may rather represent an unusual form of rejection involving endothelial cells (Boyce et al 1998).

REFERENCES

Ahsan N, Manning EC, Dabbs DJ et al (1997) Recurrent type I membranoproliferative glomerulonephritis after renal transplantation and protective role of cyclosporine in acute crescentic transformation. *Clin Transplant* 11:9–14.

Alamartine E, Boulharouz J, Berthoux F (1996) Actuarial survival rate of kidney transplants in patients with IgA glomerulonephritis: a one-center study. *Transplant Proc* 26:272–274.

Alexander SR, Arbus GS, Butt KMH et al (1990) The 1989 report of the North American Pediatric Renal Transplant Cooperative study. *Pediatr Nephrol* 4:542–553.

Allen AR, Thompson EM, Williams G et al (1996) Selective renal transplantation in primary hyperoxaluria type 1. *Am J Kidney Dis* 27:891–895.

Andresdottir MB, Assmann KJ, Hojitsma AJ et al (1997) Recurrence of type I membranoproliferative glomerulonephritis after renal transplantation: analysis of the incidence, risk factors and impact on graft survival. *Transplantation* 63:1628–1633.

Andresdottir MB, Assmann KJ, Koene RA, Wetzels JF (1998) Immunohistological and ultrastructural differences between recurrent type I membranoproliferative glomerulonephritis and chronic transplant glomerulopathy. *Am J Kidney Dis* 32:582–588.

Antignac C, Hinglais N, Gubler MC et al (1988) De novo membranous glomerulonephritis in renal allografts in children. *Clin Nephrol* 30:1–6.

Artero M, Biava C, Amend W (1992) Recurrent focal glomerulosclerosis. Natural history and response to therapy. *Am J Med* 92:375–383.

Baid S, Pascual M, Williams WW Jr et al (1999) Renal thrombotic microangiopathy associated with anticardiolipin antibodies in hepatitis C positive renal allograft recipients. *J Am Soc Nephrol* 10:146–153.

Banfi G, Colturi C, Montagnino G, Ponticelli C (1990) The recurrence of focal segmental glomerulosclerosis in kidney transplant patients treated with cyclosporine. *Transplantation* 50:594–596.

Bansal VK, Koseny GA, Fresco R et al (1986) De novo membranous nephropathy following transplantation between conjoint twins. *Transplantation* 41:404–408.

Basadonna G, Matas AJ, Najarian JS et al (1992) Transplantation in diabetic patients: the University of Minnesota experience. *Kidney Int* 42:S193–S198.

Berger J, Janewa H, Nabarra B et al (1995) Recurrence of mesangial deposition of IgA after renal transplantation. *Kidney Int* 7:232–241.

Bohman SO, Tyden G, Wilczek H et al (1985) Prevention of kidney graft diabetic nephropathy by pancreas transplantation in man. *Diabetes* 34:306–308.

Boyce NW, Hayes K, Gee D et al (1988) Cytomegalovirus infection complicating renal transplantation and its relationship to acute transplant glomerulopathy. *Transplantation* 45:706–709.

Briggs JD, Jones E (1999a) Recurrence of glomerulonephritis following renal transplantation. *Nephrol Dial Transplant* 14:564–565.

Briggs JD, Jones E (1999b) Renal transplantation for uncommon diseases. *Nephrol Dial Transplant* 14:570–575.

Bumgardner GL, Amend WC, Ascher NL, Vincenti EG (1998) Single-center long-term results of renal transplantation for IgA nephropathy. *Transplantation* 65:1053–1060.

Cameron JS (1982) Glomerulonephritis in renal transplants. *Transplantation* 34:237–245.

Cameron JS (1991) Recurrent primary disease and de novo nephritis following renal transplantation. *Pediatr Nephrol* 5:412–421.

Cochat P, Schell M, Ranchin B et al (1996) Management of recurrent nephrotic syndrome after kidney transplantation in children. *Clin Nephrol* 46:17–20.

Coppo R, Amore A, Curina P et al (1995) Characteristics of IgA and macromolecular IgA in sera from IgA nephropathy transplanted patients with and without IgAN recurrence. *Contrib Nephrol* 111:85–92.

Cosio FG, Roche Z, Agarwol A et al (1996) Prevalence of hepatitis C in patients with idiopathic glomerulopathies in native and transplant kidneys. *Am J Kidney Dis* 28:752–758.

Cosyns JP, Couchoud C, Pouteil-Noble C et al (1998) Recurrence of membranous nephropathy after renal transplantation: probability, outcome and risk factors. *Clin Nephrol* 50:144–153.

Crown AL, Woolfson RG, Griffiths MH et al (1994) Recurrent systemic Henoch–Schönlein purpura in an adult following renal transplantation. *Nephrol Dial Transplant* 9:423–425.

Cruzado JM, Gil-Vernet S, Ercilla G et al (1996) Hepatitis C virus-associated membranoproliferative glomerulonephritis in renal allografts. *J Am Soc Nephrol* 7:2469–2475.

Dantal J, Bigot E, Bogers E et al (1994) Effect of plasma protein adsorption on protein excretion in kidney transplant recipients with recurrent nephrotic syndrome. *N Engl J Med* **330**:7–14.

Dantal J, Godfrin Y, Koll R et al (1998) Antihuman immunoglobulin affinity immunoadsorption strongly decreases proteinuria in patients with relapsing nephrotic syndrome. *J Am Soc Nephrol* **9**:1709–1715.

Davison AM, Johnston PA (1992) Allograft membranous nephropathy. *Nephrol Dial Transplant* 7(Suppl 1):114–118.

Diaz-Tejeiro R, Maduell F, Diez J et al (1990) Loss of renal graft due to recurrent IgA nephropathy with rapidly progressive course: an unusual clinical evolution. *Nephron* **54**:431–433.

Dogu E, Waiser J, Böhler T et al (1999) Renal failure from diabetic glomerulosclerosis three decades after allograft transplantation. *Nephrol Dial Transplant* **14**:974–976.

Donati D, Novario R, Gastaldi L (1987) Natural history and treatment of uremia secondary to Fabry's disease: a European experience. *Nephron* **46**:353–359.

Doutrelepont J, Abramowicz D, Flonquin S et al (1998) Early recurrence of hemolytic uremic syndrome in a renal transplant recipient during prophylactic OKT3 therapy. *Transplantation* **53**:1378–1383.

Ehrich JHH, Brodehl J, Byrd DJ et al (1991) Renal transplantation in 22 children with nephropathic cystinosis. *Pediatr Nephrol* **5**:708–714.

Ehrich JHH, Loirat C, Brunner EP et al (1992) Report on management of renal failure in children in Europe XXII, 1991. *Nephrol Dial Transplant* 7(Suppl 2):36–48.

First MR, Mendoza N, Maryniak RK, Weiss MA (1984) Membranous glomerulopathy following kidney transplantation: association with renal vein thrombosis in two of nine cases. *Transplantation* **38**:603–607.

Franz M, Regele H, Schmaldienst S et al (1998) Posttransplant hemolytic uremic syndrome in adult retransplanted kidney graft recipients: advantage of FK506 therapy? *Transplantation* **66**:1258–1262.

Frascà GM, Neri L, Martello M et al (1996) Renal transplantation in patients with microscopic polyartheritis and antimyeloperaxidase antibodies: report of three cases. *Nephron* **72**:82–85.

Gallay BJ, Alpers CE, Davis CL et al (1995) Glomerulonephritis in renal allografts associated with hepatitis C infection: a possible relationship with transplant glomerulopathy in two cases. *Am J Kidney Dis* **26**:662–667.

Gerlag PGG, Koene RAP, Berden JHM (1986) Renal transplantation in light chain nephropathy: case report and review of the literature. *Clin Nephrol* **25**:101–104.

Glassock RJ (1997) Crescentic glomerulonephritis. In: Ponticelli C, Glassock RJ (eds). *Treatment of Primary Glomerulonephritis*. Oxford: Oxford University Press, pp. 234–254.

Grinyó JM, Caralps A, Carreras L et al (1988) Apparent recurrence of hemolytic uremic syndrome in azathioprine-treated allograft recipients. *Nephron* **49**:301–304.

Grünfeld JP, Knebelmann B (1998) Alport's syndrome. In: Davison AM, Cameron JS, Grünfeld JP, Kerr DNS, Ritz E, Winearls Ch G (eds). *Oxford Textbook of Clinical Nephrology*. Oxford: Oxford Medical Publications, pp. 2427–2437.

Habib R, Gagnadoux M, Broyer M (1987) Recurrent glomerulonephritis in renal transplanted children. *Contrib Nephrol* **55**:123–125.

Hammoud H, Haem J, Laurent B et al (1996) Glomerular disease during HCV infection in renal transplantation. *Nephrol Dial Transplant* **11**(Suppl 4):54–55.

Hariharan S, Savin V (1999) Recurrent and de novo glomerular diseases after renal transplantation. *Graft* 2(Suppl 2):S113–S118.

Hariharan S, Smith RD, Viero R et al (1996) Diabetic nephropathy after renal transplantation. *Transplantation* **62**:632–635.

Hariharan S, Peddi VR, Savin VJ et al (1998) Recurrent and de novo renal disease after renal transplantation. A report from the Renal Allograft Disease Registry. *Am J Kidney Dis* **31**:928–931.

Hartmann A, Holdaast H, Fauchald P et al (1992) Fifteen years experience with renal transplantation in systemic amyloidosis. *Transplant Int* **5**:15–19.

Hartung R, Livingston B, Excell L (1995) Recurrence of IgA deposits/disease in grafts. *Contrib Nephrol* **111**:13–17.

Hasegawa A, Kawamura T, Ito H et al (1989) Fate of renal grafts with recurrent Henoch–Schönlein purpura nephritis in children. *Transplant Proc* **21**:2130–2133.

Hastin D, Guillemin F, Castin N et al (1998) Pretransplant hepatitis C virus infection. *Transplantation* **65**:741–744.

Hebert D, Kim EM, Sibley RK et al (1991) Post-transplant outcome of patients with haemolytic uraemic syndrome: update. *Pediatr Nephrol* **5**:162–169.

Heering P, Kutkuhm B, Brenzel H et al (1989) Renal transplantation in amyloid nephropathy. *Int Urol Nephrol* **21**:339–343.

Heidet L, Gagnadoux MF, Beziau A et al (1994) Recurrence of de novo membranous glomerulonephritis on renal grafts. *Clin Nephrol* **41**:314–318.

Ingulli E, Tejani A (1991) Incidence, treatment and outcome of recurrent focal segmental glomerulosclerosis posttransplantation in 42 allografts in children: a single center experience. *Transplantation* **51**:401–405.

Ingulli E, Singh A, Bagi N et al (1995) Aggressive, long-term cyclosporine therapy for steroid-resistant focal segmental glomerulosclerosis. *J Am Soc Nephrol* **5**:1820–1826.

Josephson MA, Spargo B, Hollandsworth DO, Thistlewait MD (1994) The recurrence of membranous glomerulopathy in a renal transplant recipient: case report and literature review. *Am J Kidney Dis* **24**:873–878.

Kalluri R, van den Heuvel LP, Smeets HJM et al (1995) A COL4A3 gene mutation and post-transplant anti-α 3(IV) collagen autoantibodies in Alport syndrome. *Kidney Int* **47**:1199–1204.

Kessler M, Hiesse Ch, Hestin D et al (1996) Recurrence of immunoglobulin A nephropathy after renal transplantation in the cyclosporine era. *Am J Kidney Dis* **28**:99–104.

Kim EM, Striegel J, Kim Y et al (1994) Recurrence of steroid-resistant nephrotic syndrome in kidney transplants is associated with increased acute renal failure and acute rejection. *Kidney Int* **45**:1440–1445.

Kim YS, Jeong HJ, Choi KH et al (1996) Renal transplantation in patients with IgA nephropathy. *Transplant Proc* **28**:1543–1544.

Kimata N, Tanabe K, Ishikawa N et al (1996) Correlation between proteinuria and prognosis of transplant IgA nephropathy. *Transplant Proc* **28**:1537–1539.

Lai KN, Li PKT, Lui SF et al (1991) Membranous nephropathy related to hepatitis B virus. *N Engl J Med* **324**:1457–1463.

Laine J, Jalanko H, Holthöfer H et al (1993) Post-transplantation nephrosis in congenital nephrotic syndrome of the Finnish type. *Kidney Int* **44**:867–874.

Le Mao G, Rostaing L, Modesto A et al (1996) Recurrence of ANCA-associated microscopic polyangiitis after cadaveric renal transplant. *Transplant Proc* **28**:2803–2804.

Lee G, Glassock RJ (1997) Immunoglobulin A nephropathy. In: Ponticelli C, Glassock RJ (eds). *Treatment of Primary Glomerulonephritis*. Oxford: Oxford Medical Publications, pp. 186–217.

Lim EC, Chia D, Terasaki PI (1991) Studies of sera from IgA nephropathy patients to explain high kidney graft survival. *Hum Immunol* **32**:81–86.

Livneh A, Zemer D, Siegal B et al (1992) Colchicine prevents kidney transplant amyloidosis in familial Mediterranean fever. *Nephron* **60**:418–422.

Marangella M (1999) Transplantation strategies in type 1 primary hyperoxaluria: the issue of pyridoxine responsiveness. *Nephrol Dial Transplant* **14**:301–303.

Marcen R, Mampso F, Tervel JL et al (1996) Membranous nephropathy: recurrence after kidney transplantation. *Nephrol Dial Transplant* **11**:1129–1133.

Maschio G, Cagnoli L, Claroni F et al (1994) ACE-inhibition reduced proteinuria in normotensive patients with IgA nephropathy: a multicentre, randomized, placebo controlled study. *Nephrol Dial Transplant* 9:265–269.

Mathew TH (1991) Recurrent disease after renal transplantation. *Transplant Rev* 51:1–15.

Meulders Q, Pirson Y, Cosyns JP et al (1994) Course of Henoch–Schönlein nephritis after renal transplantation. *Transplantation* 58:1172–1186.

Miles AMV, Sumrani N, Horowitz R et al (1998) Diabetes mellitus after renal transplantation. *Transplantation* 65:380–384.

Montagnino G, Colturi C, Banfi G et al (1989) Membranous nephropathy in cyclosporine-treated renal transplant patients. *Transplantation* 47:725–727.

Morales JM, Martinez MA, Munoz de Bustillo E et al (1997) Recurrent type III membranoproliferative glomerulonephritis after kidney transplantation. *Transplantation* 63:1186–1188.

Mosnier JF, Degott C, Bedrossian J et al (1991) Recurrence of Fabry's disease in a renal allograft 11 years after successful renal transplantation. *Transplantation* 51:759–762.

Mourad G, Djamali A, Turc-Baron C, Cristol JP (1998) Lipoprotein glomerulopathy: a new cause of nephrotic syndrome after renal transplantation. *Nephrol Dial Transplant* 13:1292–1294.

Müller T, Sikora P, Offner G et al (1998) Recurrence of renal disease after kidney transplantation in children: 24 years of experience in a single center. *Clin Nephrol* 49:82–90.

Najarian JS, Surtherland DER, Simmons RL et al (1979) Ten year experience with renal transplantation in juvenile onset diabetes. *Ann Surg* 197:487–500.

Nast CC, Ward HJ, Koyle MA, Cohen AH (1987) Recurrent Henoch–Schönlein purpura following renal transplantation. *Am J Kidney Dis* 9:39–43.

Nissenson AR, Port FK (1989) Outcome of end-stage renal disease in patients with rare causes of renal failure. I. Inherited and metabolic disorders. *Q J Med* 73:1055–1062.

Nossent HC, Swaak TJG, Berden JHM (1991) Systemic lupus erythematosus after renal transplantation: patient and graft survival and disease activity. *Ann Intern Med* 114:183–188.

Nyberg G, Blohmé I, Persson H et al (1992) Recurrence of SLE in transplanted kidneys: a follow-up transplant biopsy study. *Nephrol Dial Transplant* 7:1116–1123.

Obermiller LE, Hoy WE, Eversole M, Sterling WA (1985) Recurrent membranous glomerulonephritis in two renal transplants. *Transplantation* 40:100–103.

Odorico JS, Knechtle SJ, Rayhill SC et al (1996) The influence of native nephrectomy on the incidence of recurrent disease following renal transplantation for primary glomerulonephritis. *Transplantation* 61:228–234.

Odum J, Peh C, Clarkson A et al (1994) Recurrence of mesangial IgA nephritis following renal transplantation. *Nephrol Dial Transplant* 9:309–312.

Ohmacht Ch, Kliem V, Burg M et al (1997) Recurrent immunoglobulin A nephropathy after renal transplantation. *Transplantation* 64:1493–1496.

Okada K, Takishita Y, Shimomura H et al (1996) Detection of hepatitis C virus core protein in the glomeruli of patients with membranous glomerulonephritis. *Clin Nephrol* 45:71–76.

Ponticelli C, Banfi G (1997) Focal and segmental glomerulosclerosis. In: Ponticelli C, Glassock RJ (eds). *Treatment of Primary Glomerulonephritis.* Oxford: Oxford Medical Publications, pp. 108–145.

Ponticelli C, Passerini P (1997) Membranous nephropathy. In: Ponticelli C, Glassock RJ (eds). *Treatment of Primary Glomerulonephritis.* Oxford: Oxford Medical Publications, pp. 146–185.

Pronovost PH, Brady HR, Gunning ME et al (1996) Clinical features, predictors of disease progression and results of renal transplantation in fibrillary/immunotactoid glomerulopathy. *Nephrol Dial Transplant* 11:837–842.

Ramos E, Tisher CC (1994) Recurrent disease in kidney transplant. *Am J Kidney Dis* 24:142–154.

Rao KV, Hafner GP, Crary GS (1994) De novo immunotactoid glomerulopathy of the renal allograft: possible association with cytomegalovirus infection. *Am J Kidney Dis* 24:97–103.

Richardson WP, Colvin RP, Cheeseman SH et al (1981) Glomerulopathy associated with cytomegalovirus viremia in renal allografts. *N Engl J Med* 705:57–62.

Roth D, Cirocco R, Zucker K et al (1995) De novo membranoproliferative glomerulonephritis in hepatitis C virus-infected renal allograft recipients. *Transplantation* 59:1676–1682.

Saborio P, Scheinman JJ (1999) Transplantation for primary hyperoxaluria in the United States. *Kidney Int* 56:1095–1100.

Saito T, Sato H, Oikawa S (1995) Lipoprotein glomerulopathy: a new aspect of lipid-induced glomerular injury. *Nephrology* 1:14–24.

Savin VJ, Sharma R, Sharma M et al (1996) Circulating factor associated with increased glomerular permeability to albumin in recurrent focal segmental glomerulosclerosis. *N Engl J Med* 334:878–883.

Scheinman JI (1991) Primary hyperoxaluria: therapeutic strategies for the nineties. *Kidney Int* 40:389–399.

Schmitt WH, Haubitz M, Mistry N et al (1993) Renal transplantation in Wegener granulomatosis. *Lancet* 342:860 (letter).

Schwarz A, Krause PH, Offermann G, Keller F (1991) Recurrent and de novo renal disease after kidney transplantation with or without cyclosporine A. *Am J Kidney Dis* 17:524–531.

Schwarz A, Krause PH, Offermann G, Keller F (1994) Impact of de novo membranous glomerulonephritis on the clinical course after kidney transplantation. *Transplantation* 58:650–654.

Senguttuvan P, Cameron JS, Hartley RB et al (1990) Recurrence of focal segmental glomerulosclerosis in transplanted kidneys: analysis of incidence and risk factors in 59 allografts. *Pediatr Nephrol* 4:21–28.

Shimizu T, Tanabe K, Oshima T et al (1998) Recurrence of membranoproliferative glomerulonephritis in renal allografts. *Transplant Proc* 30:3910–3913.

Stone JH (1998) End-stage renal disease in lupus: disease activity, dialysis, and the outcome of transplantation. *Lupus* 7:654–659.

Stone JH, Amend WJ, Criswell LA (1997) Outcome of renal transplantation in systemic lupus erythematosus. *Semin Arthritis Rheum* 27:17–26.

Swaak AJ, Nossent JC, Bronsveld W et al (1989) Systemic lupus erythematosus: II. Observations on the occurrence of exacerbations in the disease course. Dutch experience with 110 patients studied prospectively. *Ann Rheum Dis* 48:455–460.

Tarantino A, Moroni G, Banfi G et al (1994) Renal replacement therapy in cryoglobulinemic nephritis. *Nephrol Dial Transplant* 9:1426–1430.

Tejani A, Stablein DH (1992) Recurrence of focal segmental glomerulosclerosis posttransplantation: a special report of the North America Pediatric Renal Transplant Cooperative Study. *J Am Soc Nephrol* 2(Suppl):S258–S263.

Toussaint Ch, De Pauw L, Vienne A et al (1993) Radiological and histological improvement of oxalate osteopathy after combined liver–kidney transplantation in primary hyperoxaluria type 1. *Am J Kidney Dis* 21:54–63.

Trimarchi HM, Triong LD, Brennan S et al (1999) FK506-associated thrombotic microangiopathy. *Transplantation* 67:539–544.

Truong L, Gelfand J, D'Agati V et al (1989) De novo membranous glomerulonephropathy in renal allografts: a report of 10 cases and review of the literature. *Am J Kidney Dis* 14:131–144.

Van Buren D, Van Buren CT, Flechner SM et al (1985) De novo hemolytic uremic syndrome in renal transplants immunosuppressed with cyclosporine. *Surgery* 98:54–58.

Wrenger E, Pirsch JD, Cangro CB (1997) Single-center experience with renal transplantation in patients with Wegener's granulomatosis. *Transplant Int* 10:152–156.

13 INFECTIONS

For many years infections have been the most frequent cause of death in kidney transplant recipients. More recently, improved methods of immunosuppression and progress in the diagnosis and treatment of infection have led to a consistent decline in the incidence of fatal infections. However, even today, infection still occurs in most transplant recipients and remains one of the leading causes of death, especially in the early months after transplantation.

Since the consequences of infection in immunosuppressed patients can be devastating, all efforts should be made to prevent infection. If an infection develops, it is important to establish the etiologic diagnosis as quickly as possible and to institute an effective therapeutic regimen rapidly.

PROPHYLAXIS

Prevention of infections is one of the primary goals in the management of renal transplant recipients. Theoretically, the best chance of prevention is represented by low immunosuppression; however, avoiding rejection exposing the patient to infection remains a difficult task even with modern immunosuppressive therapy. A number of measures may be taken to prevent infections (Table 13.1). To lower the risk of postoperative infections, the use of drainage catheters, indwelling stents, vein catheters and other foreign bodies should be reduced to a minimum. Apart from careful nursing and strict hygiene of the patients, some general measures should be taken during hospitalization. These include removal of plants from around the patient to prevent fungal infections, hot water supply decontamination to prevent aspergillosis (Weiland et al 1983), and protection from other potentially infected patients. There should be regular inspection of air conditioning, and shower baths should be recommended, to prevent the risk of legionnaires' disease (Tobin et al 1980). Many transplant centers use a cephalosporin for 1–3 days to prevent wound infection. Oral washing with nystatin to prevent oral or gastrointestinal fungal infections is usually recommended, although there is no clear evidence of a prophylactic effect (Tollemar 1999). It is current practice to administer one tablet of trimethoprim 160 mg and sulfamethoxazole 800 mg every 24 or 48 hours, for 6–12 months after transplantation in order to reduce the risk of urinary infections

Reducing the risk of postoperative infections
    Minimize the presence and duration of drainage catheters, stents, vein catheters and other foreign bodies

Reducing environmental exposure during hospitalization
    Removal of plants from around the patient (fungi, bacteria)
    Hot water supply decontamination (legionellosis)
    Air filtration (aspergillosis)
    Protection from infected patients (tuberculosis, listeriosis etc.)

Antimicrobial prophylaxis
    Cephalosporins (perioperative) (wound infections)
    Nystatin mouth washing (candidiasis)
    Trimethoprim–sulfamethoxazole (pneumosytosis, listeriosis)
    Bactericidal antibiotics (nocardiosis, urinary tract infections)
    Antiviral prophylaxis (infected donor)
    Acyclovir–ganciclovir (CMV infections)
    Acyclovir (EBV infections)

Vaccine
    Influenza
    Varicella
    Zoster immunoglobulins

Table 13.1. Prevention of infection in renal transplant recipients

(Cuvelier et al 1985), and of infections caused by *Pneumocystis carinii* (Centers for Disease Control 1995; Fishman 1995), *Listeria*, *Nocardia* and *Toxoplasma* (Simmons and Migliori 1988; Rubin and Tolkoff-Rubin 1993). At these doses, the nephrotoxicity of trimethoprim–sulfamethoxazole is rare, but a mild increase in serum creatinine is possible. Prophylaxis with isoniazide (INH), 100 mg a day, has been suggested for patients with a history of tuberculosis or in patients who are positive for tuberculin. However, a positive tuberculin test with no additional risk factors carries a very low risk of reactivation. Moreover, it must be pointed out that there are more and more forms of INH-resistant tuberculosis. Finally, INH is often poorly tolerated and can reduce the bioavailability of cyclosporine, tacrolimus and corticosteroids (Langhoff et al 1983).

As many as 70–80% of kidney transplant recipients may show laboratory evidence of cytomegalovirus (CMV) infection after transplant, and a significant number of patients develop tissue invasive disease with considerable morbidity and occasional mortality (Rubin 1993; Murray et al 1997). Therefore, prophylaxis with antiviral therapy has been recommended in patients at risk. There is agreement that all recipients treated with antilymphocyte antibodies should receive prophylaxis independently of the seropositivity of the recipient and the donor (Jassal et al 1998). It is still questionable whether prophylaxis with antiviral therapy should be recommended for seronegative recipients on conventional immunosuppression who receive a kidney from a seropositive donor. In seronegative patients receiving a seronegative kidney and in seropositive recipients, the risk of CMV disease is low. Therefore, no antiviral therapy is required. Immunoglobulins, acyclovir, ganciclovir and valacyclovir have been used for prevention of CMV infection in organ transplant patients. A significant reduction in the incidence of CMV infection and disease has been obtained with intravenous immunoglobulins (Patel et al 1996). A drawback of immunoglobulins is that treatment should be prolonged for at least 16 weeks (Jassal et al 1998). Other disadvantages of using immunoglobulins are the cost of treatment and the heterogeneity of the preparation. Oral acyclovir is generally administered at a dose of 3.2 g per day for 12 weeks. Intravenous ganciclovir is given at doses ranging between 5 and 10 mg/kg per day for 10–14 days. Both drugs require adjustment in case of renal dysfunction (Table 13.2). Oral ganciclovir is given at doses of 1.5–2.0 g per day for 14–90 days. A recent meta-analysis of 13 controlled trials showed that prophylactic treatment with acyclovir or ganciclovir could significantly reduce the risk of CMV disease and infection, with no difference between the two agents (Couchoud et al 1998). However, a prospective randomized trial showed that oral acyclovir for 3 months provides effective prophylaxis only for recipients of seronegative donor kidneys while oral ganciclovir for 3 months protected the recipients of seropositive donor kidneys from CMV infection (Flechner et al 1998). Valacyclovir, 2 g four times per day for 90 days, also proved to be a safe and effective way to prevent CMV disease after renal transplantation (Lowance et al 1999). The doses of valacyclovir should also be adjusted according to renal function (Table 13.2).

Most transplant recipients have preformed antibodies against the Epstein–Barr virus (EBV). A few seronegative patients carry a high risk of receiving an EBV positive kidney with the consequent risk of infection. While in some patients EBV infection causes a benign polyclonal hyperplasia, in other transplant recipients, a monoclonal lymphoproliferative reaction can occur (Hanto 1992; Preiksaitis 1992). Thus, EBV seronegative patients should not be treated with antilymphocyte antibodies that expose them to an increased risk of viral infection. In addition, they should be carefully monitored in order to give a quick antiviral treatment in case of EBV infection (Hibberd and Rubin 1991). A recent study showed a significant reduction of posttransplant lymphoma when patients given antilymphocyte antibody therapy were given preemptive treatment with acyclovir or ganciclovir (Darenkov et al 1997).

Vaccination against varicella is recommended in transplant candidates without humoral immunity. Zoster immune globulins and antiviral prophylaxis should be administered to the recipient if some relative is infected with varicella. Influenza vaccine is also recommended by some authorities (Peterson and Anderson 1986).

A special problem is represented with kidneys coming from bacteremic donors. In the case of bacteremia caused by bland organisms, such as Enterobacteriaceae, *Streptococcus viridans* or penicillin-sensitive pneumococci and meningococci, a short course of

Creatinine clearance ml/min	Acyclovir	Intravenous ganciclovir	Foscarnet	Valacyclovir
>70	5.0–15 mg/kg every 8 h	5.0 mg/kg every 12 h	60–100 mg/kg every 8–12 h	30 mg/kg every 6 h
50–69	5.0–15 mg/kg every 12 h	2.5 mg/kg every 12 h	30–50 mg/kg every 8–12 h	20–25 mg/kg every 6 h
25–49	5.0–15 mg/kg every 12 h	2.5 mg/kg every 24 h	15–25 mg/kg every 8–12 h	20 mg/kg every 8 h
10–24	5.0–15 mg/kg every 24 h	1.5 mg/kg every 24 h	7.5–12.5 mg/kg every 8–12 h	20 mg/kg every 12 h
<10	2.5–5.0 mg/kg every 24 h	1.25 mg/kg every 48 h	Avoid	20 mg/kg every 24 h
Dialysis	5.0 mg/kg after dialysis	1.25 mg/kg after dialysis	50 mg/kg after dialysis	

Table 13.2. Dose adjustment of the principal antiviral agents according to creatinine clearance levels

bactericidal antibiotics may be sufficient to eradicate the microorganism. In the case of infections caused by *Staphylococcus aureus, Pseudomonas aeruginosa* or penicillin-resistant streptococci, a minimum of 2 weeks of bactericidal therapy is required. Blood cultures should remain negative over a period of a week after antibiotic therapy. Donors with infections caused by vancomycin-resistant enterococcal infections, salmonella, fungal, nocardial or active mycobacterial infection should be excluded (Rubin and Fishman 1998).

TIMETABLE FOR INFECTION AFTER TRANSPLANTATION

In the transplant recipient, infections can be caused by nosocomial microorganisms, opportunistic microorganisms or microorganisms of the community. The type, frequency and severity of the infection are roughly related to the level of immunosuppression, and the duration of immunosuppressive therapy.

According to Rubin et al (1981), there is a relatively stereotypical pattern in the timetable of posttransplant infections. In the first month following transplantation, most infections are accounted for by nosocomial microorganisms. In the period between the first and the sixth month, opportunistic infections derived from endogenous flora are frequent. After the sixth month, the type of infection is similar to that observed in the general population (Table 13.3). However, patients with poor allograft function or

0–1 month	
Bacterial:	wound infection, pneumonia, urinary tract infection, pyelitis, bacteremia
Viral:	Herpes simplex, hepatitis
1–6 months	
Viral:	CMV, Epstein–Barr, Varicella–zoster
Fungal:	*Candida, Aspergillus, Cryptococcus*
Bacterial:	*Listeria, Legionella, Nocardia*
Protozoa:	*Pneumocystis carinii*
>6 months	
Bacterial:	Community microorganism, mycobacteriosis
Viral:	Hepatitis B or C, CMV chorioetinitis

Table 13.3. Timetable of infections in renal transplant recipients

vigorous immunosuppression are still exposed to an increased risk of viral and opportunistic infections.

Infection in the first month

During the first month after transplantation, opportunistic infections are rare. Some patients have a recurrence of infection that was present in the donor or the recipient but was unrecognized or insufficiently treated (Fishman 1999). Most infections occurring in this period are nosocomial bacterial or candidal infections of the surgical wound, lungs, urinary tract, or vascular devices (Rubin 1993). Active infection is rarely transmitted when the allograft comes from a donor with bacteremia or fungemia. Such infections can seed at the vascular suture lines, leading to the formation of mycotic aneurysms causing arterial disruption (Rubin and Fishman 1998).

Infections 1–6 months after transplantation

After the first month, the combination of sustained immunosuppression and infections with immunomodulating viruses (particularly CMV, but also EBV, other herpes viruses and hepatitis viruses) opens the possibility for opportunistic infections due to *P. carinii*, *Aspergillus, Listeria monocytogenes, Cryptococcus*, and *Candida*. Particularly frequent in this period are the infections caused by CMV, which account for most of the cases of 'unexplained fever'. Lung, central nervous system, retina, urinary tract and the gastrointestinal tract are the most frequent sites of infection.

Infections after the sixth month

For most patients, problems with infection later than 6 months after transplantation are similar to those of the general community and are primarily respiratory. Urinary tract infections are frequent but are usually benign.

In 5–10% of cases, chronic rejection and intensive immunosuppressive therapy can expose the patient to opportunistic infections. Lifelong prophylaxis with trimethoprim–sulfamethoxazole and/or antifungal prophylaxis has been recommended for these patients (Fishman and Rubin 1998). Another 10% of renal transplant recipients have chronic infection with CMV, EBV, hepatitis B or C virus or papillomavirus. These infections may be progressive and lead to chorioretinitis, lymphoma, liver failure or squamous-cell cancer. Leishmaniasis, ehrlichiosis and other rare infectious diseases may also occur.

APPROACH TO THE FEBRILE RENAL TRANSPLANT PATIENT

Although fever is not always present in an infected immunosuppressed patient, the most common manifestation of an infection in a transplant patient is fever. A number of clinical, laboratory and radiological investigations is recommended in the febrile transplant patient. The first differential diagnosis should be between infection and rejection (Table 13.4). Usually an acute rejection causing fever is easy to detect because it is associated with typical signs and symptoms, such as rapid increase in plasma creatinine, oliguria, proteinuria, and tenderness of the allograft. However, a similar clinical picture can be

Rejection	Infection
PI, creatinine	Hemocrome (differential count)
Urinalysis	Mucosal plugging
(sodium, protein, sediment)	Cultures (blood, urine, secretions)
Graft ultrasonography	CMV antigenemia
Fine needle aspiration	Anti-legionella, candida,
Renal biopsy	mycoplasm antibodies
	Pulmonary
	Chest X-ray (bronchial lavage)
	Cardiac
	Echocardiogram
	Urinary
	Graft, native kidneys,
	bladder and prostate
	ultrasonography
	Neurological
	Liquor
	Cerebral TC
	Intestinal–hepatic
	Stool culture
	Liver and pancreas ultrasonography
	Serodiagnosis

Table 13.4. Investigations in a renal transplant recipient with fever

present in the case of pyelitis, perirenal hematoma, lymphocele, urinary fistula or stenosis. Ultrasonography of the kidney, ureter and bladder is usually sufficient for a correct diagnosis, but in the most difficult cases intravenous urography, computed tomography or renal biopsy may be required.

A vigorous search for the focus of infection is imperative. Although localized sites of infection can be identified in many cases, some infections manifest themselves with signs and symptoms of a systemic disease without findings of a focal infection. This is particularly frequent in the case of CMV infection, but may also occur in febrile patients with bacteremia or fungemia. While waiting for the results of blood culture, the history, the site of infection, and the time of infection can orientate the empiric antibacterial therapy (Table 13.5). It must be remembered that septicemia in renal transplant patients is usually due to a Gram-negative organism and more rarely to *Staph. aureus* and *L. monocytogenes* (Petersen and Andersen 1986). In all patients with severe infection, exogenous immunosuppression must be reduced as much as possible.

VIRAL INFECTIONS

Cytomegalovirus

Human cytomegalovirus (CMV) is a double-stranded DNA virus belonging to the family of betaherpes viridae. It is also called human herpes virus 5. Replication of CMV involves three types of genes: immediate early genes coding for IE proteins; early genes coding for E antigens; and late genes coding for L antigens. The H65 matrix is a late antigen.

CMV is the most frequent virus infecting renal transplant recipients. There are three forms of CMV infection in transplant patients: primary infection, secondary or reactivated infection and superinfection.

The primary infection is the most severe. Some 30–50% of adults are seropositive for CMV. The virus can reside in the kidney, and it is through the allograft that seronegative transplant recipients become infected. It has been estimated that seronegative recipients from seropositive donors have a greater than 50% risk of symptomatic disease (Rubin 1994). Reactivation occurs in a patient who is already a carrier of the virus. Activation from latency can be induced by several factors: therapy with antilymphocyte antibodies or other immunosuppressive agents; allogeneic reactions; and systemic infections. Systemic inflammation can reactivate CMV from latency through intracellular messengers stimulated by proinflammatory cytokines (Rubin 1990; Fietze et al 1994). Superinfection occurs when the donor and the recipient are both seropositive and the virus of donor origin reactivates.

The typical CMV disease manifests itself with fever, myalgias and malaise, that usually occur between 4 and 10 weeks after transplantation. It may be associated with anemia, leukopenia, thrombocytopenia, mild lymphocytosis and mild hepatitis. Some patients, particularly those affected by primary infection, may develop pneumonitis, encephalitis or myocarditis (Table 13.6). On the other hand, it must be noted that a

	Virus	Bacteria	Fungi	Protozoa
Pneumonia	CMV (1–4 months)	S. pneumoniae (0 months–years) H. influenzae P. aeruginosa (0–3 months) M. pneumoniae (2 months–years) Legionella sp. (1–8 weeks) Nocardia (1–6 months) M. tuberculosis (3 months–years)	H. capsulatum (2 months–years) C. neoformans Aspergillus sp. (1–3 months) Candida sp. (1–3 months)	P. carinii (1–6 months) S. stercoralis (endemic areas) C. neoformans T. gondii (3–8 months)
Mental confusion	CMV (1–4 months)	L. monocytogenes (1–6 months)		
Diarrhea	CMV (1–4 months)	Salmonella Shigella Campylobacter C. difficile	H. capsulatum (2 months–years)	E. histolytica G. lamblia Cryptosporidium Microsporidium
Unknown fever	CMV (1–4 months) EBV (2–6 months)	M. tuberculosis (3 months–years)	H. capsulatum (2 months–years)	P. carinii (1–5 months)

Table 13.5. Etiologies of some syndromes in renal transplant recipients

Signs and symptoms

    Fever, malaise, myalgias

    Leukopenia, anemia, thrombocytopenia, increase in transaminases

    Pneumonitis (pulmonary interstitial infiltrates)

    Myocarditis, pancreatitis, gastrointestinal tract

    Encephalitis

Complications

    Opportunistic infections (*Pneumocystis carinii*, aspergillosis)

    Allograft rejection

    Epstein–Barr virus; associated lymphoproliferative disorders

Table 13.6. Main signs and symptoms and possible complications of posttransplant CMV infections

reactivated and, less frequently, a primary infection may be asymptomatic, but may render the patient more susceptible to opportunistic infections, such as *P. carinii* pneumonia or invasive aspergillosis (Rubin 1994; Fishman 1995; Hadley and Karchmer 1995). While powerful antirejection therapy increases viral replication, CMV infection may, in turn, favor the development of acute rejection (Reinke et al 1994; Kashyap et al 1999). More controversial and still unproven is the possibility that CMV infection may expose patients to an increased risk of chronic rejection. CMV infection may also expose patients to an increased risk of lymphoproliferative disorders, both directly and by favoring the development of EBV infection (Fishman and Rubin 1998).

Serology viral culture, shell vial assay detection of viral genetic material by polymerase chain reaction (PCR), and detection of CMV antigenemia were employed to obtain an early and correct diagnosis of CMV infection in order to guide prophylactic and therapeutic strategies (Table 13.7). Each technique has a different diagnostic meaning and clinic impact. Serology is a useful method to ascertain whether or not patients have a history of CMV. However, a significant rise in IgG or IgM titers usually occurs late after the onset of CMV syndrome. Moreover, immunosuppressive therapy may prevent a rise in antiCMV antibodies. Therefore, serology is helpful for detecting previous CMV infections, however it cannot be used for early diagnosis and does not provide relevant clinical information (Morris et al 1990; Tanabe et al 1997). Viral culture of peripheral blood leukocytes (PBL) provides a direct demonstration of the presence of CMV. However, this technique takes a long time in order to obtain the final results and cannot be used for early diagnosis. The shell vial modification of the conventional buffy coat culture technique, which shortens the time of viral culture, was developed a few years ago. However, it is not useful for early diagnosis (Erice et al 1992; Murray et al 1997) and is not correlated with the clinical course of the infection

	Diagnosis	Sensitivity	Specificity	Correlation with clinical course
Antigenemia assay	Early	Good	Good	Good
PCR assay	Early	Good	Good	Poor
Shell vial assay	Late	Good	Good	Poor
Serology	Late	Poor	Good	Poor
DNA in leukocytes	Early	Good	Good	Good

Table 13.7. Main characteristics of the tests available for confirming the diagnosis of CMV infection

(Tanabe et al 1997). The CMV antigen test is an immunocytochemical method that, by using a monoclonal antibody specific for the pp65 CMV matrix protein, allows detection and quantification of positive PBL directly on a buffy coat preparation. This protein is abundantly produced in excess during viral replication at different body sites, and is picked up by PBL. High levels of CMV antigenemia have been found in patients with overt disease, whereas low levels correlate with asymptomatic infections (Van der Berg et al 1989). In order to identify the patients at higher risk of overt disease as early as possible, and to define preemptive strategies, threshold values of antigenemia have been determined. In one study, a threshold of 100 pp65-positive/200 000 PBL has been chosen in solid-organ recipients (Grossi et al 1995). Slightly different thresholds have been suggested in other studies (Murray et al 1997), likely due to technical reasons and to underlying clinical circumstances, such as the level of immunosuppression. PCR can also be used to detect CMV DNA in the plasma or leukocytes of the patient (Jiwa et al 1989). This test has a good sensitivity and specificity (Mendez et al 1998) and can detect the presence of viremia even before the onset of symptoms (The et al 1992). The quantitative determination of viral DNA in leukocytes (not in plasma) has recently been proposed as the assay of choice in monitoring solid organ recipients at high risk (Gerna et al 1998). It proved to correlate more closely with clinical symptoms in high-risk population than antigenemia. This could be due to the fact that CMV DNA in leukocytes is the only genuine expression of viral replication occurring at different sites, while the pp65 matrix protein is produced in excess during viral replication and assembly.

Treatment of clinical CMV disease requires administration of intravenous ganciclovir for a minimum of 2–4 weeks. Ganciclovir is a guanosine analog that, after intracellular, phosphorylation, inhibits DNA polymerase activity and is incorporated in the viral DNA with consequent inhibition of the synthesis of the chain (Faulds and Heel 1990). Ganciclovir should be administered at dose of 5 mg/kg every 12 hours with adjustment in case of renal dysfunction (Table 13.2). In order to prevent relapses or resistance, treatment should be continued until clearance of viremia before intravenous administration is documented. It is still unclear whether 2–3 months of oral ganciclovir, following intravenous administration, may be useful in preventing relapses or may rather expose the patient to resistance because of the low serum levels (Fishman and Rubin 1998). Serious side-effects of ganciclovir are infrequent and include reversible neutropenia in 25–40% of patients, thrombocytopenia in about 20% of patients, irritation at infusion site, and rarely a dose-dependent deterioration of renal function, probably due to crystallization of the drug in renal tubules (Dunn et al 1991). Generalized seizures have been reported in patients who received concomitantly imipenem–cilastatin and ganciclovir. Occasionally, allergic reactions may also occur. In cases of overt CMV infection, a decrease of immunosuppressive therapy and trimethoprim–sulfamethoxazole administration to prevent *P. carinii* infection are also recommended. Some centers also add human immunoglobulins to the treatment of severe or relapsing disease. Human immunoglobulins are available in two preparations: nonspecific globulin derived from a pool of healthy blood donors and CMV-specific hyperimmune globulins derived from selected donors with high CMV antibody titer. Both preparations are administered intravenously. It is still controversial as to whether there are significant differences with either preparation. It is also difficult to evaluate whether the addition of immunoglobulins can be helpful in ganciclovir-treated patients. A meta-analysis showed a trend of increasing benefit to organ transplant recipients (Wittes et al 1996). However, the studies taken into consideration were often inadequate for a correct statistical evaluation.

Some patients may develop resistance to ganciclovir which is manifested by a progression of CMV disease and persistence of viremia in spite of therapy. The resistance may be caused either by a reduction of intracellular phosphorylation or by a mutation of viral DNA polymerase (Hayden and Douglas 1990). Ganciclovir-resistant CMV usually responds to foscarnet. This agent is an analog of pyrophosphate that inhibits the viral DNA polymerase and interferes with the exchange of pyrophosphate from phosphorylated deoxynucleotides (Crumpacker 1992). Foscarnet must be given intravenously for 14–21 days. The initial dose is 60 mg/kg every 8 hours but the dose should be adjusted according to the renal function, as the drug is eliminated by glomerular filtration rate and tubular secretion. The maintenance dose is 120 mg/kg per day. Again, the dosage should be modified according to the creatinine clearance (Table 13.2). Foscarnet may be responsible for several side-effects: fever, nausea, anemia, diarrhea, vomiting, headache, seizures. The most severe side-effect is renal toxicity. The drug may cause a substantial increase in plasma creatinine values and may be responsible for acute tubular necrosis (Deray et al 1989) or crystalline glomerulonephritis with nephrotic syndrome (Zanetta et al 1999). The administration of saline infusion, 2.5 l/day throughout treatment with foscarnet, minimizes the risk of nephrotoxicity. Other nephrotoxic drugs, such as cyclosporine, tacrolimus, amphotericin B and aminoglycosides should be stopped or their dosage reduced, during foscarnet administration. Electrolyte imbalance, especially hypocalcemia, is also common under foscarnet therapy (Balfour 1999). Recently, a new antiCMV molecule, cidofovir, has been licensed. Its nephrotoxicity, however, is much feared.

Epstein–Barr virus

Epstein–Barr virus infection may cause a mononucleosis syndrome. However, the most worrying effect is represented by the pathogenetic role of EBV infection in lymphoproliferative disorders ranging from a benign, reversible, polyclonal B-cell proliferation to malignant lymphoma. EBV replication in the oropharynx results in infection, transformation and immortalization of B cells. In the normal subject these transformed B cells are eliminated by specific cytotoxic cells. In the immunosuppressed renal transplant recipient, this surveillance mechanism may be impaired, thus making possible the development of a lymphoproliferative disorder. The role of acyclovir in treating EBV infection is still under discussion. Controlled trials in nonimmunosuppressed patients showed only a mild benefit in the clinical course of infectious mononucleosis (Anderson and Ernberg 1988). Chemoprophylaxis with acyclovir in EBV-negative transplant recipients has been given in order to prevent lymphoproliferative disorders, but the results are not convincing. The role of a very early and prolonged intravenous administration of ganciclovir is under investigation (Green et al 1998).

Varicella zoster virus

The dermatosomal zoster is about 10 times more common in renal transplant recipients than in healthy individuals. Herpes zoster tends to follow a more protracted course in the immunosuppressed patient, but visceral dissemination rarely occurs. Oral acyclovir (800 mg four times a day for 7 days) or intravenous acyclovir in the most severe cases (250–500 mg/m^2 every 8 hours for 7 days) may halt the progression of herpes zoster in an immunocompromised host. High-dose acyclovir may rarely cause renal dysfunction because of crystallization of the drug in renal tubules (Balfour 1999). Valacyclovir, an L-valine ester of acyclovir, exhibits better oral bioavailability. Controlled trials in immunocompetent patients with herpes zoster showed that valacyclovir, at a dose of 1000 mg three times a day for 7–14 days, significantly reduced the median pain duration and decreased the proportion of patients with pain persisting for 6 months when compared to acyclovir (Beutner et al 1995; Grant et al 1997). A rare, severe, and still unexplained complication of valacyclovir is represented by thrombotic microangiopathy (Balfour 1999).

A much more serious occurrence is chickenpox. In renal transplant patients, varicella may be a devastating disease causing encephalitis, pneumonia, hepatitis, pancreatitis, disseminated intravascular coagulation and gastrointestinal ulcerations. If a patient without antibodies to varicella zoster is exposed to chickenpox then varicella zoster immune globulins should be given within 72 hours of exposure. The usual dose for intramuscular administration is 125 U/10 kg by weight in children, up to a maximum of 625 U. Adults are given a cumulative dose of 625 U. If chickenpox develops, intravenous acyclovir should be promptly instituted (10 mg/kg every 8 hours for 7–10 days, with dosage decreases for renal dysfunction).

Herpes simplex virus

Reactivation of herpes simplex virus infection is common in renal transplant recipients. Infection usually involves the orolabial region and less commonly the anogenital area, the conjunctiva, or the cornea. Occasionally, fatal hepatitis, pneumonitis or encephalitis occur.

Topical acyclovir is ineffective and is not recommended (Whitley and Gnann 1992). Most patients respond well to oral acyclovir (200–400 mg five times per day for 7–14 days). In the case of encephalitis or other visceral localization, high-dose intravenous acyclovir (10 mg/kg every 8 hours for 10–14 days) is the treatment of choice (Keating 1992).

Human herpes virus 6 (HHV-6)

Human herpes virus 6 infection occurs in 31–55% of organ transplant recipients, usually 2–4 weeks after transplant as a result of reactivation caused by intense immunosuppression. In many cases there is a coinfection or a reactivation of HHV-6 and CMV together (Ratnamohan et al 1998). Two variants have been identified: A and B. Renal transplant patients are infected almost exclusively with variant B. The clinical sequelae of HHV-6 may range from a self-limited febrile viral syndrome to tissue invasive disseminated disease. Bone marrow suppression, meningoencephalitis, interstitial pneumonitis, and a mononucleosis syndrome are the most commonly reported types of clinical disease. Apart from direct morbidity, the immune dysregulation triggered by HHV-6 may facilitate superinfections with other opportunistic pathogens. Human HHV-6 responds to ganciclovir and foscarnet, but it is resistant to acyclovir (Singh and Carrigan 1996).

Human herpes virus 8 (HHV-8)

In the last few years, solid evidence linking Kaposi's sarcoma (both in endemic and in nonendemic form, in HIV and transplant-associated forms) to HHV-8 infection has been produced (Cathomas et al 1997). Human herpes virus 8 is a novel virus, sharing biochemical and biological properties with the herpesviridae family, namely the ability to establish a latent infection that may reactivate with immunosuppression. Kaposi's sarcoma may develop in transplant recipients either as a consequence of a reactivated infection in a seropositive patient or as a primary infection in a patient without HHV-8-specific antibodies. In the latter case, a primary infection may be transmitted from the donor through the graft (Regamey et al 1998). It is likely that factors other than immunosuppression are required for Kaposi's sarcoma to develop. A response to treatment with an antiviral agent, cidofovir, has been reported in posttransplant Kaposi's sarcoma.

Polyoma virus (PV)

The polyoma viruses (PVs: BK, JC, SV40) are classified as 'slow' viruses. PVs are usually acquired in childhood and remain latent in the kidney. PVs may be found, by cytology, in the urine of about 20% of renal transplant recipients (Figure 13.1). The clinical significance of this finding remains unclear as in many patients PV does not cause significant morbidity. Recently, however, several cases of reactivation of PV infection have been reported in renal transplant recipients given vigorous immunosuppression (Binet et al 1999). PV infection may cause ureteral stenosis, hemorrhagic cystitis, and interstitial nephritis (Figure 13.2) with progressive graft loss. There is no specific treatment for PV infection. Reduction of immunosuppression may stabilize renal function in a few cases.

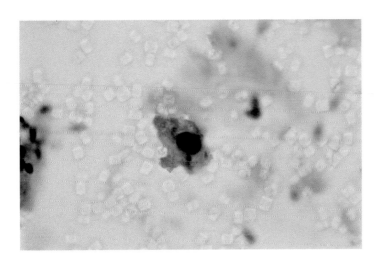

Figure 13.1. Polyoma virus in the urinary sediment. Light micrograph of urine cytology showing a tubular epithelial cell with characteristic intranuclear inclusion. (Courtesy of Dr F Egidi, University of Tennessee.)

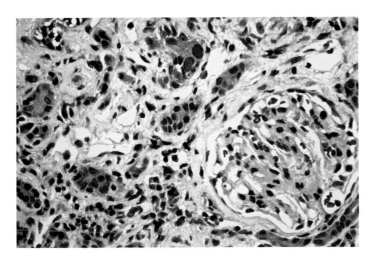

Figure 13.2. Renal biopsy. Interstitial nephritis caused by polyoma virus. The infiltrate is mainly composed of plasma cells and lymphocytes with interstitial fibrosis. (Courtesy of Dr F Egidi, University of Tennessee.)

SEPSIS

Sepsis is a syndrome defined by the presence of two or more features of systemic inflammation such as: fever or hypothermia, leukocytosis or leukopenia, tachycardia and tachypnea or supranormal minute ventilation (Bone et al 1992). Sepsis is relatively frequent in the immunosuppressed host and is usually severe. The lung is the most common site of infection, followed by the urinary tract and the abdomen, but in several cases a definite site of infection cannot be recognized. Pleural, peritoneal and paranasal sinus infections can easily be overlooked even with the use of computed tomography (Wheeler and Bernard 1999). In about 20–30% of patients, cultures are sterile.

The prognosis of sepsis largely depends on organ involvement. The average risk of death increases by 15–20% with failure of each organ. In addition to the number of organ failures, the severity of each failure worsens the prognosis (Wheeler and Bernard 1999).

Antimicrobial therapy should be guided by the isolation of the etiologic microorganism. When the pathogen is not identified, broad antibiotic coverage is usually started, narrowing the therapy when microbiological data are available. In some cases, antimicrobial therapy may paradoxically precipitate sepsis syndrome by liberating microbial products. In order to prevent renal dysfunction and other organ failure, the first approach usually consists of trying to restore hemodynamic stability by correct fluid administration. In the case of hypotension sustained by low systemic vascular resistance, alpha-adrenergic drugs may be helpful. Dopamine is usually the preferred agent as it may improve, or at least not worsen, the renal blood flow. Beta-adrenergic stimulation may be tried in the case of depressed myocardial contractility. Unfortunately, impaired microcirculation due to ischemia may not benefit from increased flow because of faulty vasoregulation.

PNEUMONITIS

Although the incidence of pneumonia has declined in recent years, pulmonary infection remains the most serious infectious disease in renal allograft recipients. Given the diverse group of potential infectious disease etiologies (Table 13.8) and the frequent lack of specificity of clinical and radiological findings (Table 13.9), an aggressive diagnostic approach is often indicated. Fiberoptic bronchoscopy with transbronchial biopsy and bronchoalveolar lavage are the most frequently used invasive techniques. Open lung biopsy and transthoracic needle aspiration may be needed in the most difficult cases.

Bacterial pneumonia

In the first month after transplantation, Gram-negative bacilli (*E. coli*, *P. aeruginosa*, *K. pneumoniae*) and *Staph. aureus* are the most frequent causes of pneumonia. While

Bacteria	Viruses
Pneumococcus	Cytomegalovirus
H. influenzae	Fungi
Staph. aureus	*Aspergillus* sp.
Legionella sp.	*Candida* sp.
Mycobacterium sp.	*Criptococcus*
Nocardia sp.	Parasites
E. coli	*P. carinii*
P. aeruginosa	*S. stercoralis*
K. pneumoniae	
Chlamydia	

Table 13.8. Main etiologic agents of pulmonary infections

Radiographic abnormality	Acute development	Chronic development
Nodular infiltrate	Bacteria	Fungi, *N. asteroides*, Tuberculosis, *P. carinii*
Cavitation	Bacteria (*Legionella*), fungi	Tuberculosis
Peribronchovascular abnormality	Bacteria, viruses (influenza)	CMV, *P. carinii*, fungi, *N. asteroides*, tuberculosis
Consolidation	Bacteria (*Legionella*)	Fungi, *N. asteroides*, Tuberculosis, viruses, *P. carinii*
Diffuse interstitial infiltrates		CMV, *P. carinii*, fungi (rare)

Table 13.9. Radiologic findings in posttransplant pneumonia. (Modified from Fishman and Rubin 1998.)

waiting for culture results, a third generation cephalosporin with or without an amino-glycoside can be given. Imipenem, ciprofloxacin or vancomycin may be administered in resistant cases.

Legionella pneumonia

Legionella has become one of the most frequent causes of nosocomial pneumonia. Chest X-ray films show irregular, nodular shadows that progress to a lobar or diffuse consolidation. Cavitation can also occur (Figure 13.3; Gombert et al 1984). Identification of the organism may be obtained with direct immunofluorescent staining and it may be grown from sputum, biopsy samples or by urine antigen assay. Elevated antibody titers develop only in an advanced phase of the disease. An increase of four times the titer to 1:128 is diagnostic of a recent exposure. A single titer of 1:256 or more indicates a recent infection caused by a *Legionella* microorganism. Erythromycin, clarithromycin or azithromycin are the antibiotics of choice for legionellosis. It must be remembered that these agents can significantly increase the blood levels of cyclosporine or tacrolimus (Ptachinski et al 1985). Rifampin is also effective and can be added to erythromycin in severe cases. As opposed to macrolides, rifampin significantly decreases the blood levels of cyclosporine or tacrolimus (Langhoff et al 1983). Fluoroquinolones (ciprofloxacin and levofloxacin) and doxycycline are also quite effective (Bartlett et al 1998).

Nocardia pneumonia

Pulmonary nocardiosis is difficult to recognize. The infection can be acute and fulminant or may have a chronic course for weeks or months. The diagnosis must be suspected in any case of chronic pneumonitis that does not respond to antibiotic therapy. The association of pneumonia with central nervous system and/or cutaneous involve-

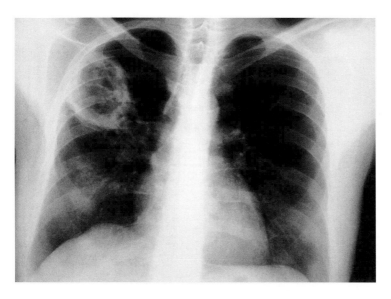

Figure 13.3. *Legionella* pneumonia. Multiple foci in the right lung with cavitation.

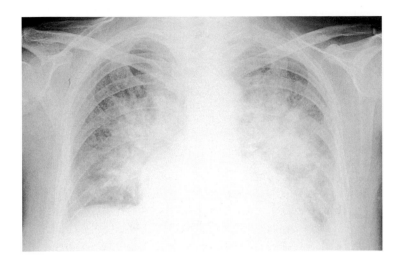

Figure 13.4. *Nocardia* pneumonia. Bilateral hilar and perihilar thickenings of different density.

ment is highly suggestive for diagnosis. The radiologic findings are variable and not specific (Figure 13.4). Computed tomography can be useful to determine the extent of infection and the response to therapy. Usually, the etiologic diagnosis requires the use of invasive procedures such as transtracheal aspiration, pulmonary needle aspiration or biopsy. Treatment with trimethoprim–sulfamethoxazole is usually successful when initiated early and continued for 6–12 months (Simpson et al 1981). Alternative agents are ciprofloxacin, cephalosporins, imipenem, and aminoglycosides.

Community pneumonia

Pneumonia occurring after the sixth month is usually caused by community micro-organisms (mainly pneumococci, influenzal virus, *S. aureus*, *K. pneumoniae*, mycoplasma or chlamydias) and should be treated accordingly. Macrolides, fluoroquinolones or doxicyclin are the antibiotics of first choice in the outpatient, while a third generation cephalosporin or a beta-lactamic agent can be associated with a macrolide or a fluoroquinolone agent in hospitalized patients (Bartlett et al 1998).

Tuberculosis

The incidence of tuberculosis is more common in transplant recipients than in the general population. Treatment should be the routine antitubercular therapy. Although short-term (9 months) therapy with INH plus rifampin may be sufficient, some patients may require an additional 9 months of treatment with INH plus ethambutol (Peterson and Anderson 1986). Both rifampin and INH may accelerate the metabolism of cyclosporine, tacrolimus and corticosteroids (Langhoff et al 1983). Therefore, the dose of immunosuppressive agents should be closely monitored. Pyrazinamide may be substituted for rifampin in cyclosporine-treated patients (Coward et al 1985), but liver function should be monitored in view of the hepatotoxicity of pyrazinamide.

Cytomegalovirus pneumonia

The diagnosis of CMV pneumonitis should be suspected in transplant patients with radiologic abnormalities between 1 and 4 months after transplantation. The suspicion of CMV is stronger if the patient was seronegative and received the kidney from a seropositive donor and/or if the patient was treated with antilymphocyte antibodies. The diagnosis may be confirmed by the presence of elevated CMV antigenemia and/or by the typical histopathologic changes (cytomegaly, intracellular inclusions with peripheral chromatin clumping, intracytoplasmic inclusions) seen with bronchoscopy or in open lung biopsy specimens.

Pneumocystis carinii pneumonia

This is a frequent complication in transplant patients treated either with cyclosporine (Hardy et al 1984) or with rapamycin (Kahan et al 1996). However, the incidence of *P. carinii* pneumonia has become rare in those centers using trimethoprim–sulfamethoxazole prophylaxis (Peterson et al 1982).

The patient with *P. carinii* pneumonia usually presents with fever and dyspnea. Physical signs are usually absent on examination. Radiographic abnormalities are variable and not specific. However, interstitial pneumonia is frequent (Figure 13.5). Severe hypoxemia is usually present. High dose trimethoprim–sulfamethoxazole is the treatment of choice. The recommended dose is 15 mg/kg of trimethoprim, divided into 3–4 doses. A treatment of 14 days is usually sufficient. In patients allergic to sulfonamides slow intravenous infusion of pentamidin, at doses ranging between 3 and 4 mg/kg per day according to the severity of the disease, may be indicated (Sattler and Feinberg 1992). Alternative treatment includes clindamycin, 900 mg every 8 hours, plus primaquine, 15 mg by mouth every day.

Fungal pneumonia

The four major fungal etiologies of pneumonia in renal transplant recipients are *Aspergillus* species, *Histoplasma capsulatum*, *Coccidioides immitis*, and *Cryptococcus neoformans* (Peterson and Andersen 1986). Because of the increased risk of fungal pneumonia, renal transplant patients with pulmonary infiltrates should have sputum specimens

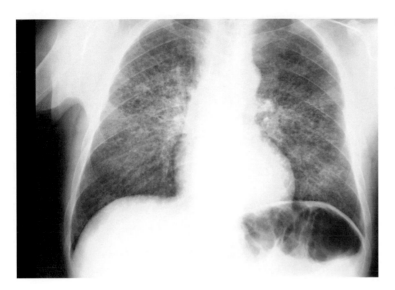

Figure 13.5.
Pneumocystis carinii
pneumonia. Interstitial
pneumonitis with hilar and
perihilar reticulonodular
thickenings.

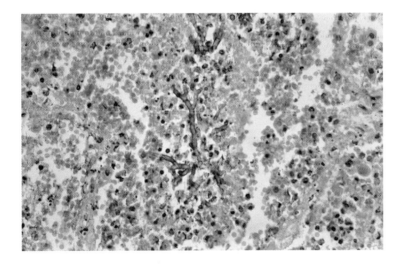

Figure 13.6. Postmortem
tissue from a case of
invasive pulmonary
aspergillosis: hyphae of
Aspergillus fumigatus,
septate, uniform In width
(3–6 μm), with dichotomous
branches, infiltrating the
necrotic tissue. H & E ×40.
(Courtesy of Dr MA Viviani,
Ospedale Maggiore, Milan.)

examined and cultured for fungi. Recovery of *H. capsulatum*, *C. neoformans* and *C. immitis* can be regarded as diagnostic. *Aspergillus* species can be found as saprophytes but the presence of hyphae at direct microscopy of the sample (Figure 13.6) and growth in culture of the fungus in a renal transplant patient with unexplained pneumonia is highly clinically significant (Peterson and Andersen 1986). Serologic tests can be of value in diagnosing disseminated mycoses. Invasive procedures may be required in difficult cases.

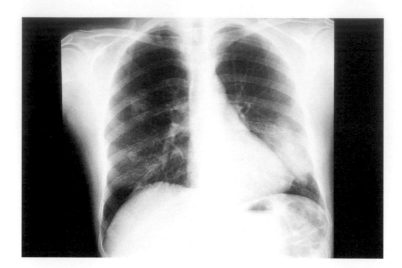

Figure 13.7. *Aspergillus* pneumonia. Patchy consolidation with faded margins.

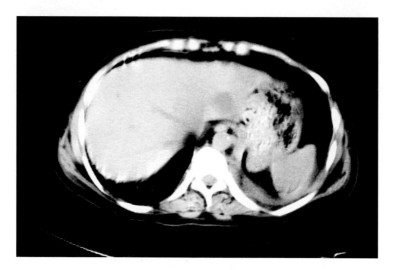

Figure 13.8. Diffuse aspergillosis. Localization in the liver. Hypodense lesion with sharp margins.

Aspergillus species cause a patchy infiltration followed by consolidation and abscess formation (Figure 13.7). Pneumonia occurs usually between 1 and 5 months after transplantation sometimes in the course of a disseminated disease (Figure 13.8). The mortality is extraordinarily high. Successful treatment depends on three factors: early diagnosis; aggressive antifungal therapy; and ability to reduce immunosuppression (Paterson and Singh 1999). Amphotericin B at doses ranging between 0.8 and 1.0 mg/kg per day is the drug of choice (Peacock et al 1993). A major disadvantage of amphotericin B is its nephrotoxicity. Recently, a lipid-based amphotericin B has been made commercially

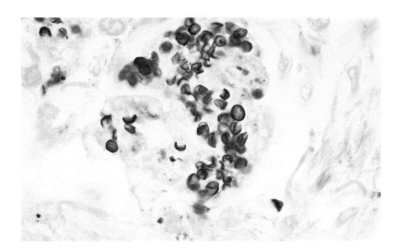

Figure 13.9. Disseminated histoplasmosis: alveolar macrophages packed with round to oval yeast-like cells of *Histoplasma capsulatum* var *capsulatum*, 2–4 μm in diameter. GMS ×100. (Courtesy of Dr MA Viviani, Ospedale Maggiore, Milan.)

available. With this lipid-soluble compound, higher doses of amphotericin B can be administered with a lower risk of nephrotoxicity (Ng and Denning 1995). Because of these characteristics, lipid-based amphotericin is currently regarded as the first line of therapy for invasive aspergillosis in transplant patients (Zak and Kusne 1998). Itraconazole at a dose of 200 mg three times per day for 3 days, followed by a maintenance dose of 200–400 mg per day, may be used in patients who do not tolerate amphotericin B. New antifungal agents such as voriconazole and the echinocandins are currently under investigation.

Histoplasmosis is relatively frequent in endemic areas (Americas, Africa). It usually presents with fever, malaise, myalgias, nonproductive cough, arthralgias and erythematosus skin lesions. Chest radiograph shows hilar adenopathy and small, irregular and disseminated infiltrates that may eventually accumulate calcium. Chronic pneumonia usually manifests as an interstitial pneumonitis, but in 20% of the cases, can produce cavitation. Recovery of *H. capsulatum* in the lung biopsy (Figure 13.9) is diagnostic. An antibody titer higher than 1:32 or a four-fold increase over the basal can also be regarded as diagnostic. Amphotericin B is the drug of choice for cases of acute pneumonitis. Itraconazole (400 mg per day) or ketoconazole (400 mg per day) for at least 6 months can cure some 65–80% of cases (Wheat 1994).

Cryptococcal pneumonia presents with cough, chest pain, mucopurulent expectoration, hemoptysis and dyspnea. Fever may be absent. Chest radiograph may show a single nodule or focal or lobar infiltrates (Perfect 1989). The treatment is amphotericin B, occasionally associated with flucytosine, 25–37.5 mg every 6 hours. The role of azoles with or without flucytosine in cryptococcal pneumonia is still under discussion.

Coccidioid pneumonia presents with nonspecific symptoms such as fever, malaise, dry cough, headache and dyspnea. Eosinophilia and erythematosus skin lesions may be found in a few patients. Radiologic findings show segmental pneumonitis, mild infiltrates, hilar adenopathy and pleural effusion. Cavitation and solitary nodules (coccidioidoma) may develop in oligosymptomatic patients. Itraconazole (400 mg per day) is particularly effective in coccidioidomycoses. Amphotericin B may be used in the few nonresponders (Galgiani 1993).

URINARY TRACT INFECTIONS

Urinary tract infection is the most common bacterial infection following renal transplantation, although the advent of effective prophylaxis with low-dose trimethoprim–sulfamethoxazole has reduced the incidence (Tolkoff-Rubin et al 1982; Cuvelier et al 1985).

Infections occurring in the first 4–6 months after transplantation are commonly associated with transplant pyelonephritis, bacteremia and frequent relapse after standard antibiotic therapy for 10–14 days, even in the absence of urologic abnormalities. Asymptomatic bacteriuria requires an antibacterial treatment for at least 10 days, then a new urine culture should be controlled. Acute pyelonephritis and/or positive bacteremia require antibiotic treatment for 4–6 weeks. As most cases of urosepsis are caused by Gram-negative bacteria, the initial treatment may be based on a cephalosporin, third- or fourth-generation imipenem, meropenem, aztreonam or in the most severe cases, aminoglycosides. Candidal infections usually respond to fluconazole and do not require amphotericin B administration.

In the late period, urinary tract infections are usually asymptomatic or oligosymptomatic and respond easily to antibacterial treatment. If a stone or obstruction is present pyelonephritis and bacteremia may develop.

CENTRAL NERVOUS SYSTEM INFECTIONS

Infections of the central nervous system (CNS) in renal transplant recipients typically present between 1 and 12 months following transplantation. The presentation of CNS infection in transplant patients may be different from that in normal patients. The onset may be subacute and systemic signs may be lacking. The most reliable symptoms that may demonstrate the presence of a CNS infection are headache and unexplained fever. Patients with such an array of symptoms, should receive computed tomography of the head and a lumbar puncture (Hooper et al 1982).

Listeria monocytogenes, C. neoformans and *A. fumigatus* account for most cases of CNS infections in transplant patients (Table 13.10). According to Fishman and Rubin (1998), CNS infection has four distinct patterns. (1) Acute meningitis is usually caused

Syndrome	Most frequent etiological agents	Clinical characteristics
Acute meningitis	*L. monocytogenes*	Signs of meningeal infection may be nonspecific
Chronic meningitis	*C. neoformans*	Occurs late. Presentation nonspecific. Concomitant lung or skin infection in some cases
Focal brain abscess	*A. fumigatus*	Seizures. Focal neurologic abnormalities. *Aspergillus* not found free in cerebrospinal fluid. Concomitant lung, skin, kidney involvement in many cases
Multifocal leukoencephalopathy	Papovavirus JC	Progressive dementia

Table 13.10. Main neurologic syndromes in renal transplant with CNS infection

by *L. monocytogenes*. It must be pointed out that in *Listeria* meningitis fever, altered sensorium and headache are the most common symptoms but some 40% of patients have no meningeal signs on admission. In cerebrospinal fluid, a high leukocyte count and a high protein concentration may be lacking. One-third of patients have focal neurologic findings and a quarter develop seizures. The prognosis is more severe in these patients. Ampicillin for 14–21 days with an aminoglycoside for 7–10 days remains the treatment of choice (Mylonakis et al 1998). (2) Subacute or chronic meningitis is characterized by fever and headache over several days or weeks. It may be associated with an altered state of consciousness. The disease is usually caused by *C. neoformans* and tends to be seen relatively late in the transplantation course. Other etiological microorganisms include *L. monocytogenes*, *H. capsulatum*, *N. asteroides*, *S. stercoralis* or *M. tuberculosis*. (3) Focal brain infections may present with seizures or focal neurologic abnormalities: the most frequent cause is a metastatic *Aspergillus* infection. *Listeria monocytogenes*, *T. gondii* or *N. asteroides* (Figure 13.10) are other possible causes of this syndrome. (4) Progressive dementia, with or without focal abnormalities, may be caused by papovavirus (namely JC virus), or more rarely herpes simplex virus, CMV or EBV, which lead to progressive multifocal leukoencephalopathy.

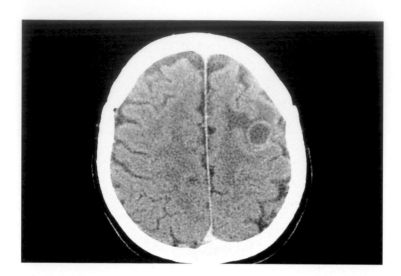

Figure 13.10. Cerebral *Nocardia* infection. Hypodense lesion surrounded by halo in the left parietal area of the brain.

WOUND INFECTIONS

In the past, wound infections were quite frequent but they are now rare in most centers. The reduced incidence may be attributed to improved surgical techniques and to the use of intraoperative antibiotics (Novick 1981; Judson 1984). Important predisposing factors are wound hematomas, urine leaks and lymphocele. The treatment should consist of surgical drainage. Antibiotic therapy is advisable, but deep wound infections are often polymicrobial in origin and difficult to treat.

REFERENCES

Anderson J, Ernberg I (1988) Management of Epstein–Barr virus infections. *Am J Med* **85**:107–109.

Balfour HH Jr (1990) Antiviral drugs. *N Engl J Med* **340**:1255–1268.

Bartlett JG, Breiman RF, Mandell LA et al (1998) Community-acquired pneumonia in adults: guidelines for management. *Clin Infect Dis* **26**:811–838.

Beutner KR, Friedman DJ, Forszpamiak C et al (1995) Valaciclovir compared with acyclovir for improved therapy for herpes zoster in immunocompetent adults. *Antimicrob Agents Chemother* **39**:1546–1553.

Binet I, Nickeleit V, Hirsch HH (1999) Polyomavirus disease under immunosuppressive drugs. *Transplantation* **67**:918–922.

Bone RC, Balk RA, Cerra FB et al (1992) Definition for sepsis and organ failures and guidelines for the use of innovative therapies in sepsis. *Chest* **101**:1644–1655.

Cathomas G, Tamm M, McGandy CE et al (1997) Transplantation-associated malignancies: restriction of human herpesvirus 8 to Kaposi's sarcoma. *Transplantation* 64:175–178.

Centers for Disease Control (1995) USPHS/IDSA guidelines for the prevention of opportunistic infections in persons infected with human immunodeficiency virus. A summary. *Morb Moral Wkly Rep* 44(RR-8):1–34.

Couchoud C, Cucherat M, Haugh M, Pouteil-Noble C (1988) Cytomegalovirus prophylaxis with antiviral agents in solid organ transplantation. *Transplantation* 65:641–647.

Coward RA, Raftery AT, Brown CB (1985) Cyclosporin and antituberculous therapy. *Lancet* ii:1342–1343.

Crumpacker CS (1992) Mechanism of action of foscarnet against viral polymerase. *Am J Med* 92(Suppl 2A):3S-7S.

Cuvelier R, Pirson Y, Alexandre G (1985) Late urinary tract infection after renal transplantation. *Nephron* 40:76–78.

Darenkov IA, Marcarelli MA, Basadonna GP et al (1997) Reduced incidence of Epstein–Barr virus-associated post-transplant lymphoproliferative disorder using preemptive antiviral therapy. *Transplantation* 64:848–852.

Deray G, Martinez F, Katalama C et al (1989) Foscarnet nephrotoxicity: mechanism, incidence and prevention. *Am J Nephrol* 9:316–321.

Dunn DL, Mayoral JL, Gillingham KJ, Loeffler CM (1991) Treatment of invasive CMV disease in solid organ transplant patients with ganciclovir. *Transplantation* 51:98–102.

Erice A, Holm MA, Gill P et al (1992) Cytomegalovirus (CMV) antigenemia assay is more sensitive than shell vial culture for rapid detection of CMV in polymorphonuclear blood leukocytes. *J Clin Microbiol* 30:2822–2825.

Faulds D, Heel RC (1990) Ganciclovir: a review of its antiviral activity, pharmacokinetic properties and therapeutic efficacy in cytomegalovirus infections. *Drugs* 39:597–606.

Fietze E, Prosch S, Reinke P et al (1994) Cytomegalovirus infection in transplant recipients: the role of tumor necrosis factor. *Transplantation* 58:675–680.

Fishman JA (1995) *Pneumocystis carinii* and parasitic infections in transplantation. *Infect Dis Clin N Am* 9:1005–1044.

Fishman JA (1999) Infection in the organ transplant recipient. *Graft* 2(Suppl II):S96–S100.

Fishman JA, Rubin RH (1998) Infection in organ-transplant recipients. *N Engl J Med* 338:1741–1751.

Flechner SM, Avery RK, Fisher R et al (1998) A randomized prospective trial of oral acyclovir versus oral ganciclovir for cytomegalovirus prophylaxis in high-risk kidney transplant recipients. *Transplantation* 66:1682–1688.

Galgiani JN (1989) Coccidioidomycosis: clinical update. *Rev Infect Dis* 11:897–912.

Gerna G, Zavattoni M, Baldanti F et al (1998) Human cytomegalovirus (HCMV) leukoanaemia correlates more closely with clinical symptoms than antigenemia and viremia in heart and heart–lung transplant recipients with primary HCMV infection. *Transplantation* 65:1378–1385.

Gombert ME, Josephson A, Goldstein EJC et al (1984) Cavitary Legionnaires' pneumonia: nosocomial infection in renal transplant recipients. *Am J Surg* 147:402–405.

Grant DM, Mauskopf JA, Bell L, Austin R (1997) Comparison of valacyclovir and acyclovir for the treatment of herpes zoster in immunocompetent patients over 50 years of age: a cost–consequence model. *Pharmacotherapy* 17:333–341.

Green M, Reyes J, Rowe D (1998) New strategies in the prevention and management of Epstein–Barr virus infection and posttransplant lymphoproliferative disease following solid organ transplantation. *Curr Opin Organ Transplant* 3:143–147.

Grossi P, Minoli L, Percivalle E et al (1995) Clinical and virological monitoring of human cytomegalovirus infection in 294 heart transplant recipients. *Transplantation* 59:847–852.

Hadley S, Karchmer AW (1995) Fungal infections in solid organ transplant recipients. *Infect Dis Clin N Am* 9:1045–1074.

Hanto DW (1992) Polyclonal and monoclonal posttransplant lymphoproliferative disease (LPD). *Clin Transplant* 6:227–234.

Hardy AM, Wajszczuk CP, Suffredini AF et al (1984) *Pneumocystis carinii* pneumonia in renal-transplant recipients treated with cyclosporine and steroids. *J Infect Dis* 149:143–148.

Hayden FG, Douglas RG (1990) Antiviral agents. In: Mandell GL, Douglas RG, Bennett JE (eds). *Principles and Practice of Infectious Disease*, 3rd edn. New York: Churchill Livingstone, pp. 370–393.

Hibberd PL, Rubin RH (1992) Antiviral therapy. An anti-malignant strategy for transplant recipients? *Clin Transplant* 6:240–245.

Hooper DC, Pruitt AA, Rubin RB (1982) Central nervous system infections in the chronically immunosuppressed. *Medicine (Baltimore)* 61:166–188.

Jassal SV, Roscoe JM, Zaltzman JS et al (1998) Clinical practice guidelines: prevention of cytomegalovirus disease after renal transplantation. *J Am Soc Nephrol* 9:1697–1708.

Jiwa NM, Van Gemert GW, Raap AK et al (1989) Rapid detection of human cytomegalovirus DNA in peripheral blood leukocytes of viremic transplant recipients by the polymerase chain reaction. *Transplantation* 48:72–76.

Judson RT (1984) Wound infection following renal transplantation. *Aust N Z J Surg* 54:223–224.

Kahan BD, Pescovitz M, Julian B et al (1996) Multi-center phase II trial of Sirolimus (SRL) in renal transplantation: six-month result. *XVI International Congress Transplantation Society*, Barcelona, August 25–30 1996 Book of Abstracts, Barcelona: AOPC, p. 75.

Kashyap R, Shapiro R, Jordan M, Randhawa PS (1999) The clinical significance of cytomegaloviral inclusions in the allograft kidney. *Transplantation* 67:98–103.

Keating MR (1992) Antiviral agents. *Mayo Clin Proc* 67:160–168.

Langhoff E, Madsen S (1983) Rapid metabolism of cyclosporin and prednisolone in a kidney transplant patient receiving tuberculostatic treatment. *Lancet* ii:1031 (letter).

Lowance D, Neumayer HH, Legendre CM et al (1999) Valacyclovir for the prevention of cytomegalovirus disease after renal transplantation. *N Engl J Med* 340:1462–1470.

Mendez J, Espy M, Smith Th et al (1988) Clinical significance of viral load in the diagnosis of cytomegalovirus disease after liver transplantation. *Transplantation* 65:1477–1481.

Morris DJ, Fox AJ, Klapper PE (1990) Diagnosis of cytomegalovirus infection in cyclosporin-treated renal allograft recipients. *J Med Virol* 32:124–131.

Murray BM, Amsterdam D, Gray V et al (1997) Monitoring and diagnosis of cytomegalovirus infection in renal transplantation. *J Am Soc Nephrol* 8:1448–1457.

Mylonakis E, Hohmann EL, Calderwood SB (1988) Central nervous system infection with *Listeria monocytogenes*: 33 years experience at a general hospital and review of 776 episodes from the literature. *Medicine (Baltimore)* 77:313–336.

Ng TTC, Denning DW (1995) Liposomal amphotericin B (AmBisome) therapy in invasive fungal infections: Evaluation of United Kingdom compassionate use data. *Arch Intern Med* 155:1093–1098.

Novick AC (1981) The value of intraoperative antibiotics in preventing renal transplant wound infections. *J Urol* 125:151–152.

Patel R, Snydman DR, Rubin RH et al (1996) Cytomegalovirus prophylaxis in solid organ transplant recipients. *Transplantation* 61:1279.

Paterson DL, Singh N (1999) Invasive aspergillosis in transplant recipients. *Medicine* 78:123–138.

Peacock JE Jr, Herrington DA, Cruz JM (1993) Amphotericin B: past, present and future. *Infect Dis Clin Pract* 2:81–86.

Perfect JR (1989) Cryptococcosis. *Infect Dis Clin N Am* **51**:277–289.

Peterson PK, Anderson RC (1986) Infection in renal transplant recipients. *Am J Med* **81**(Suppl 1A):2–10.

Peterson PK, Ferguson R, Fryd DS et al (1982) Infectious diseases in hospitalized renal transplant recipients: a prospective study of a complex and evolving problem. *Medicine (Baltimore)* **61**:360–372.

Preiksaitis JK (1992) Lymphoproliferative disorders in renal transplant recipients: urologic aspects. *Clin Transplant* **6**:235–239.

Ptachinski RJ, Carpenter BJ, Burckart GJ et al (1985) Effect of erythromycin on cyclosporine levels. *N Engl J Med* **313**:1416–1417.

Ratnamohan VH, Chapman J, Howse H et al (1998) Cytomegalovirus and human herpesvirus 6 both cause viral disease after renal transplantation. *Transplantation* **66**:877–882.

Regamey N, Tamm M, Wernli M et al (1998) Transmission of human herpesvirus 8 from renal transplant donors to recipients. *N Engl J Med* **339**:1358–1363.

Reinke P, Fietze E, Ode-Hakim S et al (1994) Late acute renal allograft rejection and symptomless cytomegalovirus infection. *Lancet* **i**:1737–1738.

Rubin RH (1990) Impact of cytomegalovirus infection on organ transplant recipients. *Rev Infect Dis* **12**(Suppl 7):S754–S766.

Rubin RH (1993) Infectious disease complications of renal transplantation. *Kidney Int* **44**:221–236.

Rubin RH (1994) Infections in the organ transplant recipient. In: Rubin RH, Young LS (eds). *Clinical Approach to Infection in the Compromised Host*, 3rd edn. New York: Plenum Publishing, pp. 629–705.

Rubin RH, Tolkoff-Rubin NE (1993) Antimicrobial strategies in the care of organ transplant recipients. *Antimicrob Agents Chemother* **37**:619–624.

Rubin RH, Fishman JA (1998) A consideration of potential donors with active infection is this a way to expand the donor pool? *Transplant Int* **11**:333–335.

Rubin RH, Wolfson JS, Cosimi AB, Tolkoff-Rubin NE (1981) Infection in the renal transplant recipient. *Am J Med* **70**:405–411.

Sattler FR, Feinberg J (1992) New developments in the treatment of *Pneumocystis carinii* pneumonia. *Chest* **101**:451–458.

Simmons RL, Migliori RJ (1988) Infection prophylaxis after successful organ transplantation. *Transplant Proc* **20**:7–11.

Simpson GL, Stinson EB, Egger MJ, Remington JS (1981) Nocardial infections in the immunocompromised host: a detailed study in a defined population. *Rev Infect Dis* **3**:492–507.

Singh N, Carrigan DR (1996) Human herpesvirus-6 in transplantation: an emerging pathogen. *Ann Intern Med* **124**:1065–1071.

Tanabe K, Tokumoto T, Ishikawa N et al (1997) Comparative study of cytomegalovirus (CMV) antigenemia assay, polymerase chain reaction, serology, and shell vial assay in the early diagnosis and monitoring of CMV infection after renal transplantation. *Transplantation* **64**:1721–1725.

The TH, Van der Ploege M, Van den Berg AP et al (1992) Direct detection of cytomegalovirus in peripheral blood leukocytes. A review of the antigenemia assay and polymerase chain reaction. *Transplantation* **54**:193–198.

Tobin JO'H, Beare J, Dunnill MS et al (1980) Legionnaires' disease in a transplant unit: isolation of the causative agent from shower baths. *Lancet* **i**:118–121.

Tolkoff-Rubin NE, Cosimi AB, Russell PS, Rubin RH (1982) A controlled study of trimethoprim–sulfamethoxazole prophylaxis of urinary tract infection in renal transplant recipients. *Rev Infect Dis* **4**:614–620.

Tollemar J (1999) Prophylaxis against fungal infections in transplant recipients: possible approaches. *Bio Drugs* **11**:309–318.

Van der Berg APM, Van der Bij W, Van Son WJ et al (1989) Cytomegalovirus antigenemia as a useful marker of symptomatic cytomegalovirus infection after renal transplantation: a report of 130 consecutive patients. *Transplantation* **48**:991–995.

Van der Bij W, Torensma R, Van Son WJ et al (1988) Rapid immunodiagnosis of acute cytomegalovirus infection by monoclonal antibody staining of blood leukocytes. *J Med Virol* **25**:179–188.

Wheat J (1994) Histoplasmosis: recognition and treatment. *Clin Infect Dis* **19**(Suppl 1):S19–S26.

Weiland D, Ferguson RM, Peterson PK et al (1983) Aspergillosis in 25 renal transplant patients. *Ann Surg* **198**:622–629.

Wheeler AP, Bernard GR (1999) Treating patients with severe sepsis. *N Engl J Med* **340**:207–214.

Whitley RJ, Gnann JW Jr (1992) Acyclovir: a decade later. *N Engl J Med* **327**:382–387.

Wittes JT, Kelly A, Plante KM (1996). Meta-analysis of CMVIG studies for the prevention and treatment of CMV infection in transplant patients. *Transplant Proc* **28**(Suppl 2):17–24.

Zak MB, Kusne S (1998) Should liposomal amphotericin B products be first line therapy for invasive aspergillosis in solid organ transplant recipients? *Curr Opin Organ Transplant* **3**:127–129.

Zanetta G, Maurice-Estepa L, Mousson C et al (1999) Foscarnet-induced crystalline glomerulonephritis with nephrotic syndrome and acute renal failure after kidney transplantation. *Transplantation* **67**:1376–1378.

14 CARDIOVASCULAR DISEASE AND ITS CAUSES

*In collaboration with A Elli**

The term cardiovascular disease includes several disorders, mostly of atherogenic nature, which may affect heart, brain, and/or lower limbs (Table 14.1). Cardiovascular complications now represent the leading cause of mortality in renal transplant recipients. In Europe, cardiovascular disease accounts for 36% of the total mortality in transplant patients, while infections account for 22% of deaths (Raine et al 1992). In the US the annual death rate from cardiovascular disease is 0.54% in transplant patients, approximately twice (0.28%) that observed in the general population (Foley et al 1998). Moreover, it has been estimated that cardiovascular disease develops approximately 20 years earlier in renal transplant recipients than in the general population (Aakhus et al 1999). Among the different cardiovascular complications, ischemic heart disease is by far the most frequent cause of mortality, accounting for more than half of deaths (Lindholm et al 1995).

Cardiac diseases
    Ischemic heart disease
    Congestive heart failure
    Left ventricular hypertrophy

Cerebrovascular diseases
    Thrombosis
    Hemorrhage

Peripheral vascular diseases
    Obliterative arterial disease of the limbs

Table 14.1. The most frequent cardiovascular diseases in renal transplant recipients

*Division of Nephrology and Dialysis, Ospedale Maggiore, Milan

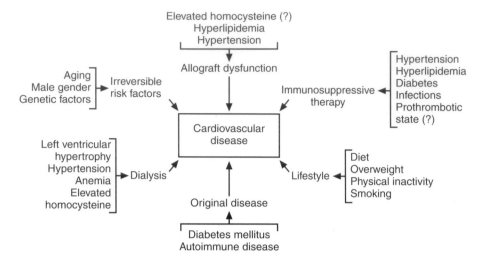

Figure 14.1. Risk factors for cardiovascular disease in transplant patients.

A number of factors may expose the transplant recipients to an increased risk of cardiovascular complications (Figure 14.1). Besides the risk factors that may also affect the general population, the renal transplant patient is exposed to the atherogenic risk related to the previous dialysis and to the use of immunosuppressive drugs (Raine 1994). Recent epidemiologic data suggest that a number of new molecules may also be associated with an increased risk of cardiovascular complications. They include homocysteine, cell adhesion molecules, infection, inflammation, abnormal coagulation and fibrinolysis, which may all be altered in renal transplantation (Frishman 1998).

DIABETES MELLITUS

Cardiovascular disease represents a major cause of death in diabetic patients, with the risk being higher in women than in men (Barrett-Connor 1997). Improvement in diagnosis, prevention and treatment has considerably improved the life expectancy for renal transplant patients with diabetes in the last few years. Nevertheless, the risk of cardiovascular death remains higher for diabetic than nondiabetic transplant recipients (Aakhus et al 1999; Tyden et al 1999). Insulin resistance and the resultant compensatory hyperinsulinemia may increase the risk of cardiovascular diseases (Stern 1995; Howard 1996). Hyperinsulinemia may cause hypertrophy of blood vessel walls (Mediratta et al 1995) and may favor the occurrence of other atherogenic risk factors, such as hypertriglyceridemia, increased plasma levels of low-density lipoprotein (LDL), decreased plasma levels of high-density lipoprotein (HDL) and arterial hypertension (Reaven 1995).

Cardiac infarct is the leading cause of death in diabetics. In this regard, it must be remembered that silent myocardial infarct is relatively frequent in diabetic transplant patients (Carlström et al 1999). This complication should be suspected whenever symptoms of left ventricular failure appear suddenly. Cardiomyopathy may also develop in diabetics with an apparently normal heart and with normal coronarography. Peripheral obliterative arteriopathy is also frequent. Apart from cardiovascular complications, diabetes may also expose transplant patients to retinopathy, neuropathy, foot ulcers and infections. Finally there is a deleterious impact of diabetes on graft survival. In spite of an increased morbidity and mortality in diabetics, some studies have reported that the graft survival rate was similar in diabetic and nondiabetic transplant patients followed for 5–6 years (Sumrani et al 1991; Vesco et al 1996). However, with longer follow-up the results were poorer. In a prospective study, the 12-year graft survival was significantly lower in diabetic (48%) than in nondiabetic patients (70%). The risk of graft loss was 3.7 times greater for diabetics, independent of age, sex and race (Miles et al 1998). Impaired graft function in diabetics was attributed to more severe hypertension, use of lower doses of immunosuppressive agents, and the development of diabetic renal disease.

After transplantation pre-existing diabetes may be aggravated or a de novo diabetes may develop. Posttransplant diabetes is mainly related to the use of corticosteroids and/or calcineurin inhibitors. Steroid-dependent diabetes is strongly related to the dose of corticosteroids (Hjelmesaeth et al 1997), the risk being higher in patients with familial predisposition, in African-American males, in patients with HLA A30 and Bw42 antigens, and in elderly subjects (Sumrani et al 1991). The direct effect of producing insulin resistance and the increase in body weight are probably the two main mechanisms by which corticosteroids may induce diabetes mellitus (Jindal 1994). Besides corticosteroids, cyclosporine (CsA) and tacrolimus may also favor the development of diabetes. The prevalence of posttransplant diabetes varied from 5 to 10% before the introduction of CsA (Markell et al 1994), while it ranges between 2.5 and 20% in the CsA-treated patients (Hjelmesaeth et al 1997). Cyclosporine may exert a diabetogenic effect through different mechanisms. In the rat, calmodulin can interfere with the insulin secretory capacity (Krausz et al 1980); moreover cyclosporine may directly inhibit the insulin production by β cells (Gillison et al 1991); finally CsA can reduce the catabolism of corticosteroids by competing with these agents for the common cytochrome P450 metabolic pathway (Ponticelli and Opelz 1995). Tacrolimus has the same diabetogenic effects. In addition, however, tacrolimus may also exert a direct toxicity on islet cells (Tamura et al 1995). The diabetogenic activity of tacrolimus is dose-dependent and may even be superior to that of CsA (Pirsch et al 1997). A multivariate analysis assessed the risk of cardiovascular complications in posttransplant diabetes. When compared to nondiabetic transplant recipients, diabetics had a relative risk of 2.2 for ischemic heart disease, 2.9 for cerebrovascular disease and 25.7 for peripheral vascular disease (Kasiske et al 1996).

Treatment

In patients with type II diabetes, hypocaloric/hypolipidic diet, physical activity and weight loss should be encouraged. If there is a moderate fasting hyperglycemia (140–230 mg/dl), an oral hypoglycemic agent should be prescribed. The most commonly used agent is sulfonylurea, an insulin secretagogue. One of the limits of this agent is represented by the possibility that in the long term the overstimulated pancreatic β cells may show a progressive reduction in insulin production. Other oral agents include biguanides, which inhibit gluconeogenesis and glucose absorption while stimulating glycolysis; the α-glucosidase inhibitors, which reduce gastrointestinal absorption of carbohydrates; and the thiazolidinediones, a new class of compounds that act by reducing insulin resistance. However, about 50% of patients require insulin treatment. The dose and the type of insulin should be decided on an individual basis as insulin requirements depend on the patient's diet, amount of exercise, and renal function. Tapering of corticosteroids also requires an adjustment of insulin dosage. In establishing the treatment one should recall that the target levels for glucose controls largely vary among diabetologists. Probably it is safer to obtain acceptable glucose levels rather than insist on 'ideal' lower glucose levels (Table 14.2). In nonexpert hands, the latter policy might expose the patient to hypoglycemia, which may be dangerous and, if frequent, portends a serious and even fatal outcome. For the same reason, attention should be paid to the Somogyi effect and the dawn phenomenon.

A further approach may consist of modifying the immunosuppressive treatment. In view of the diabetogenic role of corticosteroids, a steroid-free immunosuppression may be considered for patients with pre-existing diabetes before transplantation. Many patients may be treated with cyclosporine alone (Ponticelli et al 1997) or with a combination of a calcineurin inhibitor and mycophenolate mofetil without corticosteroids (Birkeland 1998). For patients who develop diabetes after transplantation, reduction or even complete withdrawal of corticosteroids may be tried in difficult cases. The withdrawal of corticosteroids may be followed by an easier control of diabetes as well as by improvement of hyperlipidemia and hypertension. However the potential benefits of a steroid-free immunosuppression should be weighed against the risk of precipitating

	mg/dl	mmol/l
Fasting	70–120	3.9–6.66
Preprandial	70–120	3.9–6.66
Postprandial (1–2 h)	<200	<11.1
Early morning (3–4 am)	>65	>3.6

Table 14.2. Acceptable blood glucose concentration in a diabetic patient

rejection (Hricik et al 1993). Some studies reported that after stopping corticosteroids there was an increased incidence of acute rejection that could be handled easily without consequences to the allograft function (Ponticelli and Opelz 1995), but a multicenter Canadian trial reported that patients who stopped corticosteroids were exposed to an increased risk of chronic rejection and graft failure in the long term (Sinclair 1992). Other approaches may consist of reducing the doses of CsA or tacrolimus. The introduction of mycophenolate mofetil might allow reduction of the dosage of diabetogenic drugs in difficult diabetics with stable allograft function, without an increased risk of late graft dysfunction.

ARTERIAL HYPERTENSION

Arterial hypertension is frequent in renal transplant recipients. In the precyclosporine era hypertension was found in approximately 50–70% of kidney transplant patients (Kasiske 1987; Ponticelli and Montagnino 1987). The introduction of calcineurin-inhibitor drugs has increased the prevalence of hypertension to 70–80% of adults with renal transplant (Ponticelli et al 1993; Zeier et al 1998). No significant difference in hypertension was found between cyclosporine- and tacrolimus-treated patients in controlled trials (Mayer et al 1997; Pirsch et al 1997).

Several factors may contribute to the development of posttransplant hypertension (Table 14.3). Allograft artery stenosis accounts only for a minority of cases, 2–10% in the different series (Van Ypersele de Strihou and Pochet 1992). There are three main locations for graft artery stenosis: (1) at the site of anastomosis, probably as a consequence of the surgical technique; (2) at the distal site of anastomosis, the cause of which is still ill defined; and (3) at the distal arterial branches, where multiple stenoses can be seen, probably as an expression of a chronic rejection (Roberts et al 1989). The diagnosis of graft artery stenosis may be suspected in the presence of severe hypertension, if there is a bruit at the auscultation and/or in the case of a rapid deterioration of renal function after administration of angiotensin-converting enzyme (ACE) inhibitors.

Cause	Treatment
Renal artery stenosis	Revascularization
Native kidneys	Nephrectomy
Calcineurin inhibitors	Reduce the doses
Corticosteroids	Reduce the doses
Graft dysfunction	Antihypertensive agents

Table 14.3. Potential causes and treatments of posttransplant hypertension

Echo Doppler of the allograft artery and renography with captopril may be useful (Rengel et al 1998) but the final diagnosis should be done with angiography. A rare cause of de novo hypertension is represented by a postbiopsy arteriovenous fistula. The diversion of blood flow from normal renal structures, caused by the abnormal communication between artery and vein, may result in local ischemia and renin-mediated hypertension.

Apart from these rare cases, posttransplant hypertension may be caused by several mechanisms. Inappropriate renin output from native kidneys, the use of calcineurin inhibitors and corticosteroids, allograft dysfunction and transplantation of a predisposed kidney are the most important etiopathogenetic factors. The role of native kidneys has been outlined by multivariate analyses (Kasiske 1987; Ponticelli et al 1993) that identified the presence of the native kidneys and pretransplant hypertension as independent variables associated with posttransplant hypertension. It is possible to speculate that the native kidneys may still produce renin which, although normal in absolute, might be inappropriately elevated in the presence of an increased extracellular volume. Cyclosporine may cause renal vasoconstriction through several mechanisms (Table 14.4). As a consequence, there is a reduction of glomerular filtration rate and of renal blood flow. In turn, these functional abnormalities lead to a retention of salt and water, to an increase in extracellular fluids and to an increased cardiac output (Figure 14.2). Once again the normal production of renin by the allograft and by the native kidneys could be inappropriately elevated in a setting characterized by extracellular fluid expansion (Curtis 1990; Luke 1991). Corticosteroids may further aggravate hypertension through hemodynamic modifications, hormonal changes and further retention of water and salt. Logistic regression analyses showed that corticosteroids are independently associated with posttransplant hypertension (Ponticelli et al 1993; Ratcliffe et al 1996), the effect largely depends on the dosage. In fact, a maintenance dose of prednisone of less than 10 mg/day appears to have little if any role in contributing to posttransplant hypertension (First et al 1994; Ratcliffe et al 1996). There is general agreement that allograft dysfunction represents a major cause of hypertension (Ponticelli et al 1993; Ratcliffe et

Increased production of endothelin-1

Activation of renin–angiotensin system

Reduced production of nitric oxide

Increased production of TGF-β_1

Prostaglandin imbalance

Increased sympathetic activity

Table 14.4. Potential mechanisms responsible for renal vasoconstriction caused by cyclosporine

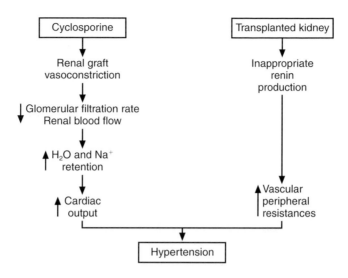

Figure 14.2. Pathogenesis of cyclosporine-induced hypertension.

al 1996, Curtis 1997). It has also been shown that patients who received the kidney from a subject of a hypertensive family have a higher probability of developing arterial hypertension after transplantation than patients who received a kidney from a member of a normotensive family (Guidi et al 1996).

Arterial hypertension is a strong risk factor for cardiovascular disease, in particular coronary heart disease and stroke. Angiotensin II, which is often elevated in patients with hypertension, can contribute to atherogenesis by stimulating the growth of smooth muscle cells and lipoxygenase activity which, in turn, can increase inflammation and oxidation of LDL. Hypertension also has proinflammatory actions on endothelium with increased formation of hydrogen peroxide and free radicals in plasma (Ross et al 1999). In a retrospective analysis we found more cardiac infarcts in hypertensive than in normotensive transplanted patients (Ponticelli et al 1993). In a study of Kasiske et al (1996), when all cardiovascular events were considered together, hypertension was found to be significantly associated with posttransplant vascular disease. A major consequence of hypertension is left ventricular hypertrophy, which is an important risk factor for a variety of cardiovascular sequelae, such as angina pectoris, myocardial infarction, stroke, heart failure, arrhythmias and sudden death (Chambers 1995). The mechanisms by which left ventricular hypertrophy is associated with the increased risk of cardiovascular complications are not fully understood (Mosterd et al 1999), but it must be pointed out that an adequate treatment with antihypertensive drugs may obtain regression of left ventricular hypertrophy (Schmieder et al 1996) and reduce the risk of cardiovascular disease (Verdecchia et al 1998). Hypertension can also be harmful for the long-term kidney graft outcome. A retrospective study on thousands of renal transplant recipients showed that increased levels of systolic and diastolic blood pressure after transplantation were significantly associated with an increased risk of graft failure. Hypertension was an independent risk factor for graft failure, even when serum creatinine concentrations were normal and when patients had never been treated for rejection crisis (Opelz et al 1998).

Treatment

In any transplant patient, nonpharmacologic measures to control blood pressure and to minimize premature cardiovascular morbidity and mortality should be recommended. These measures include weight control, a diet with a moderate sodium restriction and a low fat intake, physical exercise and cessation of smoking.

As both calcineurin inhibitors and corticosteroids cause a salt- and water-dependent hypertension, salt restriction appears to be a rational therapeutic maneuver. However, too severe a salt restriction, especially if coupled with diuretic therapy, may cause a drop in glomerular filtration rate because of the impaired capacity of hemodynamic adaptation of the transplanted kidney (Schweitzer et al 1991). Moreover diuretics may synergize with CsA in causing hypomagnesemia.

In patients with sustained blood pressure of more than 140/90 mmHg, antihypertensive agents should be started. Since increased renal vascular resistance is a prominent feature of posttransplant hypertension, drugs that lower systemic blood pressure and increase renal blood flow may have a specific indication. At least in theory, calcium antagonists could be the drugs of choice by protecting from calcineurin inhibitor nephrotoxicity (First et al 1994). In fact by modulating calcium flux, calcium antagonists may diminish the vascular smooth muscle reactivity to vasoconstrictive stimuli, so reversing the increase in renal vascular resistance induced by CsA. This effect is particularly evident at the preglomerular level, where CsA exerts vasoconstriction (English et al 1987). On the other hand, calcium antagonists can cause severe peripheral edema, and may concur with CsA in inducing gingival hyperplasia (Bencini et al 1984). When given at high doses, nifedipine might be associated with increased mortality, at least in patients with severe heart disease (Furberg et al 1995), while nondihydropyridinic calcium antagonists, such as amlodipine, verapamil, diltiazem, and nicardipine etc., can increase the blood levels of CsA (Pesavento et al 1996).

Angiotensin-converting enzyme inhibitors may be as effective as calcium antagonists in reducing blood pressure in renal transplant patients (Mourad et al 1993). They may worsen renal function in patients with transplant artery stenosis, and rarely also in patients without any evidence of transplant artery or arteriolar stenosis (Curtis et al 1993). Moreover, ACE inhibitors may cause hyperkalemia, may produce a dry cough and may induce anemia (Curtis et al 1997). On the other hand, ACE inhibitors do not affect CsA blood levels and do not cause edema. From a theoretical point of view ACE inhibitors might be helpful in preventing the progression of chronic allograft nephropathy. In fact, by interfering with the formation of angiotensin II (Egido 1996), these agents reduce the intraglomerular pressure, decrease the urinary protein excretion and inhibit the production of matrix protein and of transforming growth factor β_1 (TGFβ_1), an important mediator of interstitial fibrosis which may be involved in the development of chronic allograft nephropathy (Bennett et al 1996). On the other hand, TGFβ_1 also has a powerful immunosuppressive and anti-inflammatory activity. Its suppression might, therefore, expose the patient to an increased risk of chronic rejection. Only well-designed, prospective, randomized trials could show whether ACE inhibitors may preserve graft function by preventing fibrosis without increasing the risk of rejection or vice versa. Recently, the antagonists of angiotensin II receptors (AT1) have been made available. They are as effective as calcium antagonists, beta-blockers and ACE inhibitors in lowering blood pressure. These agents have comparable effects with ACE inhibitors on systemic and renal hemodynamic properties (Burnier and Brunner 1998). AT1 receptor antagonists are well tolerated. Unlike ACE inhibitors, they do not interfere with bradykinin production and can therefore be used in patients with dry cough caused by ACE inhibitors.

In many cases several drugs have to be used simultaneously to achieve good control of posttransplant hypertension. Besides diuretics, calcium antagonists and ACE inhibitors or AT1 receptor antagonists, β-blockers, centrally acting drugs and α-adrenergic receptor blocking drugs may be used either alone or in various combinations. In

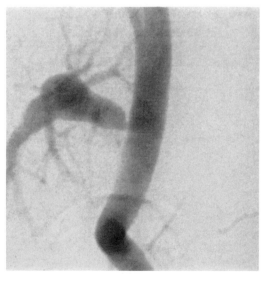

(a)

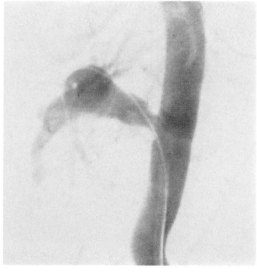

(b)

Figure 14.3. (a) Transplant artery stenosis at the beginning of the artery. (b) Correction of stenosis by PTA. (Courtesy of Dr A Nicolini, Ospedale Maggiore, Milan.)

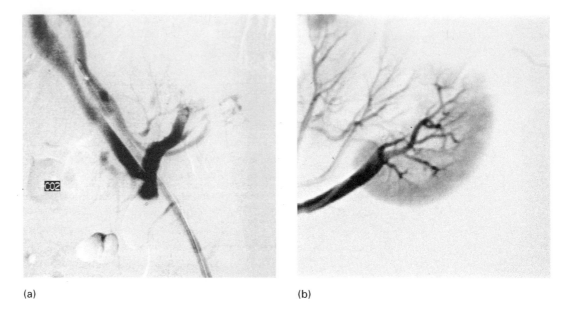

(a)   (b)

Figure 14.4.   (a) Postbiopsy arteriovenous fistula in a transplanted kidney (angiography with CO_2 technique). (b) Correction of fistula by embolization. (Courtesy of Dr A Nicolini, Ospedale Maggiore, Milan.)

the most severe cases, the powerful vasodilator minoxidil can be added to control refractory hypertension.

Bilateral nephrectomy may be considered in patients with a history of severe hypertension before transplantation. Whenever possible, reduction of cyclosporine, tacrolimus, or corticosteroids should be taken into account if other measures are ineffective.

In proven transplant artery stenosis, percutaneous transluminal angioplasty (PTA) or surgery are indicated if stenosis narrows the artery by more than 80%. In most cases PTA represents the first approach (Figure 14.3). Percutaneous transluminal angioplasty in combination with stenting using expandable metallic stents has been used successfully for recurrent stenosis (Newman-Sanders et al 1995). Because of the risks of graft loss associated with surgical intervention, surgery should be considered a second option in patients in whom PTA or stenting has failed. Embolization may repair an arteriovenous fistula with improvement of hypertension (Figure 14.4).

HYPERLIPIDEMIA

Hyperlipidemia is common after renal transplantation. It occurs as early as 3 months after transplantation and does not remit spontaneously (Markell et al 1994). In most cases hyperlipidemia persists in the late posttransplant period even 10 or more years after transplantation (Drueke et al 1991).

The posttransplant lipoprotein profile is characterized by an increase in total and LDL cholesterol, as well as in very low-density lipoproteins (VLDL) and triglycerides. Interestingly, HDL cholesterol levels are usually normal or even high, although the composition of HDL may be abnormal (Kobashigawa and Kasiske 1997). In addition LDL appears to be more susceptible to oxidation, while antioxidant levels are lower in renal transplant patients treated with CsA (Sutherland et al 1995). Lipoprotein(a) levels have been found to be normal in patients who were not receiving CsA (Webb et al 1993) and elevated in patients treated with CsA (Hilbrands et al 1993).

Several factors may favor the development of posttransplant hyperlipidemia. Because hyperlipidemia occurs early after transplantation it is likely that increased appetite, more liberal diet, and alcohol consumption can play some role in posttransplant hyperlipidemia. The roles of genetic factors, proteinuria, renal dysfunction, and diabetes mellitus are well recognized. The use of diuretics and β-blockers may also expose the patient to hyperlipidemia. Some immunosuppressive drugs such as corticosteroids, cyclosporine (Vathsala et al 1989) and rapamycin (Groth et al 1999) are also implicated in the development of hyperlipidemia, usually in a dose dependent fashion (Table 14.5). Corticosteroids may enhance the activity of acetyl-coenzyme A carboxylase and free fatty acid synthetase, increase hepatic synthesis of VLDL, downregulate LDL receptor activity of 3-hydroxy-3-methylglutaryl coenzyme A (HMG-CoA) reductase, and inhibit lipoprotein lipase (Kobashigawa and Kasiske 1997). The final result is an increased level of VLDL, total cholesterol and triglycerides and a decreased level of high-density lipoproteins. Cyclosporine may inhibit the enzyme 26-hydroxylase, so decreasing the synthesis of bile acids from cholesterol and the transport of cholesterol to the intestines. Cyclosporine binds to the LDL receptor, which results in increased serum levels of LDL-cholesterol. Cyclosporine also impairs the clearance of VLDL and LDL by decreasing lipoprotein lipase activity (Kobashigawa and Kasiske 1997). Of note, hypercholesterolemia is significantly less frequent in transplant patients given tacrolimus than in those treated with cyclosporine (Pirsch et al 1997; Satterthwaite et al 1998). Rapamycin can also increase serum cholesterol and triglyceride levels (Groth et al 1999). The mechanisms for hyperlipidemia caused by rapamycin are still unknown, although an interference with lipoprotein lipase may be speculated.

A large number of epidemiologic studies have documented the relation between elevated total cholesterol, triglycerides, LDL and the development of cardiovascular disease. Low levels of HDL are also associated with an increased cardiovascular risk (Ross et al 1999). The oxidative metabolism of LDL appears to be the final common pathway in the relation between hyperlipidemia and the development of atherosclerosis (Griendling and Alexander 1997). Moreover, oxidized LDL are involved in a number of other

Diabetes
Allograft dysfunction
Proteinuria
Hypoalbuminemia
Age
Obesity
Diet
Corticosteroids
Cyclosporine
Rapamycin
Diuretics
Beta-blockers

Table 14.5. Possible causes of posttransplant hyperlipidemia

atherogenic processes, including activation of the coagulation cascade (O'Keefe et al 1995). An atherogenic role for lipid disturbances has also been recognized in transplant patients (Abdulmassih et al 1992). Some studies reported an association between hyperlipidemia and chronic renal allograft rejection (Dimény et al 1993; Isoniemi et al 1994; Massy and Kasiske 1996), suggesting that lipoprotein abnormalities may influence the progression of chronic renal allograft nephropathy. However, the association between chronic renal allograft rejection and hyperlipidemia may be the consequence rather than the cause of renal failure. In fact, renal dysfunction, proteinuria and the additional immunosuppression often used in patients with chronic allograft nephropathy may explain the association with hyperlipidemia without implicating lipid abnormalities in the pathogenesis of chronic rejection.

Treatment

As hyperlipidemia occurs early in most renal transplant patients, the clinical assessment and treatment of hyperlipidemia should be initiated soon after transplantation. Potential strategies include physical exercise, dietary therapy, reduced doses of immunosuppressive agents and lipid lowering agents.

Transplant recipients with hypertriglyceridemia should be placed on a hypocaloric diet that restricts the intake of simple sugars and alcohol in addition to limiting fat intake to less than 30% of total daily calories. This diet may obtain weight loss and resolution or improvement of hypertriglyceridemia (Ponticelli et al 1978). Dietary modifica-

General measures
(1)   Physical exercise
(2)   Low calorie intake

Hypertriglyceridemia
(1)   Avoid alcohol and simple sugars. Limit fat intake
(2)   Use fibrates or fish oil
(3)   Reduce corticosteroids or cyclosporine

Hypercholesterolemia
(1)   Avoid saturated fats (milk, cheese, butter, chocolate, shellfish, fatty meat).
        Use polyunsaturated fats (corn oil, safflower oil)
(2)   Use statins or bile acid sequestrants
(3)   Reduce corticosteroids or cyclosporine

Table 14.6.   Main general approaches for treating posttransplant hyperlipidemia

tion is also the safest form of treatment for elevated LDL cholesterol. Patients should be placed on a hypocaloric diet low in cholesterol and in saturated fats but high in polyunsaturated fats (Table 14.6). A similar diet given for 10–12 weeks obtained a 10% reduction of plasma LDL cholesterol levels (Barbagallo et al 1999). Unfortunately, many hyperlipidemic renal transplant recipients show poor compliance to the diet in the long term (Moore et al 1990).

As the association of CsA and steroids may increase the risk of hyperlipidemia, avoiding or reducing the doses of corticosteroids can help in minimizing hyperlipidemia (Versluis et al 1987; Hricik et al 1992). A controlled study reported that renal transplant patients receiving cyclosporine alone have a lower risk of hyperlipidemia and of cardiovascular complications than patients given CsA and steroids (Ponticelli et al 1997). In a study comparing different treatments, therapy with CsA alone showed the lowest levels of plasma triglycerides, cholesterol and plasma cholesterol LDL levels when compared to regimens based on CsA plus steroids or azathioprine plus steroids. However, patients on CsA monotherapy also had the lowest levels of cholesterol HDL (Montagnino et al 1994). If steroid-free immunosuppression is considered unsafe in a particular patient, prednisone may be replaced by less hyperlipemic corticosteroids. Deflazacort, an oxazoline derivative of prednisolone, is a new glucocorticoid not yet available in the United States. This compound is at least as potent as the glucocorticoids commonly used but induces less hyperglycemia and hyperlipidemia (Elli et al 1993). Conversion from CsA to tacrolimus can also lower cholesterol, LDL and apolipoprotein B (McCune et al 1998).

	Treatment initiation level (mg/dl (mmol/l))	Goal level (mg/dl (mmol/l))	Concomitant risk factors
LDL cholesterol	≥190 (≥4.9)	≤160 (≤4.1)	Absent
LDL cholesterol	≥160 (≥4.1)	≤130 (≤3.4)	Two or more

Table 14.7. Initiation of treatment and goal levels according to NCEP guidelines. Risk factors are age (>45 years in men; >55 years in women); family history of premature coronary heart disease; smoking; hypertension; diabetes mellitus; HDL cholesterol <35 mg/dl (0.91 mmol/l)

According to the national Cholesterol Education Program, hypolipidemic drugs may be considered when LDL-cholesterol exceeds 190 mg/dl or even at lower levels if there are other risk factors (Table 14.7). There are three major cholesterol-lowering drug classes: the HMG-CoA reductase inhibitors (or statins), the bile acid sequestrants, and nicotinic acid. Probucol is suggested only for those patients who were either intolerant or refractory to the other cholesterol-lowering drugs. Fibric acid derivatives are indicated only for patients with very high triglyceride levels.

The statins (lovastatin, pravastatin, simvastatin, fluvastatin) are the most effective cholesterol-lowering agents (Table 14.8). These drugs may reduce LDL cholesterol concentrations by roughly 35–40% at optimal dosage. This reduction of LDL cholesterol is accompanied by an increase in HDL cholesterol concentration of about 10% and, frequently, by a slight decrease in triglyceride concentration (Arnadottir and Berg 1997). Statins are generally well tolerated, but potential interactions with immunosuppressive regimens should be considered when used in transplant recipients. The combination of lovastatin at relatively high doses with CsA was found to increase the risk of rhabdomyolysis, which in some cases was severe enough to cause acute renal failure (Tobert 1988). However, by adjusting the statin dosage, patients receiving CsA could be treated safely (Kupin et al 1992; Capone et al 1999). Lovastatin, simvastatin and pravastatin may cause myopathy. This side-effect is dose-dependent and is potentiated by CsA, which retards the biliary elimination of statins and prolongs their half-life (Arnadottir et al 1993). Avoiding inappropriately high concentrations of CsA, avoiding medications known to increase the risk of myopathy (gemfibrozil, nicotinic acid), and performing regular check-ups of creatinine kinase concentrations allows safe treatment of cyclosporine-treated renal transplant recipients with different statins (Arnadottir and Berg 1997). There is also interference between the statins and CsA metabolism, with the degree varying among the different statins. In fact in combination with CsA the area under the curve (AUC) of fluvastatin increases two-fold compared with 10-fold for simvastatin (Schrama et al 1998). Some authors reported a 10-fold increase of the AUC for pravastatin also (Schrama et al 1998); others, however, did not find any interference of

Drug	Suggested dose	Side-effects
HMG-CoA reductase inhibitors		
Fluvastatin	20–40 mg/day	Rhabdomyolysis
Lovastatin	10–20 mg/day	Myopathy
Pravastatin	10–20 mg/day	Increase of transaminases
Simvastatin	10–20 mg/day	Interference with cyclosporine metabolism
Bile acid resin		
Cholestiramine	4–6 g/day	Flatulence, constipation,
Colestipol	5–15 g/day (space dose by 2 h with interacting drugs)	hypersensitivity, interaction with fat-soluble drugs
Nicotinic acid	250–500 mg/day	Flushing, gastrointestinal disturbance, glucose intolerance, gout, liver damage, cyclosporine and steroids may exacerbate side-effects

Table 14.8. Cholesterol-lowering drugs

CsA with the AUC of pravastatin (Knopp 1999). Of much importance, in order to prevent any possible side-effect, the doses of statins should not exceed 10–20 mg/day for lovastatin and pravastatin, 10–20 mg/day for simvastatin and 20–40 mg/day for fluvastatin (Goldberg and Roth 1996; Kobashigawa and Kasiske 1997). Statins could also protect graft function by enhancing the immunosuppression, by inhibiting monocyte chemotaxis, and by decreasing natural killer cell cytotoxicity (Arnadottir and Berg 1997). In a randomized study, kidney transplant patients randomly allocated to pravastatin had a lower incidence of acute rejection (25 versus 64%) and needed less courses of OKT3 and methylprednisolone than patients not receiving pravastatin (Katznelson et al 1996). Since the rate of endogenous cholesterol synthesis is higher at night, the statins should be given at night. Lovastatin is better absorbed with food and should be taken with a meal. However, pravastatin should be taken on an empty stomach or at bedtime, as food decreases its absorption (Knopp 1999)

Cholestyramine and colestipol bind with bile acid, interrupt bile acid recirculation, and increase hepatic bile acid synthesis and LDL receptor activity (Grundy 1994). These agents are effective in lowering cholesterol when administered at adequate doses, but adequate doses are difficult to achieve due to frequent gastrointestinal side-effects. Although these agents may interfere with the absorption of lipid-soluble drugs, with a consequent decreased CsA concentration, such an effect was not found in a study on renal transplant patients (Jensen et al 1995). At any rate, drugs should be taken 2 hours before or 4–6 hours (minimum 2 hours) after the ingestion of cholestiramine or colestipol.

Nicotinic acid reduces LDL, increases HDL cholesterol levels, and reduces triglyceride levels (Grundy 1994). This drug may have many adverse effects which limit its clinical use. They include flushing, gastrointestinal disturbances, altered glucose tolerance, and increased incidence of gout in cyclosporine-treated patients.

Probucol slightly reduces both total and LDL cholesterol levels and does not produce a significant change in the ratio of LDL cholesterol to HDL cholesterol. Its use can be justified, however, because probucol interferes with the oxidative processes fighting the adverse effects of LDL on the arterial wall. There is an interaction with CsA causing fluctuation in blood CsA concentrations. Other side-effects are flatulence, loose stools, prolonged QT interval, and decreased HDL (Sundararajan et al 1991).

Clofibrate, bezafibrate, fenofibrate, ciprofibrate and gemfibrozil induce a reduction in hepatic VLDL synthesis and an increase in lipoprotein lipase activity, thereby causing a reduction in triglyceride concentrations and an increase in HDL cholesterol concentration. Plasma LDL cholesterol concentration falls as well, but not as markedly as with statin treatment. Thus, fibrates may be indicated in patients with hypertriglyceridemia, not in those with hypercholesterolemia. Fibrates may cause myopathy and rhabdomyolysis. These side-effects are dose-dependent and are more frequent in patients with renal insufficiency or in those given statins. Gemfibrozil has been reported to be a safe and effective lipid-lowering drug in renal transplant recipients (Chan et al 1994), but a number of patients may show a mild, reversible increase in plasma creatinine levels during treatment with fibrates. Still, it is not clear whether fibrates increase (Boissonnat et al 1994) or lower (Fehrman-Ekholm et al 1996) the plasma CsA levels. To be on the safe side, in transplant patients we prefer not to exceed a daily dose of 900 mg for gemfibrozil, 400 mg for bezafibrate or 200 mg for fenofibrate.

Fish oil may obtain a decrease in the serum triglyceride levels by reducing hepatic triglyceride production. Fish oil may also have beneficial effects on platelet aggregation, blood pressure and graft function (Homan Van der Heide et al 1993). It can be used for cases of isolated hypertriglyceridemia or as a complement to a statin in the cases of combined hyperlipidemia.

In summary, lipid-lowering measures are indicated in transplant patients with multiple risk factors for cardiovascular disease, particularly in those with pre-existent cardiovascular disease. Hyperlipidemia may be prevented by exercise and by reducing the doses of corticosteroids and cyclosporine whenever possible. Besides weight reduction and a low-fat diet, a low dose of HMG-CoA reductase inhibitor appears to be the best therapeutic choice for reducing LDL cholesterol levels. If a predominant hypertriglyceridemia is present, low calorie intake, low-fat diet and, in some cases, fish oil may help to reduce triglyceride levels. Gemfibrozil may also lower triglyceride levels but the dose should be reduced in patients with decreased renal function.

SMOKING

There is abundant evidence that in the general population smokers have an increased risk of cardiovascular disease compared with nonsmokers. In renal transplant patients a history of smoking is associated with a high prevalence of cardiovascular morbidity (Kasiske 1993). A history of smoking correlates with decreased patient survival after kidney transplantation: the magnitude of the negative impact of smoking is quantitatively similar to that of diabetes (Cosio et al 1999).

HYPERHOMOCYSTEINEMIA

Homocysteine is a sulfur-containing amino acid that results from the demethylation of methionine (Ueland and Refsum 1989). Homocysteine is toxic to endothelium, is prothrombotic, increases collagen production and decreases the availability of nitric oxide (Ross 1999).

After assays of serum homocysteine had been developed (Refsum et al 1985), several studies showed that hyperhomocysteinemia is an independent risk factor for coronary, cerebral and peripheral vascular diseases (Verhoef and Stampfer 1995). Patients with chronic renal failure, including dialysis patients, have total serum homocysteine levels two- to four-fold above normal (Massy et al 1994). Hyperhomocysteinemia is also common in renal transplant recipients (Bostom et al 1997; Arnadottir et al 1998; Dimény et al 1998) and might contribute to their increased risk for cardiovascular disease.

The mechanisms of hyperhomocysteinemia in renal transplant recipients have not been completely elucidated. Neither age nor gender influence serum homocysteine levels in renal transplant recipients (Massy et al 1994). Deficiencies of vitamin B12 or folate have been found to be associated with hyperhomocysteinemia (Ueland and Refsum 1989), but the plasma levels of these substances have been reported to be within the normal range in renal transplant recipients (Wilcken et al 1981). Instead, pyridoxal phosphate concentration deficiency, which is associated with postmethionine-loading hyperhomocysteinemia, has been found in renal transplant recipients (Lacour et al 1983). Impaired renal function is an important cause of hyperhomocysteinemia. Serum homocysteine levels are positively correlated with serum creatinine concentration and mild decrements of glomerular filtration rate are strongly and independently associated with linear increases in fasting total homocysteine levels (Bostom and Culleton 1999); however, vitamin status has a relatively marginal influence on homocysteine levels (Bostom et al 1999). Since both degradation pathways of homocysteine by either remethylation or cystathionine formation (Figure 14.5) consume serine, the decreased plasma serine found in renal transplant patients (Wilcken et al 1981) might explain the high levels of homocysteine. But low serine levels appear to be a consequence rather than a cause of increased homocysteine serum levels because of the enhancement of its catabolism which involves serine (Dudman et al 1987). The cumulative dosage of corticosteroids has been correlated with total homocysteine level (Massy et al 1994). The role

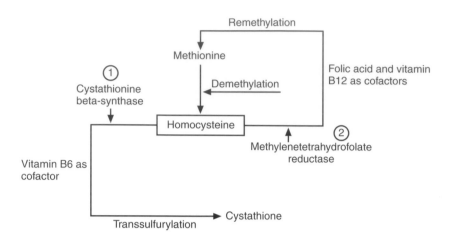

Figure 14.5. Homocysteine metabolism. Homocysteine is formed by the demethylation of the essential amino acid methionine. Two enzymes are particularly important: (1) cystathionine beta-synthase converts homocysteine to cystathione using vitamin B6 as cofactor via transsulfurylation. (2) Methylenetetrahydrofolate reductase remethylates homocysteine to methionine using folic acid and vitamin B12 as cofactors via remethylation.

of CsA is more uncertain. In one study cyclosporine-treated patients had significantly higher levels of homocysteine than those treated with azathioprine and prednisolone (Arnadottir et al 1996). In contrast both multivariate regression modeling (Bostom et al 1997) and matched analyses (Ducloux et al 1998) showed that after appropriate adjustment for renal function indices, age, and gender, CsA was not an independent determinant of total homocysteine levels in renal transplant recipients. In 1995, a common genetic variant of the gene encoding for methylenetetrahydrofolate-reductase (MTHFR) involved in the enzymatic remethylation and therefore elimination of homocysteine was described (Frosst et al 1995). This variant, consisting of a cytosine (C) to thymidine (T) transition at nucleotide position 677 (C677T variant) leading to the exchange of a highly conserved alanine to valine in the mature protein, has been associated with reduced activity and increased thermolability of this enzyme in lymphocyte extracts (Kang et al 1991). This mutation increases total plasma homocysteine both in patients with normal and impaired kidney function (Födinger et al 1997), and lowers the levels of the active form of folate (Frosst et al 1995). Also in renal transplant recipients the homozygosity for C677T transition in the MTHFR gene can significantly increase total homocysteine concentration and can lower folate levels even in patients with excellent renal function (Födinger et al 1999).

The vascular lesions found in patients with elevated plasma homocysteine are characterized by fibromuscular thickening of small arterial vessels (McCully 1969) and resemble those found in chronic allograft injury (Solez 1994), suggesting that elevated plasma homocysteine may adversely influence the long-term renal graft survival by promoting vascular sclerosis in the kidney allograft. However, in a 5-year follow-up study neither pre- nor posttransplant homocysteine plasma levels were found to influence patient or graft survival, graft function or histopathology (Dimény et al 1998). In long-term renal allograft survivors with an average graft survival of 156 months the C677T mutation of the MTHFR gene was not an important determinant of renal transplant survival (Liangos et al 1998). It is possible that other determinants of chronic transplant rejection including late acute rejection, hypertension, proteinuria, infection, delayed graft function or obesity may have stronger effects on transplant survival, thereby masking any effect attributable to the MTHFR-C677T genotype in this setting.

Treatment

Because plasma folate and vitamin B12 levels are inversely related to fasting plasma total homocysteine levels, whereas plasma vitamin B6 levels are inversely associated with a postmethionine-loading increase in plasma total homocysteine levels, supplementation with these vitamins might theoretically improve the homocysteine metabolism. Data of open-label studies were conflicting (Wilcken et al 1981; Arnadottir and Hultberg 1997). Recently, a placebo-controlled study in 29 clinically stable renal transplant recipients demonstrated that in patients with mild hyperhomocysteinemia a combination of folic acid (5.0 mg/day), vitamin B6 (50 mg/day) and vitamin B12 (0.4 mg/day), given for 6 weeks, could reduce fasting and postmethionine loading total homocysteine levels by at least 25%, with 75% of patients achieving normalization of their total homocysteine levels (Bostom et al 1997).

Further studies are needed to show whether a combination of folic acid, vitamin B12 and vitamin B6 should be included in the routine treatment of renal transplant patients.

Dialysis

Even before dialysis uremic patients may be affected by left ventricular hypertrophy, dilated cardiomyopathy and congestive heart failure. The cardiovascular state may worsen with time on dialysis. Hypertension, anemia, chronic fluid overload, hyperlipidemia and glucose intolerance may contribute to worsen this cardiovascular profile. Recent studies (Montagnino et al 1997; Cosio et al 1998) pointed out that there is a relationship between time on dialysis and patient mortality. Cosio et al (1998) pointed out that increasing time on dialysis increased the prevalence of both left ventricular hypertrophy and cardiomegaly and these relationships were statistically independent of other risk factors.

HYPERURICEMIA

An association between elevated serum uric acid and cardiovascular disease has been suspected for many years but never demonstrated. The problem was recently revisited in the Framingham Heart Study sample (Culleton et al 1999). A careful analysis of 117 376 person-years of follow-up indicated that uric acid does not have any causal role in the development of coronary heart disease, death from cardiovascular disease, or death from all causes. Thus, the frequently observed hyperuricemia should no longer be regarded as a cardiovascular risk factor in transplant patients.

COAGULATION FACTORS

There is now good evidence that elevated plasma levels of fibrinogen, factor VII, and von Willebrand factor are associated with an increased risk of acute stroke and coronary artery disease in the general population (Frishman et al 1998). These factors are elevated in renal transplant patients, being higher in those who had cardiovascular events than in those who had not (Irish and Green 1997). An impaired fibrinolysis, with increased risk of thrombosis, may also occur in some renal transplant patients as a consequence of the elevated plasminogen activator inhibitor levels found in patients treated with CsA, in diabetics and in hypercholesterolemic patients (Verpooten et al 1996). Both cyclosporine and tacrolimus significantly enhance platelet aggregation and secretion in response to physiological agonists (Babinska et al 1998). Rapamycin may also enhance platelet aggregation and secretion through a direct dose-dependent effect on platelet function (Babinska et al 1998). All these abnormalities might realize a prothrombotic state in renal transplant recipients that may contribute to atherogenesis, cardiovascular complications and to the development of a chronic allograft nephropathy.

CELL ADHESION MOLECULES

Adhesion molecules play a key role in thrombosis, restenosis after percutaneous translu-minal coronary angioplasty, atherosclerosis and reperfusion injury (Price and Loscalzo 1999). These molecules act by mediating the interaction of circulating mononuclear leukocytes with the vascular endothelium. Elevated levels of cell adhesion molecules are associated with hyperlipidemia and there may be a link between smoking and the expression of cell adhesion molecules (Hackman et al 1996; Shen et al 1996). P-selectin, E-selectin, intercellular adhesion molecule-1 (ICAM-1) and vascular cell adhesion mole-cule-1 (VCAM-1) are upregulated and strongly expressed on intertubular capillaries, proximal tubules, and endothelium of transplanted kidney (Fuggle et al 1993), in particular during episodes of acute rejection and in chronic rejection (Fuggle and Koo 1998).

INFECTION AND INFLAMMATION

Several reports have shown a correlation between the incidence of atherosclerosis and the presence of specific pathogens including *Chlamydia pneumoniae*, *Helicobacter pylori*, cytomegalovirus (CMV) and herpes class viruses (Frishman et al 1998). The potential mechanisms arise from the inflammatory response to infection. Bacterial infection and endotoxin release stimulate monocytes, increase the secretion of interleukin-1 (IL-1) and tumour necrosis factor (TNF), increase thrombocyte adherence, reduce levels of antithrombin III and induce downregulation of the fibrinolytic system (Nieminen et al 1993). Endotoxin may also raise levels of thromboxane 2, inhibit tissue plasminogen activation, decrease lipoprotein lipase activity and damage endothelial cells. The infection also impairs glucose and lipid metabolisms. These metabolic consequences may contribute to increased cardiovascular risk.

Cytomegalovirus (CMV) may produce atherogenic effects by several mechanisms. Cytomegalovirus induces elevation of perivascular infiltrate of monocytes/macrophages, which are known to play a role in the development of atherosclerotic lesions (Li et al 1998). It may also cause endothelial injury that precipitates intimal lesion development in human atherosclerosis (Li et al 1995). The cytokines released during a response to CMV-infected cells have the capacity to increase the expression of ICAM-1 and VCAM-1 on endothelial cells (Fuggle and Koo 1998). In turn, these molecules mediate the interaction of circulating mononuclear leukocytes with the vascular endothelium, an early event in atherosclerosis (Frishman et al 1998).

OBESITY

There is a close relationship between excessive accumulation of body fat and premature cardiovascular morbidity and mortality. Obesity is often associated with lipoprotein abnormalities, elevated concentrations of plasminogen activator inhibitor-1, insulin resistance, increased left ventricular mass, left ventricular wall thickness, and left ventricular cavity size (Abate 1999).

In obese transplant patients (body mass index greater than 30 kg/m^2) cardiac events represent the leading cause of deaths (Modlin et al 1997). The great incidence of post-transplant diabetes may contribute to the elevated cardiovascular risk in this population. The high mortality in obese recipients results in the major difference in graft loss when compared with a nonobese group, with a diminished 5-year graft survival of nearly 20% (Modlin et al 1997). Because of elevated mortality after transplantation, a thorough evaluation of cardiovascular state and appropriate dietetic measures are recommended in obese candidates for transplantation.

CONCLUSIONS

The risk factors for cardiovascular disease can be grouped into two broad categories: (1) unmodifiable factors such as age, male gender and family history of premature heart disease; (2) potentially modifiable factors such as cigarette smoking, physical inactivity, overweight, diabetes, high blood pressure, high blood cholesterol level and immunosuppressive regimens. There is today evidence that the risk of cardiovascular disease falls significantly if a patient quits smoking, reduces excess alcohol, has an active lifestyle, reduces weight and receives aggressive treatment for elevated blood pressure and cholesterol level. Thus any effort should be made to convince the transplant patient to modify diet and lifestyle and to adhere to drug prescriptions. Reduction of cardiovascular morbidity can improve not only the life-expectancy and the quality of life of the transplant recipient but also their allograft function and survival.

REFERENCES

Aakhus S, Dahl K, Widerne TE (1999) Cardiovascular morbidity and risk factors in renal transplant patients. *Nephrol Dial Transplant* **54**:648–654.

Abate N (1999) Obesity as a risk factor for cardiovascular disease. *Am J Med* **107** (suppl 2A): 125–135.

Abdulmassih Z, Chevalier A, Bader C et al (1992) Role of lipid disturbances in the atherosclerosis of renal transplant patients. *Clin Transplant* **6**:106–113.

Arnadottir M, Berg AL (1997) Treatment of hyperlipidemia in renal transplant recipients. *Transplantation* **63**:339–345.

Arnadottir M, Hultberg B (1997) Treatment with high-dose folic acid effectively lowers plasma homocysteine concentration in cyclosporine-treated renal transplant recipients. *Transplantation* **64**:1087.

Arnadottir M, Erikson LD, Thysell H, Karkas JD (1993) Plasma concentration profiles of simvastatin 3-hydroxy-3-methyl-glutaryl-coenzyme A reductase inhibitory activity in kidney transplant recipients with and without cyclosporine. *Nephron* **65**:410–413.

Arnadottir M, Hultberg B, Vladov V et al (1996) Hyperhomocysteinemia in cyclosporine treated renal transplant recipients. *Transplantation* **61**:509–512.

Arnadottir M, Hultberg B, Wahlberg J et al (1998) Serum total homocysteine concentration before and after renal transplantation. *Kidney Int* **54**:1380–1384.

Babinska A, Markell MS, Salifu MO et al (1998) Enhancement of human platelet aggregation and secretion induced by rapamycin. *Nephrol Dial Transplant* **13**:3153–3159.

Barbagallo CM, Gefalù AB, Gallo S et al (1999) Effects of Mediterranean diet on lipid levels and cardiovascular risk in renal transplant recipients. *Nephron* **82**:199–204.

Barrett-Connor E (1997) Sex differences in coronary heart disease. Why are women so superior? The 1995 Ancel Keys Lecture. *Circulation* **95**:252–264.

Bencini PL, Crosti C, Sala F et al (1984) Gingival hyperplasia by nifedipine. *Acta Derm Venereol (Stockh)* **65**:362–365.

Bennett WM, De Mattos A, Meyer MM et al (1996) Chronic cyclosporine nephropathy: the Achille's heel of immunosuppressive therapy. *Kidney Int* **50**:1089–1100.

Birkeland SA (1998) Steroid-free immunosuppression after kidney transplantation with antithymocyte globulin induction and cyclosporine and mycophenolate mofetil maintenance therapy. *Transplantation* **66**:1207–1210.

Boissonnat P, Salen P, Guidollet J et al (1994) The long-term effects of the lipid-lowering agent fenofibrate in hyperlipidemic heart transplant recipients. *Transplantation* 58:245–247.

Bostom AG, Culleton BF (1999) Hyperhomocysteinemia in chronic renal disease. *J Am Soc Nephrol* 10:891–900.

Bostom AG, Gohl RY, Beaulieu A et al (1999) Determinants of fasting plasma total homocysteine levels among chronic stable renal transplant recipients. *Transplantation* 68:257–261.

Bostom AG, Gohl RY, Tsai MY et al (1997) Excess prevalence of fasting and postmethionine-loading hyperhomocysteinemia in stable renal transplant recipients. *Arterioscler Thromb Vasc Biol* 17:1894–1900.

Burnier M, Brunner HR (1998) Angiotensin II receptor antagonists in hypertension. *Kidney Int* 54(Suppl 68):S107–S111.

Capone D, Stanziale P, Gentile A et al (1999) Effects of simvastatin and pravastatin on hyperlipidemia and cyclosporine blood levels in renal transplant recipients. *Am J Nephrol* 19:411–415.

Carlström J, Nordén G, Mjörnstedt L, Nyberg G (1999) Increasing prevalence of cardiovascular disease in kidney transplant patients with type 1 diabetes. *Transplant Int* 12:176–181.

Chambers J (1995) Left ventricular hypertrophy. *Br Med J* 311:273–274.

Chan TM, Cheng IKP, Tam SCF (1994) Hyperlipidemia after renal transplantation: treatment with gemfibrozil. *Nephron* 63:317–323.

Cosio FG, Alamir A, Yim S et al (1998) Patient survival after renal transplantation: I. The impact of dialysis pre-transplant. *Kidney Int* 53:767–772.

Cosio FG, Falkentrain MF, Pesavento TE et al (1999) Patient survival data after renal transplantation: II. The input of smoking. *Clin Transplant* 13:336–341.

Culleton BF, Larson MG, Kannel WB, Levy D (1999) Serum uric acid and risk for cardiovascular disease and death: the Framingham Heart Study. *Ann Intern Med* 131:7–13.

Curtis JJ (1990) Cyclosporine and hypertension. *Clin Transplant* 4:337–340.

Curtis JJ (1997) Treatment of hypertension in renal allograft patients: does drug selection make a difference? *Kidney Int* 63(Suppl):S75–S77.

Curtis JJ, Laskow PA, Jones PA et al (1993) Captopril-induced fall in glomerular filtration rate in cyclosporine-treated hypertensive patients. *J Am Soc Nephrol* 3:1570–1574.

Diményi E, Fellstrom B, Larsson E et al (1993) Hyperlipoproteinemia in renal transplant recipients: is there a linkage with chronic vascular rejection? *Transplant Proc* 25:2065–2066.

Diményi E, Hultberg B, Wahlberg J et al (1998) Serum total homocysteine does not predict outcome in renal transplant recipients. *Transplantation* 12:563–568.

Drueke TB, Abdulmassih Z, Lacour B et al (1991) Atherosclerosis and lipid disorders after renal transplantation. *Kidney Int* 39(Suppl 31):S24–S28.

Ducloux D, Fournier V, Rebibou JN et al (1998) Hyperhomocysteinemia in renal transplant recipients with and without cyclosporine. *Clin Nephrol* 49:232–235.

Dudman NPB, Tyrrell PA, Wilcken DEL (1987) Homocysteinemia: depressed plasma serum levels. *Metabolism* 36:198–202.

Egido J (1996) Vasoactive hormones and renal sclerosis. *Kidney Int* 49:578–597.

Elli A, Rivolta R, Quarto Di Palo F et al (1993) A randomized trial of deflazacort versus 6-methylprednisolone in renal transplantation. Immunosuppressive activity and side effects. *Transplantation* 55:209–212.

English J, Evan A, Houghton D, Bennett W (1987) Cyclosporine induces acute renal dysfunction in the rat. Evidence of arteriolar vasoconstriction with preservation of tubular function. *Transplantation* 44:135–141.

Fehrman-Ekholm I, Jogestraud T, Angelin B (1996) Decreased cyclosporine levels during gemfibrozil treatment of hyperlipidemia after kidney transplantation. *Nephron* 72:483.

First MR, Neylan JF, Rocher LL, Tejani A (1994) Hypertension after renal transplantation. *J Am Soc Nephrol* 4(Suppl 1):S30–S36.

Födinger M, Wölfe G, Fischer G et al (1999) Effect of MTHFR 677C>T on plasma total homocysteine levels in renal graft recipients. *Kidney Int* 55:1072–1080.

Foley RN, Parfrey PS, Sarnak MJ (1998) Epidemiology of cardiovascular disease in chronic renal disease. *J Am Soc Nephrol* 4:S16–S23.

Frishman WH (1998) Biologic markers as predictors of cardiovascular disease. *Am J Med* 104:S18–S27.

Frosst P, Blom HJ, Milos R et al (1995) A candidate genetic risk factor for vascular disease. A common mutation in methylenetetrahydrofolate reductase. *Nat Genet* 10:111–113.

Fuggle SV, Koo DDH (1998) Cell adhesion molecules in clinical renal transplantation. *Transplantation* 65:763–769.

Fuggle SV, Sanderson JB, Groy DW et al (1993) Variation in expression of endothelial adhesion molecules in pretransplant and transplanted kidneys: correlation with intragraft events. *Transplantation* 55:117–123.

Furberg CD, Psaty BM, Meyer JV (1995) Nifedipine: dose-related increase in mortality in patients with coronary heart disease. *Circulation* 92:1326–1331.

Gillison SL, Bartlett ST, Curry DL (1991) Inhibition by cyclosporine of insulin secretion: a β cell specific alteration of islet tissue function. *Transplantation* 52:890–895.

Goldberg R, Roth D (1996) Evaluation of fluvastatin in the treatment of hypercholesterolemia in renal transplant recipients taking cyclosporine. *Transplantation* 62:1559–1564.

Griendling KK, Alexander RW (1997) Oxidative stress and cardiovascular disease. *Circulation* 96:3264–3265.

Groth CG, Backman L, Morales JM et al (1999) Sirolimus (rapamycin)-based therapy in human renal transplantation: similar efficacy and different toxicity compared with cyclosporine. Sirolimus European Renal Transplant Study Group. *Transplantation* 67:1036–1042.

Grundy SM (1994) National Cholesterol Education Program. Second report of the expert panel on detection, evaluation, and treatment of high blood cholesterol in adults (Adult Treatment Renal II). *Circulation* 99:1329.

Guidi E, Menghetti D, Milani S et al (1996) Hypertension may be transplanted with the kidney in humans: a long-term historical prospective follow-up of recipients grafted with kidney coming from donors with or without hypertension in their families. *J Am Soc Nephrol* 7:1131–1138.

Hackman A, Yasunori A, Insull W Jr et al (1996) Levels of soluble cell adhesion molecules in patients with dyslipidemia. *Circulation* 93:1334–1338.

Hilbrands LB, Demacher PNM, Hoitsma AJ (1993) Cyclosporine and serum lipids in renal transplant recipients. *Lancet* 341:765–766.

Hjelmesaeth J, Hartman A, Kofstad J et al (1997) Glucose intolerance after renal transplantation depends upon prednisolone dose and recipient age. *Transplantation* 64:979–983.

Homan Van der Heide JJ, Bilo HJG, Donker JM et al (1993) Effect of dietary fish oil on renal function and rejection in cyclosporine-treated recipients of renal transplants. *N Engl J Med* 329:769–773.

Howard BV (1996) Risk factors for cardiovascular disease in individuals with diabetes. The strong heart study. *Acta Diabetol* 33:180–184.

Hricik DE, Schulak JA (1993) Metabolic effects of steroid withdrawal in adult renal transplant recipients. *Kidney Int* 44:S26–S29.

Hricik DE, Bartucci MR, Mayes JT, Schulak JA (1992) The effects of steroid withdrawal on the lipoprotein profiles of cyclosporine-treated kidney and kidney–pancreas transplant recipients. *Transplantation* 54:868–871.

Hricik DE, Schulak JA, O'Toole MA, Herson J (1993) Steroid free immunosuppression in cyclosporine-treated renal transplant recipients: a meta-analysis. *J Am Soc Nephrol* 4:1300–1305.

Irish AB, Green FR (1997) Environmental and genetic determinants of the hypercoagulable state and cardiovascular disease in renal transplant recipients. *Nephrol Dial Transplant* 12:167–173.

Isoniemi H, Nurminen M, Tikkanen MJ et al (1994) Risk factors predicting chronic rejection of renal allografts. *Transplantation* 57:68–72.

Jensen RA, Lal SM, Diaz-Arias A et al (1995) Does cholestyramine interfere with cyclosporin absorption? A prospective study in renal transplant patients. *ASAIO J* 41:M704–M706.

Jindal RM (1994) Posttransplant diabetes mellitus. A review. *Transplantation* 58:1289–1298.

Kang SS, Passen EL, Ruggie N et al (1991) Thermolabile defect of methylenetetrahydrofolate reductase. An inherited risk factor for coronary artery disease. *Am J Hum Genet* 48:536–545.

Kasiske BL (1987) Possible causes and consequences of hypertension in stable renal transplant patients. *Transplantation* 44:639–643.

Kasiske BL (1993) Risk factors for cardiovascular disease after renal transplantation. *Min Electrolyte Metab* 19:186–195.

Kasiske BL, Guijarro C, Massy ZA et al (1996) Cardiovascular disease after renal transplantation. *J Am Soc Nephrol* 7:158–165.

Katznelson S, Wilkinson AH, Kobashigawa JA et al (1996) The effect of pravastatin on acute rejection after kidney transplantation: a pilot study. *Transplantation* 61:1469–1474.

Knopp RM (1999) Treatment of lipid disorder. *N Engl J Med* 341:498–511.

Kobashigawa JA, Kasiske BL (1997) Hyperlipidemia in solid organ transplantation. *Transplantation* 63:331–338.

Krausz Y, Wolheim CB, Siegal E, Sharp GWG (1980) Possible role for calmodulin in insulin release: studies with trifluoperazine in the rat pancreatic islets. *J Clin Invest* 66:603–607.

Kupin WL, Venkat KK, Mozes M (1992) Long-term efficacy and safety of lovastatin in the treatment of hypercholesterolemia in renal transplant recipients. *J Am Soc Nephrol* 3:865.

Lacour B, Parry C, Drüeke T et al (1983) Pyridoxal 5-phosphate deficiency in uremic undialyzed, hemodialyzed and non-uremic kidney transplant patients. *Clin Chim Acta* 127:205–215.

Li F, Grauls G, Yin M, Bruggeman CA (1995) Initial endothelial injury and cytomegalovirus infection accelerate the development of allograft arteriosclerosis. *Transplant Proc* 27:3552–3554.

Li F, Yin M, Van Dam JG et al (1998) Cytomegalovirus infection enhances the neointima formation in rat aortic allografts. *Transplantation* 65:1298–1304.

Liangos O, Kreutz R, Beige J et al (1998) Methylenetetrahydrofolate reductase gene C 677 T variant and kidney transplant survival. *Nephrol Dial Transplant* 13:2351–2354.

Lindholm A, Albrechtsen D, Frödin L et al (1995) Ischemic heart disease. Major cause of death and graft loss after renal transplantation in Scandinavia. *Transplantation* 60:451–457.

Luke RG (1991) Pathophysiology and treatment of post-transplant hypertension. *J Am Soc Nephrol* 2(Suppl 1):S37–S44.

Markell MS, Armenti V, Danovitch G, Sumrani N (1994) Hyperlipidemia and glucose intolerance in the post-renal transplant patient. *J Am Soc Nephrol* 4:S37–S47.

Massy ZA, Kasiske BL (1996) Post-transplant hyperlipidemia: mechanisms and management. *J Am Soc Nephrol* 7:971–977.

Massy ZA, Chadefaux-Vekemans B, Chevalier A et al (1994) Hyperhomocysteinemia: a significant risk factor for cardiovascular disease in renal transplant recipients. *Nephrol Dial Transplant* 9:1103–1108.

Mayer AD, Dimitrewski J, Squifflet JP et al (1997) Multicenter randomized trial comparing tacrolimus (FK 506) and cyclosporine in the prevention of renal allograft rejection: a report of the European Tacrolimus Multicenter Renal Study Group. *Transplantation* 64:436–443.

McCune TR, Thacker LR, Peters TG et al (1998) Effects of tacrolimus on hyperlipidemia after successful renal transplantation. *Transplantation* 65:87–92.

McCully KS (1969) Vascular pathology of homocysteinemia. Implications for the pathogenesis of atherosclerosis. *Am J Pathol* 56:111–128.

Mediratta S, Fozailoff A, Frishman WH (1995) Insulin resistance in systemic hypertension: pharmacotherapeutic implications. *J Clin Pharmacol* 35:943–956.

Miles AMV, Sumrani N, Horowitz R et al (1998) Diabetes mellitus after renal transplantation. *Transplantation* 65:380–384.

Modlin CS, Flechner SM, Goormastic M et al (1997) Should obese patients lose weight before receiving a kidney transplant? *Transplantation* 64:599–604.

Montagnino G, Tarantino A, Aroldi A et al (1994) Lipid profile in renal transplant recipients under various immunosuppressive regimens. *Transplant Proc* 26:2634–2636.

Montagnino G, Tarantino A, Cesana B et al (1997) Prognostic factors of long-term allograft survival in 632 CyA-treated recipients of a primary renal transplant. *Transplant Int* 10:268–275.

Moore RA, Callahan MF, Cody M et al (1990) The effect of the American Heart Association Step I. Diet on hyperlipidemia following renal transplantation. *Transplantation* 49:60–62.

Mosterd A, D'Agostino RB, Silbershatz H et al (1999) Trends in the prevalence of hypertension, antihypertensive therapy and left ventricular hypertrophy from 1950 to 1989. *N Engl J Med* 340:1221–1227.

Mourad G, Ribstein J, Mimran A (1993) Converting-enzyme inhibitor versus calcium antagonist in cyclosporine-treated renal transplants. *Kidney Int* 43:419–425.

Newman-Sanders AP, Gedroyce WG, Kutoubi MA et al (1995) The use of expandable metal stents in transplant renal artery stenosis. *Clin Radiol* 1995:50:245–250.

Nieminen MS, Mattila K, Valtonen V (1993) Infection and inflammation as risk factors for myocardial infarction. *Eur Heart J* 14(Suppl K):12–16.

O'Keefe JH Jr, Lavie CJ Jr, McCallister BD (1995) Insights into the pathogenesis and prevention of coronary artery disease. *Mayo Clin Proc* 70:69–79.

Opelz G, Wujciak T, Ritz E (1998) Association of chronic kidney graft failure with recipient blood pressure. *Kidney Int* 53:217–222.

Pesavento TE, Jones PA, Julian BA, Curtis JJ (1996) Amlodipine increases cyclosporine levels in hypertensive renal transplant patients. Results of a prospective study. *J Am Soc Nephrol* 7:831–835.

Pirsch JD, Miller J, Deierhoi MH et al (1997) A comparison of tacrolimus (FK 506) and cyclosporin for immunosuppression after cadaveric renal transplantation. *Transplantation* 63:977–983.

Ponticelli C, Montagnino G (1987) Cause of arterial hypertension in kidney transplantation. *Contrib Nephrol* 54:226–230.

Ponticelli C, Opelz G (1995) Are corticosteroids really necessary in renal transplantation? *Nephrol Dial Transplant* 10:1587–1591.

Ponticelli C, Barbi GL, Cantaluppi A et al (1978) Lipid disorders in renal transplant recipients. *Nephron* 20:189–195.

Ponticelli C, Montagnino G, Aroldi A (1993) Hypertension after transplantation. *Am J Kidney Dis* 21(Suppl 2):S73–S78.

Ponticelli C, Tarantino A, Segoloni GP et al (1997) A randomized study comparing three cyclosporine-based regimens in cadaveric renal transplantation. *J Am Soc Nephrol* 8:638–646.

Price DT, Loscalzo J (1999) Cellular adhesion molecules and atherogenesis. *Am J Med* 107:85–97.

Raine AEG (1994) Cardiovascular complications after renal transplantation. In: Morris PJ (ed.). *Kidney Transplantation. Principle and Practice*, 4th edn. London: WB Saunders, pp. 339–355.

Raine AEG, Margreiter R, Brunner FP et al (1992) Report on management on renal failure in Europe XXII, 1992. *Nephrol Dial Transplant* 7(Suppl 2):7–35.

Ratcliffe PJ, Dudley CRK, Higgins RM et al (1996) Randomized controlled trial of steroid withdrawal in renal transplant recipients receiving triple immunosuppression. *Lancet* 348:643–648.

Reaven GM (1995) Pathophysiology of insulin resistance in human disease. *Physiol Rev* 75:473–486.

Refsum H, Helland S, Ueland PM (1985) Radioenzymic determination of homocysteine in plasma and urine. *Clin Chem* 31:624–628.

Rengel M, Gomes-da-Silva G, Incháustegui L et al (1998) Renal artery stenosis after kidney transplantation: diagnostic and therapeutic approach. *Kidney Int* 54(Suppl 68):S99–S106.

Roberts JP, Ascher NL, Feyd DS et al (1989) Transplant artery stenoses. *Transplantation* 48:580–583.

Ross R (1999) Atherosclerosis. An inflammatory disease. *N Engl J Med* 340:115–126.

Satterthwaite R, Aswad S, Sunga V et al (1998) Incidence of new-onset hypercholesterolemia in renal transplant patients treated with FK506 or cyclosporine. *Transplantation* 65:446–449.

Schmieder RE, Martus P, Klingbeil A (1996) Reversal of ventriculum hypertrophy in essential hypertension: a meta-analysis of randomized double-blind studies. *JAMA* 275:1507–1513.

Schrama YC, Hené RJ, De Jonge N et al (1998) Efficacy and muscle safety of fluvastatin in cyclosporine-treated cardiac and renal transplant recipients. *Transplantation* 66:1175–1181.

Schweitzer E, Matas AJ, Gillingham KG et al (1991) Cause of renal allograft loss. Progress in the 1980s, challenges for the 1990s. *Ann Surg* 214:679–688.

Shen Y, Rattan V, Sultana C, Kalra VK (1996) Cigarette smoke condensate-induced adhesion molecule expression and transendothelial migration of monocytes. *Am J Physiol* 270:H1624–H1633.

Sinclair NR for the Canadian Multicentre Transplant Study Group (1992) Low-dose steroid therapy in cyclosporine-treated renal transplant recipients with well-functioning grafts. *Can Med Assoc J* 147:645–655.

Solez K (1994) International standardization of criteria for histologic diagnosis of chronic rejection in renal allograft. *Clin Transplant* 8:345–350.

Stern MP (1995) Perspectives in diabetes: diabetes and cardiovascular disease. The common soil hypothesis. *Diabetes* 44:369–374.

Sumrani NB, Delaney V, Ding Z et al (1991) Diabetes mellitus after renal transplantations in the cyclosporine era. An analysis of risk factors. *Transplantation* 51:343–347.

Sundararajan V, Cooper DKC, Muchmore J et al (1991) Interaction of cyclosporine and probucol in heart transplant patients. *Transplant Proc* 28:2028–2032.

Sutherland WHF, Walker RJ, Ball MJ et al (1995) Oxidation of low density lipoproteins from patients with renal failure and renal transplants. *Kidney Int* 48:227–236.

Tamura K, Fujimura T, Tsutmi T et al (1995) Transcriptional inhibition of insulin by FK506 and possible involvement of FK506 binding protein-12 in pancreatic β cell. *Transplantation* 59:1606–1613.

Tobert JA (1988) Rhabdomyolysis in patients receiving lovastatin after cardiac transplantation (letter). *N Engl J Med* 318:48.

Tyden G, Bolinder J, Solders G et al (1999) Improved survival in patients with insulin-dependent diabetes mellitus and end-stage diabetic nephropathy 10 years after combined pancreas and kidney transplantation. *Transplantation* 67:645–648.

Ueland PM, Refsum R (1989) Plasma homocysteine, a risk factor for vascular disease: plasma levels in health, disease, and drug therapy. *J Lab Clin Med* 114:473–501.

Van Ypersele de Strihou C, Pochet JM (1992) Hypertension in the transplant patient. In: Cameron JS, Davison AM, Kerr D, Grünfeld JP, Ritz E (eds). *Oxford Textbook of Clinical Nephrology.* Oxford: Oxford University Press, pp. 1594–1602.

Vathsala A, Weinberg RB, Shoenberg L et al (1989) Lipid abnormalities in cyclosporine-treated renal transplant recipients. *Transplantation* 48:37–43.

Verdecchia P, Schillaci G, Borgioni C (1998) Prognostic significance of serial changes in left ventricular mass in essential hypertension. *Circulation* 97:48–54.

Verhoef P, Stampfer MJ (1995) Prospective studies of homocysteine and cardiovascular disease. *Nutr Rev* 53:283–288.

Verpooten GA, Cools FJ, Van der Planken MG et al (1996) Elevated plasminogen activator inhibitor levels in cyclosporine-treated renal allograft recipients. *Nephrol Dial Transplant* 11:347–351.

Versluis DJ, Wenting GJ, Derky FH et al (1987) Who should be converted from cyclosporine to conventional immunosuppression in kidney transplantation and why. *Transplantation* **44**:387–389.

Vesco L, Busson M, Bedrossian J et al (1996) Diabetes mellitus after renal transplantation. *Transplantation* **61**:1475–1478.

Webb AT, Reaveley DA, O'Donnell M et al (1993) Does cyclosporine increase lipoprotein(a) concentrations in renal transplant recipients? *Lancet* **341**:268–270.

Wilcken DEL, Gupta VJ, Betts AK (1981) Homocysteine in the plasma of renal transplant recipients: effects of cofactors for methionine metabolism. *Clin Sci* **61**:743–749.

Zeier M, Mandelbaun A, Ritz E (1998) Hypertension in the transplanted patient. *Nephron* **80**:257–268.

15 MALIGNANCY

*In collaboration with G Montagnino**

Much of what we know about neoplasias in renal allograft recipients derives from the pioneering studies of Penn in the late sixties (Penn et al 1969) and by the subsequent institution of the Cincinnati Transplant Tumor Registry (CTTR). Since the first reports on the association between cancer and immunosuppression in renal allograft recipients (McKahnn 1969; Penn et al 1969), an increasing awareness of the predisposing effect of immunosuppression for the development of tumors has arisen. This holds true for de novo cancers occurring after transplantation, for the evolution of pre-existing tumors in the allograft recipient and for the transmission of cancer from the donor to the recipient.

DE NOVO CANCERS

Epidemiology

The prevalence of de novo cancers in renal transplantation ranges between 1 and 6% (Cockburn and Krupp 1989; Sheil et al 1993; Penn 1994), similar to the 4% reported in individuals with genetically determined immunodeficiency disease (Spector et al 1978). In our experience at Ospedale Maggiore in Milan (Montagnino et al 1996), taking into account only cancers occurring at least 1 year after transplantation, the prevalence of neoplasias was 8.9%. The incidence of neoplasias as a whole is about 3–4 times more frequent among transplant recipients than in an age-matched control population (Kinlen 1985; Sheil et al 1993). According to Penn (1994, 1996), some neoplasias, which are common among the general public (carcinoma of the prostate, breast, lung, colon, rectum, bladder and uterus), have a lower incidence among transplant recipients, while in situ cervical carcinomas of the uterus have a similar incidence rate among the general population (37%) and allograft recipients (31%). On the contrary, non-Hodgkin's lymphomas, Kaposi's sarcomas and carcinomas of the kidney, liver, skin, lip, vulva and perineum are much more frequent among transplant recipients, with an incidence varying from 6 to 0.5% (Table 15.1). These data are at odds with two other

*Division of Nephrology and Dialysis, Ospedale Maggiore, Milan

Higher incidence

    Kaposi's sarcoma (400–1000 times)

    Skin carcinomas (100 times)

    Vulvar, anal carcinomas (100 times)

    Non-Hodgkin's lymphoma (28–49 times)

    Hepatic carcinoma (20–38 times)

    Labial carcinoma (29 times)

    Renal carcinoma (8.9 times)

Lower incidence

    Breast carcinoma

    Prostate carcinoma

    Lung carcinoma

    Colon carcinoma

    Bladder carcinoma

    Uterus carcinoma

    Rectum carcinoma

Table 15.1. Comparison between the incidence of cancer in renal transplant recipients and in general population

major registries, the Nordic Renal Transplant Registry (NRTR) (Birkeland et al 1995) and the Australian and New Zealand Transplant Registry (ANZTR) (Sheil et al 1979, 1993), showing an increased incidence of nearly all types of cancers in renal transplant recipients. This might be explained by differences in the studied population, differences in the criteria for cancer inclusion and in the average age of patients at transplantation (Penn 1999).

After transplantation, the risk of developing Kaposi's sarcomas increases by 400–1000 times, vulvar and anal carcinomas by 100 times, non-Hodgkin's lymphomas by 28–49 times (Kinlen 1985), hepatocellular carcinomas by 20–38 times and labial carcinomas by 29 times. In situ cervical uterine carcinomas increase from 3.3 (Fairley et al 1994) to 16 times (Penn 1990), while renal carcinomas increase by 8.9 times (Sheil et al 1993). Skin cancers and lip cancers account for 36–46% of the total cancers (Penn 1994; Montagnino et al 1996) and are particularly frequent in sunny countries (Sheil et al 1993).

The incidence of posttransplant lymphoproliferative disease (PTLD) seems to be disturbingly high in the series from the USA. This difference is probably accounted for by the large use of sequential immunosuppression with antilymphocyte antibodies in the USA (Penn 1995a), while sequential immunosuppression is used more rarely in Europe (London et al 1995). Some tumors, such as Kaposi's sarcoma, have a racial distribution and are frequently reported in Arabic, Jewish and Mediterranean populations (Akhtar et al 1984; Montagnino et al 1994), while reports from large series of renal transplant recipients from Northern countries did not report a single case of Kaposi's sarcoma (Vogt et al 1990).

Etiology and pathogenesis

Several factors may favor the development of posttransplant cancer (Table 15.2). Immunosuppressive therapy is one of the most important causative factors. The risk of tumor is clearly related to the intensity of immunosuppression, while there is no evidence that immunosuppressive drugs exert a specific oncogenic effect. In spite of a recent study suggesting that cyclosporine (CsA) can promote cancer progression by a direct cell-autonomous effect via transforming growth factor-β (TGF-β) stimulation, independent of its effect on the host's immune system (Hojo et al 1999), several studies found no difference in the incidence of neoplasia between transplant patients treated with azathioprine (Aza) and those treated with CsA, at least up to 10 years (Penn 1990; London et al 1995; Montagnino et al 1996). An exception is Kaposi's sarcoma, which is 400–500 times more frequent among graft recipients treated with azathioprine and steroids than in general population (Harwood et al 1979) and about 1000 times more frequent among CsA-treated renal transplant recipients (Cockburn and Krupp 1989) While the incidence of cancer is similar in patients treated with CsA or Aza, the time of appearance of cancer after transplantation may change in patients given CsA or Aza (Penn 1990). Neoplasias tend to develop after a relatively short period of time in transplanted patients treated with CsA, in mean 60–67 months after transplantation (Penn 1986; Montagnino et al 1996). Kaposi's sarcomas and lymphomas have the shortest mean time of appearance (21 and 33 months respectively) while hepatobiliary and vulvar/perineal carcinomas the longest (82 and 112 months respectively; Penn 1996). There is evidence that the use of antilymphocyte antibodies increases the risk of posttransplant lymphoproliferative disorders (see later). Once again, it seems that this effect is related to the more powerful immunosuppression caused by these agents rather than to a specific oncogenic effect. An indirect confirmation of the role played by the intensity of immunosuppression is given by the observation that living-donor recipients and well-matched HLA transplant recipients have a lower incidence of posttransplant cancer (G Opelz, personal communication).

A disturbing feature with posttransplant neoplasias is their tendency to increase with time. This can be explained by the length of continuous antigenic stimulation, by the natural aging process of the grafted population and/or by the increased time of exposure to immunosuppressive agents and viral pathogens. In a series, the cumulative risk of tumors was 18% at 10 years and 50% at 20 years (Gaya et al 1995). In an Australian review of 6596 patients, the actuarial probabilities of developing a tumor were 66% at 24 years for cutaneous neoplasias, 27% for noncutaneous neoplasias and 72% overall (Sheil et al 1993). It has to be pointed out, however, that the incidence of cutaneous

Immunosuppression
Chronic antigenic stimulus
Virus
Age
Environment
Duration of uremia
Genetic diversity
Duration of transplant

Table 15.2. Risk factors for posttransplant cancer

neoplasias is highly influenced by sun exposure, leading to possible overestimations in the Australian series. In an Italian experience on 854 renal transplant recipients, the probabilities of developing a cancer of whatever origin, including basal cell carcinomas, after 20 years from transplantation was 32% (Montagnino et al 1996), almost half that reported by the Australian registry (Sheil et al 1993). However, Italian data mostly referred to patients immunosuppressed with azathioprine and steroids.

Chronic antigenic stimulation by the allograft (Gleichmann et al 1975) and viral infections (Klein and Klein 1997) are recognized as important causes of neoplastic tissue development. At least 15% of all cancers are associated with viral infections (zur Hausen 1991). Human papilloma virus (HPV) has been implicated in various skin, oropharynx, esophagus and bladder cancers (Arendt et al 1997; Bavinck and Berkhout 1997). Epstein–Barr virus (EBV) is the main etiologic agent in the genesis of posttransplant lymphoproliferative diseases (Ho et al 1988). The role of hepatitis virus B and C in hepatocellular carcinoma is well recognized.

HPV16 has been implicated in uterine cervical cancer and HTLV-1 and 2 in human T cell leukemia. Finally, human herpes virus 8 (HHV-8) has been found by polymerase chain reaction in all forms of Kaposi's sarcoma (Moore and Chang 1995; Shalling et al 1995; Table 15.3).

Besides viruses, attention has also been focused on other microbial agents such as *Helicobacter pylori*, which might be implicated in the induction of lymphomas associated with the gastric mucosa (Wotherspoon et al 1993; Eidt et al 1995).

The pathogenetic mechanisms linking viruses to lymphomas have been recently thoroughly reviewed by Birkeland (1998; Table 15.3). Epstein–Barr virus generates a polypeptide analogous in structure and bioactivity to natural interleukin-10. This cytokine has been suggested to have an important role in EBV-induced PTLD and graft tolerance by inducing anergy to donor-specific alloantigens through its suppressive effects on macrophage and T lymphocyte functions (Birkeland and Bendtzen 1996; Birkeland et al 1999). Other potential mechanisms that may trigger cell proliferation

Cancer	Virus
Lymphoma	Epstein–Barr virus, CMV (?)
Kaposi's sarcoma	Human herpes virus-8
Vulva, perineum carcinoma	Human papilloma virus
Liver carcinoma	Hepatitis B and C virus
Oropharynx, esophagus carcinoma	Human papilloma virus
Bladder carcinoma	Human papilloma virus
Leukemia	HTLV 1 and 2
Cervix carcinoma	Human papilloma virus
Skin cancer	Human papilloma virus

Table 15.3. Etiologic role of viruses in posttransplant cancers

may derive from apoptosis, oncogenes and tumor suppressor genes. It has been suggested that apoptosis is a protective host response to eliminate virus infected cells. Some viruses (such as cytomegalovirus and EBV) can modulate apoptosis by inhibition, thus allowing the virus to complete its replication cycle before the cell dies. Bcl-2 proto-oncogene, which regulates the effector phase of apoptosis and positively promotes cell proliferation, is strongly expressed in patients with PTLD (Chetty et al 1996). Epstein–Barr virus upregulates Bcl-2, thereby promoting cell survival and viral replication (Nunez et al 1989). Other genes can interact with tumorigenesis, such as TP53, which encodes for p53, a protein that regulates the progression of cell cycle in the G_1-S stage. In the absence of mutations, p53 behaves as an oncosuppressor gene. However, if mutations occur, as it has been documented in most Burkitt's lymphomas (Cherney et al 1997) as well as in cutaneous lesions (Gibson et al 1997), p53 becomes a dominant oncogene. Normal cells with DNA damage show an upregulation of p53 and stop at this stage for repair, while cells with mutant p53 let damaged DNA proceed, leaving random oncogenetic changes to occur (Fisher 1994). Some oncogenic adenoviruses and human papilloma viruses produce proteins capable of downregulating p53 protein. Natural killer cells, cytokines and cell adhesion molecules may also collaborate in the development of tumor lesions. Natural killer cell adhesion to endothelial cells is facilitated by vascular endothelial growth factors and their activity is mediated through interleukin-2 (IL-2). Some tumoral cells, such as Kaposi's sarcoma spindle cells, depend on angiogenic factors for their proliferation (Ziegler 1990). They produce autocrine and paracrine angiogenic factors that induce the proliferation of other endothelial cells (Nakamura et al 1988). In HIV-positive patients, it has been postulated that one of these factors might be of retroviral origin (Gallo 1990). Some angiogenic factors may moreover facilitate lymphocyte recognition of angiogenic vessels, whereas others may protect vessels from cytotoxic lymphocytes (Melder et al 1996). Finally, it has been proposed that host–donor microchimerism might favor PTLD development (Nalesnik and Starzl 1997) and that microchimerism might be one explanation for the preferential occurrence of malignancies in the transplanted graft itself, arising from donor cells (Goldstein et al 1996). However, an alternative pathogenetic role for the local effect of cytokines or other tumor-promoting interactions (T lymphocytes and vessels) in the site of the grafted organ cannot be excluded.

Another possible predisposing role for cancer development may be played by the prolonged uremic status before transplantation. Some tumors, such as hepatic, thyroid or colon adenocarcinomas, are as frequent among dialysis patients as in transplanted population (Brunner et al 1988, 1995), and other malignancies also, such as anogenital cancers, seem to have a similar incidence among dialysis patients and transplant recipients (Fairley et al 1994). Birkeland (1998) reported a series of possible predisposing factors for the development of tumors in patients with end-stage renal disease: (1) uremia, which may be considered a state of immune deficiency (Kramer et al 1985); (2) a possible linkage between kidney disease and the risk of cancer; (3) previous immunosuppression used to treat many kidney diseases such as primary glomerulonephritis, lupus nephritis, vasculitis, mixed connective tissue diseases, etc.; and (4) the prolonged use of potentially oncogenic drugs, such as analgesic drugs (phenacetin). Further etiologic factors include age, environmental factors, genetic predisposition and duration of the allograft. The risk of tumors is related to the age of the recipient: the older the age the higher the risk of tumor (Montagnino et al 1996). Aging is characterized by a reduced reparative cell proliferation and DNA repair after exposure to environmental factors, such as ultraviolet radiation (Wei et al 1993; Moriwaki et al 1996). Moreover, the longer the exposition to oncogenic factors (iatrogenic and viral) the higher the probability of developing a neoplasia. Some tumors may have a genetic and ethnic diversity. Some HLA antigens, such as B27 and DR7, have been found to be associated with a higher incidence of skin cancer in organ transplant recipients (Bouwes-Bavinck et al 1991). Kaposi's sarcoma is more frequent in Mediterranean countries (Qunibi et al 1988; Montagnino et al 1994) and in first and second generation immigrants coming from those countries (AGR Sheil, personal communication). On the other hand, environmental factors might be equally important in the induction of Kaposi's sarcoma, since its increased incidence among Mediterranean transplant recipients might be related to the increased incidence of HHV-8 infection in these populations (Parravicini et al 1997).

Lymphomas

Non-Hodgkin's lymphomas (NHL) are the second most common malignancies after skin and lip cancers, while Hodgkin's disease is only slightly more common in transplanted patients than in the general population (Birkeland et al 1995). The development of PTLD may be preceded by the appearance of a monoclonal Ig peak. In liver transplant recipients 23% of patients showing a persistent monoclonal band developed a

PTLD after 3.8 months on average (Pageaux et al 1998). On the other hand, most kidney transplant recipients showing monoclonal peaks did not develop any PTLD after years of follow-up (Radl et al 1985).

The incidence of PTLD varies according to the organ transplanted, being 1.4–2.5% among adult kidney transplant recipients, 2.1–2.8% in liver, 1.8–6.3% in heart and 4.5–10% in lung transplant recipients (Starzl et al 1984; Leblond et al 1995; Walker et al 1995; Swinnen 1997). Heart and lung allograft recipients are indeed usually treated with a stronger immunosuppression (Penn 1995a). In a report of the Transplant Collaborative Study (Opelz and Henderson 1993) on 452 141 renal transplant patients followed for at least 1 year after transplantation, the incidence of PTLD was 224/100 000 in the first year, 54/100 000 in the second year, then remaining elevated through the sixth year (31/100 000). The incidence of NHL in the normal population was of 27/100 000. A clear increase in PTLD was observed in patients who received antilymphocyte globulins or OKT3 monoclonal antibodies (Swinnen et al 1990).

Epstein–Barr virus has been demonstrated by DNA hybridization studies in biopsy specimens from patients with PTLD (Saemundsen et al 1981). B cells acutely infected by EBV express about 90 transformation-associated viral genes which may serve as targets for the immune system. Acute infection is kept under control by natural killer (NK) cells and by EBV-specific $CD4^+$ or $CD8^+$ cytotoxic T lymphocytes (CTL). Latently infected B cells express only a limited number of genes: EBV nuclear antigen 1 (EBNA) and latent membrane protein 2 (LMP-2). This restricted gene expression is a mechanism through which the virus evades host responses. Moreover, EBNA-1 is required for the viral DNA to maintain itself in actively dividing lymphocytes and can reduce the surface expression of MHC class I and adhesion molecules, while LMP-2 allows the virus to limit its gene expression in the latency phase (Cohen 1997). These latently infected B lymphocytes are immortalized through the production of an EBV-encoded gene, BCRF1 which has more than 80% amino acid identity with IL-10 (Moore et al 1990), which inhibits the synthesis of interferon-γ (IFN-γ) by lymphocytes and NK cells. The inhibition of IFN-γ can favor the outgrowth of EBV-transformed B cells. All these factors impair the ability of the immune system to eliminate the virus and lead to the development of polyclonal polymorphic hyperplasia that may evolve into a more malignant monoclonal tumor.

Of interest, the incidence of PTLD is increased 7–10-fold in patients who had symptomatic cytomegalovirus (CMV) disease. In addition, EBV replication is regularly observed in patients with CMV infection (Tolkoff-Rubin and Rubin 1998). In CsA-treated patients the incidence of PTLD is related to the doses of CsA (Calne et al 1981; Gaya et al 1995). The addition of azathioprine to full doses of CsA may increase the risk of lymphoma (Wilkinson et al 1989). While the risk of PTLD development with tacrolimus seems to be comparable with that observed with CsA in some series (Armitage et al 1993), Cox et al (1995) reported a 2.9% prevalence of PTLD after liver transplantation in CsA-treated children, which increased to 19% in those who received tacrolimus, similar to the 22% incidence in the series by Reding et al (1994) in tacrolimus treated pediatric liver transplant recipients. A peculiar feature of PTLD is the

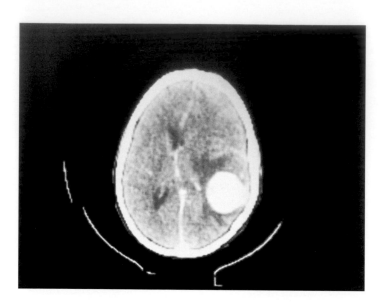

Figure 15.1. Cerebral right parietal lymphoma in a 26-year-old woman transplanted 4 years earlier. The mass, revealed by contrast medium, displaces lateral ventricula.

high incidence in the pediatric population, where PTLD represent 53% of malignancies, while in adults, PTLD represent 15% of neoplasias (Penn 1998b). The increased incidence of PTLD in the pediatric population has been attributed to the higher rate of primary EBV infection after transplantation (Dror et al 1999) and to the higher amount of lymphoid tissue than in adults.

After the introduction of CsA, the pattern of distribution of lesions has changed, with a higher extranodal involvement than in general population (Penn and First 1986). About 70% of PTLD occur in extranodal localizations (Penn 1998a), particularly in the liver, lungs, central nervous system (CNS), bowel, kidneys and spleen. Central nervous system involvement is associated with lymphoid infiltration in other organs in 10–15% of cases, while in 12–14% of cases brain (Figure 15.1) is the only involved site versus a 1–2% prevalence of unique CNS localization in the general population. In 12–23% of cases the kidney is affected by lymphomatous cells, which may erroneously be misinterpreted as rejection infiltrates. The clinical presentation is variable (Table 15.4). In some cases lymphoma presents as a benign infectious mononucleosis-like syndrome. Sometimes the patient complains of progressive weight loss. In other cases, the presentation is dramatic, because of intestinal perforation. Posttransplantation lymphoproliferative diseases may involve multiple organs or cause extranodal masses in the brain, gastrointestinal system (Figure 15.2) or in lungs (Figure 15.3). About 85% of lymphomas are of B cell lineage. Morphological classification has defined three main features for PTLD: (1) polymorphic diffuse B cell hyperplasia, characterized by the presence of differentiated plasmacytes and by the absence of atypia or necrosis; (2) polyclonal polymorphic B cell

Presentation	Percentage (%)
Clinical symptoms	
Fever	52
Lymphoadenopathy	28
Tonsillitis	28
Intestinal perforation	16
Weight loss	8
Localization	
Multiple organs	51
Small intestine	47
Large bowel	6
Brain	22–27
CNS only	12
Other organs	10
Lungs	15–38
Kidney	12–23

Table 15.4. Clinical presentation of posttransplant lymphoproliferative disorders

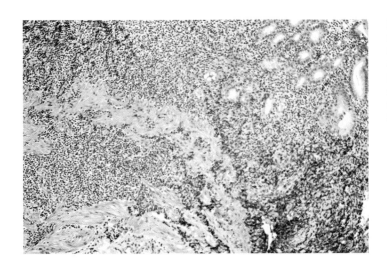

Figure 15.2. Marginal zone extranodal lymphoma (MALT-associated) localized to the antral gastric region. Observe the infiltration through the muscolaris mucosae. (Courtesy of Professor R Buffa, University of Milan.)

lymphomas, characterized by nuclear atypia of the large cells and extensive necrosis; and (3) monoclonal polymorphic B cell lymphomas (Table 15.5). While polymorphic lesions may be polyclonal, monomorphic lesions are always monoclonal (Nalesnik et al

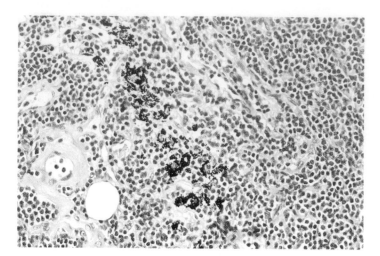

Figure 15.3. Low-grade, non-Hodgkin's B lymphoma in lung parenchyma. The general architecture is completely substituted by proliferation of lymphoid infiltrate. (Courtesy of Professor R Buffa, University of Milan.)

Polymorphic diffuse B cell hyperplasia (retention of the underlying architecture)

    Affects mostly children and adolescents

    Develops shortly after transplantation

    Is polyclonal

    Multiple EBV infections

    Good prognosis

    Often regresses after stopping immunosuppression

Polyclonal polymorphic B cell lymphomas (obliteration of the underlying architecture)

    Extranodal diffusion

    Mean age 40 years

    Develops shortly after transplantation

    Polyclonal or monoclonal

    Single EBV infection

Monoclonal polymorphic B cell lymphomas (architecture similar to usual lymphoma)

    Frequent in lymph nodes, but also extranodal

    Mean age 55 years

    Develops late after transplantation

    Always monoclonal

    Single EBV infection

Table 15.5. Categories of posttransplant lymphoproliferative disorders

Early lesions

    Reactive plasmacytic hyperplasia

    Infectious mononucleosis-like

Polymorphic PTLD

    Polyclonal

    Monoclonal

Monomorphic PTLD

    B cell lymphoma

        (1) Diffuse large-cell lymphoma (immunoblastic, centroblastic, anaplastic)

        (2) Burkitt's/Burkitt's-like lymphoma

    T cell lymphoma

        (1) Peripheral T cell lymphoma, unspecified type (usually large-cell)

        (2) Anaplastic large-cell lymphoma (t or null)

        (3) Other types (e.g. T-NK)

Other

    T cell-rich/Hodgkin's disease-like large B cell lymphoma

    Plasmacytoma-like

    Myeloma

Table 15.6. Categories of posttransplant lymphoproliferative disorders according to the Society for Hematopathology Workshop (Harris et al 1997)

1988; Whiting and Hanto 1998), although this has been recently challenged (Dror et al 1999). Less frequent are Hodgkin's lymphomas and T cell lymphomas. Classification of PTLD has been reviewed by the Society for Hematopathology in a recent workshop (Harris et al 1997; Table 15.6).

Whiting and Hanto (1998) suggested that all patients with PTLD should be determined for the clonality of lymphoproliferation through cell typing of surface and cytoplasmic immunoglobulins, cytogenetic analysis of metaphase preparations, immunoglobulin gene rearrangement analysis by blot hybridization and analysis of tandem repeats of EBV genomes. Clonality is an important prognostic factor, since polyclonal lesions respond better to treatment. Also, clonal cytogenetic abnormalities (gene rearrangements) revealed by metaphase examination of biopsy specimens (Hanto et al 1989) may disclose malignant transformation of benign polyclonal B cell proliferation into malignant monoclonal lymphoma.

T cell lymphomas represent only 12–14% of PTLD in transplanted patients, with a high mortality rate and a rapid onset after transplantation, despite reduction in immunosuppression (Van Gorp et al 1994).

Therapy

A sequential treatment approach has been suggested, according to the stage of the disease (Davis et al 1998; Whiting and Hanto 1998; Table 15.7). Polymorphic diffuse B cell hyperplasia still seems dependent upon active viral replication. In this case, the use of acyclovir or valacyclovir, which inhibit EBV DNA replication, may be sufficient to treat the disease. However, acyclovir has no effect on latent EBV genome in nonproducer cell lines (Hanto et al 1982): EBV replication in these cells occurs only during host cell proliferation and depends on host DNA polymerase and is presumably unaffected by acyclovir (Birkeland et al 1999). In these cases, as well in cases with cytogenetic abnormalities, reduction or withdrawal of immunosuppression is the first therapeutical step (Swinnen et al 1995). This maneuver may lead to regression of PTLD in 25–42% of cases (Starzl et al 1984). A second approach is the introduction of interferon-α 2b, which is capable of increasing the activity of cytotoxic T lymphocytes against EBV. Interferon-α 2b does not increase infections, but may expose to an increased risk of rejection. Interferon-α gives a rapid response—within 3 weeks in approximately 50% of patients (Davis et al 1998)—so enabling decisions about alternative treatments to be made quickly. Chemotherapy with various schemes is indicated when interferon-α 2b fails or when the disease has a rapid progression. Chemotherapy associated with radiation therapy or with resection of localized disease plus withdrawal of immunosuppression is mandatory in patients with monoclonal lesions containing clonal cytogenetic abnormalities in most cells. With this sequential approach, up to 76% of patients have been successfully treated in one series (Davis at al 1998), while in a pediatric series (Dror et al 1999), up to 80% of patients, including those with monomorphic or monoclonal lesions, achieved complete or partial remission without receiving systemic chemotherapy. Alternative treatments with anti-B cell antibody therapy such as anti-CD21 plus anti-CD24 antibodies (Fischer et al 1991) or anti-CD38 antibodies (Antoine et al 1996) have been of some value in patients with polyclonal tumors unable to undergo a reduction in immunosuppression, but are not effective in patients with monoclonal lymphoma.

As a conclusion, it seems that a high percentage of PTLD occurring in patients treated with cyclosporine may be prevented through the use of antiviral agents, such as acyclovir, valacyclovir or ganciclovir or may undergo resolution by stopping immunosuppression and adding interferon-α, sometimes without subsequent rejection of the grafts, in contrast to the lethal course in the absence of immunosuppression withdrawal (Starzl et al 1984).

(1) Stop immunosuppression and antiviral treatment
(2) Interferon-α
(3) Chemotherapy and/or radiation therapy and/or resection of localized mass
(4) Anti-B cell antibody treatment

Table 15.7. Possible sequential treatment approach in patients with PTLD

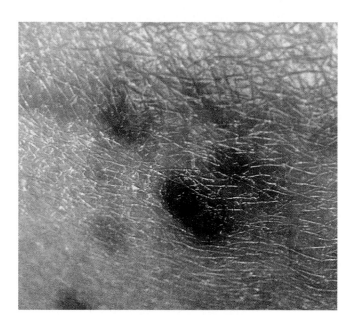

Figure 15.4. Nodular Kaposi's sarcoma: the elementary lesions consist of violaceous nodules, elevated upon the skin surface.

Kaposi's sarcoma

Kaposi's sarcoma (KS) is a multicentric vascular tumor, probably of viral etiology. Identification of herpes virus-like DNA sequences has been documented in AIDS-associated KS lesions (Chang et al 1994). A study in healthy blood donors revealed a positivity for HHV-8 in about 4% of cases, which turned out to increase to 100% in transplant recipients with KS (Gao et al 1996). In another study (Parravicini et al 1997), most transplant patients who developed KS were found to be infected by HHV-8 before transplantation, suggesting that in most cases, KS was due to viral reactivation.

Kaposi's sarcoma is characterized by an angioproliferation of the upper dermis constituted by a mixed cellular population, comprising infiltrating lymphocytes, proliferating fibroblasts, endothelial cells and characteristic eosinophilic 'spindle cells.' It can manifest with papular or nodular red-bluish cutaneous lesions (Figure 15.4). Lesions may be single (Figure 15.5), or may occur both in the skin and in the oropharyngeal mucosa and, in its more severe manifestations, also in the visceral mucosae. About 27% of patients with visceral localization of KS may not display any cutaneous lesions, but in 13% the presence of lesions in the oral mucosa may favor the diagnosis.

Kaposi's sarcoma is a rare tumor, representing 0.01–0.06% of tumors in the general population, but its prevalence increases with immunosuppression, being higher among transplant recipients treated with CsA than in those given Aza and steroids. Kaposi's sarcoma shows a geographic distribution, with a prevalence of 4–7.8% among Arab and Mediterranean renal transplant patients (Akhtar et al 1984; Qunibi et al 1988) and of 0.4% among transplanted patients from northern and western countries (Odajnyk and

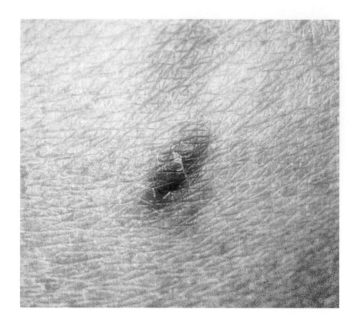

Figure 15.5. Epidemic-like type of Kaposi's sarcoma: this kind of lesion is frequently observed in CsA-treated patients. Lesions consist of oval and fusiform maculae, distributed along the lines of skin cleavage. A single lesion may be present.

Muggia 1985). In Italian renal transplant recipients with more than 6 months of follow-up, there was a prevalence of 1.6% and an incidence of 22.1/100 000 patients/year versus an incidence of 0.16/100 000 patients/year in a genetically comparable control population (Montagnino et al 1994). The risk ratio for KS among 6596 Australian recipients of cadaver donor renal allografts has been calculated to be more than 1000 (Sheil et al 1993), while in an Italian experience the risk ratio for KS was 224.7 (Montagnino et al 1994). The male/female ratio, which is usually 9–15:1 in the general population, decreases after transplantation to 2.2–3:1. The age of onset is much younger among transplant recipients than in the general population. Kaposi's sarcoma generally occurs after a short period since transplantation (38.7 ± 38.3 months in our series), usually earlier in CsA-treated than in azathioprine-treated patients. In its disseminated form or with a mucovisceral involvement, KS is generally more aggressive than the forms with an exclusive cutaneous localization. About 53% of patients with isolated cutaneous lesions can heal versus 27% of patients with mixed lesions. The development of disseminated mucovisceral lesions implies a high risk of death. Thus, transplanted patients with suspect cutaneous lesions should be seen by a dermatologist in order to have an early diagnosis and prompt therapeutic measures (Montagnino and Bencini 1994).

Therapy

The role of immunosuppressive treatment in both the induction and management of KS is of paramount importance. The only risk factors for KS development in a series of 854 kidney transplant recipients were CsA treatment and 10 or more high-dose intravenous methylprednisolone pulses for treatment of rejection (Montagnino et al 1996). According to Penn (1980), approximately 25% of patients with nonvisceral lesions have complete or partial remission of KS following cessation or reduction of immunosuppressive therapy. In a single center series (Montagnino et al 1994), the prognosis was even better as 11 of 13 patients had a regression or complete healing of their lesions after reduction of immunosuppression and 9 of 13 (69%) maintained their graft function after a mean follow-up of 41.9 ± 21.7 months since Kaposi's sarcoma diagnosis and immunosuppressive therapy withdrawal (mean plasma creatinine at the end of follow-up: 1.8 ± 0.4 mg/dl). Therefore, this maneuver should be tempted as a first-line treatment in all cases. Circumscribed lesions usually stop or heal simply by reducing CsA dosage. More widespread and severe cutaneous lesions, in the presence of oral mucosa localizations, require complete CsA withdrawal. The reintroduction of immunosuppression at low doses should be cautious and only after healing has been documented. In fact, the reintroduction or the increase of immunosuppressive therapy can result in a fatal reactivation with visceral involvement after a partial regression of KS.

The recent introduction of new antiviral agents has prompted new therapeutic options in these patients. Adefovir, an acyclic nucleoside phosphonate (ANP) with both antiretrovirus and antiherpes virus activity, was shown to effectively block HHV-8 DNA replication in vitro (Neyts and De Clercq 1997). The ANP analog cidofovir and phosphonoformic acid (PFA-foscarnet) are the two other agents which have shown potent antiHHV-8 activity, both in vitro (Medveczky et al 1997) and in vivo (Robles et al 1999), while ganciclovir showed an intermediate strength against HHV-8. However, the clinical relevance of these new agents in the prevention and treatment of KS still requires confirmation in prospective trials (Boulanger 1999).

In order to exclude visceral involvement, a complete staging should be performed, through a chest radiograph examination, abdominal ultrasound scan or computed tomography, gastroscopy and colonoscopy. In case of visceral lesions, immunosuppressive agents should be gradually withdrawn, while maintaining only small doses of prednisone. Interferon should be started in cases which do not respond to cessation of immunosuppression. Vincristine, vinblastine, bleomycin and doxorubicin, alone or in combination, have also been used with comparable efficacy (Shepherd et al 1997) and their use should be restricted to very aggressive mucovisceral lesions, not responsive to both immunosuppression withdrawal and local radiotherapy.

Cutaneous cancers

These lesions are also described in Chapter 17. We will only comment here on their incidence in the transplant population and on their etiology. Cutaneous cancers represent the most common type of neoplasia after organ transplantation (36% according to the CTTR), being more common in countries with a high sunlight exposition and in patients with light complexion.

A number of factors may predispose to skin cancer (Table 15.8). The ultraviolet component of sunlight may modify the DNA of keratinocytes and may favor a cellular proliferation by interfering with the local immune response. Ultraviolet B radiation is mostly responsible for the formation of DNA lesions, through the production of pyrimidine dimers and pyrimidine (6–4) pyrimidone photoproducts (Freeman et al 1989; Mitchell and Nairn 1989), which can lead to mutations if incorrectly repaired (Mitchell and Nairn 1989; Moriwaki et al 1996). The effect of sunlight is enhanced by immunosuppressive therapy, through a depletion of cells committed to immune surveillance against tumor (Galvao et al 1998). Moreover, azathioprine may exert an additive action through the inhibition of DNA synthesis and through the strong photo-oxidative properties of its two major metabolites, 6-mercaptopurine and methyl-nitro-thio-imidazole, which may cause photosensitization. In areas with reduced sunlight exposure, transplantation increases the occurrence of cutaneous tumors by 4–7 times versus an increase of 21 times in southern countries (Hardie et al 1980). In some populations an increased frequency of cutaneous neoplasias has been found among patients homozygous for HLA-B27 and HLA-DR7 while the risk for skin cancer is reduced in graft recipients homozygous for HLA-A11 (Bouwes-Bavinck et al 1991). Viruses may be another etiologic factor: cutaneous tumors may develop from papilloma virus-induced warts, through a neoplastic transformation induced by sunlight exposure and prolonged immunosuppression (Koranda et al 1974; Mullen et al 1976). Squamous cell carcinomas are the most frequent lesions in the transplanted population, with an increase of 40–250 times the reported incidence in the general population. Cancer is often preceded by precancerous lesions such as keratoacanthosis, epidermodysplasia verruciformis or actinic porokeratosis, or by extensive atrophic cutaneous areas. These lesions should therefore be accurately evaluated by a dermatologist in order to prevent their evolution into malignant lesions. Especially in patients under long-term immunosuppression, sun exposure of areas affected by these precancerous conditions should be strongly contraindicated. These lesions may appear in multiple parts of the body, either exposed to sunlight or not. While in the general population cancerous lesions develop around the seventh to eighth decade of life, in transplant recipients they tend to appear around the fourth to fifth decade, with a more aggressive evolution than in the general population. According to the CTTR, lymph nodal metastases are observed in 5.8% of cutaneous neoplasias, 75% of them being due to squamous cell carcinomas. Moreover, 5.1% of patients with cutaneous tumors die, 60% of deaths being caused by squamous cell carcinoma, only 33% by malignant melanomas.

Basal cell carcinomas are the second most frequent cutaneous neoplastic lesions in

Ultraviolet B radiation

Modification of keratinocyte DNA. Production of pyrimidine dimers and pyrimidine–pyrimidone photoproducts causing mutations

Immunosuppressive therapy

Depletion of cells committed in immune surveillance

Azathioprine

Inhibition of DNA synthesis. Photosensitization through 6-mercaptopurine and methyl-nitro-thio-imidazole

Genetic factors

Increased frequency in patients homozygous for HLA-B27 and HLA-DR7. Reduced frequency in patients homozygous for HLA-A11

Viruses

Papilloma virus-induced warts. Human herpes virus-8 (KS)

Predisposing cutaneous lesions

Keratoachanthosis, porokeratosis, epidermodysplasia verruciformis

Aging
Atrophic cutaneous areas

Table 15.8 Predisposing factors and mechanisms of induction of cutaneous cancers

transplanted patients, occurring 10 times more frequently than in the normal population. In normal subjects, basal cell carcinomas usually outnumber squamous cell carcinomas by 5:1, while in the transplant population the opposite has been observed (Penn 1990), with a squamous to basal cell carcinoma ratio of 1.8:1. In Milan, the incidence was 34/10 000 patients/year and the incidence of basal cell carcinoma was 19/10 000 patients/year. An age at transplantation greater than 40 years was the unique risk factor for the development of squamous cell carcinoma in our series, while no risk factor was observed for basal cell carcinoma development (Montagnino et al 1996).

Melanomas represent 5.3% of all skin cancers in transplant recipients (Penn 1994), occurring 1.7–5 times more frequently than in the general population (Sheil et al 1993; Birkeland et al 1995). While in the general population melanomas are rarely observed in youth, in the CTTR experience 54% of melanomas occurred in pediatric recipients, at a mean age of 12 years. Melanomas appear in mean 61 months after transplantation (Euvrard et al 1998) and usually have a poor prognosis, with a 24–30% mortality. A predisposing condition is represented by cutaneous nevi (Grob et al 1996). Melanomas occurring before transplantation have a recurrence rate of about 20%, even if the primary lesion appeared 10 years before grafting (Euvrard et al 1998). Unlike squamous cell and basal cell carcinomas, which are correlated with total cumulative exposure to ultraviolet radiation, melanomas are associated with intense intermittent sun exposure (Holman et al 1986; Bentham and Aase 1996, Gilchrest et al 1999), being most common in patients with indoor occupations who occasionally expose themselves to high sun radiation during vacations.

Therapy

Preventive measures are important. Transplant patients should be advised to avoid excessive sun exposure and to apply sun-protective lotions to the most exposed areas (forehead, neck, forearms, hands and shoulders). Most squamous and basal cell carcinomas usually heal after surgical removal. However, most patients with cutaneous neoplasias also display multiple precancerous lesions, which should be treated in order to prevent recurrence of carcinomas. Whenever possible, a gradual reduction of immunosuppression may be considered. Systemic retinoids may slow down the progression of dysplastic lesions to cancer (McKenna and Murphy 1999). Retinoids do not interfere with immunosuppression, but may be burdened by undesired untoward effects such as liver toxicity and hyperlipidemia and should be therefore prescribed only in cases of widespread precancerous lesions.

Renal carcinomas

Most renal carcinomas occur in the native kidneys, although about 9% of them may involve the transplanted kidney. Some 5–10% of renal neoplasias are carcinomas of the renal pelvis. According to the CTTR they represent 14% of all tumors (Penn 1995). This elevated prevalence may be explained by the high number of patients undergoing renal transplantation because of analgesic abuse nephropathy. Acquired cystic disease (ACD) of native kidneys is another predisposing factor for the development of renal carcinomas, being observed in up to 73% of patients with renal cell carcinoma (Kliem et al 1997). It is observed in 30–95% of patients undergoing regular dialytic treatment and is characterized by an incidence of neoplasias 30–40 times higher than in the general population. Some authors, however (Ishikawa 1992; Tajima et al 1998), reported a tendency of ACD to regress after renal transplantation.

Carcinomas of the vulva and perineum

According to the CTTR, these carcinomas occur at an earlier age than in the general population (42 versus 50–70 years). About one-third of patients have in situ lesions. The cancer is often preceded by condilomas or papilloma virus infections. These carcinomas may be multifocal, with involvement of the vulva and perineum, but also of the vagina and uterine cervix (Penn 1986). Carcinomas of the uterine cervix represent 11% of neoplasias among transplant recipients in the CTTR. Sillman et al (1984) reported an incidence of uterine neoplasias 14–16 times higher in transplant recipients than in the general population. This outlines the importance of an accurate gynecological screening in order to diagnose any precancerous lesion early.

A gynecological examination performed every 3 years is fundamental for an early diagnosis of papilloma virus infections and genital dysplasias. The visit should include a pap-test, a colposcopy and a histological evaluation of anogenital dysplastic lesions. Since a pap-test may give a high proportion of false-positive reactions, an annual colposcopy with epithelial dyeing with acetic acid and toluidine blue should be performed. All abnormal areas should be biopsied and the dysplastic or papilloma virus-infected areas should be treated with a laser vaporization or an electroresection or with 5-fluorouracyl topical ointments.

Miscellaneous tumors

A number of neoplasias (hepatomas, adenocarcinomas of the colon, histiocytomas, fibrosarcomas, mesotheliomas, etc.) have too low an incidence to be correctly evaluated from a statistical point of view. The Australian and New Zealand Registry reported an increased incidence of endocrinous carcinomas (289 times), leukemia (5.6 times), carcinomas of the digestive system (2.5 times) and respiratory system (2 times) as compared to the general population (Sheil et al 1993).

General recommendations

In order to reduce the increased risk of cancer in transplant recipients some guidelines should be followed. They include regular surveillance, dietetic measures, style of life and appropriate treatment of viral infections (Table 15.9).

PRE-EXISTING CANCERS

A recent review of the recurrence rates of 1297 pre-existing tumors in renal transplant recipients has been published by the CTTR (Penn 1997a). The recurrence rate was 21% for cancers treated before, and 33% for those treated after transplantation. Some tumors (incidental renal, uterine body, tumor of the testis, carcinoma of the cervix, thyroid) showed low recurrence rates (1–7%), other tumors (Hodgkin's lymphoma, Wilm's tumor, prostate carcinoma, melanoma) showed an intermediate recurrence rate (11–21%), while tumor of the breast, symptomatic renal carcinoma, cancer of the

Regular surveillance (once a year)
- Dermatological evaluation
- Gynecological evaluation (colposcopy)
- Prostatic evaluation (PSA, ultrasonography)
- Native kidney ultrasonography
- Occult blood in the stools

Life habits
- Stop smoking
- Minimize sun exposure
- Reduce the intake of fats
- Minimize salt-cured and smoked food
- Use alcohol in moderation
- Self-examination of breasts and testes
- Do not underevaluate febrile episodes (viral infections?)

Table 15.9. Main recommendations to a transplant recipient for prevention or early detection of cancers

bladder, nonmelanoma skin cancer and myeloma had a recurrence rate of 23%. Factors contributing to low recurrence rates were a favorable histology (in situ carcinomas or low-grade malignancy) and a long time interval between treatment of malignancy and transplantation (more than 5 years). In the tumors treated after transplantation, 39% of recurrences were from nonmelanoma skin cancers, followed by carcinoma of the prostate (12%), incidental renal carcinomas (8%) and symptomatic renal carcinoma (5%).

For cancers with a high recurrence rate, a waiting period of at least 5 years before transplantation is recommended, due to the possibility that immunosuppression may stimulate the growth of dormant metastases.

TRANSMISSION OF CANCER FROM DONORS

The CTTR recruited data on 270 patients who received organs from donors with malignancies (Penn 1997b). The most frequent neoplasms of the 163 studied cadaver donors were primary brain tumor (46 cases), carcinomas of the kidney (46 cases), lung (30), malignant melanoma (12), choriocarcinoma (6), hepatobiliary (5) and breast cancers (4). Of the 30 living donors studied, the most frequent tumors were: carcinomas of the kidney (9 cases), colon (4), cervix (3) and breast (3). A local spread of tumor was observed in six cases and distant metastases in 66 transplant recipients.

In case of malignancies confined to the allograft, prompt identification and excision of the lesion at the time of surgery has allowed no recurrence of malignancy after a mean follow-up of 79 months. In 12 other cases with no apparent tumor at harvesting, a transplant nephrectomy was performed after a mean of 3 months in 10 patients, with no recurrence in any recipient after a mean follow-up of 78 months.

Allograft nephrectomy, discontinuation of immunosuppression and local radiation therapy gave good results in most cases of local spread of tumor, while 67% of recipients with widespread metastases died of cancer and only 27% of them had complete remission following treatment.

Malignant melanomas and choriocarcinomas are the most dangerous donor neoplasms, with high rates of distant metastases and mortality in the recipient. Primary brain tumors and renal carcinomas also have high rates of transmission and of distant metastases. For this reason, donors with intracranial bleeding, but no evidence of hypertension, intracranial aneurysm or arteriovenous malformation, should be carefully screened in order to exclude the presence of cerebral metastases from occult primary neoplasias. Moreover, donors with brain cancers who have received radiotherapy, chemotherapy, craniotomies, ventriculoatrial or ventriculoperitoneal shunts should be used with great caution, because of the possibility of dissemination deriving from such maneuvers. Measurement of beta-human chorionic gonadotropin is useful in order to exclude the presence of choriocarcinomas in female donors with menstrual irregularities following pregnancy or abortion.

Transmission of HHV-8 virus from the donor with potential risk of Kaposi's sarcoma for the recipient has been recently demonstrated (Regamey et al 1998).

REFERENCES

Akhtar M, Bunuan H, Ashraf M, Godwin JT (1984) Kaposi's sarcoma in renal transplant recipients. *Cancer* 53:258–266.

Antoine C, Garnier JL, Duboust A et al (1996) Successful treatment of posttransplant lymphoproliferative disorder with renal graft preservation by monoclonal antibody therapy. *Transplant Proc* 28:2825–2826.

Arendt MJ, Benton EC, McLaren KF et al (1997) Renal allograft recipients with high susceptibility to cutaneous malignancy have an increased prevalence of human papillomavirus DNA in skin tumors and a greater risk of anogenital malignancy. *Br J Cancer* 75:722–728.

Armitage JM, Fricker FJ, DelNido P et al (1993) A decade (1982 to 1992) of pediatric cardiac transplantation and the impact of FK 506 immunosuppression. *J Thorac Cardiovasc Surg* 105:464–472.

Bavinck JNB, Berkhout RJM (1997) HPV infections and immunosuppression. *Clin Dermatol* 15:427–437.

Bentham G, Aase A (1996) Incidence of malignant melanoma of the skin in Norway, 1955–1989: associations with solar ultraviolet radiation, income and holidays abroad. *Int J Epidemiol* 25:1132–1138.

Birkeland SA (1998) Malignancies occurring de novo after transplantation. *Curr Opin Organ Transplant* 3:82–89.

Birkeland SA, Bendtzen K (1996) Interleukin-10 and Epstein–Barr virus induced post transplant lymphoproliferative disorder. *Transplantation* 61:1425–1426.

Birkeland SA, Storm HH, Lamm LU et al (1995) Cancer risk after renal transplantation in the Nordic countries, 1964–1986. *Int J Cancer* 60:183–189.

Birkeland SA, Bendtzen K, Møller B et al (1999) Interleukin-10 and posttransplant lymphoproliferative disorder after kidney transplantation. *Transplantation* 67:876–881.

Boulanger E (1999) Human herpesvirus 8 (HHV8). II. Pathogenic role and sensitivity to antiviral drugs. *Ann Biol Clin* 57:19–28.

Bouwes-Bavinck JN, Vermeer BJ, Van der Woude FJ et al (1991) Relation between skin cancer and HLA antigens in renal transplant recipients. *N Engl J Med* 325:843–848.

Brunner FP, Fassbinder W, Broyer C (1988) Combined report on regular dialysis and transplantation in Europe. XVIII 1987. *Nephrol Dial Transplant* 2(Suppl 1):5–32.

Brunner FP, Landais P, Selwood NH on behalf of the EDTA-ERA Registry Committee (1995) Malignancies after renal transplantation: the EDTA-ERA registry experience. *Nephrol Dial Transplant* 10 (Suppl 1):74–80.

Calne RY, Rolles K, White DJG et al (1981) Cyclosporin-A in clinical organ grafting. *Transplant Proc* 13:349–358.

Chang Y, Cesarman E, Pessin MS et al (1994) Identification of herpes-virus-like DNA sequences in AIDS-associated Kaposi's sarcoma. *Science* 266:1865–1869.

Cherney BW, Bhatia KG, Sgadari C et al (1997) Role of the p53 tumor suppressor gene in the tumorgenicity of Burkitt's lymphoma cells. *Cancer Res* 57:2508–2515.

Chetty R, Biddolph S, Kaklamanis L et al (1996) Bcl-2 proteins strongly expressed in posttransplant lymphoproliferative disorders. *J Pathol* 180:254–258.

Cockburn IT, Krupp P (1989) The risk of neoplasms in patients treated with cyclosporine. *J Autoimmun* 2:723–731.

Cohen JI (1997) Epstein–Barr virus and the immune system. Hide and seek. *JAMA* 278:510–513.

Cox KL, Lawrence-Miyasaki LS, Garcia-Kennedy R et al (1995) An increased incidence of Epstein–Barr virus infection and lymphoproliferative disorder in young children on FK506 after liver transplantation. *Transplantation* 59:524–529.

Davis CL, Wood BL, Sabath DE et al (1998) Interferon-α treatment of posttransplant lymphoproliferative disorder in recipients of solid organ transplants. *Transplantation* 66:1770–1779.

Dror Y, Greenberg M, Taylor G et al (1999) Lymphoproliferative disorders after organ transplantation in children. *Transplantation* 67:990–998.

Eidt S, Bayerdörffer E, Stolte M (1995) Treat the infection and cure the cancer. *Lancet* 345:874–875.

Euvrard S, Kanitakis J, Pouteil-Noble C (1998) Skin cancers in organ transplant recipients. *Curr Opin Organ Transplant* 3:96–104.

Fairley CK, Sheil AGR, McNeil JJ et al (1994) The risk of anogenital malignancies in dialysis and transplant patients. *Clin Nephrol* 41:101–105.

Fischer A, Blanche S, Le Bidois J et al (1991) Anti B cell monoclonal antibodies in the treatment of severe B cell lymphoproliferative syndrome following bone marrow and organ transplantation. *N Engl J Med* 324:1451–1456.

Fisher DE (1994) Apoptosis and cancer. *Cell* 8:539–542.

Freeman SE, Hacham H, Gange RW et al (1989) Wavelength dependence of pyrimidine dimer formation in DNA of human skin irradiated in situ with ultraviolet light. *Proc Natl Acad Sci USA* 86:5605–5609.

Gallo RC (1990) Mechanisms of disease induction by HIV. *J AIDS* 3:380–389.

Galvao MM, Sotto MN, Kihara SM et al (1988) Lymphocyte subsets and Langerhans cells in sun-protected and sun-exposed skin of immunosuppressed renal allograft recipients. *J Am Acad Dermatol* 38:38–44.

Gao SJ, Kingsley L, Li M et al (1996) KSHV antibodies among Americans, Italians and Ugandans with and without Kaposi's sarcoma. *Nat Med* 8:925–928.

Gaya SBM, Rees AJ, Lechler RI et al (1995) Malignant disease in patients with long-term renal transplants. *Transplantation* 59:1705–1709.

Gibson GE, O'Grady A, Kay EW et al (1997) p53 tumor suppressor gene protein expression in premalignant and malignant skin lesions of kidney transplant recipients. *J Am Acad Dermatol* 36:924–931.

Gilchrest BA, Eller MS, Geller AC, Yaar M (1999) The pathogenesis of melanoma induced by ultraviolet radiation. *N Engl J Med* 340:1341–1348.

Gleichmann E, Gleichmann H, Schwartz RS (1975) Immunologic induction of malignant lymphoma: identification of donor and host tumors in the graft-versus-host model. *J Natl Cancer Inst* 54:107–116.

Goldstein DJ, Austin JHM, Zuech N et al (1996) Carcinoma of the lung after heart transplantation. *Transplantation* 62:772–775.

Grob JJ, Bastuji-Garin S, Vaillant R et al (1996) Excess of nevi related to immunodeficiency: a study in HIV-infected patients and renal transplant recipients. *J Invest Dermatol* 107:694–697.

Hanto DW, Frizzera G, Gajl-Peczalska KJ et al (1982) Epstein–Barr virus induced B-cell lymphoma after renal transplantation. Acyclovir therapy and transition from a polyclonal to a monoclonal B-cell proliferation. *N Engl J Med* 306:913–918.

Hanto DW, Birkenbach H, Frizzera G et al (1989) Confirmation of the heterogeneity of posttransplant Epstein–Barr virus associated B-cell proliferations by immunoglobulin gene rearrangement analyses. *Transplantation* 47:458–464.

Hardie IR, Strong RW, Hartley LJ et al (1980) Skin cancer in caucasian renal allograft recipients living in a subtropical climate. *Surgery* 87:177–183.

Harris NL, Ferry JA, Swerdlow SH (1997) Post transplant lymphoproliferative disorders: summary of Society for Hematopathology Workshop. *Semin Diagn Pathol* 14:8–14.

Harwood AR, Osoba D, Hofstader S et al (1979) Kaposi's sarcoma in recipients of renal transplants. *Am J Med* 76:759–765.

Ho M, Jaffe R, Miller G et al (1988) The frequency of Epstein–Barr virus infection and associated lymphoproliferative syndrome after transplantation and its manifestation in children. *Transplantation* 45:719–727.

Hojo M, Morimoto T, Maluccio M et al (1999) Cyclosporine induces cancer progression by a cell-autonomous mechanism. *Nature* 397:530–534.

Holman CDJ, Armstrong BK, Heenan PJ (1986) Relationship of cutaneous malignant melanoma to individual sunlight-exposure habits. *J Natl Cancer Inst* 76:403–414.

Ishikawa I (1992) Acquired cysts and neoplasms of the kidneys in renal allograft recipients. *Contrib Nephrol* 100:245–268.

Kinlen LJ (1985) Incidence of cancer in rheumatoid arthritis and other disorders after immunosuppressive therapy. *Am J Med* 78(Suppl 1A):44–49.

Klein G, Klein E (1977) Immune surveillance against virus-induced tumors and non-rejectability of spontaneous tumors: contrasting consequences of host versus tumor evolution. *Proc Natl Acad Sci USA* 74:2121–2125.

Kliem V, Kolditz M, Behrend M et al (1997) Risk of renal cell carcinoma after kidney transplantation. *Clin Transplant* 11:255–258.

Koranda FC, Dehmel EM, Kahn G, Penn I (1974) Cutaneous complications in immunosuppressed renal homograft recipients. *JAMA* 229:419–424.

Kramer P, Broyer M, Brunner FP et al (1985) Combined report on regular dialysis and transplantation in Europe, XIV 1983. *Proc Eur Dial Transplant Assoc* 21:2–65.

Leblond V, Sutton L, Dorent R et al (1995) Lymphoproliferative disorders after organ transplantation: a report of 24 cases observed in a single institution. *J Clin Oncol* 13:961–968.

London NJ, Farmey SM, Will EJ et al (1995) Risk of neoplasia in renal transplant patients. *Lancet* 346:403–406.

McKahnn CF (1969) Primary malignancy in patients undergoing immunosuppression for renal transplantation. *Transplantation* 8:209–212.

McKenna DB, Murphy GM (1999) Skin cancer chemophylaxis in renal transplant recipients. 5 years' experience using low-dose acitretin. *Br J Dermatol* 140:656–660.

Medveczky MM, Horvath E, Lund T, Medveczky PG (1997) In vitro antiviral drug sensitivity of the Kaposi's sarcoma-associated herpesvirus. *AIDS* 11:1327–1332.

Melder RJ, Koenig GC, Witwer BP et al (1996) During angiogenesis, vascular endothelial growth factor and basic fibroblast growth factor regulate natural killer cell adhesion to tumor endothelium. *Nat Med* 2:992–997.

Mitchell DL, Nairn RS (1989) The biology of the (6–4) photoproduct. *Photochem Photobiol* 49:805–819.

Montagnino G, Bencini PL (1994) Cutaneous and mucosal nodules in a transplant patient. *Nephrol Dial Transplant* 9:1503–1504.

Montagnino G, Bencini PL, Tarantino A et al (1994) Clinical features and course of Kaposi's sarcoma in kidney transplant patients: report of 13 cases. *Am J Nephrol* 14:121–126.

Montagnino G, Lorca E, Tarantino A et al (1996) Cancer incidence in 854 kidney transplant recipients from a single institution: comparison with normal population and with patients under dialytic treatment. *Clin Transplant* 10:461–469.

Moore KW, Vieira P, Fiorentino DF et al (1990) Homology of cytokine synthesis inhibitory factor (IL-10) to the Epstein–Barr virus gene BCRF1. *Science* 248:1230–1234.

Moore PS, Chang Y (1995) Detection of herpesvirus-like DNA sequences in Kaposi's sarcoma in patients with and without HIV infection. *N Engl J Med* 332:1181–1185.

Moriwaki S, Ray S, Tarone RE et al (1996) The effect of donor age on the processing of UV-damaged DNA by cultured human cells: reduced DNA repair capacity and increased DNA mutability. *Mutat Res* 364:117–123.

Mullen DL, Silverberg RG, Penn I, Hammond WS (1976) Squamous cell carcinoma of the skin and lip in renal homograft recipients. *Cancer* 37:729–734.

Nakamura S, Salahuddin SZ, Biberfeld P et al (1988) Kaposi's sarcoma cells: long-term culture with growth factor from retrovirus-infected CD4⁺ T-cells. *Science* 242:426–430.

Nalesnik MA, Starzl TE (1997) On the crossroad between tolerance and posttransplant lymphoma. *Curr Opin Organ Transplant* 2:30–35.

Nalesnik MA, Jaffe R, Starzl TE et al (1988) The pathology of posttransplant lymphoproliferative disorders occurring in the setting of cyclosporine A-prednisone immunosuppression. *Am J Pathol* 133:173–191.

Neyts J, De Clercq E (1997) Antiviral drug susceptibility of human herpesvirus 8. *Antimicrob Agents Chemother* 41:2754–2756.

Nunez G, Seto M, Seremetis S et al (1989) Growth- and tumor-promoting effects of deregulated Bcl-2 in human B-lymphoblastoid cells. *Proc Natl Acad Sci USA* 86:4589–4593.

Odajnyk C, Muggia FM (1985) Treatment of Kaposi's sarcoma: overview and analysis by clinical setting. *J Clin Oncol* 3:1277–1285.

Opelz G, Henderson R for the Collaborative Transplant Study (1993) Incidence of non-Hodgkin lymphoma in kidney and heart transplant recipients. *Lancet* 342:1514–1516.

Pageaux G-P, Bonnardet A, Picot M-C et al (1998) Prevalence of monoclonal immunoglobulins after liver transplantation. Relationship with posttransplant lymphoproliferative disorders. *Transplantation* 65:397–400.

Parravicini C, Olsen SJ, Capra M et al (1997) Risk of Kaposi's sarcoma-associated herpes virus transmission from donor allografts among Italian posttransplant Kaposi's sarcoma patients. *Blood* 1997,**90**:2826–2829.

Penn I (1980) Some contributions of transplantation to our knowledge of cancer. *Transplant Proc* **12**:676–680.

Penn I (1986) Cancers of anogenital region in renal transplant recipients. Analysis of 65 cases. *Cancer* **58**:611–616.

Penn I (1990) Cancers complicating organ transplantation. *N Engl J Med* **323**:1767–1769.

Penn I (1994) Occurrence of cancers in immunosuppressed organ transplant recipients. In: **Terasaki PI**, Cecka JM (eds). *Clinical Transplants 1994*. Los Angeles: UCLA Tissue Typing Laboratory, pp. 99–109.

Penn I (1995a) Malignancy after immunosuppressive therapy: how can the risk be reduced? *Clin Immunother* **9**:207–218.

Penn I (1995b) Primary kidney tumors before and after renal transplantation. *Transplantation* **59**:480–485.

Penn I (1996) Epidemiology of cancer in transplant patients. In: Touraine JL, Traeger J, Bétuel H et al (eds). *Cancer in Transplantation. Prevention and Treatment*. London: Kluwer Academic, pp. 3–15.

Penn I (1997a) Evaluation of transplant candidates with pre-existing malignancies. *Ann Transplant* **2**:14–17.

Penn I (1997b) Transmission of cancer from organ donors. *Ann Transplant* **2**:7–12.

Penn I (1998a) De novo cancers in organ allograft recipients. *Curr Opin Organ Transplant* **3**:188–196.

Penn I (1998b) The role of immunosuppression in lymphoma formation. *Semin Immunopathol* **20**:343–355.

Penn I (1999) Posttransplant malignancies. *Transplant Proc* **31**:1260 1262.

Penn I, First MR (1986) Development and incidence of cancer following cyclosporine therapy. *Transplantation* **18**:210–215.

Penn I, Hammond W, Brettschneider L, Starzl TE (1969) Malignant lymphomas in transplant patients. *Transplant Proc* **1**:106–112.

Qunibi W, Akhtar M, Sheth K et al (1988) Kaposi's sarcoma: the most common tumor after renal transplantation in Saudi Arabia. *Am J Med* **84**:225 232.

Radl J, Valentijn RM, Haaijman JJ, Paul LC (1985) Monoclonal gammopathies in patients undergoing immunosuppressive treatment after renal transplantation. *Clin Immunol Immunopathol* **37**:98–102.

Reding R, Wallemacq PE, Lamy ME et al (1994) Conversion from cyclosporine to FK506 for salvage of immunocompromised pediatric liver allografts. Efficacy, toxicity and dose regimen in 23 children. *Transplantation* **57**:93–100.

Regamey N, Tamm M, Wernli M et al (1998) Transmission of human herpesvirus 8 infection from renal transplant donors to recipients. *N Engl J Med* **138**:301–303.

Robles R, Lugo D, Gee L, Jacobson MA (1999) Effect of antiviral drugs used to treat cytomegalovirus end-organ disease on subsequent course of previously diagnosed Kaposi's sarcoma in patients with AIDS. *AIDS Res Hum Retroviruses* **20**:34–38.

Saemundsen AK, Purtilo DT, Sakamoto K et al (1981) Documentation of Epstein–Barr virus (EBV) infection in immunodeficient patients with life-threatening lymphoproliferative disease by EBV complementary RNA/DNA and viral DNA/DNA hybridization. *Cancer Res* **41**:4237–4242.

Shalling M, Ekman M, Kaaya E (1995) A role for a new herpes virus (KSHV) in different forms of Kaposi's sarcoma. *Nat Med* **1**:707–708.

Sheil AGR, Mahony JF, Horvath JS et al (1979) Cancer and survival after cadaveric donor renal transplantation. *Transplant Proc* **11**:1052–1054.

Sheil AGR, Disney APS, Mathew TH, Amiss N (1993) De novo malignancy emerges as a major cause of morbidity and late failure in renal transplantation. *Transplant Proc* **25**:1383–1384.

Sheil AGR, Disney APS, Mathew TH (1997) Lymphoma incidence, cyclosporine, and the evolution and major impact of malignancy following organ transplantation. *Transplant Proc* **29**:825–827.

Shepherd RA, Maher E, Cardella C et al (1997) Treatment of Kaposi's sarcoma after solid organ transplantation. *Clin Oncol* **15**:2371–2377.

Sillman F, Stank A, Sedlis A et al (1984) The relationship between human papilloma virus and lower genital intraepithelial neoplasia in immunosuppressed women. *Am J Obstet Gynecol* **150**:300–308.

Spector BD, Perry GSI, Kersey JH (1978) Genetically determined immunodeficiency disease (GDID) and malignancy. Report from the Immunodeficiency Cancer Registry. *Clin Immunol Immunopathol* **11**:12–29.

Starzl TE, Nalesnik MA, Porter KA et al (1984) Reversibility of lymphomas and lymphoproliferative lesions developing under cyclosporin-steroid therapy. *Lancet* **323**:583–587.

Swinnen LJ (1997) Treatment of organ transplant-related lymphoma. *Hematol Oncol Clin North Am* **11**:963–973.

Swinnen LJ, Costanzo-Nordin MR, Fisher SG et al (1990) Increased incidence of lymphoproliferative disorders after immunosuppression with the monoclonal antibody OKT3 in cardiac-transplant recipients. *N Engl J Med* **323**:1723–1728.

Swinnen LJ, Mullen GM, Carr TT (1995) Aggressive treatment for postcardiac transplant lymphoproliferation. *Blood* **86**:3333–3340.

Tajima E, Aikawa A, Ohana T et al (1998) Effect of kidney transplantation on acquired cystic lesions in native kidneys. *Transplant Proc* **30**:3060–3061.

Tolkoff-Rubin NE, Rubin RH (1998) Viral infections in organ transplantation. *Transplant Proc* **30**:2060–2063.

Van Gorp J, Doornewaard H, Verdonck LF et al (1994) Posttransplant T-cell lymphoma. Report of three cases and a review of the literature. *Cancer* **73**:3064–3072.

Vogt P, Frei U, Repp H et al (1990) Malignant tumors in renal transplant recipients receiving cyclosporin: survey of 598 first kidney transplantations. *Nephrol Dial Transplant* **5**:282–288.

Walker RC, Marshall WF, Stickler JG et al (1990) Pretransplant assessment of the risk of lymphoproliferative disorders. *Clin Infect Dis* **20**:1346–1353.

Wei Q, Matanoski GM, Farmer ER (1993) DNA repair and aging in basal cell carcinoma: a molecular epidemiology study. *Proc Natl Acad Sci USA* **90**:1614–1618.

Whiting JF, Hanto DW (1998) Cancer in recipients of organ allografts. In: Racusen LC, Solez K, Burdick JF (eds). *Kidney Transplant Rejection.* New York: Marcel Dekker, pp. 577–604.

Wilkinson AH, Smith JL, Hunsicker LG et al (1989) Increased frequency of posttransplant lymphomas in patients treated with cyclosporine, azathioprine and prednisone. *Transplantation* **47**:293–296.

Wotherspoon AC, Doglioni C, Diss TC et al (1993) Regression of primary low-grade B-cell gastric lymphoma of mucosa-associated lymphoid tissue type after eradication of *Helicobacter pylori*. *Lancet* **342**:575–577.

Ziegler JL (1990) Kaposi's sarcoma: introduction and overview. *J AIDS* **3**(Suppl):S1–S3.

zur Hausen H (1991) Virus in human cancers. *Science* **254**:1167–1173.

16 GASTROINTESTINAL, PANCREATIC AND HEPATOBILIARY COMPLICATIONS

GASTROINTESTINAL COMPLICATIONS

The incidence of gastrointestinal complications in renal transplantation is relatively high. These complications may be severe and may lead to graft loss and even patient death. The most frequent gastrointestinal complications in renal transplant recipients include oral lesions, esophagitis, peptic ulcer, colon hemorrhage or perforation and pancreatitis.

Oral lesions

Aphthous ulcers are frequent and often recur in the same patient. They are well defined circles and may be single or multiple. Ulcers can be found on all areas of the oral mucosa, except the hard palate, gingiva, and vermilion border.

Herpes simplex may cause cold sores or a gingivostomatitis often accompanied by fever, malaise and lymphadenopathy. Mucosal vesicles may be also caused by Varicella-zoster virus.

Leukoplakia, characterized by white plaques, and histologically by benign hyperkeratosis, may occur in any area of the mouth. This lesion may transform into squamous cell carcinoma. Oral warts are more frequent than in the normal population. Kaposi's sarcoma may present as a red, purple, brown or bluish macule or nodule (Figure 16.1).

Oral candidiasis is frequent in renal transplant recipients. It can be the result of the immunosuppression or may develop after vigorous antibiotic treatment. It may cause irregular or widespread erythema, erosive changes, or a typical creamy surface. Nystatin suspension or clotrimazole may be effective but should be administered several times a day with the contact time with the oral mucosa being short.

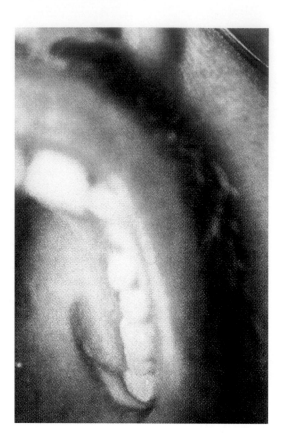

Figure 16.1. Oral Kaposi's sarcoma localized at palate.

Esophageal disorders

The commonest esophageal disorder in renal transplant recipients is represented by candidal esophagitis. This usually occurs within 6 months after transplantation and is particularly frequent in leukopenic or overimmunosuppressed patients as well as in patients debilitated from infections or other complications. A role for omeprazole has also been hypothesized (Mosimann 1993). Usually esophagitis is associated with candidal stomatitis and epiglottitis. Occasionally, esophagitis may be complicated by fungemia. Milder cases may be treated with local nystatin. Most patients respond to a treatment of intravenous amphotericin B for 2–6 days (Frick et al 1998).

Stomach and duodenum disorders

Peptic ulcer was a frequent cause of mortality until a few years ago, accounting for about 4% of deaths after transplantation (Kestens and Alexandre 1988). More recently, however, the prognosis has improved and mortality or graft loss due to peptic ulcer have

History of previous peptic ulcer
Elevated gastric acid secretion
H. pylori colonization
High-dose corticosteroids
Emotional stress
Cigarette smoking

Table 16.1.   Main etiologic factors for posttransplant peptic ulcer

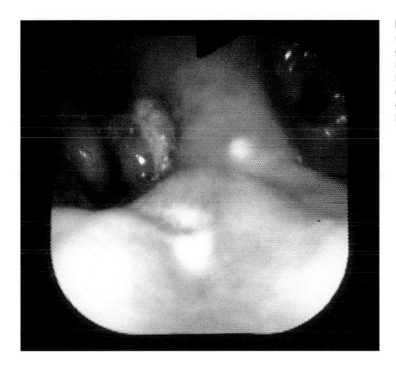

Figure 16.2.   Two peptic ulcers of the angulus at gastroscopy in a transplant recipient with a previous history of peptic ulcer during dialysis treatment. (Courtesy of Dr A Carrara, Ospedale Maggiore, Milan.)

become exceptional. Several factors may contribute to the development of posttransplant peptic ulcer disease (Table 16.1). An important risk factor is a history of peptic ulcer disease (Benoit et al 1993; Figure 16.2). In this regard, it must be remembered that although the prevalence of peptic ulcer is not increased in dialysis patients, almost 50% of them suffer from dyspepsia and show an elevated gastric acid secretion (Kang 1993). Moreover, about half of renal transplant recipients have *Helicobacter pylori* colonization of the stomach (Teenan et al 1993). The role of corticosteroids is still controversial (Conn and Poynard 1994) but it is likely that high doses of corticosteroids may have an ulcerogenic effect (Faro and Corry 1979), as several cases of hemorrhagic ulcers

645

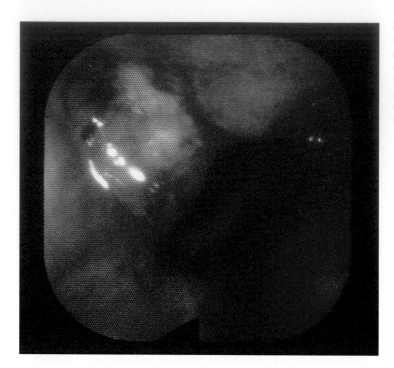

Figure 16.3. Duodenal ulcer with signs of bleeding developed after treatment of acute rejection with intravenous high-dose steroid pulses. (Courtesy of Dr A Carrara, Ospedale Maggiore, Milan.)

in transplant patients occurred during or immediately after the administration of intravenous high-dose methylprednisolone pulses (Figure 16.3). The emotional stress caused by the operation and by possible complications may also play an important role, although the mechanisms by which stress contributes to ulcer disease are still uncertain. Finally, cigarette smoking may lead to ulceration by reducing the pyloric sphincter pressure and decreasing pancreatic bicarbonate secretion.

At present the incidence of peptic ulcer has declined substantially. This is mainly due to the fact that transplant candidates are actively screened for evidence of peptic ulcer before transplantation. Patients with pre-existing ulcer are usually treated with H_2-receptor antagonists and appropriate antibiotic therapy directed to eradicate *H. pylori*. Moreover, the doses of corticosteroids have been considerably reduced in comparison with the past. The incidence of rejection and other complications is also reduced. Today, many transplant groups use prophylactic H_2-receptor antagonists for all patients after operation. The utility of this routine prophylaxis may be challenged but it is a common experience that the mortality due to gastroduodenal perforation or hemorrhage fell to almost zero after the constant use of preventive antiulcer therapy. At any rate, there are no doubts that patients with a history of a previous ulcer should be given H_2-receptor antagonists for the first few months after transplantation. Considering the excellent results of nonoperative ulcer therapy in transplant patients (Troppman et al 1995), surgery should be limited to exceptional, complicated cases.

Small bowel disorders

An increased incidence of ischemia and obstruction of small bowel has been reported in patients with polycystic kidney disease, possibly as a consequence of circulating active secretagogues produced by extrarenal cysts (Andreoni et al 1999).

Ulcers of the small intestine represent a rare but dreadful complication of renal transplantation, development of which may be favored by corticosteroids, cytomegalovirus (CMV) infections and intestinal ischemia. About 75% of the ulcers are located in the ileum and 25% in the jejunum (Komorowski et al 1986). The clinical picture consists of periumbilical colicky pain, nausea and vomiting. Frequently the patient presents with small bowel obstruction, bleeding, or perforation. The diagnosis is difficult. Plain films of the abdomen may show signs of obstruction or perforation. Endoscopy may reveal ulcers in the high jejunum. If the involved segment is perforated, stenotic or bleeding, it should be resected.

Colon disorders

There is an increased risk of colonic complications in renal transplant recipients, particularly in aged subjects and in patients with polycystic kidney disease (Domínguez Fernández et al 1998). Caecum or ascending colon hemorrhage can occur in association with severe CMV infection. Colon perforation may complicate a diverticular disease. Abdominal pain, fever, tenderness and leukocytosis are the most frequent signs, but the clinical presentation may be atypical with vague abdominal symptoms in immunosuppressed patients. Pneumoperitoneum may occur in about one-third of cases. Plain abdominal X-ray films, CT scan and/or colonoscopy are helpful for a correct diagnosis. The prognosis is particularly severe, with a mortality rate ranging between 20% (Benoit et al 1993) and 66% (Pollak et al 1985). However, aggressive diagnostic evaluation and treatment improved the prognosis in a recent series (Lederman et al 1998). Treatment should consist of early surgery under a broad spectrum of antibiotics and reduction of immunosuppressive therapy.

Pseudomembranous enterocolitis is a severe disease which may complicate antimicrobial treatments. Its incidence is increased in pediatric kidney transplant recipients, in females, and after treatment with monoclonal antilymphocyte antibodies (West et al 1999). Symptoms may begin at any time during the course of antimicrobial treatment or even after antimicrobial agents have been stopped. *Clostridium difficile* is the pathogen responsible in most cases. Colitis is the result of a toxin-mediated enteric disease while there is no microbial invasion of the intestinal mucosa. The most common symptom is diarrhea, often associated with fever. Dehydration, hypoalbuminemia, electrolyte disturbances and colonic perforation, due to necrotizing colitis with gangrene, are the most frequent complications. Colonoscopy, showing a typical pseudomembranous colitis, and the identification of *C. difficile* in the stool may confirm the diagnosis. Treatment consists of vancomycin given orally, 125–500 mg four times daily for 7–14 days. Cholestyramine, 1 g three times daily for 5 days, may bind the toxin and may be used in milder cases.

ACUTE PANCREATITIS

Posttransplantation pancreatitis is an infrequent complication with a high risk of mortality. The incidence of acute pancreatitis in renal transplant recipients ranges around 1% (Fernandez-Cruz et al 1989; Chapman et al 1991).

Several factors may contribute to the pathogenesis of pancreatitis after transplantation (Table 16.2). There is a well-known association between end-stage renal disease and acute pancreatitis with radiological findings ranging from normal anatomy to fulminant necrotizing pancreatitis (Van Dyke et al 1986). Secondary hyperparathyroidism may cause inflammatory changes in the pancreas (Sitges-Serra et al 1988). Many dialysis patients have a silent gallstone disease (Badalamenti et al 1994), which may increase the risk of acute pancreatitis either by obstruction or by reflux of biliary or duodenal contents, which stimulate the pancreatic secretion. Corticosteroids (Truhan and Ahmed 1989), azathioprine (Guillaume et al 1984) and cyclosporine (Lorber et al 1987) can all be responsible for pancreatitis. Changes consistent with the presence of cytomegalovirus in the gland have been seen in patients with posttransplant pancreatitis suggesting a possible role for viral infection (Joe et al 1989). Hypertriglyceridemia, which may be frequent in transplant patients, has been considered as a predisposing factor for pancreatitis (Toskes 1990).

Acute pancreatitis usually has a rapid onset, with upper abdominal pain, vomiting, fever, tachycardia, leukocytosis and elevation of serum levels of pancreatic enzymes. The histological picture may vary from interstitial edema to necrosis. Computed tomography shows an enlarged pancreas (Figure 16.4) and portions of the pancreas without contrast enhancement in the case of pancreatic necrosis. At endoscopic retrograde cholangiopancreatography (ERCP), intraparenchymal extravasation due to necrosis can be seen (Figure 16.5).

End-stage renal failure
Secondary hyperparathyroidism
Gallstone disease
Corticosteroids
Azathioprine
Calcineurin inhibitors
Cytomegalovirus infection
Hypertriglyceridemia

Table 16.2. Factors predisposing to posttransplant acute pancreatitis

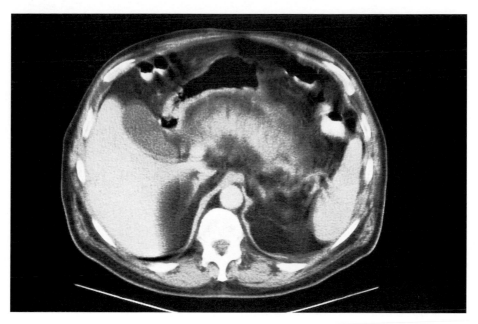

Figure 16.4. Acute pancreatitis. A diffusely enlarged pancreas with loss of cleavage plan. Exudative peripancreatic collection.

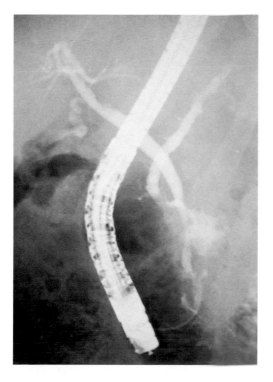

Figure 16.5. ERCP. Acute pancreatitis of the head of the pancreas with intraparenchymal extravasation due to necrosis and compression of the choledocus. (Courtesy of Dr A Carrara, Ospedale Maggiore, Milan.)

Systemic
   Acute renal failure
   Acute respiratory distress syndrome
   Shock
   Coagulopathy
   Hyperglycemia
   Hypocalcemia
   Gastrointestinal bleeding
   Alcohol consumption

Local
   Pancreatic abscesses
   Pancreatic pseudocysts

Table 16.3. Complications of acute pancreatitis

If pancreatitis remains sterile the overall mortality is about 10%, while it ranges between 30 and 40% if there is an infected necrosis. The differential diagnosis may be made by CT-guided fine-needle aspiration of pancreatic and peripancreatic tissue. In renal transplant recipients acute pancreatitis may follow a fulminating course. Early death is due to a multisystem organ failure with development of adult respiratory distress syndrome, renal failure, upper gastrointestinal bleeding, disseminated intravascular coagulation and shock. In other patients death occurs later, usually from infection. In surviving patients a number of systemic and local complications may occur (Table 16.3). Necrosis, edema and hemorrhage in the pancreatic bed and surrounding tissues may lead to formation of phlegmon or pseudocyst, which can be differentiated by ERCP (Figure 16.6) ultrasonography or computed tomography (Figure 16.7). A serious complication of either phlegmon or pseudocyst is pancreatic abscess, characterized by increased pain, hectic fever and leukocytosis. Another possible complication is represented by chronic pancreatitis (Figure 16.8).

Specific interventions for acute pancreatitis have generally not been helpful. Resting the pancreas has not changed the course of the disease. Enzyme inhibitors, total parenteral nutrition, and peritoneal lavage did not affect morbidity or mortality (Steinberg and Tenner 1994). As somatostatin may inhibit pancreatic secretion, trials with somatostatin or octreotide have been performed, but with little success (Lamberts et al 1996). Severe acute pancreatitis requires intensive management of cardiovascular, pulmonary, renal and septic complications. Imipenem is probably the antibiotic of choice for the latter complication (Steinberg and Tenner 1994). Endoscopic retrograde cholangiopancreatography and sphincterotomy in gallstone pancreatitis (Figure 16.9) results in reduced biliary sepsis. The timing and types of intervention in patients with acute

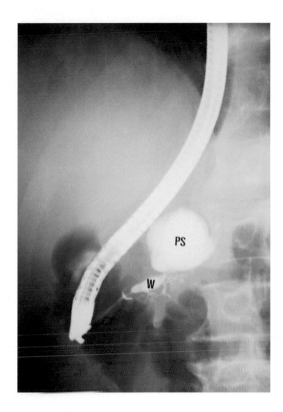

Figure 16.6. ERCP. Pancreatic pseudocyst (PS) communicating with the Wirsung duct. (Courtesy of Dr A Carrara, Ospedale Maggiore, Milan.)

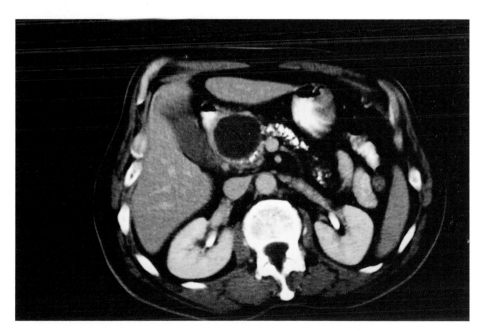

Figure 16.7. Pseudocyst of the head of pancreas at computed tomography.

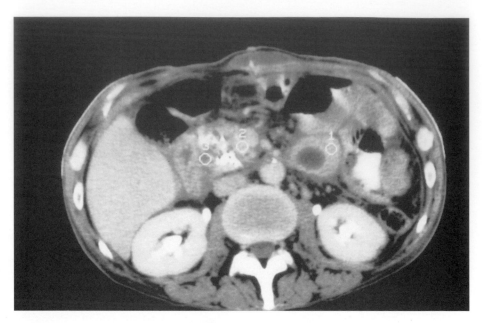

Figure 16.8. Chronic pancreatitis. Calcification of the head.

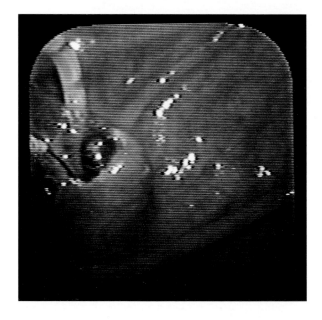

Figure 16.9. Endoscopic view of a papillosphincterotomy with removal of an ampullary impacted stone causing pancreatitis. (Courtesy of Dr A Carrara, Ospedale Maggiore, Milan.)

necrotizing pancreatitis are controversial. Supportive medical therapy is generally recommended in patients with sterile acute pancreatitis, which carries a relatively low mortality. Conversely, as infected necrotizing pancreatitis is almost universally fatal without intervention, debridement and resection of infected necrosis should be undertaken soon after confirmation of infected necrosis. Alternative methods of debridement are aggressive irrigation and drainage through large percutaneous catheters, and transgastric or transduodenal drainage and irrigation (Baron and Morgan 1999).

LIVER COMPLICATIONS

Hepatitis viruses

Hepatitis virus infection is one of the major causes of morbidity and mortality in renal transplantation. Apart from liver disease the viruses may cause extrahepatic complications including hematologic, cutaneous, musculoskeletal and renal disorders (such as glomerulonephritis and thrombotic microangiopathy). Most patients acquire hepatitis viruses before transplantation mainly through blood transfusions. In a few cases, however, the infection can be transmitted via the allograft from donors with actively replicating viruses.

Hepatitis B (HBV) infection

Hepatitis B virus is a DNA virus. Some 20 years ago the incidence of HBV infection was high in dialysis patients. More recently, however, only exceptionally does a dialysis patient become infected with HBV. There are several reasons for this reduced incidence of HBV infection. (1) In most dialysis units HBV carriers are isolated and prophylactic measures are taken. (2) Hepatitis B virus-negative patients receive systemic vaccination against HBV. (3) The use of blood transfusion in dialysis patients is considerably reduced since recombinant human erythropoietin has been made available. (4) There is a rigorous control for hepatitis virus in the blood to be transfused.

After renal transplantation the spontaneous disappearance of HB antigens and HBV DNA is very rare, around 3% (Fornairon et al 1996). On the contrary, immunosuppressive therapy generally favors viral replication. Hepatitis B virus-positive patients may remain asymptomatic for years, with a moderate elevation of alanine-aminotransferase (Pol et al 1990; Aroldi et al 1992; Morales 1998). However, in spite of good clinical conditions and mild biologic abnormalities, most patients show a progressive worsening of histologic lesions from mild chronic hepatitis (Figure 16.10) to cirrhosis (Figure 16.11). In a study with iterative liver biopsies after a mean follow-up of 66 months, cirrhosis was found in 28% of patients and chronic active hepatitis in another 42% (Fornairon et al 1996). Older age, female sex, and the presence of chronic active hepatitis were found to be significantly associated with the risk of developing cirrhosis (Rao et al 1993). Other investigators found that patients with positive HBV DNA or HbeAg at transplantation had the highest risk of developing severe liver disease (Fairley et al 1991). At any rate, the risk of cirrhosis and death increases with the time, being around 4% per patient year (Parfrey et al 1985). In the very long term there is a high rate of active viral replication and diabetes. Many patients die of either extrahepatic sepsis or

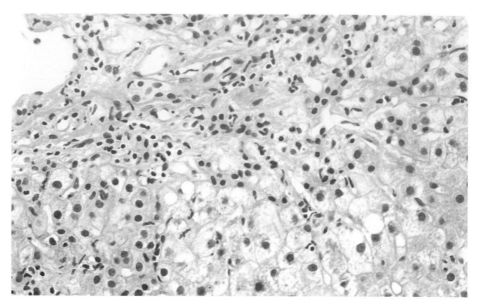

Figure 16.10. Liver biopsy in a 34-year-old HBV-positive kidney transplant recipient. Portal area shows scarce mixed inflammatory infiltrates and ductal proliferation. Periportal hepatocytes show clear cytoplasms due to cholate stasis and some tubular arrangement with perisinusoidal fibrosis. (H & E ×75)

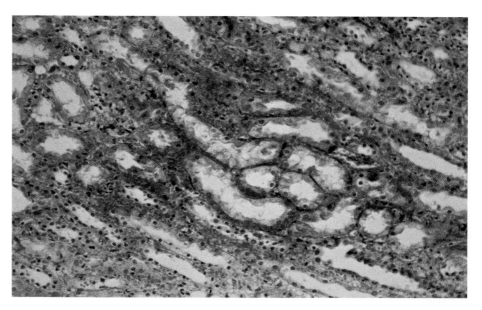

Figure 16.11. Chronic hepatitis and cirrhosis. Broad bands of fibrous tissue due to centroportal bridging necrosis, separate two parenchymal nodules. Chronotrope-anilin ×25. (Courtesy of Dr MF Donato, Ospedale Maggiore, Milan.)

Creatinine clearance (ml/min)	Daily dose of lamivudin (mg)
>50	100
30–50	50
15–30	25
5–15	15
5	10
Hemodialysis	10

Table 16.4. Doses of lamivudin in patients with renal insufficiency

liver failure (Aroldi et al 1998; Younossi et al 1999). In a few cases the accumulation of HBV stimulates immune response in spite of immunosuppression, leading to fibrosing cholestatic hepatitis and rapid progression to liver failure (Figure 16.12).

The treatment of hepatitis B was disappointing until recently. In liver transplant patients, intra- and postoperative administration of immunoglobulins has not benefited patients with viral replication (Konig et al 1994). Treatment with ganciclovir (Singh et al 1995), interferon-alpha (Marcellin et al 1994), and reduced immunosuppression gave equivocal results. Recently the new antiviral, lamivudine, proved able to improve the manifestations of HBV involvement and to maintain most transplant patients free of viral recurrence (Rostaing et al 1997; Goffin et al 1998). The daily dose in patients with normal renal function ranges between 100 and 150 mg. In patients with renal insufficiency the dose should be modified according to the values of creatinine clearance (Table 16.4). Treatment is usually well tolerated even when given uninterruptedly for up to 2 years. Unfortunately, some 20–30% of patients develop resistance to the drug within 8–12 months, due to viral mutation. Moreover, withdrawal of the drug may result in biochemical and virological relapse. In vitro studies showed a very potent activity of the new antiviral adefovir.

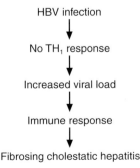

HBV infection

↓

No TH$_1$ response

↓

Increased viral load

↓

Immune response

↓

Fibrosing cholestatic hepatitis

Figure 16.12. A possible mechanism for rapid progression liver failure in HBV-positive transplant patients.

655

Hepatitis C (HCV) infection

Contrarily to HBV, HCV is an RNA virus. The prevalence of HCV infection in hemodialysis patients ranges between 15 and 30% (Vosnides 1997), while it ranges between 0 and 25% in home hemodialysis and peritoneal dialysis patients (Pereira and Levey 1997). Several genotypes of HCV have been recognized. The carriers of genotype 1a and 1b have significantly higher probability of developing chronic liver disease than patients with other genotypes (Nousbaum et al 1995; Aroldi et al 1998; Prieto et al 1999). Alcohol consumption may also accelerate the progression of liver disease. Coinfection with HBV worsens the course of HCV-positive patients (Pouteil-Noble et al 1995; Aroldi et al 1998).

About 50–80% of renal allograft recipients with HCV infection may remain asymptomatic and with normal serum transaminase levels for 5 years and sometimes even more (Roth 1995). However, these data should be interpreted with caution as more than half of patients with normal liver function may show chronic liver disease at histological examination (Berthoux 1995; Orloff et al 1995). Moreover, iterative liver biopsies showed a progressive worsening of fibrosis with progression to cirrhosis in most patients (Vosnides 1997). On the other hand, even liver biopsy may show wide variations in the severity of the lesions, depending on the indications to biopsy (mild or severe biochemical abnormalities) and on the timing of biopsy, an early biopsy usually showing milder lesions (Figure 16.13) than a late biopsy. Clinical studies showed that

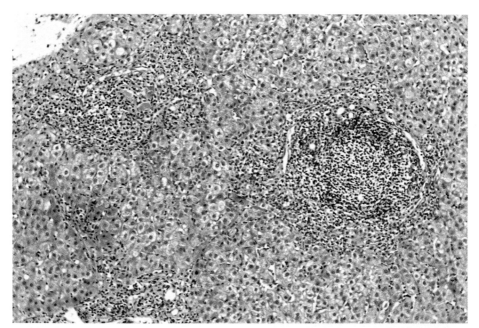

Figure 16.13.   Liver biopsy taken in a 42-year-old HCV-positive woman 8 months after renal transplantation. Mild chronic active hepatitis. Enlarged portal tracts with lymphoid follicles with germinal centers and bile ducts lesions. Mild periportal piecemeal necrosis is present. In the lobule there are small foci of liver cell necrosis with modest lymphocytic reaction. H & E ×25. (Courtesy of Dr MF Donato, Ospedale Maggiore, Milan.)

when patients are followed for at least 10 years more than 50% of HCV-positive transplant patients show chronic liver disease (Vosnides 1997). In a few cases, a fibrosing cholestatic hepatitis may develop (Figure 16.14), usually with rapid evolution to liver failure (Munoz de Bustillo 1998; Toth et al 1998).

Some studies reported that renal allograft and patient survival are similar in HCV-positive and in HCV-negative transplant recipients (Stempel et al 1993; Kliem et al 1996; Vosnides 1997). However, the results are strongly influenced by the length of the follow-up. In our experience, although the 14-year graft survival was similar in HCV-positive and HCV-negative patients (55% versus 59%), the patient survival was significantly lower in HCV-positive patients (Aroldi et al 1998). Extrahepatic sepsis, liver failure and cardiovascular disease accounted for most deaths in HCV-positive renal transplant recipients. Recent reports confirmed a significantly higher mortality in HCV-positive than in HCV-negative renal transplant recipients followed for 10–20 years (Hanafusa et al 1998; Legendre et al 1998; Mathurin et al 1999). These data suggest an ominous impact of HCV status in the long term for renal allograft recipients. On the other hand, when the outcome of renal transplant patients was compared with that of dialysis patients on a waiting list the risk of death was considerably lower, after the first postoperative period, in HCV-positive patients who received a renal allograft (Port et al 1993; Knoll et al 1997; Pereira et al 1998).

The treatment of HCV infection in renal transplant patients is still disappointing. Reduction of immunosuppression and withdrawal of corticosteroids might theoretically

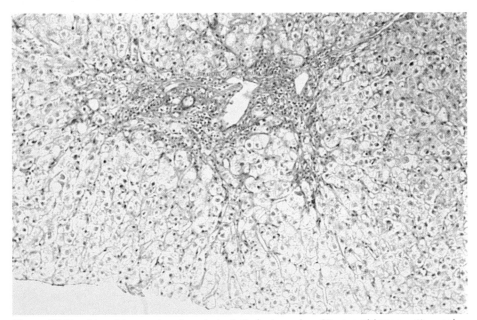

Figure 16.14. Liver biopsy showing cholestatic features in a 35-year-old man with renal transplant. Enlarged portal tract with some ductal proliferation. Periportal interface shows perihepatocytic fibrosis spreading into the lobule. PAS ×25. (Courtesy of Dr MF Donato, Ospedale Maggiore, Milan.)

reduce the virus replication, but there are no controlled trials supporting this hypothesis. On the other hand, such an approach may expose the patient to an increased risk of acute rejection, as HCV may upregulate MHC class II antigens in the allograft (Roth 1995). Interferon-alpha is not particularly effective in eradicating the virus, may be poorly tolerated and can also increase the expression of HLA antigens and induce acute rejection (Rostaing et al 1995). However, good renal tolerance and effective prevention of HCV-RNA replication has been reported with interferon in patients infected with genotype 2a and without cirrhosis (Yasamura et al 1997). The association of interferon-alpha with ribavirin, an antiviral agent, proved to be superior to interferon alone in obtaining a sustained virologic response and histologic improvement in nontransplant patients with chronic HCV (McHutchison et al 1998). Ribavirin is usually well tolerated. However the drug accumulates in the membrane of erythrocytes, leading to membrane fragility and in some cases to hemolysis and anemia. Ribavirin-induced anemia is dose-dependent and is more frequent in patients with renal failure. It is, however, reversible after stopping ribavirin. In spite of the increased risk of rejection caused by interferon, the combined treatment with ribavirin may be suggested for patients with progressive liver disease.

Hepatitis GB virus (HGBV) infection

Patients on maintenance hemodialysis are at increased risk for HGBV infection, which may be transmitted by transfusions or other means (Sampietro et al 1997). However, there is evidence that HGBV per se is not associated with acute or chronic hepatitis. Even in renal transplant recipients the positivity of HGBV does not affect the outcome (Murthy et al 1998; Rostaing et al 1999).

Liver hemosiderosis

Normal ferritin levels range between 15 and 200 ng/ml in males and between 12 and 150 ng/ml in females. Iron overload, caused by repeated blood transfusions or by inadequate parenteral iron supplementation, may lead to massive iron deposits in parenchymal cells that are stored as insoluble granular, gold-brown aggregates known as hemosiderin (Figure 16.15). In this case the serum ferritin level usually exceeds 800 ng/ml. In the liver, with advancing hemosiderosis, fibrosis increases and cirrhosis may develop.

In renal transplant recipients the prevalence of hemosiderosis ranges between 4 and 38% (Rao and Anderson 1985), the differences being accounted for by the different criteria used for defining hemosiderosis, by the different duration of dialysis, and by different transfusion policies. It is likely that since the introduction of human recombinant erythropoietin the incidence of hemosiderosis in dialysis and transplant patients has reduced. After transplantation, the rise in hemoglobin levels is accompanied by a

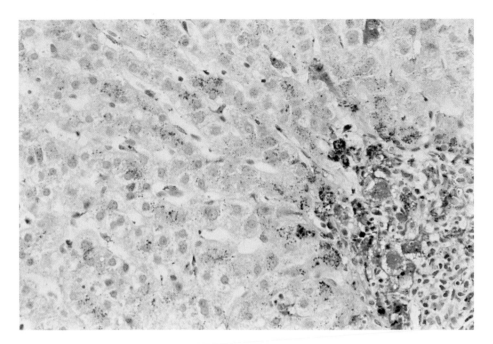

Figure 16.15. Iron overload in a 50-year-old male transplant recipient submitted to multiple transfusions before transplantation. Portal tracts and periportal areas show aggregates of iron-laden macrophages together with a moderate amount of hemosiderin in the parenchymal cells. Perl's ×75. (Courtesy of Dr MF Donato, Ospedale Maggiore, Milan.)

decrease in serum ferritin levels, which are lowest at the sixth month. After this time ferritin levels increase, their evolution depending on the iron status at transplantation (Teruel et al 1989). In exceptional cases a complete histologic resolution may occur after transplantation (Kadry et al 1992), but in most patients iron overload is difficult to remove, particularly if serum ferritin levels exceed 800 ng/ml. Hemosiderosis can cause tissue fibrosis and progressive liver failure, and many patients die either from liver failure or concomitant sepsis (Rao and Anderson 1985).

Treatment consists of periodic phlebotomies. The removal of 300 ml of blood depletes the body of 200–250 mg of iron. An early treatment may obtain a normalization of serum ferritin (which is usually higher than 800 ng/ml) and serum transaminases. However, if hepatic fibrosis has developed, treatment is usually ineffective. Thus, particularly in polytransfused patients, a regular monitoring of serum ferritin after transplantation is recommended. Magnetic resonance imaging of the liver may be a useful guide for deciding the intensity of treatment (Park et al 1994).

Hepatic veno-occlusive disease

This is a nonthrombotic obliterative process of the central or sublobular hepatic veins. The disease may be caused by pyrrolizidine alkaloids, chemotherapy or irradiation. A score of cases have been reported in renal transplant recipients all treated with azathioprine and prednisone (Read et al 1986; Liano et al 1989). However, the relationship of azathioprine with hepatic veno-occlusive disease remains poorly understood. A possible role for a hepatotropic viral infection has been hypothesized as the association with cytomegalovirus infection or viral hepatitis is frequent. The clinical picture is characterized by ascites, hepatomegaly, cholestasis and portal hypertension. The prognosis is poor. Most patients die a few months after the discovery of the disease.

Interruption of azathioprine has led to clinical improvement in occasional cases. Anticoagulant therapy and portacaval shunt have also been tried with some success (Eisenhauer et al 1984). Liver transplantation should be considered for patients who fail to respond to these measures.

Nodular regenerative hyperplasia

This is an unusual liver disease, histologically characterized by a diffuse nodular involvement of the liver and by the absence of fibrosis. The disease may lead to intrahepatic portal hypertension and/or chronic anicteric cholestasis.

A few cases of nodular regenerative hyperplasia of the liver have been reported in renal transplant patients, some associated with peliosis hepatitis or veno-occlusive disease (Buffet et al 1989). Stenosis and thromboses of small portal vessels might be responsible for the disease, leading to abnormal liver perfusion with atrophy of hypoperfused areas and regenerative hyperplasia of hyperperfused areas. A pathogenetic role for azathioprine or viral infections may by suspected (Jones et al 1989). Azathioprine withdrawal was followed by the disappearance of biochemical and clinical abnormalities in a few cases (Buffet et al 1989).

CHOLELITHIASIS AND CHOLEDOCOLITHIASIS

There is an increased risk of cholelithiasis in transplant patients (Figure 16.16). This may be due to the high prevalence of gallstones in dialysis patients (Badalamenti et al 1994) as well as to the use of cyclosporine (Kahan 1989), which augments the lithogenicity of the bile and may also induce cholestasis by inhibiting the ATP-dependent bile salt transport (Kadmon et al 1993).

The administration of ursodeoxycholic acid (5–10 mg/kg per day) may dissolve cholesterol and mixed gallstone and reduce cholestasis (Kallinowski et al 1991). Under treatment, the blood levels of cyclosporine should be checked as improvement of cholestasis and enhanced absorption of cyclosporine may increase the blood levels of the drug (Sharobeem et al 1993).

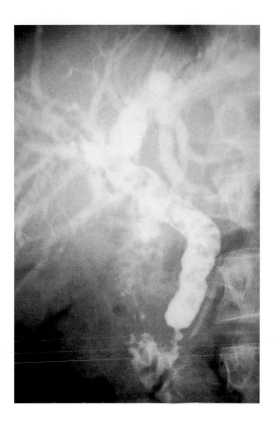

Figure 16.16. ERCP. Massive calcolosis of the biliary tract in a transplant patient. (Courtesy of Dr A Carrara, Ospedale Maggiore, Milan.)

As cholelithiasis and choledocolithiasis may expose the patient to the risk of severe complications, including cholecystitis, cholangitis, obstructive jaundice and pancreatitis, some surgeons recommend prophylactic cholecystectomy. It is also recommended for asymptomatic patients who do not respond to medical therapy. Surgery is certainly indicated in patients with frequent symptoms, in patients with prior complications of gallstone disease, as well as in patients at high risk of complications (large gallstones, calcified gallbladder etc.). Endoscopic sphincterotomy followed by stone extraction is a possible alternative in patients with common duct stones.

REFERENCES

Andreoni KA, Pelletier RP, Elkhammas EA et al (1999) Increased incidence of gastrointestinal surgical complications in renal transplant recipients with polycystic disease. *Transplantation* **67**:262–266.

Aroldi A, Tarantino A, Montagnino G et al (1992) Renal transplant recipients and chronic liver disease: statistical evaluation of predisposing factors. *Nephron* **61**:290–292.

Aroldi A, Lampertico P, Elli A et al (1998) Long-term evolution of anti-HCV positive renal transplant recipients. *Transplant Proc* **30**:2076–2078.

Badalamenti S, De Fazio C, Castelnovo C et al (1994) High prevalence of silent gallstone disease in dialysis patients. *Nephron* **66**:225–227.

Baron TH, Morgan DE (1999) Acute necrotizing pancreatitis. *N Engl J Med* **340**:1412–1417.

Benoit G, Moukarzel M, Verdelli G et al (1993) Gastrointestinal complications in renal transplantation. *Transpl Int* **6**:45–49.

Berthoux F (1995) Hepatitis C virus infection and disease in renal transplantation. *Nephron* **71**:386–394.

Buffet C, Cantarovich M, Pelletier G et al (1988) Three cases of nodular regenerative hyperplasia of the liver following renal transplantation. *Nephrol Dial Transplant* **3**:327–330.

Chapman WC, Nylander WA, Williams LF Sr, Richie RE (1991) Pancreatic pseudocyst formation following renal transplantation. *Clin Transplant* **5**:86–89.

Conn HO, Poynard T (1994) Corticosteroids and peptic ulcer: meta-analysis of adverse events during steroid therapy. *J Intern Med* **236**:619–632.

Domínguez Fernández E, Albrecht KH, Heemann U et al (1998) Prevalence of diverticulosis and incidence of bowel perforation after kidney transplantation in patients with polycystic kidney disease. *Transpl Int* **11**:28–31.

Eisenhauer T, Hartman H, Rumpf KW et al (1984) Favourable outcome of hepatic veno-occlusive disease in a renal transplant patient receiving azathioprine, treated by portacaval shunt. *Digestion* **30**:185–190.

Fairley CK, Mijch A, Gust ID et al (1991) The increased risk of fatal liver disease in renal transplant patients who are hepatitis B e antigen and/or HBV DNA positive. *Transplantation* **52**:497–500.

Faro RS, Corry RJ (1979) Management of surgical gastrointestinal complications in renal transplant recipients. *Arch Surg* **114**:310–312.

Fernandez-Cruz L, Targarona EM, Cugat E et al (1989) Acute pancreatitis after transplantation. *Br J Surg* **76**:1132–1135.

Fornairon S, Pol S, Legendre Ch et al (1996) The long-term virologic and pathologic impact of renal transplantation on chronic hepatitis B infection. *Transplantation* **62**:297.

Frick T, Fryd DS, Goodale RL et al (1988) Incidence and treatment of candida esophagitis in patients undergoing renal transplantation. Data from the Minnesota prospective randomized trial of cyclosporine versus antilymphocyte globulin-azathioprine. *Am J Surg* **155**:311–313.

Goffin E, Horsmans Y, Cornu C et al (1998) Lamivudine inhibits hepatitis B virus replication in kidney graft recipients. *Transplantation* **66**:407–409.

Guillaume P, Grandjean E, Male PJ (1984) Azathioprine-associated acute pancreatitis in the course of chronic active hepatitis. *Dig Dis Sci* **29**:78–79.

Hanafusa T, Ichikawa H, Kyo M et al (1998) Retrospective study on the impact of hepatitis C virus infection on kidney transplant patients over 20 years. *Transplantation* **66**:471–476.

Joe L, Ansher AF, Gordin FM (1989) Severe pancreatitis in an AIDS patient in association with cytomegalovirus infection. *South Med J* **82**:1444–1445.

Jones MC, Best PV, Catto GRD (1988) Is nodular regenerative hyperplasia of the liver associated with azathioprine therapy after renal transplantation? *Nephrol Dial Transplant* **3**:331–333.

Kadmon M, Klünemann C, Böhme M et al (1993) Inhibition by cyclosporin A of adenosine triphosphate-dependent transport from the hepatocyte to bile. *Gastroenterology* **104**:1507–1514.

Kadry Z, Yang HC, Gifford RR (1992) Histologic resolution of documented hemosiderosis in a renal transplant recipient. *Transpl Int* **5**:118–119.

Kahan BD (1989) Cyclosporine. *N Engl J Med* **321**:1725–1738.

Kallinowski B, Theilmann L, Zimmermann R et al (1991) Effective treatment of cyclosporine-induced cholestasis in heart-transplanted patients treated with ursodeoxycholic acid. *Transplantation* **51**:1128–1129.

Kang JY (1993) The gastrointestinal tract in uremia. *Dig Dis Sci* **38**:257–268.

Kestens PJ, Alexandre GPJ (1988) Gastroduodenal complications after transplantation. *Clin Transplant* 1988:**2**:221–226.

Kliem V, Van Den Hoff, Brunkhorst R et al (1996) The long-term course of hepatitis C after kidney transplantation. *Transplantation* **62**:1417–1421.

Knoll GA, Tankersley MR, Lee JY et al (1997) The impact of renal transplantation on survival in hepatitis C-positive end-stage renal disease patients. *Am J Kidney Dis* **29**:608–614.

Komorowski RA, Cohen EB, Kamiffman HM (1986) Gastrointestinal complications in renal transplant recipients. *Am J Clin Pathol* **86**:161–167.

Konig V, Hopf U, Neuhaus P et al (1994) Long-term follow up of hepatitis B virus-infected recipients after orthotopic liver transplantation. *Transplantation* **58**:553–559.

Lamberts SWJ, van der Lely AJ, de Herder WW, Hofland LJ (1996) Octreotide. *N Engl J Med* **334**:246–254.

Lederman ED, Conti DJ, Lempert N et al (1998) Complicated diverticulitis following renal transplantation. *Dis Colon Rectum* **41**:613–618.

Legendre C, Garriche V, Bihan L et al (1998) Harmful long-term impact of hepatitis C virus infection in kidney transplant recipients. *Transplantation* **65**:667–670.

Liano F, Moreno A, Matesanz R et al (1989) Veno-occlusive hepatic disease of the liver in renal transplantation: is azathioprine the cause? *Nephron* **51**:509–516.

Lorber MI, Van Buren CT, Flechner SM et al (1987) Hepatobiliary and pancreatic complications of cyclosporine therapy in 466 renal transplant recipients. *Transplantation* **43**:35–40.

Marcellin P, Samuel D, Areias J et al (1994) Pretransplantation interferon treatment and recurrence of hepatitis B virus after liver transplantation for hepatitis B-related end-stage liver disease. *Hepatology* **19**:6–12.

Mathurin P, Mouquet C, Poynard T et al (1999) Impact of hepatitis B and C virus on kidney transplantation outcome. *Hepatology* **29**:257–263.

McHutchison JG, Gordon SC, Schiff ER et al (1998) Interferon alfa-2b or in combination with ribavirin as initial treatment for chronic hepatitis C. *N Engl J Med* **339**:1485–1492.

Morales JM (1998) Renal transplantation in patients positive for hepatitis B or C (Pro). *Transplant Proc* **30**:2064–2069.

Mosimann F (1993) Esophageal candidiasis, omeprazole therapy and organ transplantation. A word of caution. *Transplantation* **56**:492–493.

Munoz de Bustillo E, Ibarrola C, Colina F et al (1998) Fibrosing cholestatic hepatitis in hepatitis C virus-infected renal transplant recipients. *J Am Soc Nephrol* **9**:1109–1113.

Murthy BVR, Muerhoff AS, Desai SM et al (1998) Predictors of GBV-C infection among patients referred for renal transplantation. *Kidney Int* **53**:1769–1774.

Nousbaum JB, Pol S, Nalpas B et al (1998) Hepatitis C virus type 1b (II) infection in France and Italy. *Ann Intern Med* **122**:161–168.

Orloff SL, Stempel CA, Wright TL et al (1995) Long-term outcome in kidney transplant patients with hepatitis C (HCV) infection. *Clin Transplant* **9**:119–124.

Parfrey PS, Farge D, Forbes C et al (1985) Chronic hepatitis in end-stage renal disease: comparison of HbsAg-negative and HbsAg-positive patients. *Kidney Int* **28**:959–967.

Park SB, Kim HC, Lee SH et al (1994) Evolution of serum ferritin levels in renal transplant recipients with severe iron overload. *Transplant Proc* **26**:2054–2055.

Pereira BJG, Levey AS (1997) Hepatitis C virus infection in dialysis and renal transplantation. *Kidney Int* **51**:981–999.

Pereira BJG, Natov SN, Bouthot BA et al (1998) Effect of hepatitis C infection and renal transplantation on survival in end-stage renal disease. *Kidney Int* **53**:1374–1381.

Pol S, Debure A, Degott C et al (1990) Chronic hepatitis in kidney allograft recipients. *Lancet* **335**:878–880.

Pollak R, Hav T, Mozes MF (1985) The spectrum of peritonitis in renal transplant recipients. *Ann Surg* 51:617–620.

Port F, Wolfe R, Mauger A et al (1993) Comparison of survival probabilities for dialysis patients vs cadaveric renal transplant recipients. *JAMA* 270:1339–1343.

Pouteil-Noble C, Tardy JC, Chossegros P et al (1995) Coinfection by hepatitis B virus and hepatitis C virus in renal transplantation: morbidity and mortality in 1098 patients. *Nephrol Dial Transplant* 10(Suppl 6):122–124.

Prieto M, Berenguer M, Rayon M et al (1999) High incidence of allograft cirrhosis in hepatitis C virus genotype 1b infection following transplantation: relationship with rejection episodes. *Hepatology* 29:250–256.

Rao KV, Anderson WR (1985) Hemosiderosis and hemochromatosis in renal transplant recipients. Clinical and pathological features, diagnostic correlations, predisposing factors and treatment. *Am J Nephrol* 5:419–430.

Read A, Wiesner RH, LaBrecque DR et al (1986) Hepatic veno-occlusive disease associated with renal transplantation and azathioprine therapy. *Ann Intern Med* 104:651–655.

Rostaing L, Izopet J, Baron E et al (1995) Preliminary results of treatment of chronic hepatitis C with recombinant interferon alpha in renal transplant patients. *Nephrol Dial Transplant* 10:93–96.

Rostaing L, Henry S, Cisterne JM et al (1997) Efficacy and safety of lamivudine on replication of recurrent hepatitis B after cadaveric renal transplantation. *Transplantation* 64:1624–1627.

Rostaing L, Izopet J, Arnaud C et al (1999) Long-term impact of superinfections by hepatitis G virus in hepatitis C virus-positive renal transplant patients. *Transplantation* 67:556–560.

Roth D (1995) Hepatitis C virus infection and the renal allograft recipient. *Nephron* 71:249–253.

Sampietro M, Badalamenti S, Graziani G et al (1997) Hepatitis G virus in hemodialysis patients. *Kidney Int* 5:348–352.

Sharobeem R, Baca Y, Furet Y et al (1993) Cyclosporine A and ursodeoxycholic acid interaction. *Clin Transplant* 7:223–226.

Singh N, Gayowski T (1995) Lack of sustained efficacy of combination ganciclovir and foscarnet for hepatitis B virus recurrence after liver transplantation. *Transplantation* 59:1629–1630.

Sitges-Serra A, Alonso M, de Lecea C (1988) Pancreatitis and hyperparathyroidism. *Br J Surg* 75:158–160.

Steinberg W, Tenner S (1994) Acute pancreatitis. *N Engl J Med* 330:1198–1210.

Stempel CA, Lake J, Kuo G, Vincenti F (1993) Hepatitis C—its prevalence in end stage renal failure patients and clinical course after kidney transplantation. *Transplantation* 55:273–276.

Teenan RP, Burgoyne M, Brown IL, Murray WR (1993) *Helicobacter pylori* in renal transplant recipients. *Transplantation* 56:100–102.

Teruel JL, Lamas S, Vila T et al (1989) Serum ferritin levels after renal transplantation: a prospective study. *Nephron* 51:462–465.

Toskes PP (1990) Hyperlipemic pancreatitis. *Gastroenterol Clin North Am* 19:783–791.

Toth MC, Pascual M, Chung RT et al (1998) Hepatitis C virus-associated fibrosing cholestatic hepatitis after renal transplantation. Response to interferon-alpha therapy. *Transplantation* 66:1254–1258.

Troppman C, Papalois BE, Chiou A et al (1995) Incidence, complications, treatment, and outcome of ulcers of the upper gastrointestinal tract after renal transplantation during the cyclosporine era. *J Am Coll Surg* 180:433–443.

Truhan PA, Ahmed AR (1989) Corticosteroid: a review with emphasis on complications of prolonged systemic therapy. *Ann Allergy* 62:375–388.

Van Dyke JA, Rutsky EA, Stanley RJ (1986) Acute pancreatitis associated with end-stage renal disease. *Radiology* 160:403–405.

Vosnides GC (1997) Hepatitis C in renal transplantation. *Kidney Int* 52:843–861.

West M, Pirenne J, Chavers B et al (1999) Clostridium difficile colitis after kidney and kidney–pancreas transplantation. *Clin Transplant* **13**:318–323.

Yasamura T, Nakajima H, Hamashima T et al (1997) Long-term outcome of recombinant INF-α treatment of chronic hepatitis C in kidney transplant recipients. *Transplant Proc* **29**:784–786.

Younossi ZM, Braun WE, Protiva DE (1999) Chronic viral hepatitis in renal transplant recipients with allografts functioning for more than 20 years. *Transplantation* **67**:272–275.

17 SKIN COMPLICATIONS

In collaboration with F Zorzi*

Cutaneous or mucosal complications are frequent in renal transplant recipients. The lesions are mainly related to the prolonged use of immunosuppressive drugs, but an important contributing role may also be played by exposure to sunlight and viral infections. Cutaneous complications may be subdivided into cancerous lesions, lesions caused by drugs, infections and miscellaneous lesions.

CANCEROUS LESIONS

Renal transplant recipients are exposed to a high risk of skin cancers. The spectrum of premalignant and malignant lesions includes Kaposi's sarcoma, actinic keratosis, Bowen's disease, keratoacanthoma, porokeratosis, basal cell carcinomas, squamous cell carcinomas, anogenital carcinomas and melanoma. Cross-sectional studies have reported a prevalence of skin cancer between 5 and 20% (Liddington et al 1989; Glover et al 1994). The incidence of cancer progressively increases with the duration of follow-up after intervention. In populations with heavy exposure to sunlight, such as in Australia, there is a linear increase in the incidence of cutaneous cancer, reaching 66% at 24 years posttransplantation (Sheil et al 1993). The incidence of skin neoplasms in more temperate climates is around 40% at 20 years (Hartevelt et al 1990).

Several factors may predispose to skin cancer. The oncogenic effect of ultraviolet B (UVB) light is well known. Ultraviolet B radiation may favor the initiation of cancer by modifying the DNA of keratinocytes and may favor cellular proliferation by interfering with the local immune response. Ultraviolet light has a very short penetration through garments and is thus of concern only for exposed body surfaces. A number of factors may interfere with the oncogenic risk of prolonged exposure to sunlight. It is well known that skin tumors are rare in the black population while they are frequent in patients with pale, thin skin. Genetic factors may also play a role. There is an increased risk of skin cancer in patients homozygous for HLA-B27 and HLA-DR7 (Bouwes-Bavinck et al 1991). Moreover, several members of a family may develop the same type

*Institute of Dermatology, University of Milan, Milan

of tumor in the same area. Finally there is increasing evidence that human papilloma virus (HPV) infection is involved in the development of skin cancer (Arends et al 1997; Mansat-Krzyzanowska et al 1997) and a possible role for Epstein–Barr virus has been recently hypothesized (Ternsten-Bratel et al 1998). In turn, immunosuppression amplifies the deleterious effect of UVB by causing dermal depletion of cells related to immune surveillance against tumor (Galvao et al 1998), favoring the papilloma virus infection (Pelisson et al 1996), and inactivating the tumor suppressor gene p53 protein (Gibson et al 1997).

Skin cancers in renal transplant recipients have some peculiar characteristics. While in the general population basal cell carcinomas outnumber squamous cell carcinomas, the mean ratio being 5:1, the reverse is true in renal transplant recipients with a ratio of 1:1.7 (Penn 1998). Nonmelanoma skin cancers occur in the normal population mostly in the seventh and eighth decades of life, whereas in transplant patients the average age is 30–40 years. Even if most skin cancers have a low grade of malignancy the mortality rate for skin neoplasms is about 5% in the renal transplant population, compared with 1–2% of all cancer deaths in general population, mostly cases of melanoma (Penn 1998).

To minimize the morbidity and mortality of skin cancer some preventive measures should be recommended (Table 17.1). They include diligent UV protection, frequent self-examination of the skin and regular dermatologic evaluation (Di Giovanna 1998). Unfortunately, only a minority of transplanted patients are followed-up regularly by a dermatologist (Cowen and Billingsley 1999). A recent questionnaire showed that the knowledge of transplant patients about the risk of skin cancer was not good. The use of sun protective measures such as sun avoidance and protective clothing was poor and the use of sun barrier creams was inappropriate (Seukeran et al 1998). Topical retinoids may be useful to treat solar keratoses and warts (Euvrard et al 1997). Some patients with multiple tumors may benefit from long-term, low-dose acitretin (McKenna and Murphy 1999).

Kaposi's sarcoma

Kaposi's sarcoma (KS) is a multifocal, vascular, malignant tumor that accounts for more than 5% of malignancies in transplant patients. The incidence of KS is 400–500 greater

Avoidance of sun exposure (use of appropriate clothes, use of sun-protective creams)
Avoidance of intensive sun and/or UV light exposure (risk of melanoma)
Avoidance of smoking (risk of lip cancer)
Frequent self-examination
Regular dermatological evaluation

Table 17.1 Measures to prevent the risk of skin cancer in renal transplant recipients

in renal transplant patients compared with controls of the same ethnic origin (Penn 1997). The male to female ratio is 2.8:1 in transplant patients, far less than the 10–15:1 ratio seen in the general population.

Kaposi's sarcoma-associated herpes virus, also known as human herpes virus-8 (HHV-8), is the first known human member of the genus *Rhadinovirus*. It has been regularly found by polymerase chain reaction in all forms of KS (classic KS, AIDS-KS, endemic KS and organ transplant KS), in certain types of Castleman's disease and in cavity-based B lymphoma (Gessain 1997; Ganem 1998; Mendez et al 1998). HHV-8 contains potential oncogens able to transform all lines in vitro and HHV-8 viremia and the detection of HHV-8 in all the forms of KS makes it the most attractive candidate causative agent to date (Simonart et al 1998). The precise interaction with other factors involved in the development of KS, including cytokines and antiapoptosis genes, requires further elucidation (Kennedy et al 1998). After transplantation, HHV-8 can reactivate quickly, the risk being higher in patients with strong immunosuppression (Eberhard et al 1999). Increased HHV-8 DNA levels in peripheral blood lymphocytes are associated with the development of KS (Mendez et al 1999). Of concern, HHV-8 can be also transmitted through renal allografts, representing a potential risk factor for transplantation-associated KS (Regamey et al 1988).

In the skin, KS lesions have a dark blue or purplish color, being initially almost macular and progressively more tumid (Figure 17.1). Lesions usually begin on the

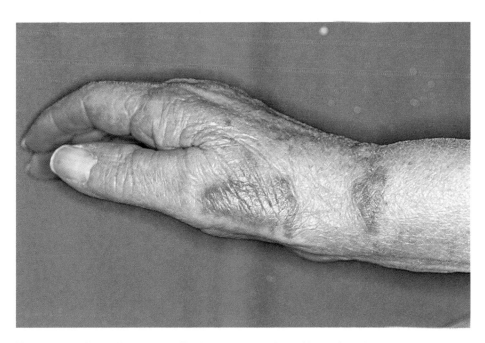

Figure 17.1. Kaposi's sarcoma. Erythematous patches of irregular, elongated shape with little infiltration. The surface is smooth, the consistency firm. These lesions are indolent and not ulcerated.

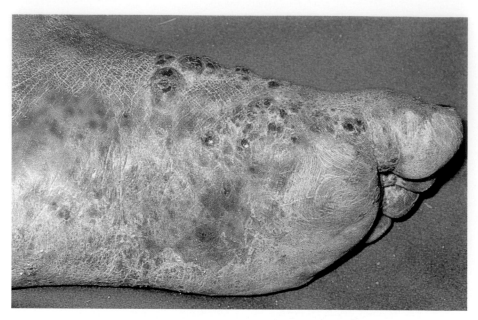

Figure 17.2. Kaposi's sarcoma. Violaceous, infiltrated, firm plaques of ecchymotic aspect on the foot with superimposed nodules. The nodules are more friable and may ulcerate. Long-standing lesions may be tender.

extremities, most commonly on the feet, with multifocal and asymptomatic development (Figure 17.2). The rate of spread is remarkably variable. Lymph nodes, mucosal surfaces and internal organs, particularly the small intestine, may all be involved as the disease progresses. About 60% of patients have a nonvisceral KS confined to the skin, conjunctiva, or oropharyngolaryngeal mucosa. Only 10% of patients do not have skin disease.

In transplant patients, withdrawal or even reduction of immunosuppression may obtain improvement and even complete recovery of KS, particularly if the lesions are limited to the skin (Montagnino et al 1994). Reduction or withdrawal of immunosuppression allows the immune system to recover sufficiently to reduce viral replication with subsequent viral persistence and low grade viral replication that coincides with clinical remission of the KS lesions. While many patients show a progressive, irreversible allograft dysfunction, other patients may maintain stable graft function with a mild immunosuppression or with small doses of prednisone alone (Montagnino et al 1994; Moose et al 1998). Because of the viral origin of KS, an antiviral treatment may be theoretically indicated. Ganciclovir (Neyts and De Clercq 1997), ciolofovix and foscarnet (Medveczky et al 1997) given at high doses could suppress clinical reactivation of KS in a few patients with AIDS but could not inhibit episomal virus DNA synthesis. When required, treatment options include excision or radiotherapy of single lesions and/or the use of cytotoxic drugs such as vincristine, cyclophosphamide, vinblastine, bleomycin, doxorubicin, or actinomycin, both intralesional and systemic.

Solar keratosis, Bowen's disease and Bowenoid papulosis

Solar keratosis, formerly known as actinic keratosis, is a premalignant condition. It is preferentially localized on sun-exposed areas and consists of round–oval well-defined erythematous patches, with dry and keratotic adherent scale that causes bleeding if detached (Figure 17.3). Long-term evolution may be toward squamous cell carcinoma. The histologic pattern is that of an in situ carcinoma. Particularly in sun exposed patients, one can find hundreds of lesions. The best treatments are liquid nitrogen or electrocurettage. Widespread lesions may be treated with oral retinoids.

Bowen's disease is a intraepithelial carcinoma, which may be located on the trunk or limbs (Figure 17.4). Its clinical and histological features are similar to those of solar keratosis. When located on the genitalia the condition is called erythroplasia of Queyrat, which presents as one or a few large plaques and histologically shows advanced dysplasia and carries significant risk of malignancy.

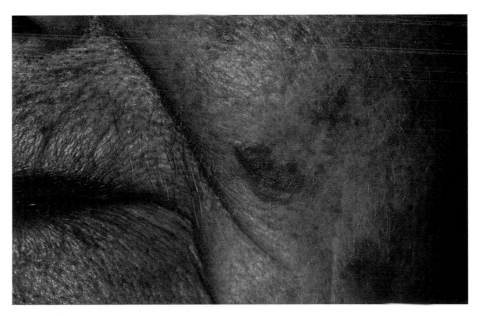

Figure 17.3. Solar keratoses: an erythematosquamous lesion on sun-exposed areas. If inflamed, the lesion can be more infiltrated and mimic a frank squamous cell carcinoma. Palpation can reveal a keratotic, rough surface.

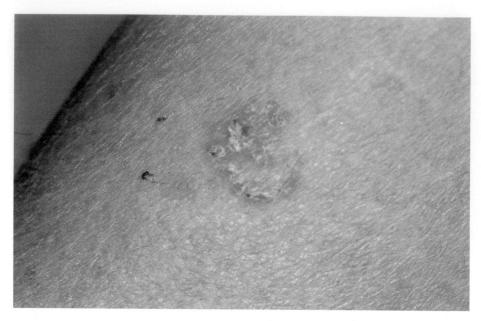

Figure 17.4. Bowen's disease. Slowly enlarging erythematosquamous patch. Hyperkeratosis and infiltration are usually not prominent.

Full thickness epidermal dysplasia of the vulva or penis is now classified as grade III vulval or penile intraepithelial neoplasia, even if the term Bowenoid papulosis is still used by many dermatologists. This neoplasia is strongly associated with HPV-16 infection. In iatrogenically immunosuppressed patients the neoplasia is refractory to treatment. The evolution to carcinoma of the vulva, perineum, scrotum, penis, perianal skin or anus is not uncommon.

Carcinomas of the vulva and perineum

The incidence of these tumors is 100-fold increased in renal transplant patients if compared with controls (Penn 1989). One-third of patients have in situ lesions. Patients with invasive lesions are much younger than their counterparts in the normal population. One-third of affected patients have a history of condylomata acuminata.

In carcinoma of the penis, the initial lesion is almost always within the preputial sac. It may be preceded by erythroplasia, or a warty excrescence that can be misdiagnosed as a wart.

Carcinoma of the vulva may develop either de novo, or from pre-existing areas of leukoplakia or Bowen's disease. The anterior vulva, and especially the labia minora, are the main areas involved. The lesion most commonly presents as an ulcerated nodule. Pre-existing Bowen's disease or leukoplakia should heighten clinical suspicion.

Squamous cell carcinoma (SCC) of the skin

This malignant tumor arises from the keratinocytes of the epidermis. Squamous cell carcinoma is the commonest malignancy in transplant patients. It usually develops on sun-exposed sites and often coexists with a background of viral warts. In such patients papilloma virus and sun exposure appear to act as cocarcinogens (Barr et al 1989). In immunosuppressed patients the malignancy of SCC is greater. Thus it is extremely important that transplant recipients are strongly recommended to avoid sun exposure. Usually SCC does not arise on healthy skin but on sunlight damaged skin (Figure 17.5). These photo-induced lesions consist of solar elastoidosis of the dermis, hyperkeratosis, irregular pigmentation and teleangiectasia of the skin, or leukokeratosis of the lips. The clinical appearance can be misleading, however. The first evidence of malignancy is induration. Thus, any indurated lesion should be submitted to histological analysis. The area may be plaque-like, verrucous, tumid or ulcerated, without sharp limits, usually extending beyond the visible margins of the lesion. The edges are an opaque yellow

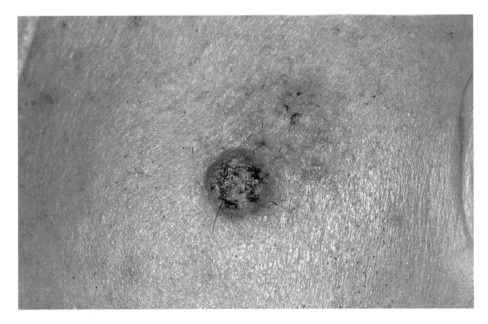

Figure 17.5. Squamous cell carcinoma. There is a photo-damaged area surrounding the tumor. The central nodule is firm, indolent, and can ulcerate.

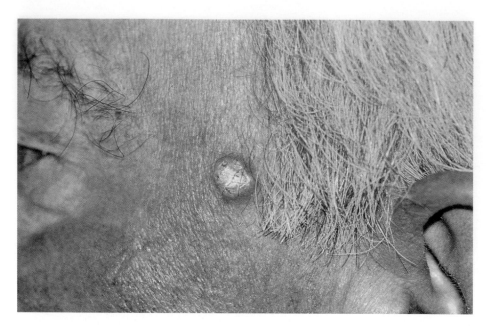

Figure 17.6. Keratoacanthoma. Keratotic nodule on the temporal area. In most cases the tumor presents as a solitary lesion. At the periphery the lesion is skin-colored to red with little teleangiectases beneath the surface. The center contains a yellowish, horny plug.

color and tissue around the tumor is inflamed. The most common sites are those more exposed to the sun: backs of the hands and forearms, the upper part of the face and, in men, the pinna. Also frequent is the localization on the lower lip, particularly in patients with smoking habits (De Visscher et al 1997). The evolution is faster than in basal cell carcinoma but much slower than in keratoacanthoma. Regional lymph nodes may become enlarged as the result of either infection or metastases. The three effective approaches to the cure of SCC are: surgery, local destruction, or radiotherapy.

Keratoacanthoma is a rapidly evolving tumor of the skin, composed of keratinizing squamous cells. The tumor is benign in most cases, with spontaneous resolution. In immunosuppressed patients, cases have been reported in association with human papillomavirus infection (Dyall Smith et al 1991) but a definite proof of a viral cause is lacking. The tumor usually presents most commonly on extremities as a firm, rounded, flesh colored or red papule that in a few weeks may become 10–20 mm across. At this nodular stage, the center contains a horny plug (Figure 17.6). As the lesion matures the accumulating keratin protrudes from the top of the lesion, resembling a crater.

The most useful clues to clinical diagnosis are well preserved symmetry of the lesion and no infiltration at the base. Spontaneous resolution is achieved in about 3 months with epidermal covering receding towards the base and the horny core being shed. Multiple lesions can also occur.

Basal cell carcinoma

This is a malignant tumor which rarely metastasizes. Basal cell carcinoma is composed of pluripotential cells that form continuously during life and, like embrionic primary epithelial germ cells, have the potential to form hair, sebaceous glands and apocrine glands.

The presence of a large number of nevi, freckles and solar elastosis all add to the basal cell carcinoma risk, suggesting an etiologic role both for UV radiation as well for regional factors. Basal cell carcinoma may arise in skin damaged by sunlight, ionizing radiations (Patack 1991), and scars (Hendricks 1980). In immunosuppressed patients an association with HPV has been reported (Barr et al 1989).

The early tumors are small, translucent and pearly, with thin epidermis and visible teleangiectasia (Figure 17.7). As the mass of the tumor grows, ulceration can occur and may re-epithelialize and break down several times before becoming permanent. Pigment, when present, is usually unevenly distributed in the tumor. In the pagetoid variant, the basal cell carcinoma spreads only superficially, is bounded by a slightly raised thread-like margin and has a central atrophic and scaly zone (Figure 17.8). The morpheic or sclerodermiform variant shows dense fibrosis of the stroma producing a thick plaque rather than a tumor.

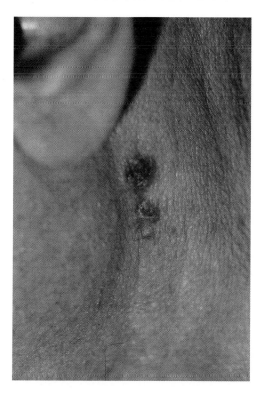

Figure 17.7. Nodular basal cell carcinoma. The lesion is firm, not tender, with a characteristic translucent aspect with waxy reflexes. When present, the pearly margin is a very useful tool for diagnosis.

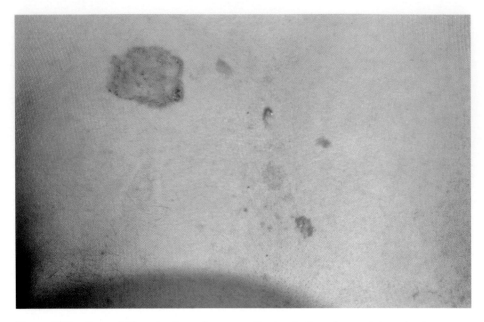

Figure 17.8. Pagetoid basal cell carcinoma on the trunk: the micronodular edge is evident. The epidermis covering the central zone is atrophic and scaly. Combined with increased vascularity, this feature gives resemblance to Paget's disease of the nipple. In poorly cared-for patients, pagetoid basal cell carcinomas may achieve a very large size.

Typically basal cell carcinoma runs a slow progressive course of peripheral extension, which procures the thread-like margins, the nodule with a central depression or an expanding rodent ulcer. A patient who has one basal cell carcinoma should always be followed, both because new tumors may develop elsewhere and because there is some risk of local recurrence.

Surgery, cryosurgery, Mohs' surgical technique with pathological control of excision margins and radiotherapy are all good therapeutic options.

Melanoma

This highly malignant tumor arises from epidermal melanocytes. Melanomas usually develop in areas exposed to the sun intermittently and are more common in persons with intense intermittent exposure to ultraviolet radiation (Gilchrest et al 1999). The incidence of melanoma in renal transplant is three to six-fold higher than in other immunosuppressed patients (Penn 1996). Racial (melanoma in the black population is one-tenth that in the white population), phenotypic (fair skin, total number of melanocytic nevi), and genetic factors (abnormalities on chromosome 9p11, the locus of

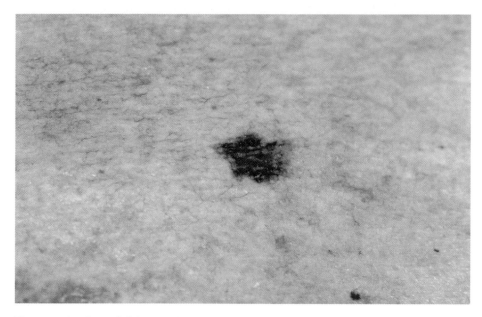

Figure 17.9. Superficial spreading melanoma. Pigmented and almost nonpalpable lesion. Asymmetry, irregular borders, irregularity in color distribution, and a diameter of 0.5 cm or more are all suspect features for a malignant lesion.

the p16 gene, which codes for the cyclin-dependent kinase inhibitor 2A, are probably involved in the etiology (Koh 1991; Monzon et al 1998).

Clinicopathologically there are several forms of melanoma. Superficial spreading melanoma is an irregularly shaped brown lesion usually still macular and only later palpable, with variations in brown and black pigmentation (Figure 17.9). Regression may cause pigment loss. The essential pathological features are focuses of malignant melanoma cells in the dermis with areas of in situ, that is intraepithelial, malignant changes in the adjacent epidermis. Nodular melanoma (Figure 17.10) is most commonly located on the trunk and is an elevated, dome-shaped polypoid or even pedunculated structure often totally or partially devoid of pigment (amelanotic melanoma). Histologically, there is a focus of invasive melanoma cells in the dermis in direct contact with epidermis but without abnormalities of the adjacent epidermis on either side of the nodule. Lentigo maligna melanoma is a flat, variously pigmented, irregularly shaped lesion most commonly located on the face. With time, a raised central nodule develops. Histologically, after a long phase of in situ involvement, invasion into the underlying dermis will take place. Acral lentiginous melanoma (and subungueal melanoma), found mainly on the sole of the foot, is a large macular, lentiginous pigmented area around an invasive raised tumour. The histologic pattern consists of an extensive area of lentiginous changes in the epidermis around the focus of invasive melanoma.

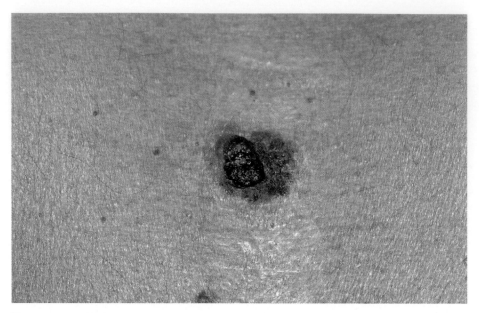

Figure 17.10. Nodular melanoma. These lesions often ulcerate. The nodular component is not in the center of the lesion, giving a more asymmetric aspect to the lesion. Color is variable from dark brown to light brown, red, blue, and black. A whitish color is sometimes visible. Amelanotic melanomas are especially difficult to diagnose clinically.

Epiluminescence, which allows the examination of the surface of the pigmented lesion at moderate magnifications with a small and simple handheld device, may be a useful tool for diagnosis.

Whenever possible, adequate surgical excision is the basic principle of treatment. Sentinel lymph node biopsy, that is the biopsy of the lymph node into which drains the dye or the radiolabelled material injected in the site of the tumor, allows, if negative, avoidance of unnecessary full lymph node disection (Brady and Coit 1997).

Merkel-cell carcinoma (MCC)

Merkel-cell carcinoma is an uncommon tumor most commonly affecting elderly Caucasians. Usually the tumor manifests as a solitary painless erythematous nodule, sometimes ulcerated, located on the head or neck. More than half of patients develop local lymph node metastases and almost half develop distant metastases. The mortality rate is 25–35% within 2 years.

Sporadic cases of MCC have been reported in renal transplant recipients (Formica et al 1994; Williams et al 1998) suggesting an increased incidence in immunosuppressed patients.

LESIONS CAUSED BY DRUGS

The immunosuppressive agents used to prevent rejection may be responsible for several lesions of the skin or mucosae (Table 17.2).

Corticosteroids

Renal transplant recipients given corticosteroid treatment may show the typical Cushingoid appearance, with facial and neck fullness, buffalo hump, increased supraclavicular and suprasternal fat, and trunkal obesity. These features are usually dose-dependent and

---

Corticosteroids
- Full-moon facies
- Acne
- Facial erythrosis
- Neck fullness
- Buffalo hump
- Maldistribution of fat
- Bateman's purpura
- Atrophy of the skin
- Striae rubrae

Azathioprine
- Thinning of the hair
- Hair loss

Cyclosporine
- Hypertrichosis
- Alopecia
- Skin hyperpigmentation
- Sebaceous hyperplasia
- Epidermal cysts
- Pilar keratosis
- Gum hyperplasia

Tacrolimus
- Alopecia

Table 17.2 Skin lesions caused by immunosuppressive agents

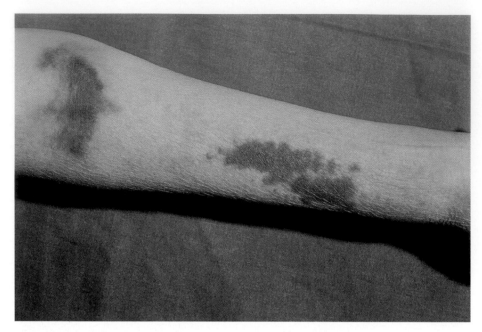

Figure 17.11. Bateman's purpura in a transplant patient receiving long-term steroid therapy

are caused by abnormalities in fat distribution. Cushingoid features are particularly frequent in the initial posttransplant period, when higher doses of corticosteroids are used. In the long term, some lesions may spontaneously disappear. However, some 40% of patients still maintain a Cushingoid appearance in spite of the low dosage of prednisone.

The most frequent complication of corticosteroids is acne, which is usually dose-related. Acne occurs early on the cheeks, forehead, chin and chest. Rarely the lesions may progress to nodulocystic transformation (acne conglobata). Doxicycline, 100 mg daily, may be effective in reducing acne. Severe cases can be successfully treated with isotretinoin or acitretin, a second-generation retinoid used also for progressive solar keratoses, widespread warts or recurrent skin malignancies. The severity of acne tends to decrease when the doses of corticosteroids are reduced.

A complication seen particularly in patients given prolonged corticosteroid administration is the so-called Bateman's purpura (Figure 17.11). It consists of irregular purpuric areas that develop spontaneously or after minor trauma, mainly on the extensor surfaces of the hands, forearms, and legs, often with spontaneous star-shaped pseudo-scars. Striae rubrae are wide and violaceous stripes, mainly located over the abdomen, thighs, and buttocks. Facial erythrosis and rosacea can occur. Finally, the skin of corticosteroid-treated patients can become atrophic and friable. Topical retinoic acid at concentrations ranging from 0.01% to 0.05%, may reverse this complication. Some patients, however, complain of irritation. Ammonium lactate 6–12% creams are usually better tolerated. Some patients have increased hair growth mainly on the face and back.

Teleangiectases, ecchymoses and skin atrophy tend to develop or to aggravate after 10 or more years in spite of reduced doses of corticosteroids (Bencini et al 1983). It must be noted that cyclosporine and corticosteroids are both metabolized by cytochrome P450. This may cause some retention of active metabolites of both drugs, with consequent appearance of corticosteroid-related side-effects even when low doses of corticosteroids are used.

Azathioprine

Azathioprine may cause thinning of the hair and scalp hair loss. Azathioprine may also be responsible for changes of color or texture of the hair. Actinic keratoses may occur in azathioprine-treated patients particularly after extensive sunlight exposure.

Cyclosporine

The skin is one of the principal sites of accumulation of cyclosporine. The drug, which is highly lipophilic, may partly be eliminated through the sebaceous glands. This could explain the frequent pilosebaceous lesions observed in cyclosporine-treated patients.

A frequent complication of cyclosporine is represented by hypertrichosis, which is usually dose-dependent (Figure 17.12). Hypertrichosis is characterized by thick and pigmented hair appearing over the trunk, back, shoulder, arms, neck, forehead, helices, and malar areas. This complication is particularly disturbing in black-haired women and in children. A possible mechanism for cyclosporine-induced hypertrichosis is the increased activity of α-reductase, an enzyme that transforms androgens into dihydrotestosterone in peripheral tissues (Vexian et al 1990). If so, treatment with finasteride, an inhibitor of α-reductase successfully used in patients with idiopathic hirsutism (Riffmaster 1995) may be helpful.

Alopecia areata and universalis have also been observed. Accelerated male-pattern balding may occur. Skin hyperpigmentation and bullous or vegetative lesions have also been reported in cyclosporine-treated patients (Ponticelli and Bencini 1995).

Sebaceous hyperplasia, epidermal cysts, and pilar keratosis have been reported in 10–20% of patients treated with cyclosporine, but it can be difficult to discern whether these lesions should be attributed to cyclosporine, to corticosteroids, or to both drugs. Cyclosporine may also be responsible for acne. However, apart from hypertrichosis, there are no major differences in skin lesions between patients treated with cyclosporine and those treated with azathioprine at least in the early stages after transplantation. (Bunney et al 1990).

Gum hyperplasia occurs in about one-third of transplant patients treated with cyclosporine. This complication generally occurs after 3 or more months of treatment and can be worsened by the concomitant administration of calcium channel blockers or phenytoin. It is at least partially preventable with careful oral hygiene. Initially, a hyperplasia of the anterior interdental papillae occurs which subsequently spreads to the whole gum also involving the inner side (Figure 17.13). A 5-day treatment with

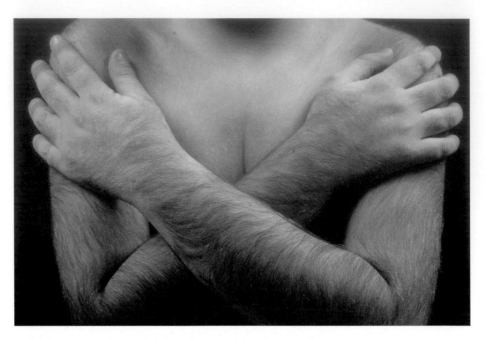

Figure 17.12. Hirsutism in a 10-year old girl given cyclosporine.

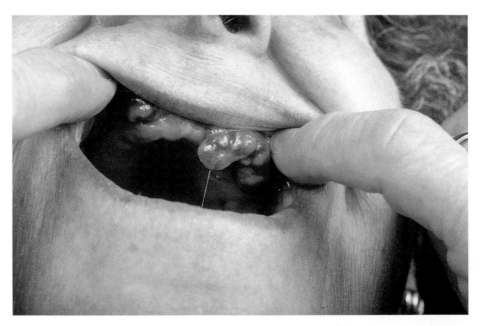

Figure 17.13. Gingival hyperplasia in cyclosporine-treated patient. Good oral hygiene can minimize this side-effect.

azythrocin, a macrolide antimicrobial agent, may improve the subjective symptoms and the clinical picture (Nash and Zaltzman 1998). It must be pointed out, however, that the macrolide may increase the blood levels of cyclosporine. The most severe cases require gingivectomy. The possibility that a gingival Kaposi's sarcoma may mimick a cyclosporine-related gingival hyperplasia should be taken into account.

Tacrolimus

In spite of the similar mechanism of inhibition of calcineurin, tacrolimus gives fewer skin abnormalities and does not cause gingival hyperplasia. Cases of alopecia have been reported in patients treated with tacrolimus (Talbot et al 1997).

INFECTIONS

Mycotic infections

Mycotic infections account for about half of the mucocutaneous infections observed in transplant patients. Candidiasis of the mouth and intertriginous areas of the skin is particularly frequent in the early posttransplant period when the dosage of immunosuppressive drugs is highest. Oral rinsing with sodium bicarbonate, nystatin or other antifungal agents may be helpful in preventing this complication.

Infections due to dermatophytes, that is ringworm-causing fungi, become increasingly frequent in the late posttransplant period. Their clinical appearance is often atypical due to the lack of the erythematous changes.

Pityriasis versicolor, caused by the lipophilic yeast *Pityrosporon ovale/orbiculare*, is the prevalent infection, affecting about 20% of transplant patients (Barba et al 1996). This complication, which can involve large areas of the trunk and flexural zones, is characterized by multiple and widespread small scaly macules either hypopigmented or hyperpigmented. The same fungus can also cause an acneiform eruption consisting of bland or mildly erythematosus follicular papules and pustules over the shoulders, chest, upper back, and arms (pityrosporum folliculitis). Patients may be treated with imidazole cream or selenium sulphate shampoo.

Primary cutaneous aspergillosis is rare. It is characterized by painful erythematous plaques, and sometimes cellulitis. Disseminated aspergillosis may produce cutaneous lesions such as papulae and pustules or subcutaneous nodules. Nocardiosis may also present with cutaneous pustules or with particularly painful subcutaneous nodules, and is easy to biopsy (Maccario et al 1998). Generalized cryptococcosis may cause erythema nodosum-like deep nodules, whereas primary cutaneous cryoptococcosis may appear as nodular, pustular, ulcerative lesions or abscesses with enlargement of lymph nodes (Figure 17.14). Subcutaneous pheohyphomicosis caused by dermatiaceous fungi is a rare

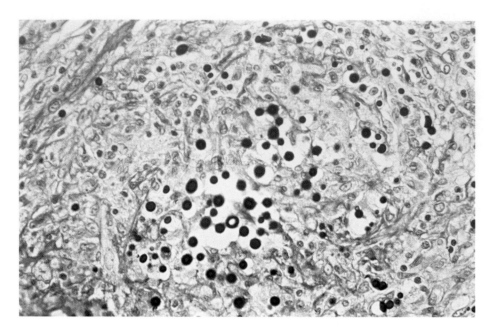

Figure 17.14. Lymphonodal cryptococcosis: pleiomorphic, single and budding yeast cells surrounded by a wide carminophilic capsule Mayer's mucicarmine. ob ×40. (Courtesy of Dr MA Viviani, Ospedale Maggiore, Milan.)

complication. Phycomycosis of the sinuses may manifest as a facial cellulitis. Dissemination of previously localized pathogenic agents, such as *Histoplasma capsulatum*, may lead to erysipela-like lesions. Early cutaneous histoplasmosis consists of painless diffuse swelling of the affected areas, whereas older lesions are represented by multiple draining ulcers (Shuttleworth et al 1987).

Cutaneous chromomycosis is characterized by scaly papules that may progress to verrucous nodules or ulcerating plaques. It is caused by pigmented fungi that are common saprophytes growing in soil, vegetation, and wood. Dermal alternariasis can manifest as fleshy papules and nodules, smooth and firm, spreading centrifugally, with an elevated crusted border and a central area slightly depressed and atrophic.

Whereas mucormycosis is one of the most common causes of opportunistic mycotic infection in immunosuppressed patients, cutaneous mucormycosis is rare. It can develop in burns and superficial wounds where spores are introduced in breaks in the skin. Clinical appearance is an erythematous macula that develops central vesiculation and necrosis. The demonstration of nonseptate hyphae in smears or by culture is the most useful tool for diagnosis.

Viral infections

Herpes simplex may have a limited extension without serious consequences but may also cause multifocal, extensive, and hemorrhagic lesions. Ulcers of the mouth and the perioral, perigenital, and perianal skin can occur in the most severe cases. Herpes zoster can be responsible for gangrenous and hemorrhagic lesions, which usually do not extend to other areas. However, atypical herpetic infection may also cause disseminated ulcerative or necrotic skin. The administration of systemic acyclovir (5 mg/kg intravenously every 8 hours for 5 days) or valacyclovir (1 g orally three times daily for 7 days) is mandatory for patients with severe lesions (Balfour 1999).

Varicella can occur in transplant patients, and can have a life-threatening course. Children awaiting a renal transplant should receive specific vaccine to prevent this complication. If varicella develops, immunosuppression should be reduced and even stopped in the most severe cases. Specific immunoglobulin infusion and acyclovir (10 mg/kg intravenously every 8 hours for 7–10 days) may improve the prognosis.

Cutaneous manifestations caused by cytomegaloviruses are very rare. These consist of exanthema with vasculitis, hyperpigmented nodules and plaques, vesicobullae, and buccal and perineal ulcerations.

Oral hairy leukoplakia, a typical Epstein–Barr virus lesion mostly observed in patients affected by AIDS, has been also reported in HIV-negative transplant recipients.

Warts and condylomata caused by human papilloma virus are frequent in long-term functioning transplant patients, approaching 85% at 5 years (Leigh and Glover 1995). They develop on sun-exposed areas, mainly in light-skinned patients (Figures 17.15 and

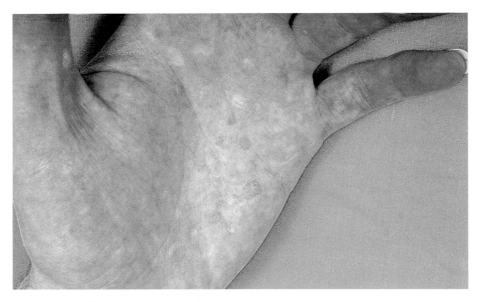

Figure 17.15. Plane warts on a hand.

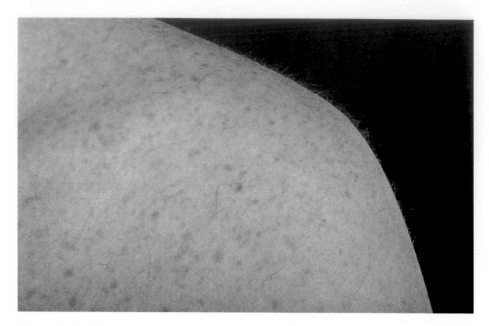

Figure 17.16. Plane warts widespread, yellow-pink, smooth-surfaced papules on limbs and trunk. Plane warts are polygonal or round in shape and may be flat or slightly elevated. Sometimes lichen planus causes difficulty in differential diagnosis.

17.16). They are usually multiple and their extension may be so widespread as to constitute general verrucosis. This is seen more frequently in long-term transplant patients (Barba et al 1997). Sunlight exposure and prolonged immunosuppressive treatment decrease the number of epidermal antigen-presenting Langerhans cells, which are important for cutaneous immunosurveillance (Hepburn et al 1994). Topical keratolytic agents or retinoic acid are the treatments of choice. Sometimes general treatment with second generation retinoids, such as acitretin, is required (Yuan et al 1995).

In immunosuppressed patients there is widespread occurrence of lesions with a clinical pattern similarly to epidermodysplasia verruciformis. This precancerous condition is characterized by several widespread viral warts and pityriasis versicolor-like lesions. The infection is caused by oncogenic human papilloma viruses.

About 20% of renal transplant patients have antibodies against virus-like particles of epidermodysplasia verruciformis (Stark et al 1998).

Extensive diffusion of condylomata acuminata or of molluscum contagiosum can also occur in renal transplant recipients.

Bacterial infections

Bacterial infections are usually trivial in the early period after transplantation, being represented almost exclusively by folliculitis (Figures 17.17 and 17.18). However, subcutaneous abscesses, erysipelas, and impetigo, caused by Gram-positive cocci, may develop in the long term (Figure 17.19). Cutaneous infections caused by atypical mycobacteria are often manifested as a spreading cellulitis around joints.

Miscellaneous lesions

Disseminated actinic porokeratosis may occur in up to 10% of transplant patients (Figure 17.20). It is caused by a proliferation of an abnormal clone of epidermal cells

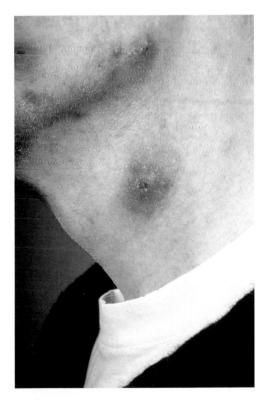

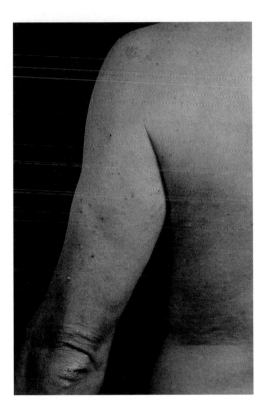

Figure 17.17. Abscessual folliculitis in a renal transplant patient. In these patients, folliculitis may be trivial, with tiny pustules on an erythematous base. However, one can see follicular abscesses, with erythematous, inflamed and exquisitely tender lesions that ulcerate and discharge pus.

Figure 17.18. Folliculitis of limbs and trunk: the most common causative agents are Gram-positive microorganisms and yeasts. Pruritus is very variable, sometimes annoying and requiring therapy. A microbiological assessment can be rarely achieved and the treatment is often empiric.

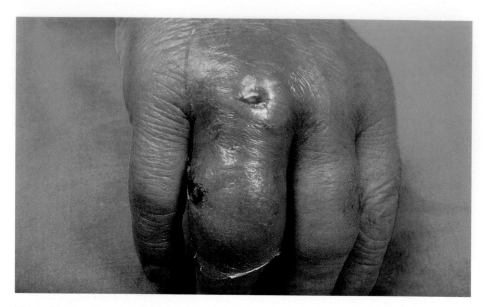

Figure 17.19. Cutaneous abscess following minor trauma in an immunosuppressed patient. Such events may have a rapid evolution and require prompt and vigorous antibiotic therapy.

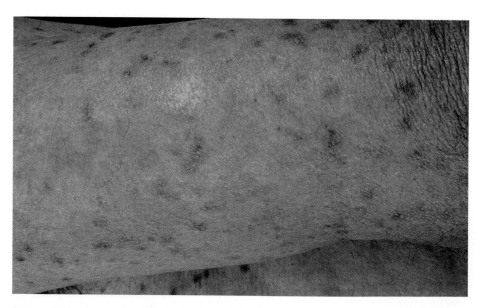

Figure 17.20. Disseminated porokeratosis. Widely disseminated, asymptomatic, flat lesions, particularly visible on sun-exposed areas, such as extensor aspects of the limbs. A careful observation may disclose a raised, fine, keratotic wall. The histological counterpart of this finding is cornoid lamella.

and clinically is characterized by annular lesions surrounded by a raised keratotic ring histologically constituted of a column of parakeratotic cells. Norwegian scabies is characterized by thick crusted plaques. Urticaria may be a cutaneous manifestation of an intestinal infestation, such as giardiasis.

Malakoplakia, the term meaning soft-plaque, is an immunodeficiency disease in which macrophages fail to phagocytose and digest bacteria adequately. It has been observed in the skin and subcutaneous tissues adjacent to the transplant scar. Histologically one can find in the skin large foamy hystiocytes with basophilic inclusion bodies, so-called Michaeli–Gutmann bodies, which are considered to represent abnormal degradation of bacteria and are pathognomonic for this disease. The origin of this disorder remains unknown, although there is some evidence suggesting a possible role of Gram-negative enteric bacilli. In transplant patients the disease is related to drug-induced immunosuppression (Barba et al 1996).

REFERENCES

Arends MJ, Benton EC, McLaren KM et al (1997) Renal allograft recipients with high susceptibility to cutaneous malignancy have an increased prevalence of human papillomavirus DNA in skin tumours and a greater risk of anogenital malignancy. *Br J Cancer* 75:722–728.

Balfour HH Jr (1999) Antiviral drugs. *N Engl J Med* 340:1255–1268.

Barba A, Tessari GB, Boschiero L, Chieregato GC (1996) Renal transplantation and skin diseases: review of the literature and results of a 5-year follow up of 285 patients. *Nephron* 73:131–136.

Barba A, Tessari G, Talamini G, Chieregato GC (1997) Analysis of risk factors for cutaneous warts in renal transplant recipients. *Nephron* 77:422–426.

Barr BBB, Benton EC, McLaren K et al (1989) Human papilloma virus infection and skin cancer in renal allograft recipients. *Lancet* i:124–128.

Bencini PL, Montagnino G, De Vecchi A et al (1983) Cutaneous manifestations in renal transplant recipients. *Nephron* 34:79–83.

Bouwes-Bavinck JNB, Vermeer BJ, Van der Woude FJ et al (1991) Relation between skin cancer and HLA antigens in renal transplant recipients. *N Engl J Med* 325:843–848.

Brady MS, Coit DG (1997) Sentinel lymph node evaluation in melanoma. *Arch Dermatol* 133:1014–1020.

Bunney MH, Benton EC, Barr BB et al (1990) The prevalence of skin disorders in renal allograft recipients receiving cyclosporin A compared with those receiving azathioprine. *Nephrol Dial Transplant* 5:379–382.

Cowen EW, Billingsley EM (1999) Awareness of skin cancer by kidney transplant patients. *J Am Acad Dermatol* 40:697–701.

De Visscher JG, Bouwes Bavinck JN, Van der Waal I (1997) Squamous cell carcinoma of the lower lip in renal-transplant recipients. Report of six cases. *Int J Oral Maxillofac Surg* 26:120–123.

Di Giovanna JJ (1998) Posttransplantation skin cancer: scope of the problem, management, and role for systemic retinoid chemoprevention. *Transplant Proc* 30:2771–2775.

Dyall Smith D, Trowell H, Dyall Smith ML (1991) Benign human papillomavirus infection and skin cancer in renal transplant recipients. *Int J Dermatol* 30:785–789.

Eberhard DK, Kliem V, Brunkhorst R (1999) Five cases of Kaposi's sarcoma in kidney graft recipients. *Transplantation* 67:180–184.

Euvrard S (1991) Cutaneous complications in renal transplant recipients. *Eur J Dermatol* 1:171–184.

Euvrard S, Kanitakis J, Pouteil-Noble C et al (1997) Skin cancers in organ transplant recipients. *Ann Transplant* 64:669–673.

Formica M, Basolo B, Funaro L et al (1994) Merkel cell carcinoma in a renal transplant recipient. *Nephron* 68:399–402.

Galvao MM, Sotto MN, Kihara SM et al (1998) Lymphocyte subsets and Langerhans cells in sun-protected and sun-exposed skin of immunosuppressed renal allograft recipients. *J Am Acad Dermatol* 38:38–44.

Ganem D (1988) Human herpesvirus 8 and its role in the genesis of Kaposi's sarcoma. *Curr Clin Top Infect Dis* 18:237–251.

Gessain A (1997) Human herpesvirus 8 and associated diseases: Kaposi's sarcoma, body cavity based lymphoma and multicentric Castleman disease: clinical and molecular epidemiology. *Bull Acad Nat Med* 181:1023–1034.

Gibson GE, O'Grady A, Kay EW (1997) p53 tumor suppressor gene protein expression in pre-malignant and malignant skin lesions of kidney transplant recipients. *J Am Acad Dermatol* 36:924–931.

Gilchrest BA, Eller MS, Geller AC, Yaar M (1999) The pathogenesis of melanoma induced by ultraviolet radiation. *N Engl J Med* 340:1341–1348.

Glover MT, Niranjan N, Kwan JTC, Leigh IM (1994) Non-melanoma skin cancer in renal transplant recipients: the extent of the problem and a strategy for management. *Br J Plast Surg* 47:86–89.

Hartevelt MM, Bouwes-Bavinck JN, Koote AM et al (1990) Incidence of skin cancer after renal transplantation in the Netherlands. *Transplantation* 49:506–509.

Hendricks WM (1980) Basal cell carcinoma arising in chickenpox scars. *Arch Dermatol* 116:1304–1305.

Hepburn DJ, Divakar D, Bailey RR, McDonald KJ (1994) Cutaneous manifestation of renal transplantation in a New Zealand population. *NZ Med J* 107:497–499.

Kennedy MM, Cooper K, Howells DD et al (1998) Identification of HHV8 in early Kaposi's sarcoma: implications for Kaposi's sarcoma pathogenesis. *Mol Pathol* 51:14–20.

Koh HK (1991) Cutaneous melanoma. *N Engl J Med* 325:171–182.

Leigh IM, Glover MT (1995) Skin cancer and warts in immunosuppressed renal transplant recipients. *Cancer Res* 139:69–86.

Liddington M, Richardson AJ, Higgins RM et al (1989) Skin cancer in renal transplant recipients. *Br J Surg* 76:1002–1005.

Maccario M, Tortorano AM, Ponticelli C (1998) Subcutaneous nodules and pneumonia in a kidney transplant recipient. *Nephrol Dial Transplant* 31:681–686.

Mansat-Krzyzanowska E, Dantal J, Hourmant M et al (1997) Frequency of mucosal HPV DNA detection (types 6/11, 16/18, 31/35/51) in skin lesions of renal transplant patients. *Transplant Int* 10:137–40.

McKenna DB, Murphy GM (1999) Skin cancer chemophylaxis in renal transplant recipients. 5 years' experience using low-dose acitretin. *Br J Dermatol* 140:656–660.

Medveczky MM, Horvath E, Lund T, Medveczky PG (1997) In vitro antiviral drug sensitivity of the Kaposi's sarcoma-associated herpesvirus. *AIDS* 11:1327–1332.

Mendez JC, Procop GW, Espy MJ et al (1998) Detection and semiquantitative analysis of human herpesvirus 8 DNA in specimens from patients with Kaposi's sarcoma. *J Clin Microbiol* 36:2220–2222.

Mendez JC, Procop WG, Espy MJ et al (1999) Relationship of HHV8 replication and Kaposi's sarcoma after solid organ transplantation. *Transplantation* 67:1200–1201.

Montagnino G, Bencini PL, Tarantino A et al (1994) Clinical features and course of Kaposi's sarcoma in kidney transplant patients: report of thirteen cases. *Am J Nephrol* **14**:121–126.

Monzon J, Liu L, Brill H et al (1998) CDKN2A mutations in multiple primary melanomas. *N Engl J Med* **338**:879–887.

Moose MR, Treurnicht FK, Van Rensburg EJ et al (1998) Detection and subtyping of human herpesvirus-8 in renal transplant patients before and after remission of Kaposi's sarcoma. *Transplantation* **66**:214–218.

Nash MM, Zaltzman JS (1998) Efficacy of azithromycin in the treatment of cyclosporine-induced gingival hyperplasia in renal transplant recipients. *Transplantation* **65**:1611–1615.

Neyts J, De Clercq E (1997) Antiviral drug susceptibility of human herpesvirus 8. *Antimicrob Agents Chemother* **41**:2754–2756

Patack MA (1991) Ultraviolet radiation and the development of non-melanoma and melanoma skin cancer: clinical and experimental evidence. *Skin Pharmacol* **4**(Suppl 1):85–94.

Pelisson I, Soler C, Chardonnet Y et al (1996) A possible role for human papillomaviruses and c-myc, c-Ha-ras, and p53 gene alterations in malignant cutaneous lesions from renal transplant recipients. *Cancer Detect Prev* **20**:20–30, 1996.

Penn I (1989) Why do immunosuppressed patients develop cancer? *CRC Crit Rev Oncogen* **1**:27–52.

Penn I (1996) Malignant melanoma in organ allograft recipients. *Transplantation* **61**:274–378.

Penn I (1997) Kaposi's sarcoma in transplant recipients. *Transplantation* **64**:669–673.

Penn I (1998) De novo cancers in organ allograft recipients. *Curr Opin Organ Transplant* **4**:188–196.

Ponticelli C, Bencini PL (1995) The skin in renal transplant recipients. In: Massry SG, Glassock RJ (eds). *Textbook of Nephrology*. Baltimore: Williams and Wilkins, pp. 1704–1706.

Regamey N, Tamm M, Wernli M et al (1998) Transmission of human herpesvirus 8 infection from renal-transplant donors to recipients. *N Engl J Med* **339**:1358–1363.

Rittmaster RS (1995) Medical treatment of androgen-dependent hirsutism. *J Clin Endocrinol Metab* **80**:2559–2563.

Seukeran DC, Newstead CG, Cunliffe WJ (1998) The compliance of renal transplant recipients with advice about sun protection measures. *Br J Dermatol* **138**:301–303.

Sheil AGR, Disney APS, Mathew TH, Amiss N (1993) De novo malignancy emerges as a major cause of morbidity and late failure in renal transplantation. *Transplant Proc* **25**:1383–1384.

Shuttleworth D, Philpot CM, Salaman JR (1987) Cutaneous fungal infection following renal transplantation: a case control study. *Br J Dermatol* **117**:585–590.

Simonart T, Noel JC, Van Vooren JP, Parent D (1998) Role of viral agents in the pathogenesis of Kaposi's sarcoma. *Dermatology* **196**:447–449.

Stark S, Petridis AK, Ghim SJ et al (1998) Prevalence of antibodies against virus-like particles of epidermodysplasia verruciformis-associated HPV8 in patients at risk of skin cancer. *J Invest Dermatol* **111**:696–701.

Talbot D, Rix D, Abusin K et al (1997) Alopecia as a consequence of tacrolimus therapy in renal transplantation. *Transplantation* **64**:1631–1632.

Ternsten-Bratel A, Kjellström C, Rickstem A (1998) Specific expression of Epstein–Barr virus in cutaneous squamous cell carcinoma from heart transplant recipients. *Transplantation* **66**:1524–1529.

Vexiau P, Fiet J, Boudou Ph et al (1990) Increase in plasma 5α-androstase-3α, 17β-diol glucuronide as a marker of peripheral andogen action in hirsutism: a side-effect induced by cyclosporine A. *J Steroid Biochem* **35**:133–137.

Williams RH, Morgan MB, Mathieson IM, Rabb H (1998) Merkel cell carcinoma in a renal transplant patient: increased incidence? *Transplantation* **65**:1396–1397.

Yuan ZF, Davis A, Macdonald K, Bailey RR (1995) Use of acitretin for the skin complications in renal transplant recipients. *NZ Med J* **108**:255–256.

18 MUSCULOSKELETAL, OCULAR AND HEMATOLOGICAL COMPLICATIONS

*In collaboration with A. Aroldi**

MUSCULOSKELETAL COMPLICATIONS

Most patients undergoing kidney transplantation already have some degree of renal osteodystrophy, a general term encompassing all histological derangements of bone that may occur in uremic patients such as hyperparathyroidism (with or without osteitis fibrosa), osteomalacia, osteosclerosis and adynamic bone disease. In some patients more than one of these conditions may be present at the same time. After successful renal transplantation some improvement of hyperparathyroidism, aluminum-related bone disease and amyloidosis may occur, but the introduction of immunosuppressive agents, particularly corticosteroids, may expose the patient to the risk of new bone complications, such as osteoporosis and osteonecrosis, as well as muscle and joint complications (Table 18.1).

Hyperparathyroidism (HPTH)

When a renal graft starts to function properly, it does so in a setting characterized by negative calcium and positive phosphate balances, low production of calcitriol, continuous stimulation of parathyroid hormone (PTH) synthesis and secretion due to the hypertrophy and hyperplasia of the parathyroid gland, and resistance to the calcemic action of PTH (Slatopolsky et al 1992). The recovery of glomerular filtration and tubular function after successful renal transplantation can correct the main causal factors of secondary HPTH, namely phosphate retention, decreased synthesis of calcitriol and hypocalcemia. But while the reversal of these abnormalities takes only few days,

Division of Nephrology and Dialysis, Ospedale Maggiore, Milan

693

Bone complications
    Hyperparathyroidism
    Aluminum associated disorders
    β2-microglobulin-related amyloidosis
    Osteoporosis
    Osteonecrosis

Muscle and joint complications
    Painful legs syndrome
    Polyarthralgias
    Myopathy
    Tendinitis
    Gout

Table 18.1. Bone, muscle and joint complications in renal transplant recipients

months may be needed before the parathyroid functional mass improves (Bonarek et al 1999).

The most important factor for the persistence of HPTH is represented by poor graft function. As serum calcitriol levels correlate with renal function (Martin-Malo 1996), normal production of calcitriol by the graft can favor the involution of HPTH, but in patients with poor renal allograft function the calcitriol production may be insufficient to inhibit parathyroid secretion. The use of drugs that impair intestinal calcium absorption (corticosteroids) or block calcitriol synthesis (ketoconazole) can also interfere with the involution of HPTH after transplantation. Thus, a secondary HPTH may persist in a proportion of patients (Cundy et al 1983; Messa et al 1998). In patients with persistent HPTH, the set-point for the calcium-controlled PTH secretion may be shifted around higher calcium values with further slowing in HPTH involution. This increase in the set-point may be the result of an underexpression of the calcium-sensing receptor (Kifor et al 1996), occurring in the hyperplastic parathyroid glands of severe HPTH. Exceptionally, it might even occur that glands with nodular hyperplasia, which have reduced density of calcitriol receptors (Korkor et al 1987), never return to normal size and function (Drueke 1995).

Generally, the time-course and degree of persistent posttransplant hyperparathyroidism are correlated with the duration and intensity of pretransplant HPTH and with the volume of parathyroid glands (McCarron et al 1982; Cundy et al 1983; Parfitt 1997). Radiographic alterations in persistent posttransplant hyperparathyroidism are similar to those seen in dialysis patients with signs of accelerated bone resorption (Figure 18.1) and osteosclerosis (Figure 18.2). Persistent mild hypercalcemia (10.5–12 mg/dl) generally resolves within a year, but in about 4–10% of recipients it continues over the

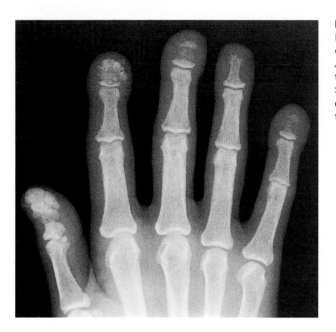

Figure 18.1. Severe hyperparathyroidism in a dialysis patient. Acroosteolysis of the terminal phalanges. Subperiostial resorption, cortical thinning and fluffy trabecular structure.

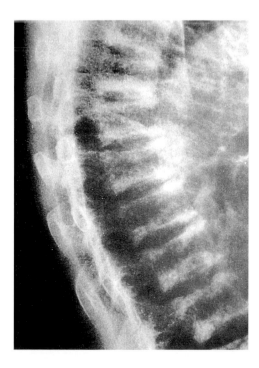

Figure 18.2. Severe hyperparathyroidism in a dialysis patient. Osteosclerosis of the thoracic spine due to sclerosis of the vertebral endplates ('rugger jersey spine'). From Bedani PL, Orzincolo C, Scutellari PN, Gilli P (eds). *Imaging dell'apparato muscoloscheletrico in nefrologia.* Milan: Wichtig, 1988. Reproduced with permission.

next 2 years and finally resolves without specific intervention. Hypophosphatemia may be another manifestation of persistent hyperparathyroidism during the first year after transplantation. It may be enhanced by the coexistence of a severe hyperphosphaturia, due to tubular dysfunction either caused by ischemia–reperfusion damage, by rejection and/or by the use of corticosteroids (Higgins et al 1990). Whether or not hypophosphatemia may be responsible for osteomalacia is still under discussion (Felsenfeld et al 1986). However hypophosphatemia may contribute to the pathogenesis of severe myopathy. Persistent hypophosphatemia may require phosphate replacement therapy or may be corrected by oral calcium and vitamin D supplements (Dumoulin et al 1995).

The serum parathyroid concentration above which hyperparathyroidism may cause severe complications has not been defined. This is an important practical problem since posttransplant parathyroid surgery may expose the patient to the risk of refractory hypocalcemia and low-turnover bone disease. Hypocalcemia in hypoparathyroid patients with restored glomerular filtration is difficult to treat, because urinary calcium excretion is enhanced in the absence of parathyroid hormone. Corticosteroids may further contribute to hypocalcemia by reducing intestinal calcium absorption. Moreover hypoparathyroid patients may develop low-turnover bone disease due to decreased parathyroid hormone-mediated turnover. The surgical choice between subtotal parathyroidectomy or total parathyroidectomy with subcutaneous autotransplantation largely depends on the experience of the surgeon. The former technique has a higher rate of persistent and recurrent hyperparathyroidism, but the latter approach exposes the patient to the risk of hypoparathyroidism due to death of the reimplanted parathyroid tissue. Because of the potential risk of severe persistent hypocalcemia, we suggest subtotal parathyroidectomy as a first-line approach for renal transplant recipients.

An autonomous pattern of PTH secretion (tertiary HPTH), caused either by enlargement of all parathyroid glands or by two- or single gland enlargement may occur after transplantation (Figure 18.3) (Kilgo et al 1990). Tertiary HPTH is usually associated with overt hypercalcemia because of the enhanced sensitivity of peripheral target organs (particularly the bone) to PTH action (Cundy et al 1983; Messa et al 1998). Rarely, hypercalcemia exceeds 13 mg/dl, becoming symptomatic. Severely hypercalcemic patients may develop polyuria, polydipsia, hypertension, pruritus, 'red eyes' and may suffer from nausea, vomiting, or neurologic disorders, including somnolence and mental confusion. Hypercalcemia may also cause an acute and reversible decline in renal function or a chronic nephropathy (Zeiden et al 1991). Rarely, hypercalcemia may cause calciphylaxis with peripheral ischemic necrosis due to vascular calcification (Figure 18.4). This syndrome may be seen in patients with severe, uncontrolled pretransplant hyperparathyroidism. Even if hypercalcemia is not so severe usually, it is mandatory to prevent fluid deprivation. Administration of agents that can worsen hypercalcemia, such as oral calcium, vitamin D supplements and thiazide diuretics should be avoided. In case of calciphylaxis parathyroidectomy is imperative.

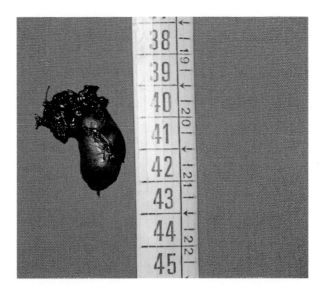

Figure 18.3. A large parathyroid adenoma removed from a transplant recipient with persistent hyperparathyroidism.

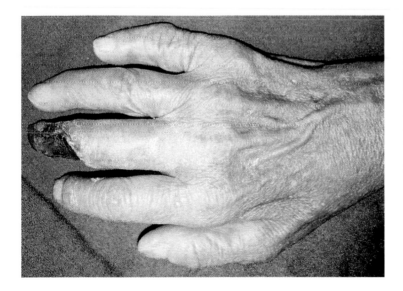

Figure 18.4. Calciphylaxis in a patient with severe hyperparathyroidism. Necrosis of the distal phalanx of the third finger. From Bedani PL, Orzincolo C, Scutellari PN, Gilli P (eds). *Imaging dell'apparato muscoloscheletrico in nefrologia.* Milan: Wichtig, 1988. Reproduced with permission.

Aluminum-associated disorders

In dialysed patients aluminum accumulation may be associated with low-turnover osteomalacia, adynamic bone disease (Smith et al 1986), proximal myopathy (Ihle et al 1986), microcytic anemia (Drueke et al 1986) and progressive dementia and seizures (Alfrey 1986). After successful renal transplantation the increased urinary excretion may reverse the aluminum accumulation with improvement of signs and symptoms. Proximal weakness and bone pain may improve quickly. The removal of the bone content of aluminum can take a longer time. However bone biopsy specimens show markedly improved histologic parameters of bone metabolism (Piraino 1988). On the basis of a study in the rat showing that citrate can increase urinary aluminum excretion (Cochran et al 1994), Massari et al (1997) administered a single dose of oral potassium citrate to eight transplant patients. A marked increase in urinary aluminum excretion was achieved. If these preliminary results were confirmed, potassium citrate administration might represent a safe way to accelerate aluminum detoxification.

β_2-microglobulin-related amyloidosis

This form of amyloidosis, caused by an accumulation of β_2-microglobulins, typically affects patients undergoing long-term dialysis (Zingraff and Druecke 1991). It is characterized by cystic bone lesions, destructive arthropathies and tenosynovitis (Figure 18.5). After transplantation, articular symptoms quickly improve, because of the anti-inflammatory effects of immunosuppressive agents. Unfortunately, since the tissue deposits of the protein cannot be mobilized, cystic bone lesions do not decrease in size and carpal tunnel syndrome does not ameliorate after transplantation despite the increased renal clearance of β_2-microglobulin.

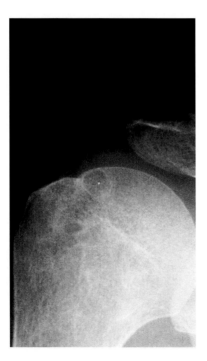

Figure 18.5. Osteoarticular amyloidosis in a patient with long-term hemodialysis. Osteolysis of the superior epiphysis. This type of lesion does not reverse after successful renal transplantation.

Osteoporosis

Osteoporosis is a systemic bone disease with reduced bone mass, altered architecture and increased fracture rate. The bone loss predominantly affects cancellous bone. Fractures involving the long bones are more common than those involving the vertebral bodies and usually occur more than 3 years after transplantation. Bone loss is greater during the first 6 months after transplantation varying from 3 to 7%, then continues at a lower rate (Julian et al 1991; Kwan et al 1992; Horber et al 1994), approximately 2% per year, in patients followed-up to 10 years after transplantation (Pichette et al 1996). The risk of osteoporotic fractures after transplantation is particularly high in diabetics and in females (Nisbeth et al 1999).

Pathogenesis

In the general population, several factors may contribute to the pathogenesis of osteoporosis, namely older age, female sex, postmenopausal status, insufficient mobilization, inadequate calcium intake, smoking, excessive alcohol consumption. The same factors may operate in renal transplant recipients. More specific factors include end-stage renal failure and genetic factors. As a matter of fact, a number of hemodialysed patients may show low bone mass (Yamaguchi et al 1996), a finding often neglected by nephrologists. Genetic factors may also play a role in the degree of bone loss. Patients with the 'favorable' bb genotype for the vitamin D receptor gene have been shown to recover more bone after renal transplantation than those with Bb and BB genotypes (Torres et al 1996). However, in renal allograft recipients the most frequent cause of osteoporosis is represented by corticosteroid treatment. The deleterious effects of corticosteroids on bone and mineral homeostasis are well recognized. Nearly all patients taking prednisone at doses in excess of 10 mg/day have substantial bone loss, regardless of age, gender or menopausal status (Lukert and Kream 1996). In renal transplant patients, the bone loss has been found to be more rapid during the first 12 months of therapy when the doses of corticosteroids are higher (Wolpaw et al 1994; Grotz et al 1995; McIntyre et al 1995). However, other studies (Julian et al 1991; Almond et al 1994; Massari et al 1994) did not find a relationship between bone loss and the dose of corticosteroids, pointing out that even small doses of prednisone (7.5 mg/day) when given for long periods of time may cause demineralization of areas rich in trabecular bone such as vertebrae, distal ends of long bones and ribs.

The pathogenesis of steroid-induced bone loss is multifactorial (Table 18.2). Pharmacological doses of corticosteroids may cause generalized defects in calcium transport across biological membranes which may concur with other, still unknown, mechanisms in reducing the net intestinal calcium absorption (Lukert and Kream 1996). Corticosteroids also cause hypercalciuria both by increasing bone resorption and urinary calcium excretion (Reid and Ibbertson 1987). In turn, a negative calcium balance stimulates parathyroid hormone secretion which further increases bone resorption (Dempster 1989). Moreover the interference of corticosteroids with gonadotropin release and the

Systemic interactions

　　Defect in Ca^{2+} transport across biological membranes

　　Hypercalciuria, negative Ca^{2+} balance, hyperparathyroidism

　　Reduced adrenal androgen and estrogen production

　　Inhibited secretion of growth hormone and skeletal growth factors

Local interactions

　　Decreased osteoblast recruitment

　　Enhanced osteoclast activity

　　Altered sensitivity of osteoclasts to PTH

Table 18.2. Pathogenesis of corticosteroid-induced osteoporosis

corticosteroid-induced suppression of adrenocorticotropic hormone cause reduced secretion of adrenal androgens and estrogens (Lukert 1996). The resulting hypogonadal state may contribute to further bone loss. Finally, corticosteroids inhibit the secretion of growth hormone and decrease the production and/or the bioactivity of some skeletal growth factors, such as insulin-like growth factor 1 and transforming growth factor-β_1. The final result is reduced bone formation and/or impaired growth. Corticosteroids also have a direct effect on bone. They decrease osteoblast recruitment and differentiation, and inhibit synthesis of type I collagen. As a consequence, there is a decrease in osteoid surface and in mineral apposition rate (Dempster 1989). Biochemically there is a low production of osteocalcin, a major noncollagenous bone matrix protein. Another direct effect on bone is represented by the enhancing effect on osteoclast activity and by the altered sensitivity of osteoclasts to parathyroid hormone. The sum of these direct effects of corticosteroids leads to bone loss. Corticosteroids may also indirectly favor the development of osteoporosis because they may cause proximal and systemic myopathy. Myopathy reduces physical activity and mobility so altering the gravitational forces on the skeleton and reducing weight-bearing activity and mobility. Myopathy may also expose the patient to fracture by increasing the propensity to fall.

The effects of other immunosuppressive agents on bone are less well known. The introduction of cyclosporine (CsA) has permitted reduction in the dosage of corticosteroids during the first period of transplantation. However, improvement in graft survival leads to a more prolonged administration of corticosteroids with increased risk of osteoporosis. Studies in rats showed that the administration of CsA at doses comparable to those used in transplantation can cause bone loss, mostly trabecular, accelerated bone turnover, increased bone resorption and bone remodeling (Movsowitz et al 1988, 1989; Schlosberg et al 1989). There is little information in humans. A transversal study in renal transplant recipients found no difference in bone mineral density between patients given CsA alone and those given CsA or azathioprine in combination with corticosteroids (Cueto-Manzano et al 1999). On the other hand, in a prospective randomized trial, renal transplant patients assigned to receive CsA alone, without steroid, had a significant improvement of bone mineral density during the first 18 months, suggesting that CsA does not interfere with bone mineralization. In the same study patients assigned to receive CsA plus steroids, after transplantation showed a significant decrease of bone mineral density (Aroldi et al 1997).

In rat, tacrolimus (FK506) causes bone loss of even greater magnitude than that described with CsA (Cvetkovic et al 1994). However there is little information about the effects of tacrolimus on bone in humans. Experimental studies in rat showed that rapamycin does not cause bone loss but may increase remodeling and decrease growth rate (Bryer et al 1995). Rapamycin may also induce testicular atrophy in rats, thereby reducing sex hormones (Morris et al 1992). This may theoretically expose the patient to osteopenia in the long term, but there is still no information available for humans. Mycophenolate mofetil has no effect upon bone volume in rat (Dissanayake et al 1998) and no data are available in humans. Azathioprine has been used for many years in transplantation. Short-term studies in rats showed no effect on bone volume, but documented an increase in the number of osteoclasts (Joffe et al 1993).

Treatment of osteoporosis

As a general rule, patients at risk of osteoporosis should be active physically, should discontinue those life-style habits (tobacco and alcohol) that are risk factors for osteoporosis, and should have a diet adequate in calcium, proteins, and vitamins (Table 18.3). Calcium administration at a dose of 1000 mg/day is an effective and inexpensive way of offsetting impaired calcium absorption and to decrease parathyroid secretion. Higher calcium administration (1500–2000 mg daily) may be indicated in postmenopausal women. However the physician should keep in mind the risk of inducing hypercalciuria or hypercalcemia in transplanted patients with persistent mild hyperparathyroidism. It is therefore necessary to monitor carefully both urinary and plasma calcium.

Oral calcium 1 g a day
Physical activity (general rule)
1,25 dihydroxyvitamin D_3 (if impaired renal function, menopause)
Calcitonin
Bisphosphonates
Estrogens (in amenorrheic or postmenopausal women)

Table 18.3. Prevention and treatment of osteoporosis

A number of drugs are employed for the prevention and treatment of osteoporosis. Vitamin D therapy may be theoretically indicated, as calcitriol may increase calcium absorption and may also stimulate the function of osteoblasts (Aloia et al 1988; Gallagher and Riggs 1990). However, the precise mechanism by which vitamin D may prevent bone loss in this setting is unknown. In a study, calcitriol treatment and adequate calcium intake reduced bone loss in corticosteroid-induced osteoporosis. However this effect was significant only within the first year. After 2 years of treatment the bone loss appeared to be even greater with vitamin D than with calcium alone (Sambrook et al 1993). Thus, there is no clear indication for vitamin D therapy in kidney transplant recipients, with the relevant exception of patients with low levels of vitamin D, since 1,25 dihydroxycholecalciferol deficiency might contribute to aggravation of secondary hyperparathyroidism. Thus, the use of vitamin D, at doses ranging between 0.25 and 0.5 μg /day, should be reserved for patients with renal allograft insufficiency or for postmenopausal women.

Calcitonin is a specific inhibitor of bone resorption. Eel and salmon calcitonin have the highest activity/weight ratio. Pig and human calcitonins have a weaker effect. Secretion of endogenous calcitonin is modulated by blood calcium levels. Calcitonin inhibits bone resorption and thereby lowers plasma calcium. The type of administration, the frequency and the amount of calcitonin for preventing and treating osteoporosis are still under investigation. The nasal bioavailability of salmon calcitonin is only 10–25% when compared with subcutaneous or intramuscular injection, but the biological effects of the nasal spray represent 40% of those observed with the injectable form (Reginster et al 1987). Conflicting results have been reported in corticosteroid-induced osteoporosis. A double-blind placebo-controlled study by Adachi et al (1997a) concluded that calcitonin spray 200 IU/day prevented early bone loss in the lumbar spine in half of the corticosteroid-treated patients. However, Sambrook et al (1993) did not show any benefit for prevention of corticosteroid-induced osteoporosis by adding calcitonin to calcitriol. As the amino acid sequence of salmon calcitonin differs from that of the human hormone, specific antibodies may develop in most patients after administration of salmon calcitonin. Whether these antibodies interfere with the activity of calcitonin is unclear, but it is well known that the long-term administration of salmon calcitonin can lead to resistance to the hormone and subsequent reduction of efficacy (Plosker and McTavish 1996). A downregulation of the skeleton receptor for calcitonin has also been hypothesized, which may provide an explanation for this 'calcitonin-escape' phenomenon (Takahashi et al 1995).

Bisphosphonates bind preferentially to bones with high turnover rates, such as trabecular bone. These agents oppose the increased bone resorption caused by corticosteroids by inhibiting osteoclast activity and by reducing the number of osteoclasts (Adachi et al 1994). Osteoclast survival may be decreased by destruction when contact is made with bone containing bisphosphonate or by apoptosis (Rodan and Fleisch 1996). As a consequence fewer osteoclasts are recruited to bone remodeling sites and differentiation of osteoclast precursor is impaired. The number of trabecular perforations, which are the cause of reduced bone strength, is decreased. A randomized trial showed that in rheumatic patients receiving high-dose steroids, the mean bone density of the lumbar spine increased in the group given etidronate for 1 year while it decreased in the placebo-treated patients who received calcium alone (Adachi et al 1997b). Recently the intravenous administration of a long-acting bisphosphonate was proposed in order to reduce the number of pills patients have to take, especially during the first posttransplant period. A combination of a cyclical intravenous administration of ibandronate (2 mg every 3 months) with a high dietary calcium intake (1000 mg/day) has been proposed in order to prevent bisphosphonate-induced hypocalcemia (Thiebaud et al 1996). A similar approach may consist of intermittent intravenous infusions of pamidronate (30 mg every 3 months) associated with 800 mg elemental calcium supplement (Fan et al 1996; Boutsen et al 1977).

Estrogen therapy effectively prevents bone loss in postmenopausal women. Although no studies regarding the effects of hormone replacement therapy in organ transplant recipients have been published, it is rational to give estrogen replacement therapy both to premenopausal women with amenorrhea and to postmenopausal women, before and after transplantation, if no contraindication exists. Progesterone must be given concomitantly to prevent endometrial hyperplasia. The recent new selective estrogen receptor modulator, raloxifene, has proved able to maintain bone mass in postmenopausal women (Hochner-Celnikier 1999). It may exert fewer uterine effects with lower risk of bleeding and, potentially, a decreased risk for breast cancer.

Human parathyroid hormone, given subcutaneously, significantly increases spinal bone mass in osteoporotic postmenopausal women taking corticosteroids and estrogen (Lane et al 1998). This treatment may be reserved for patients with previous total parathyroidectomy.

Fluoride can stimulate bone formation, and may therefore be used in corticosteroid-induced osteoporosis, in which inhibition of osteoblast function may play a pathogenetic role. Treatment with disodium monofluorophosphate, elemental calcium, and calcidiol was associated with a significant increase in bone mineral density in cardiac transplant patients with established osteoporosis (Meys et al 1993). However, increase in bone mineral density in response to fluoride is not associated with improvement in bone quality and strength, or reduction in fracture rates.

Osteonecrosis

Osteonecrosis is the death of marrow cells and the associated trabeculae and osteocytes not due to infection. This skeletal complication has also been labeled aseptic necrosis, avascular necrosis, and osteochondritis dissecans. The apparently synergistic roles of steroids and hyperparathyroid bone disease have been the focus of the pathogenesis of osteonecrosis. The development of osteonecrosis in transplanted patients treated with high-dose prednisone supports an important role for steroids (Bradford et al 1984; Lausten et al 1998). A meta-analysis of studies including transplant recipients and patients with lupus erythematosus found an association between osteonecrosis and the cumulative dosage of oral steroids, but not with methylprednisolone pulses (Felson and

Anderson 1987). It is likely that hyperparathroidism may enhance the damaging effects of steroids. Some studies showed that serum parathyroid hormone concentrations at the time of transplantation were correlated with the subsequent development of osteonecrosis (Vincenti et al 1981; Nehme et al 1989). A review of the literature including early studies showed that osteonecrosis afflicts 3–41% of kidney transplant recipients (First 1993). However, over the last few years the incidence of aseptic necrosis has decreased (Parfrey et al 1986), because of lower doses of steroid, better control of pretransplant hyperparathyroidism, and better clinical and nutritional condition of the patient at the time of transplantation.

About half of the cases present within the first 2 years after transplantation, the remaining cases may appear after 10 or more years. Osteonecrosis usually develops in weight-bearing bones, the femoral head being the most common site. Other sites affected are the femoral condyle, tibial plateau, body of the talus and humeral head. The distal tibia and humerus, proximal radius and ulna are affected less frequently (Julian et al 1992). The disease can be multifocal. The onset of osteonecrosis is insidious with stiffness and reduced mobility of the joint. Pain exacerbated by weight-bearing may precede radiographic changes. Pain may be referred from the hip to the ipsilateral knee. Effusions may develop, especially if the knee or elbow is involved.

Roentgenograms were the most frequently used method of diagnosing osteonecrosis until recently. However, computed tomography, scintigraphy combined with single-photon-emission computed tomography, computed tomography with multiplanar

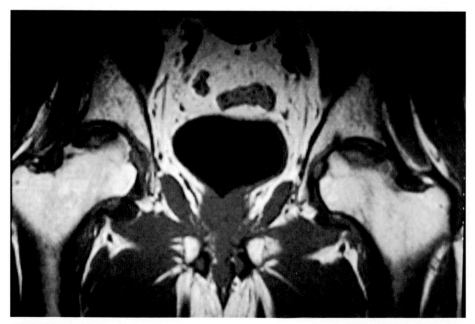

Figure 18.6.   Bilateral necrosis of femoral heads in a transplant recipient (computed tomography).

reconstructions and magnetic resonance imaging have proven to be more sensitive. At present magnetic resonance imaging is the best technique to diagnose early osteonecrosis of the femoral head (Figure 18.6). An early diagnosis may permit less invasive treatment in the early clinical course. Several stages of osteonecrosis have been recognized (Table 18.4). It is possible that steroid-free immunosuppression, the use of very low-dose prednisone or the use of corticosteroids less toxic to the bone, such as deflazacort (Gennari et al 1985), may reduce the risk of osteonecrosis. Treatment of osteonecrosis depends on the progression of the infarct. In stages I and II the benefit from purely conservative management such as limited weight-bearing and anti-inflammatory medications is short-lived. Attempts to preserve the femoral head by core decompression may be desirable. Decompression is useful in the relief of pain, but the femoral head often deteriorates further. Surgical intervention for patients with stage III or IV is inevitably contemplated. Total hip replacement in renal transplant recipients allows significantly increased activity and relief from pain (Brazil et al 1986).

Staging	Symptoms	Diagnosis
I	Asymptomatic, silent	Subtle mottled densities at MNR
II	Intermittent, aching, poorly localized	The infarct produces a rim of increased bone density at its periphery
III	Pain is activity-related in the groin area referred down the anteromedial thigh to the knee	Radiographic crescent sign of demarcation between the collapsing infarcted segment and the subchondral bone
IV	A notable limp, severe pain in the hip, limitation of motion, internal rotation being most seriously affected	Necrotic segmental collapses, producing a flattening of the femoral head
V	Symptoms indistinguishable from degenerative arthritis in the joint	Osteophyte formation at the margins of the femoral head and acetabulum. Collapse of the femoral head. Advanced degenerative arthritis with marked osteophyte formation around the femoral head
VI	Exacerbation	The acetabulum is flattened with loss of the normal curvature and containment of the femoral head. The femoral head may migrate laterally, eroding the acetabular edge because of excessive pressure from weight bearing

Table 18.4. Stages of progression of osteonecrosis

Muscular and joint complications

Painful legs syndrome

This syndrome is characterized by pain over the long bones, localized to the knees and ankles, without joint inflammation. The pain is mostly symmetrical, may interfere with walking, is not relieved by rest and may wake the patient during sleeping. The pain arises at the first month after transplant and usually resolves spontaneously in a few months. In its mild form the syndrome is common. The incidence of the severe form has been around 10% in some series (Lucas et al 1991). This syndrome does not correlate with previous hyperparathyroidism, and its pathogenesis is still unknown. Lucas et al (1991) found a relationship between the appearance of the painful legs syndrome and the initiation of cyclosporine therapy. Gauthier et al (1994) reported an improvement of the syndrome after administration of vasodilating calcium-channel blockers.

Polyarthralgias

Polyarthralgias due to diffuse myalgias and joint effusion may occur after rapid tapering of corticosteroid dosage, that is after treatment of acute rejection with high intravenous doses of methylprednisolone. The knees are the most symptomatic joints. The synovial fluid is sterile and tests for rheumatoid factors or antinuclear antibodies are negative. The syndrome is transient and seems not to be predictive of osteonecrosis.

Myopathy

Myopathy due to muscular damage after transplantation may be caused by steroid treatment and/or by severe hypophosphatemia. The legs are the most severely affected area. Moderate physical training may partially reverse the atrophy and improve exercise capacity (Horber et al 1985). Although the proximal limb muscles are painful, serum enzyme concentrations in muscles are usually normal. In contrast, diffuse pain due to rhabdomyolysis, in patients treated with hypolipemic drugs such as fibrates and hydroxymethylglutanyl-coenzyme A (HMG co-A) reductase inhibitors, is always accompanied with increased concentrations of muscle enzyme.

Tendinitis

Tendinitis and spontaneous rupture of tendons may occasionally occur after successful transplantation. Achilles tendons and extensor tendons of quadriceps and of the hand are most commonly affected. The cause remains unknown. As this complication more often develops in patients with a long history of dialysis, one may speculate a role for hyperparathyroidism or for deposits of β_2-microglobulin (dialysis amyloidosis). However, in several cases tendinitis also develops in patients with a short period of dialysis. It is possible that corticosteroids and CsA may play a pathogenetic role (Lucas et al 1991). Cases of tendinitis have also been reported in patients treated with pefloxacine or cyprofloxacine (Dekens-Konter et al 1994).

Gout

Gout is more frequent in patients under CsA or tacrolimus, which cause hyperuricemia by reducing the renal excretion of uric acid. Moreover the use of diuretics and renal dysfunction increase the plasma levels of uric acid. No therapy is required for asymptomatic hyperuricemia. The use of allopurinol, which inhibits the xanthine oxidase enzyme, should be limited to patients with uricemia higher than 10 mg/dl. The initial dose should not exceed 100 mg/day in order to avoid an exaggerated mobilization of uric acid deposits which can trigger a gout attack. As azathioprine is metabolized to inactive products by xanthine oxidase, the concomitant use of allopurinol and azathioprine causes an accumulation of 6-mercaptopurine that can lead to severe suppression of the bone marrow, with neutropenia, thrombocytopenia and anemia. Thus in the case of concomitant administration of allopurinol, the dosage of azathioprine must be reduced by 50–75% or the patient should be switched to mycophenolate mofetil. Uricosuric agents, such as probenicid or sulfinpyrazone, are less effective than allopurinol and become even less effective when creatinine clearance is lower than 80 ml/min. Moreover, uricosuric agents may favor urate stone formation. Thus, fluids should be forced and urine pH should be kept at 6 under uricosuric treatment. In the case of an acute attack of gout the agent of choice is colchicine, at a dose of 0.6–1 mg which may be repeated after 1 hour to a maximum of 3–4 mg. Colchicine may cause diarrhea. Often relief of pain and diarrhea occur simultaneously. Nonsteroidal anti-inflammatory drugs are also effective, but should be used with caution because they can lead to interstitial nephritis or renal function impairment caused by the inhibition of renal vasodilating prostaglandins.

OCULAR COMPLICATIONS

Ocular complications occur frequently in transplant recipients.

Retinopathy

Arterial hypertension may lead to typical retinal lesions characterized by arteriolar narrowing, tortuosity, and arteriovenous nicking (Figure 18.7). In the case of severe hypertension, cotton-wool spots, flame-shaped hemorrhages and hard exudates may be seen at fundoscopy. Exudative detachment, disc edema and optic atrophy may develop in patients with accelerated, uncontrolled hypertension. In patients with severe and long-standing hypertension a marked, sudden reduction of blood pressure may cause infarction of the optic nerve and visual loss. In other patients blindness may occur as a result of a cortical infarction (Leys et al 1998).

Retinal detachment (Figure 18.8) and diffuse retinal pigment epitheliopathy may occur in renal transplant recipients (Gass et al 1992). Renal failure, fluid and electrolyte imbalance, and hypertension may contribute to the pathogenesis of this disorder, but

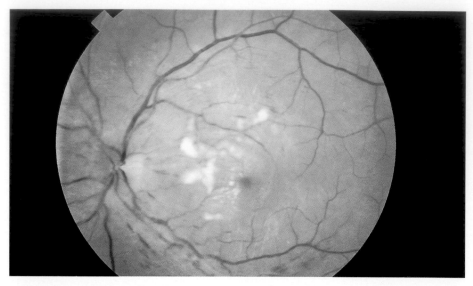

Figure 18.7. Hypertensive retinopathy with exudates, arteriolar narrowing, and tortuosity in a transplant patient. (Courtesy of Professor R Ratiglia, University of Milan.)

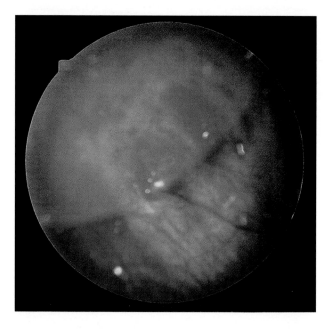

Figure 18.8. Retinal detachment in a transplant patient with severe hypertension and hypercorticism. (Courtesy of Professor R Ratiglia, University of Milan.)

the most important role is probably played by corticosteroids (Polak et al 1995). Reduction of corticosteroids and laser photocoagulation may be tried in order to improve the bad visual prognosis.

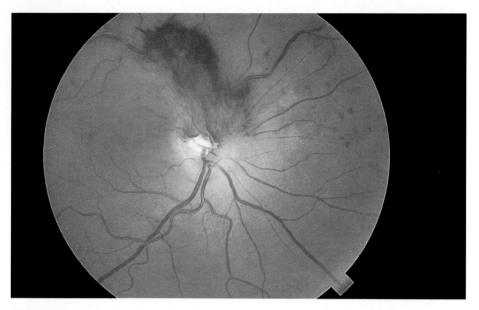

Figure 18.9. Diabetic retinopathy with retinal edema, hemorrhage, and vessel proliferation. (Courtesy of Professor R Ratiglia, University of Milan.)

Diabetic retinopathy is characterized by retinal edema, retinal ischemia and new vessel growth (Figure 18.9). This proliferative retinopathy can be accelerated by arterial hypertension. Treatment consists of panretinal photocoagulation. Vitrectomy may reduce the progression of proliferative retinopathy, by removing vitreous hemorrhage and by inducing vitreoretinal traction (Leys et al 1998).

Viral infection may lead to severe retinal complications. Cytomegalovirus may cause a hemorrhagic and necrotizing retinitis which is rapidly progressive in most cases. Varicella-zoster virus and herpes simplex virus may cause acute retinal necrosis. Prolonged antiviral treatment and reduction of immunosuppression may be tried. However the visual prognosis is usually poor.

Cataract

Cataract is the most frequent ocular complication in transplant recipients (Figure 18.10). Posterior subcapsular cataracts have been reported in 20–40% of renal transplant recipients (First 1993). The etiopathogenetic role of corticosteroids is well established and a correlation between the development of cataract and the doses of corticosteroids has been found (Hardie et al 1992). A prospective randomized trial showed that a steroid-free immunosuppression significantly reduced the risk of cataract

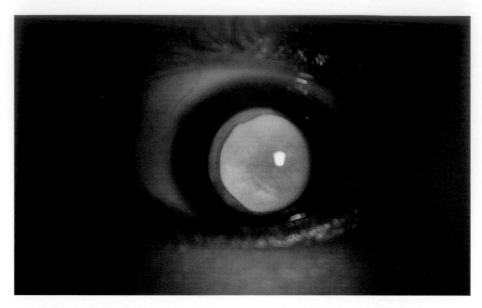

Figure 18.10. Subluxated cataract with dense central opacification. (Courtesy of Professor R Ratiglia, University of Milan.)

in cadaveric renal transplant recipients. However, a small number of patients given cyclosporine alone developed cataract, suggesting a cataractogen role for cyclosporine also (Ponticelli et al 1997).

Increase in intraocular pressure, caused by corticosteroids, can be found in 1–2% of transplant patients (Jayamanne and Porter 1998). This complication may lead to acute glaucoma in predisposed patients with increased resistance of aqueous outflow.

Miscellaneous

Bacterial and fungal infections may be responsible for rare cases of endophthalmitis (Figure 18.11). Apart from retinitis, herpes viruses may also cause keratitis. Exceptionally, ocular neoplasias may also occur in transplant patients. They include lymphoma of the vitreous, keratoacanthoma or squamous cell carcinomas of the eyelids (Leys et al 1998). Persisting hyperparathyroidism and hypercalcemia may cause corneal calcifications.

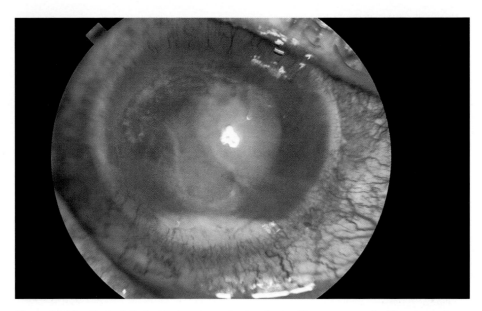

Figure 18.11. Endophthalmitis in a transplant patient with severe sepsis. (Courtesy of Professor R Ratiglia, University of Milan.)

HEMATOLOGICAL COMPLICATIONS

Anemia

After successful renal transplantation hemoglobin values gradually increase reaching normal values within 6–12 weeks. Patients with incomplete recovery of kidney allograft function may still show anemia because of an insufficient production of erythropoietin. Persistence of anemia in a patient with normal allograft function should prompt a search for occult sepsis, gastrointestinal bleeding, iron deficiency or vitamin B12 deficiency. Azathioprine mofetil mycophenolate and angiotensin-converting-enzyme (ACE) inhibitors may also cause anemia in renal transplant recipients. Anemia caused by azathioprine is usually associated with leukopenia and thrombocytopenia. Rarely, azathioprine may exert a selective erythroid toxicity with macrocytosis (McGrath et al 1975). Angiotensin-converting enzyme inhibitors can also cause anemia in renal transplant recipients, with a fall in hematocrit levels of 10% or more. Anemia is completely reversible after the cessation of the drug (Vlahakos et al 1991). The mechanism responsible for this anemia is still unclear, but it is possible that ACE-inhibitors may function by decreasing insulin-like growth factor-1 which has been demonstrated to promote erythropoiesis (Morrone et al 1997).

A microangiopathic hemolytic anemia may develop in patients with malignant

711

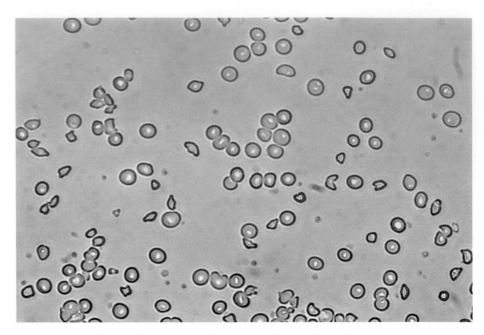

Figure 18.12. Microangiopathic hemolytic anemia in a patient with a de novo posttransplant hemolytic uremic syndrome. Note the fragmented, irregular erythrocytes.

hypertension or after the use of cyclosporine (Nizze et al 1988), tacrolimus (Trimarchi et al 1999) or OKT3 (Doutrelepont et al 1992). The presence of fragmented cells (Figure 18.12) associated with unconjugated hyperbilirubinemia, decreased or absent serum haptoglobin levels, elevated serum lactic dehydrogenase (LDH) levels, and reticulocytosis may allow a prompt diagnosis. Microangiopathic hemolytic anemia is usually associated with hypertension, acute renal failure and thrombocytopenia. Withdrawal of the offending drug and intensive treatment of hypertension may be useful for reversing or halting hemolytic anemia and renal failure. Plasma infusion can correct thrombocytopenia.

A different type of hemolytic anemia may occur in transplant recipients with minor ABO incompatibility with the donor (Povlsen et al 1990). Patients of group A receiving a kidney of group O or patients of group AB receiving a kidney of group A or B may develop hemolytic anemia in 14–20% of cases. The risk is higher in patients given cyclosporine (Ramsey et al 1991) and in patients of group A receiving a kidney of group O, probably because the titer of anti-A antibodies is higher than that of anti-B in group O persons. A possible role for autoantibodies produced by passenger lymphocytes has also been hypothesized (Elhence et al 1998). Clinically hemolytic anemia develops within 3–22 days after transplant. It may be severe enough to warrant blood transfusions. Spontaneous recovery occurs within 7–10 days (Ramsey 1991). In the most severe cases interruption of cyclosporine and high-dose prednisone treatment may be tried.

Polycythemia

About 10–15% of patients may develop erythrocytosis within 12 months after renal transplantation. In about 30–40% of cases erythrocytosis spontaneously resolves within 18–24 months (Qunibi et al 1991). Several factors may contribute to the development of posttransplant polycythemia (Table 18.5). The most frequent cause is probably represented by an overproduction of erythropoietin by the diseased native kidneys (Friman et al 1990), particularly in the case of acquired cysts, polycystic disease and diabetic nephropathy. Renal artery stenosis of the transplanted kidney is another possible cause of polycythemia while the use of diuretics may be responsible for a spurious erythrocytosis, with reduced plasma volume and normal erythrocytic volume. Recent data suggest that, as in polycythemia vera, erythrocytosis in renal transplant recipients might be mediated by an excessive production of insulin-like growth factor-1, which is an important regulator of erythropoiesis (Morrone et al 1997; Brox et al 1998).

Patients with polycythemia may suffer from headache, vertigo and blurred vision as the result of increased blood viscosity and hypervolemia. Thrombocytosis, platelet dysfunction and hyperviscosity may favor thrombotic complications, which may involve both arterial and venous occlusive events.

The goal of treatment is to reduce the hematocrit to approximately 45%, a level at which the complications of hyperviscosity and hypervolemia can be minimized.

Native kidneys
  Long duration of dialysis
  Acquired cystic disease
  Polycystic kidney disease
  Hydronephrosis

Transplanted kidney
  Renal artery stenosis
  Chronic rejection
  Hydronephrosis

Diabetes mellitus

Cystinosis

Smoking

Arterial hypertension
Diuretics (pseudopolycythemia)

Table 18.5. Main causes of posttransplant erythrocytosis

Angiotensin-converting enzyme inhibitors may be used as a first approach. In a placebo-controlled trial, the administration of enalapril at a daily dose of 2.5 mg reduced the hematocrit by 5–6%, while there was no change in the placebo group (Beckingham et al 1995). Further studies confirmed the therapeutic role of ACE inhibitors in posttransplant polycythemia. The decrease in hematocrit was correlated with the decrease in insulin-growth factor-1 but not with erythropoietin concentration, suggesting a direct effect of ACE inhibitor with this growth factor (Morrone et al 1997). Besides ACE inhibitors, the angiotensin II type 1 receptor antagonists can also lower hematocrit in posttransplant erythrocytosis (Julian et al 1998). Repeated phlebotomies may be used in patients who do not respond to ACE inhibitors. The initial phlebotomy regimen may remove 500 ml of whole blood. The same aliquot may be removed after a few days until hematocrit falls to 45%. As repeated phlebotomies may lead to iron deficiency, which prevents a rapid increase of hematocrit, some patients may maintain normal hematocrit with only two or three phlebotomies per year. Bilateral nephrectomy of the native kidneys could cure posttransplant erythrocytosis in some cases. It has been hypothesized that the ischemia of the native kidneys could be accelerated after transplantation, with consequent overproduction of erythropoietin (Friman et al 1990). Theophylline has also been used. This drug is an antagonist of adenosine which is an important mediator in the biosynthesis of erythropoietin. In one study, the administration of theophylline, at a dose of 8 mg/kg per day for 8 weeks, significantly reduced the levels of hematocrit and erythropoietin in eight patients with posttransplant erythrocytosis (Bakris et al 1990). However, in another controlled trial aminophylline proved to be ineffective (Mazzali and Filho 1998).

Leukopenia

Leukopenia may be induced by agents inhibiting the purine synthesis, such as azathioprine and mofetil mycophenolate. At the doses currently used with these agents severe leukopenia is rare, with the exception of a few patients with a genetic defect of thiopurine methyltransferase which mediates the *S*-methylation of 6-mercaptopurine (Chocair et al 1992). It is safe, however, to reduce the doses of these drugs when numbers of circulating white blood cells are lower than $5000/mm^3$ and to stop treatment transiently if leukocytes fall below $3000/mm^3$. It must be remembered that the association of allopurinol with azathioprine may expose the patient to the risk of severe granulocytopenia, as the xanthine-oxidase block caused by allopurinol causes an accumulation of active metabolites of 6-mercaptopurine.

Other drugs used in renal transplantation that may favor leukopenia are ganciclovir, trimethoprim–sulphametoxazole, penicillins and alpha-methyldopa. A number of infections, particularly viral infections and overwhelming bacterial infections, may be associated with neutropenia.

Severe granulocytopenia exposes to an increased risk of bacterial and fungal infections. The administration of granulocyte colony stimulating factor may be indicated whenever the number of neutrophils is lower than $1000/mm^3$ in a febrile patient (Dale 1993).

REFERENCES

Adachi JD, Cranney A, Goldsmith CH et al (1994) Intermittent cyclic therapy with etidronate in the prevention of corticosteroid induced bone loss. *J Rheumatol* **21**:1922–1926.

Adachi JD, Bensen WG, Bell MJ et al (1997a) Salmon calcitonin nasal spray in the prevention of corticosteroid-induced osteoporosis. *Br J Rheumatol* **36**:255–259.

Adachi JD, Bensen WG, Brown J et al (1997b) Intermittent etidronate therapy to prevent corticosteroid induced osteoporosis. *N Engl J Med* **337**:382–387.

Alfrey AC (1986) Dialysis encephalopathy. *Kidney Int* **29**(Suppl 19):S53–S57.

Aloia JF, Vaswani A, Yeh JK et al (1988) Calcitriol in the treatment of postmenopausal osteoporosis. *Am J Med* **84**:401–408.

Almond M, Kwan J, Evans K, Cunningham J (1994) Loss of regional bone mineral density in the first 12 months following renal transplantation. *Nephron* **66**:52–57.

Aroldi A, Tarantino A, Montagnino G et al (1997) Effects of three immunosuppressive regimens on vertebral bone density in renal transplant recipients. *Transplantation* **63**:380–386.

Bakris GL, Santer ER, Hussey JL et al (1990) Effects of theophylline on eythropoieten production in normal subjects and in patients with erythrocytosis after renal transplantation. *N Engl J Med* **323**:86–90

Beckingham IJ, Woodrow G, Hinwood M et al (1995) A randomized placebo controlled study of enalapril in the treatment of erythrocytosis after renal transplantation. *Nephrol Dial Transplant* **10**:2316–2320.

Bedani PL, Orzincolo C, Scutellari PN, Gilli P (eds) (1988) *Imaging dell'apparato muscoloscheletrico in nefrologia.* Milan: Wichtig.

Bonarek H, Merville P, Bonarek M et al (1999) Reduced parathyroid functional mass after successful kidney transplantation. *Kidney Int* **56**:642–649.

Boutsen Y, Jamart J, Esselinckx W et al (1997) Primary prevention of glucocorticoid-induced osteoporosis with intermittent intravenous pamidronate: a randomized trial. *Calcif Tissue Int* **61**:266–271.

Bradford DS, Szalapski EW, Sutherland DER et al (1984) Osteonecrosis in the transplant recipient. *Surg Gynecol Obstet* **159**:328–334.

Brazil M, Linderer RJ, Dickhans MJ et al (1986) Aseptic hip necrosis after renal transplantation. *Arch Surg* **121**:803–805.

Brox AG, Mangel J, Hanley JA et al (1998) Erythrocytosis after renal transplantation represents an abnormality of insulin-like growth factor-1 and its binding proteins. *Transplantation* **66**:1053–1058.

Bryer H, Isserow JA, Armstrong EC et al (1995) Azathioprine is bone sparing and does not alter cyclosporin A induced bone loss in the rat. *J Bone Miner Res* **10**:1191–1200.

Cecka M (1988) ABO blood group antigens and kidney transplantation. In: Terasaki PI (ed.). *Clinical Kidney Transplants.* Los Angeles: UCLA Tissue Typing Laboratory, pp. 189–198.

Chocair PR, Duley JA, Simmonds HA, Cameron JS (1992) The importance of thiopurine methyltransferase activity for the azathioprine in transplant recipients. *Transplantation* **53**:1051–1056.

Cochran M, Chawtur V, Phillips J, Dilena B (1994) Effect of citrate infusion on urinary aluminum excretion in the rat. *Clin Sci* **86**:223–226.

Cueto-Manzano AM, Konel S, Hutchison AJ et al (1999) Bone loss in long-term renal transplantation: histopathology and densitometry analysis. *Kidney Int* **55**:2021–2029.

Cundy T, Kanis JA, Heynen G et al (1983) Calcium metabolism and hyperparathyroidism after renal transplantation. *Q J Med* **205**:67–68.

Cvetkovic M, Mann G, Romero D et al (1994) Deleterious effects of long term cyclosporine A, cyclosporine G, and FK506 on bone mineral metabolism in vivo. *Transplantation* **57**:1231–1237.

Dale DC (1998) Potential role of colony stimulating factors in the prevention and treatment of infectious diseases. *Clin Infect Dis* **18**:S180–S181.

Dekens-Konter JA, Knol A, Olsson S et al (1994) Tendinitis of the achilles tendon caused by pefloxacin and other fluoroquinolone derivates. *Ned Tijdschr Geneeskd* **138**:528–531.

Dempster DW (1989) Bone histomorphometry in glucocorticoid-induced osteoporosis. *J Bone Miner Res* **4**:137–141.

Dissanayake I, Goodman C, Bowman A et al (1998) Mycophenolate mofetil: a promising new immunosuppressant which does not cause bone loss in the rat. *Transplantation* **65**:275–278.

Doutrelepont JM, Abramowicz D, Florquin S et al (1992) Early recurrence of hemolytic uremic syndrome in a renal transplant recipient during prophylactic OKT3 therapy. *Transplantation* **53**:1378–1383.

Drueke T (1995) The pathogenesis of parathyroid gland hyperplasia in chronic renal failure. *Kidney Int* **48**:259–272.

Drueke TB, Lacour B, Touam M et al (1986) Effect of aluminum on hematopoiesis. *Kidney Int* **29**(Suppl 19):S45–S48.

Dumoulin G, Hory B, Nguyen N et al (1995) Acute oral calcium load decreases parathyroid secretion and suppresses tubular phosphate loss in long-term renal transplant recipients. *Am J Nephrol* **15**:238–244.

Elhence P, Sharma RK, Chaudhary RK, Gupta RK (1998) Acquired hemolytic anemia after minor ABO incompatible renal transplantation. *J Nephrol* **11**:40–43.

Fan S, Almond MK, Ball E et al (1996) Randomized prospective study demonstrating prevention of bone loss by pamidronate during the first year after transplantation. *J Am Soc Nephrol* **7**:1789 (abstract).

Felsenfeld A, Gutman R, Drezner M, Llach F (1986) Hypophosphatemia in long-term renal transplant recipients: effect on bone histology and 1,25-dihydroxycholecalciferol. *Min Electrolyte Metab* **12**:333–341.

Felson DT, Anderson JJ (1987) A cross-study evaluation of association between steroid dose and bolus steroids and avascular necrosis of bone. *Lancet* **i**:902–906.

First MR (1993) Long-term complications after transplantation. *Am J Kidney Dis* **22**:477–486.

Friman S, Nyberg G, Blohmé I (1990) Erythrocytosis after renal transplantation: treatment by removal of the native kidneys. *Nephrol Dial Transplant* **5**:969–973.

Gallagher JC, Riggs BL (1990) Action of 1,25-dihydroxyvitamin D3 on calcium balance and bone turnover and its effect on vertebral fracture rate. *Metabolism* **39**(Suppl 1):S30–S34.

Gass JDM, Slamovits ThL, Fuller DG et al (1992) Posterior chorioretinopathy and retinal detachment after organ transplantation. *Arch Ophthalmol* **110**:1717–1722.

Gauthier V, Barbosa L (1994) Bone pain in transplant recipients responsive to calcium channel blockers. *Ann Intern Med* **121**:863–865.

Gennari C, Imbimbo B (1985) Effects of prednisone and deflazacort on vertebral bone mass. *Calcif Tissue Int* **37**:592–593.

Grotz W, Mundinger A, Rasenack J et al (1995) Bone loss after kidney transplantation: a longitudinal study in 115 graft recipients. *Nephrol Dial Transplant* **10**:2096–2100.

Hardie I, Matsunami C, Hilton A et al (1992) Ocular complications in renal transplant recipients. *Transplant Proc* **24**:177.

Higgins R, Richardson A, Endre Z et al (1990) Hypophosphatemia after renal transplantation: relationship to immunosuppressive drug therapy and effects on muscle detected by P nuclear magnetic resonance spectroscopy. *Nephrol Dial Transplant* **5**:62–68.

Hochner-Celnikier D (1999) Pharmacokinetics of raloxifene and its clinical application. *Eur J Obstet Gynecol Reprod Biol* **85**:23–29.

Horber FF, Scheidegger JR, Grunig BE et al (1985) Thigh muscle mass and function in patients treated with glucocorticoids. *Eur J Clin Invest* **15**:302–307.

Horber FF, Casez JP, Steiger U et al (1994) Changes in bone mass early after kidney transplantation. *J Bone Miner Res* **9**:1–9.

Ihle BU, Becker GJ, Kincaid-Smith PS (1986) Clinical and biochemical features of aluminum-related bone disease. *Kidney Int* **29**(Suppl 19):S80–S86.

Joffe I, Katz I, Sehgal S et al (1993) Lack of change of cancellous bone volume with short term use of the new immunosuppressant rapamycin in rats. *Calcif Tissue Int* **53**:45–52.

Jayamanne DGR, Porter R (1998) Ocular morbidity following renal transplantation. *Nephrol Dial Transplant* **13**:2070–2073.

Julian BA, Laskow DA, Dubovsky J et al (1991) Rapid loss of vertebral bone density after renal transplantation. *N Engl J Med* 1991 **325**:544–550.

Julian BA, Qualres LD, Niemann KMW (1992) Musculoskeletal complications after renal transplantation. *Am J Kidney Dis* **19**:99–120.

Julian BA, Brantley RR Jr, Barker CV et al (1998) Losartan, an angiotensin II type 1 receptor antagonist, lowers hematocrit in posttransplant erythrocytosis. *J Am Soc Nephrol* **6**:1104–1108.

Kilgo MS, Pirsch JD, Warner TE et al (1998) Tertiary hyperparathyroidism after renal transplantation. *Surgery* **124**:677–684.

Kifor O, Moore FD, Wang P et al (1986) Reduced immunostaining for the extracellular Ca^{2+}-sensing receptor in primary uremic hyperparathyroidism. *J Clin Endocrinol Metab* **81**:1598–1606.

Korkor A (1997) Reduced binding of [^{3}H]1,25-dihyroxyvitamin D3 in the parathyroid glands of patients with renal failure. *N Engl J Med* **316**:1573–1577.

Kwan JTC, Almond MK, Evans K, Cunningham J (1992) Changes in total body bone mineral content and regional bone mineral density in renal patients following renal transplantation. *Miner Electrolyte Metab* **18**:166–168.

Lane A, Lane NE, Sanchez S et al (1998) Parathyroid hormone treatment can reverse corticosteroid-induced osteoporosis. *J Clin Invest* **102**:1627–1633.

Lausten GS, Lemser T, Jensen PK, Egfjord M (1998) Necrosis of the femoral head after kidney transplantation. *Clin Transplant* **12**:572–574.

Leys A, Proesmans W, Devriendt K (1998) The eye and the kidney. In: Davison A, Cameron JS, Grünfeld JP, Kerr DNS, Ritz E, Winearls CG (eds). *Oxford Textbook of Clinical Nephrology*. Oxford: Oxford Medical Publications, pp. 2787–2808.

Lucas VP, Ponge L, Plougastel-Lucas M (1991) Musculoskeletal pain in renal transplant recipients. *N Engl J Med* **325**:1449 (letter).

Lukert BP (1996) Glucocorticoid-induced osteoporosis. In: Marcus R, Feldman D, Kelsey J (eds). *Osteoporosis*. New York: Academic Press, pp. 801–820.

Lukert B, Kream BE (1996) Clinical and basal aspects of glucocorticoid action in bone. In: Bilezikian JP, Raisz LG, Rodan GA (eds). *Principles of Bone Biology*. New York: Academic Press, pp. 533–548.

Martin-Malo A, Rodriguez M, Martinez ME et al (1996) The interaction of PTH and dietary phosphorus and calcium on serum calcitriol levels in the rat with experimental renal failure. *Nephrol Dial Transplant* **11**:1553–1558.

Massari PU, Garay G, Ulla MR (1994) Bone mineral content in cyclosporine-treated renal transplant patients. *Transplant Proc* **26**:2646–2648.

Mazzali M, Filho GA (1998) Use of aminophylline and enalapril in posttransplant polycythemia. *Transplantation* **65**:1461–1464.

McCarron DA, Muther RS, Lenfesty B, Bennet WM (1982) Parathyroid function in persistent hyperparathyroidism: relationship to gland size. *Kidney Int* **22**:662–670.

McGrath BP, Ibels LS, Raik E et al (1975) Erythroid toxicity of azathioprine: macrocytosis and selective marrow hypoplasia. *Q J Med* **44**:57–63.

McIntyre H, Menzies B, Rigby R et al (1995) Long-term bone loss after renal transplantation. Comparison of immunosuppressive regimens. *Clin Transplant* **9**:20–24.

Messa PG, Sindici C, Cannella G et al (1998) Persistent secondary hyperparathyroidism after renal transplantation. *Kidney Int* 54:1704–1713.

Meys E, Terreaux-Duvert F, Beaume-Six T et al (1993) Effects of calcium, calcidiol and monofluorophosphate on lumbar bone mass and parathyroid function in patients after cardiac transplantation. *Osteoporosis Int* 3:329–332.

Morris RE (1992) Rapamycins: antifungal, antitumor, antiproliferative, and immunosuppressive macrolides. *Transplant Rev* 6:39–87.

Morrone LF, Di Paolo S, Logoluso F (1997) Interference of angiotensin-converting enzyme inhibitors in erythropoiesis in kidney transplant recipients. *Transplantation* 64:913–918.

Movsowitz C, Epstein S, Fallon M et al (1988) Cyclosporine A in vivo produces severe osteopenia in the rat: effect of dose and duration of administration. *Endocrinology* 123:2571–2577.

Movsowitz C, Epstein S, Ismail F et al (1989) Cyclosporin A in the oophorectomized rat: unexpected severe bone resorption. *J Bone Miner Res* 4:393–398.

Nehme D, Rondeeau E, Paillard F et al (1989) Aseptic necrosis of bone following renal transplantation: relation with hyperparathyroidism. *Nephrol Dial Transplant* 4:123–128.

Nisbeth U, Lindh E, Liunghall S et al (1999) Increased fracture rate in diabetes mellitus and females after renal transplantation. *Transplantation* 67:1218–1222.

Nizze H, Mihatsch MJ, Zollinger HU et al (1985) Cyclosporine-associated nephropathy in patients with heart and bone marrow transplants. *Clin Nephrol* 30:248–260.

Parfitt AM (1997) The hyperparathyroidism of chronic renal failure: a disorder of growth. *Kidney Int* 52:3–9.

Parfrey PS, Ferge D, Parfrey NA et al (1986) The decreased incidence of aseptic necrosis in renal transplant recipients—a case control study. *Transplantation* 41:182–187.

Pichette V, Bonnardeaux A, Prudhomme L et al (1986) Long-term bone loss in kidney transplant recipients: a cross-sectional and longitudinal study. *Am J Kidney Dis* 28:105–114.

Piraino B, Carpenter BJ, Puschett JB (1988) Resolution of hypercalemia and aluminum bone disease after renal transplantation. *Am J Med* 85:728–730.

Plosker GL, McTavish D (1996) Intranasal salmon calcitonin: a review of its pharmacological properties and in the management of postmenopausal osteoporosis. *Drugs Aging* 8:378–400.

Polak BCP, Baarsma GS, Snyers B (1995) Diffuse retinal pigment epitheliopathy complicating systemic corticosteroid treatment. *J Ophthalmol* 79:922–925.

Ponticelli C, Tarantino A, Segoloni GP et al (1997) A randomized study comparing three cyclosporine-based regimens in cadaveric renal transplantation. *J Am Soc Nephrol* 8:638–646.

Povlsen JV, Rasmussen A, Hansen HA et al (1990) Acquired haemolytic anaemia due to isohemagglutinins of donor origin following ABO-minor incompatible kidney transplantation. *Nephrol Dial Transplant* 5:148–151.

Qunibi WY, Barri Y, Devol E et al (1991) Factors predictive of post-transplant erythrocytosis. *Kidney Int* 40:1153–1159.

Ramsey G (1991) Red cell antibodies arising from solid organ transplants. *Transfusion* 31:76–86.

Reginster JY, Denis D, Albert A et al (1987) Assessment of the biological effectiveness of nasal synthetic salmon calcitonin by comparison with intramuscular or placebo injection in normal subjects. *Bone Miner* 2:133–140.

Reid IR, Ibbertson HK (1987) Evidence of decreased tubular reabsorption of calcium in glucocorticoid-treated asthmatics. *Horm Res* 27:200–204.

Rodan GA, Fleisch HA (1996) Bisphosphonates: mechanism of action. *J Clin Invest* 97:2692–2696.

Sambrook P, Birmingham J, Kelly P et al (1993) Prevention of corticosteroid osteoporosis: a comparison of calcium, calcitriol and calcitonin. *N Engl J Med* 328:1747–1752.

Schlosberg M, Movsowitz C, Epstein S et al (1989) The effect of cyclosporin A administration and its withdrawal on bone mineral metabolism in the rat. *Endocrinology* 124:2179–2184.

Slatopolsky E, Delmez J (1992) Bone disease in chronic renal failure and after transplantation. In: Coe FL, Favus MJ (eds). *Disorders of Bone and Mineral Metabolism*. New York: Raven Press, pp. 905–917.

Smith AJ, Faugere MC, Abreo K et al (1986) Aluminum-associated bone disease in mild and advanced renal failure: evidence for high prevalence and morbidity and studies on etiology and diagnosis. *Am J Nephrol* 6:275–283.

Takahashi S, Goldring S, Katz M et al (1995) Down-regulation of calcitonin receptor mRNA expression by calcitonin during human osteoclast-like cell differentiation. *J Clin Invest* 95:167–171.

Thiebaud D, Kriegbaum H, Huss H et al (1996) Intravenous injections of ibandronate in the treatment of postmenopausal osteoporosis. *Osteoporosis* 1:321–325.

Torres A, Machado M, Concepcion Mt et al (1996) Influence of vitamin D receptor genotype on bone mass after renal transplantation. *Kidney Int* 50:1726–1733.

Trimarchi HM, Troung LD, Brennans S et al (1999) FK 506-associated thrombotic microangiopathy: report of two cases and review of the literature. *Transplantation* 67:539–543.

Vincenti F, Hattner R, Amend WJ et al (1981) Decreased secondary hyperparathyroidism in diabetic patients receiving hemodialysis. *JAMA* 245:930–933.

Vlahakos DV, Canzanello VJ, Madaio MP et al (1991) Enalapril-associated anemia in renal transplant recipients treated for hypertension. *Am J Kidney Dis* 17:199–205.

Wolpaw T, Deal C, Fleming-Brooks S et al (1994) Factors influencing vertebral bone density after renal transplantation. *Transplantation* 58:1186–1189.

Yamaguchi T, Kannoe E, Tsubota J et al (1996) Retrospective study on the usefulness of radius and lumbar bone density in the separation of hemodialysis patients with fractures from those without fractures. *Bone* 19:549–555.

Zeiden B, Shabtal M, Waltzer WC et al (1991) Improvement in renal transplant function after subtotal parathyroidectomy in a hypercalcemic kidney allograft recipient *Transplant Proc* 23:2285–2288.

Zingraff J, Drueke T (1991) Can the nephrologist prevent dialysis related amyloidosis? *Am J Kidney Dis* 18:1–11.

19 GYNECOLOGIC AND OBSTETRIC CONSIDERATIONS

*In collaboration with Vaseem Ali, Pamela D Berens, and Allan R Katz**

INTRODUCTION

A substantial number of renal transplants occur in females, and approximately 80% of transplanted women are under the age of 55 years (Cecka and Terasaki 1993). The USRDS 1999 annual report (National Institutes of Health 1999) indicates that a preponderance of transplants occur in patients of reproductive age. Gynecologic concerns thus represent a frequent reason for seeking medical attention. Patients with end-stage renal disease (ESRD) may experience amenorrhea, anovulation, and infertility, in addition to the other gynecologic concerns commonly experienced by patients with normal renal function. Following transplantation, resumption of cyclic menses and return of fertility typically occurs within an average of 6 months (Abramovici et al 1971; Makowski and Penn 1976). Because renal transplant patients may experience a return of fertility, patients should be counseled on the risks of pregnancy and alternate means of contraception. Despite the presence of underlying medical conditions and the use of immunosuppressants, many transplant recipients choose to pursue pregnancy. It is estimated that 1 in 50 female transplant patients of childbearing age will become pregnant. In general, the pregnancy has little effect on long-term graft survival. Cautious prenatal care with communication among specialists, meticulous control of confounding medical complications, and antenatal fetal surveillance may help to assure the best possible outcome.

OBSTETRIC CONSIDERATIONS

Physiology of pregnancy in renal transplantation

Many physiologic changes that normally occur during pregnancy and puerperium involve the genitourinary tract and thus must be given special consideration in transplant patients. In pregnant, nontransplant patients, renal plasma flow and glomerular filtration rates (GFRs) increase as early as 3–4 weeks after conception and continue to

Department of Obstetrics, Gynecology, and Reproductive Medicine, University of Texas Medical School, Houston

rise throughout most of the pregnancy to 200–250 ml/min (approximately a 25 and a 40% increase, respectively, over baseline), decreasing to normal as term pregnancy approaches and remaining below baseline for many months during the puerperium. Because of these changes, the blood urea nitrogen (BUN) and serum creatinine values typically decrease to one-half to two-thirds of the prepregnancy values (Sims and Krantz 1958). The renal vasodilatation and increased GFR associated with pregnancy also occur in renal transplant patients who have good renal function despite the ectopic location of the kidney (Baylis 1999). In general, a slight reduction in GFR occurs in the late third trimester, and 15% of transplant recipients display significantly decreased renal function after pregnancy.

The renal transplant patient also displays similar changes in renal morphology as nontransplanted women, including a 30% increase in renal volume (Christensen et al 1989). Postpartum, transplant recipients show a 1.5-cm-greater mean kidney length (adjusted for height), as measured by intravenous pyelogram, than nonpregnant, non-transplant patients; subsequently, those in the former group lose 1 cm in length over the next 6 months (Bailey and Rolleston 1971). In addition, dilatation of the renal pelvis, calyces, and ureters, particularly on the right side, owing to mechanical issues, may persist for several months after delivery. Nonobstructive ureteral dilatation commonly occurs in normal pregnancy, persisting in the puerperium. Some of these changes may owe to compression of the ureter against the pelvic inlet by the pregnant uterus (Rubi and Sala 1968). The condition of the transplanted ureter may vary, owing to its ectopic location and resultant lack of similar compressive forces (Figure 19.1). Moreover, the elevated progesterone level during pregnancy may alter ureteral peristalsis.

The bladder undergoes structural and functional changes during normal pregnancy, producing at least a transient difficulty of incomplete emptying among 20% of postpartum women. Although the condition lasts only 3 months, many women display long-term changes. Postpartum stress urinary incontinence is reported in 21% of women undergoing spontaneous vaginal delivery and in 34% of women undergoing instrumented vaginal delivery (Meyer et al 1998). Furthermore, after delivery, the bladder neck hypermobility and functionally diminished urethral length that occurs in nontransplant patients may cause increased urinary stasis that would be expected to predispose transplant patients to an increased risk of infection.

Prepregnancy counseling

Adequate counseling is imperative before the renal transplant patient considers pregnancy; it is generally recommended that pregnancy be deferred for 18 months to 2 years after transplantation, the period of greater risk of acute rejection as well as higher doses of immunosuppressive medications.

Renal transplant patients are advised to consider pregnancy only if they fit the recommended guidelines of Davison et al (Davison et al 1976; Sturgiss and Davison 1991; Davison 1995; Davison and Lindheimer 1999): good health for at least 2 years post-

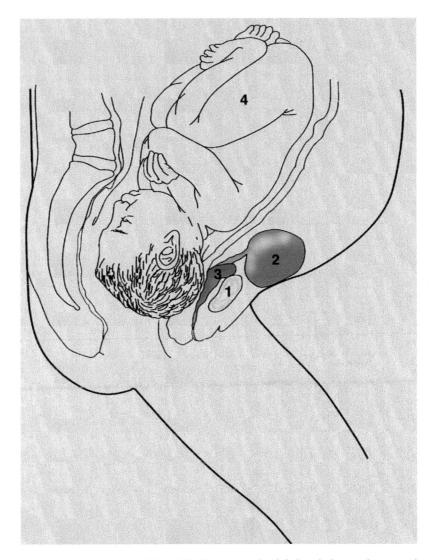

Figure 19.1. Term fetus positioned in the maternal pelvis in relation to the transplanted kidney. (1) Symphysis pubis; (2) transplanted kidney and ureter; (3) bladder; (4) fetus.

transplant; stature compatible with good obstetrical outcome; absent or minimal proteinuria; absence of hypertension; no evidence of graft rejection; absence of pelvicalyceal distention on recent intravenous urogram; stable renal function with serum creatinine no more than 2 mg/dl and preferable below 1.4 mg/dl; and minimal drug therapy, namely, prednisone (Pred) no more than 15 mg per day, azathioprine (AZA) no more than 2 mg/kg per day, and cyclosporine (CsA) no more than 5 mg/kg per day.

Strict control of diabetes and hypertension is imperative prior to pregnancy, since these medical disorders have significant implications for adverse maternal and fetal outcomes. In addition, maternal age over the age of 35 years is associated with an increased incidence of chromosomal abnormalities in the fetus; for these patients, genetic counseling and possible amniocentesis are recommended. Furthermore, potential fetal infections such as rubella, varicella, hepatitis B, cytomegalovirus (CMV), and toxoplasmosis must be evaluated. Vaccination may be offered and pregnancy delayed for 3 months if the patient is rubella nonimmune or negative for varicella. Hepatitis B vaccination can be administered prior to or during pregnancy, with no delay necessary prior to pursuing pregnancy. Smoking, alcohol, and illicit drug use should be discouraged. Prenatal folic acid 400 µg daily should be initiated at 6 weeks prior to conception.

Implications of commonly used medications for pregnancy

Prednisone

Immunosuppressant medications are maintained during the pregnancy (Table 19.1); dosage adjustments should be based on maternal indications. Although a daily Pred dosage no more than 15 mg prior to pregnancy is recommended, a recent study reported that a dosage of no more than 7.5 mg daily was the most significant predictor of a positive pregnancy outcome for renal transplant recipients (Bar et al 1997). However, studies suggest that either Pred or prednisolone has little effect on the developing fetus (Briggs et al 1998). These drugs are considered category B (Table 19.2); that is, they are compatible with pregnancy and breast-feeding. Although Cote et al (1974) report one case of temporary immunosuppression in a newborn exposed to high doses of Pred and AZA throughout pregnancy, other infants similarly exposed have not displayed this effect (Cederqvist et al 1977).

Azathioprine

Azathioprine, a category D drug, has been shown to be teratogenic in some animal studies, although no specific anomalies have been associated with its use in humans. However, neonatal leukopenia and thrombocytopenia have been reported. Maternal leukocyte count at 32 weeks gestation correlates with cord blood leukocyte count. DeWitte et al (1984) found that among patients who, at 32 weeks, displayed a leukocyte count at or below one standard deviation for normal pregnancy, a 50% dose reduction of AZA was not associated with neonatal leukopenia or thrombocytopenia. Although intrauterine growth restriction (IUGR) has also been associated with the use of AZA (Briggs et al 1998), it is difficult to determine whether the problem is caused by the drug itself or by the underlying medical conditions of patients.

Cyclosporine

Cyclosporine is classed as category C for pregnancy. Animal studies do not demonstrate a teratogenic effect, and no specific pattern of anomalies has been noted in human

Drug type	Drug	Pregnancy category	Specific associations
Immunosuppressants	Prednisone	B	Reported few if any fetal effects.
	Cyclosporine	C	IUGR? Spontaneous abortion?
	Azathioprine	D	Transient neonatal leukopenia and thrombocytopenia. IUGR?
	Tacrolimus	C	No associated anomalies reported, but limited information available.
	Mycophenolate mofetil	C	Effect on organogenesis in animal studies. Single report of use in pregnancy without adverse effects.
Antihypertensive agents	α-Methyldopa	C	Reduction in neonatal systolic blood pressure.
	Hydralazine	C	Rarely, neonatal thrombocytopenia.
	Labetolol	C/D	IUGR? Neonatal hypotension, neonatal β-blockade.
	Atenolol	D	IUGR? Neonatal hypotension, neonatal β-blockade.
	ACE inhibitors	D	Fetal hypocalvarium, renal failure, oligohydramnios, fetal and neonatal death.
	Doxazosin	B	No reports available of use of this drug in human pregnancy.
	Clonidine	C	No adverse fetal effects reported but limited information available.
	Prazosin	C	No adverse fetal effects reported but limited information available.
Diuretics	Furosemide	C	Decreased placental perfusion.
	Thiazide diuretics	D	Neonatal thrombocytopenia, hypoglycemia, hyponatremia and hypokalemia. Decreased placental perfusion? Nonspecific increased risk for congenital anomalies?
Antibiotics	Cephalosporins	B	Cephalosporins are generally considered safe in pregnancy.
	Fluoroquinolones	C	Animal studies indicate an association with fetal cartilage damage and arthropathies. Nonspecific increase risk for congenital anomalies?
	Penicillins	B	Penicillins are generally considered safe in pregnancy.
	Vancomycin	C	Generally considered safe in pregnancy, case report of hearing impairment.
	Clindamycin	B	Generally considered safe in pregnancy.
	Metronidazole	B	Conflicting information available. Use during the first trimester contraindicated. Frequently used outside first trimester.
	Nitrofurantoin	B	No adverse fetal effects appear to be associated. Due to glutathione deficiency, theoretical risk of fetal hemolytic anemia at term.
	Tetracycline	D	Adverse effects on fetal bones and teeth. Maternal liver toxicity. Congenital anomalies?
Antivirals	Gancyclovir	C	No reports of use in human pregnancy available. Embryotoxic, carcinogenic and mutagenic in animal studies.
	Acyclovir	C	No adverse fetal or neonatal effects associated. Minimal risk based on current data but limited data available.
Pain medications	ASA	C/D	Risk of neonatal hemorrhage? IUGR? Premature closure of the ductus arteriosus in late pregnancy.
	Ibuprofen	B/D	Third-trimester use associated with premature closure of the ductus arteriosus, persistent pulmonary hypertension of the newborn.
	Acetaminophen	B	Usual doses considered safe in pregnancy. High doses potentially toxic.
	Codeine	C/D	High or prolonged doses at term associated with neonatal depression and possible narcotic withdrawal.

Table 19.1. Commonly used medications in transplant patients and pregnancy category

	Experimental information	Recommendations
Category A	Controlled studies in humans fail to demonstrate risk with first trimester exposure, possibility of fetal harm is remote	Possibility of fetal harm remote
Category B	Either: Animal studies do not demonstrate fetal risk and there are no controlled studies in pregnant women Or: Animal studies show an adverse effect that was not confirmed in controlled studies in women in the first trimester	Probably safe in pregnancy
Category C	Either: Animal studies show an adverse effect and there are no controlled studies in pregnant women Or: Studies in animals and women are unavailable	Drugs should be used only if potential benefit justifies potential fetal risk.
Category D	Positive evidence of human fetal risk, but benefits may be acceptable despite the risk	Drug may be used for life-threatening situation or serious disease for which safer drugs cannot be used or are ineffective
Category X	Positive evidence of fetal risk and the use of the drug in pregnant women clearly outweighs any possible benefit	Contraindicated in pregnancy

Table 19.2. Definitions of fetal risk factors related to drug exposure (Adapted from Briggs et al (1998))

infants born to mothers treated with CsA during pregnancy. Intrauterine growth retardation has been noted in pregnancies exposed to CsA, although it is not known whether this effect is drug-related (Briggs et al 1998). One study noted an increased rate of spontaneous abortions among renal transplant recipients receiving CsA versus those receiving prednisolone and AZA (Haugen et al 1994); however, other studies have not supported this finding (Armenti et al 1997).

Antihypertensive medications

During pregnancy, patients with underlying hypertension may continue their regimen of drug treatment. Medications to control hypertension are typically used to target diastolic blood pressure below 100 mmHg; however, it has not been possible to demonstrate that maintaining the blood pressure below this level during pregnancy benefits either maternal or fetal outcome.

Only limited information is available on the use of new antihypertensive agents during pregnancy. Owing to the extensive experience with α-methyldopa, this drug is considered the first-line therapeutic agent and is classed as category C. No specific anomalies are associated with its use, although a small but clinically insignificant reduction in neonatal systolic blood pressure has been observed during the first 2 days of life (Whitelaw 1981). If α-methyldopa fails to provide adequate control, labetalol and atenolol are the preferred drugs. Labetalol is classed as a category C drug in the first trimester pregnancy and category D in the second and third trimesters, due to a possible association with growth restriction, although it is unclear whether the effect owes to the underlying hypertensive disorder or to the drug itself. Transient hypotension in the newborn has been reported (Briggs et al 1998). Atenolol is considered a category D agent that may cause IUGR, but no specific anomalies have been associated with this agent. β-blockade has been reported in some newborns, requiring that infants be closely observed over the first 24–48 hours of life (Briggs et al 1998). Hydralazine, a category C drug, is frequently used for acute hypertensive control during hospitalization.

Enzyme inhibitors

Owing to an association with fetal hypocalvarium, renal failure, oligohydramnios, and fetal or neonatal death, angiotensin-converting enzyme inhibitors should be avoided during pregnancy. Patients pursuing pregnancy should be switched to other medications. If conception occurs during use of these medications, the drugs should be discontinued immediately. In 1991, the US Food and Drug Administration (FDA) reported an association of fetal renal failure with enalapril, captopril, and lisinopril: of the 29 reported cases, 41% proved fatal. These agents are relatively contraindicated in pregnancy unless maternal well-being cannot be assured with an alternative agent.

Diuretics

Theoretically, a reduced plasma volume might decrease placental perfusion; thus, diuretics should not be instituted during pregnancy. No demonstration of improved perinatal outcome has been shown using furosemide for the treatment of hypertension during pregnancy. Thiazide diuretics, but not the category C drug furosemide, have been reported to produce neonatal thrombocytopenia (Briggs et al 1998).

727

Antibiotics

Most antibiotics can be prescribed during pregnancy with relative safety; there are no significant fetal considerations. In contrast, administration of fluoroquinolones may cause fetal cartilage damage and arthropathies in animals treated with these agents. While some information on the use of fluoroquinolones in humans suggests a major clinical concern, safer antibiotic choices are increasingly becoming available (Briggs et al 1998).

Analgesics

Pain requirements during pregnancy are best controlled with acetaminophen. If this drug is insufficient, acetaminophen with codeine is frequently prescribed. Both aspirin and ibuprofen are countraindicated, especially when used for more than a brief duration or in the third trimester of pregnancy. Demerol and morphine can both be used for short periods as needed during or after delivery to control surgically related pain.

Antepartum management

Optimal pregnancy outcome is best assured by a multidisciplinary team involving the renal transplant team, high-risk obstetrician, and internist. The renal transplant team is best positioned to monitor renal function, diagnose and treat acute or chronic rejection, and adjust immunosuppressant medications. The high-risk obstetrician is best equipped to maintain fetal surveillance and follow for signs and symptoms of pre-eclampsia. The internist may participate by managing hypertension, diabetes, and cardiovascular status.

The initial obstetrical visit includes a complete history and physical. Routine antenatal evaluation is requested and should include: complete blood count; rubella titer; screens for HbsAg and human immunodeficiency virus (HIV); screens for blood type and antibodies; Pap smear; gonorrhea and chlamydia testing as appropriate; electrolytes, BUN, and creatinine; TORCH titers as appropriate; urinalysis and urine culture; baseline 24-hour urine collection for total protein and creatinine clearance; and obstetrical ultrasound to assure accurate dating.

Other pertinent obstetric laboratory testing during pregnancy includes α-fetoprotein or triple-screen testing for neural tube defects and chromosomal abnormalities. These tests are performed at 16–20 weeks in women under age 35 years. Women 35 years and older should be offered amniocentesis and genetic counseling. Pregestational diabetic patients should be maintained on insulin during pregnancy. Oral agents should not be used, and patients should be converted to insulin either prior to or upon identification of pregnancy. Patients who are not pregestational diabetics should undergo glucose tolerance testing at 26–28 weeks gestation. Risk factors for diabetes, including prior gestational diabetes, prior macrosomic infant, strong family history of diabetes, and obesity, require additional, earlier glucose testing. Near week 36 of pregnancy, cultures should be obtained from the lower third of the vagina and perineum for group B streptococcus colonization.

In addition to an early ultrasound to assure accurate dating (Figure 19.2), an ultrasound at 20 weeks gestation is recommended to evaluate fetal anatomy. Ultrasounds should be performed every 4 weeks to monitor fetal growth, as IUGR of the fetus is more common in the transplant patient. Based on information on other patients with vascular disease, antenatal fetal surveillance should be initiated at or prior to week 32, if otherwise indicated by suggestion of growth restriction. Biophysical profiles, consisting of ultrasound assessment of fetal tone, movement and breathing motions, and measurement of amniotic fluid volume, are performed weekly, although patients with suspected growth restriction may benefit from twice-weekly testing. A nonstress test with external fetal monitoring is also performed. Each parameter is scored 2 points if normal and 0 points if abnormal, with an optimal score of 10 points. The patients should be instructed on daily assessment of fetal movements.

Low-risk obstetrical patients are seen monthly; high-risk transplant patients should be seen every 2 weeks until 32 weeks and every week from 32 weeks to delivery. The presence of underlying confounding conditions, such as diabetes or hypertension, may increase the frequency of required visits. During these visits, maternal weight; urine evaluation for protein, ketones and glucose; and blood pressure monitoring should be performed. Monthly laboratory testing includes a complete blood count with platelets; electrolytes, BUN, and creatinine and urinalysis and urine culture.

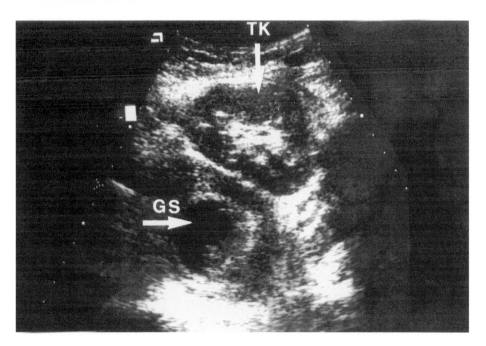

Figure 19.2. Transvaginal ultrasound examination of a female renal transplant patient in early pregnancy. TK: transplanted kidney; GS: intrauterine gestational sac.

Repeat 24-hour urine evaluation for total protein and creatinine clearance is performed in the presence of any suggestion of pre-eclampsia or increase in proteinuria based on urine dip strip testing. Thorough evaluation of abnormal Papillomavirus smears should be undertaken in the pregnant renal transplant patient, since both conditions are known to predispose to development of cervical dysplasia. Urinary tract infections and asymptomatic bacteria should be promptly treated, and frequent episodes suggest the need for suppressive antibiotics.

Renal transplant patients have an increased incidence of preterm delivery. Discussion of signs and symptoms of premature labor from 20 weeks onward is beneficial. Frequent pelvic examinations may assist with early diagnosis of premature labor.

Antenatal complications

Registries tracking the outcome of pregnancy in transplant patients are ongoing in North America, Europe, and Japan (Armenti et al 1994; Ehrich et al 1996; Davison and Redman 1997). Most of the available information is from the National Transplantation Pregnancy Registry (NTPR) which, since 1991, has maintained an ongoing database of pregnant transplant patients from the US, Canada, and Puerto Rico. A 1994 evaluation of the database reported the outcome of 156 pregnancies as follows: ectopic, 1%, therapeutic abortion, 12%; spontaneous abortion, 16%; stillbirth, 2.6%; and live birth, 68.6%. Prematurity, defined as delivery before 37 weeks, occurred in 56% of pregnancies in renal transplant recipients, compared to 11% in the overall population. Low birth weight, defined as less than 2500 g, occurred in 49.5% of pregnancies (Armenti et al 1994). Furthermore, transplant patients frequently experience an increased occurrence of pregnancy complications (Framarino et al 1993).

Most of the available information on pregnancy in renal transplant recipients pertains to patients treated during pregnancy with CsA Sandimmune-based immunosuppressant regimes (Gaughan et al 1996). A recent study in CsA-treated patients demonstrated a relationship between high creatinine levels ($\geq$2.5 mg/dl) before and during pregnancy, with an increased incidence of renal graft loss postpartum (Armenti et al 1998). Hypertension and a history of multiple pregnancies were not independently associated with graft loss. Although no increase in the overall fetal anomaly rates has been reported among patients treated with CsA Neoral or tacrolimus (TRL), only fragmentary information is available.

In 1994, the NTPR reported the incidence of rejection during pregnancy and the first 3 months after delivery to be 14.5% in the CsA-based group and 5.7% in the non-CsA (primarily AZA-based) group (Armenti et al 1994). Within 2 years of delivery, 17% of CsA-treated patients experienced graft loss and an increased risk of low birthweight (Armenti et al 1997). Among the other patients, pregnancy does not substantially affect renal allograft survival or long-term renal function (First et al 1995; Sturgiss and Davison 1995). Though only 23 pregnancies were evaluated, no cases of graft loss were reported among Neoral- or TRL-treated patients (Armenti et al 1997).

Pregestational diabetes

Patients with underlying diabetes require meticulous glucose control prior to pursuing pregnancy, since poor glycemic control correlates with an increased risk of fetal congenital malformations. Optimized glycemic control includes evaluation of finger stick glucose values four times daily. This test is typically performed fasting and 2 hours postprandially, maintaining fasting levels at no more than 90 mg/dl, and 2-hour postprandial levels below 120 mg/dl. Glycosylated hemoglobin levels of at least 10% at conception seem to correlate with the risk of congenital malformations. Fetal echocardiography at 22 weeks may assist with detection of fetal cardiac defects in this population.

Patients with pregestational diabetes are frequently managed with weekly antenatal visits to assist with glucose control and to ensure dietary compliance to an intake of 30–35 kcal/kg of ideal body weight throughout the pregnancy. Oral hypoglycemic agents are not used in pregnancy, since they cross the placenta, possibly resulting in fetal hyperinsulinemia, and since they are associated with an increased incidence of congenital malformations.

Owing to an increased risk of stillbirth in the diabetic patient, delivery should be accomplished near term. If delivery is planned prior to 39 weeks without a confounding indicator other than the diabetes, assessment of fetal lung maturity by amniocentesis is performed (Cunningham et al 1997). Frequent assessment of glucose is required during labor and is typically performed every 1–2 hours of active labor. Elevated maternal glucose levels pass to the fetus, thus increasing insulin production and possibly causing hypoglycemia of the infant after delivery; an insulin infusion drip is frequently employed during labor to manage glucose elevations.

Chronic hypertension

Although severe chronic hypertension requires therapy, this treatment has not been shown to improve pregnancy outcomes of pre-eclampsia or perinatal mortality (Cunningham et al 1997). Patients affected by chronic hypertension and maintained on antihypertensive agents display an outcome similar to that of patients expectantly managed during pregnancy, with intervention only if values are greater than 160 mmHg systolic or greater than 110 mmHg diastolic. Indeed, the data raise controversy whether patients treated with antihypertensives have an increased incidence of fetal growth restriction.

Owing to extensive experience with α-methyldopa in pregnancy, this agent is the most frequently used initial therapy when medical management of hypertension is performed during pregnancy. Labetalol is another frequently used antihypertensive agent. ACE-inhibitors should be avoided in pregnancy, and patients maintained on these agents should discontinue use upon diagnosis of pregnancy. For patients who are expectantly managed during pregnancy, reinitiation of therapy is necessary when systolic pressure exceeds 160 mmHg or diastolic blood pressure exceeds 105 mmHg. Normal physiologic changes of pregnancy tend to decrease the blood pressure during the second trimester, with subsequent reversal in the third trimester to a level similar to the baseline values. Left lateral bed rest maximizes placental perfusion.

Prenatal care of the pregnant patient with underlying chronic hypertension necessitates baseline evaluation of a 24-hour urine collection at the initial obstetrical visit, with repeat evaluation if the urinalysis shows proteinuria or worsening hypertension. Weekly obstetrical visits are prudent in the presence of any increase in blood pressure or proteinuria. Maternal weight is important in assessing fluid retention. The increased incidence of IUGR necessitates serial ultrasound evaluation for assessment of fetal growth. Weekly antenatal fetal testing should begin by 32 weeks, or sooner in the presence of any indication of poor fetal growth or other concern for fetal well-being.

Patients with severe chronic hypertension, especially in the presence of underlying renal disease, are at an increased (approaching 50%) risk for superimposed pregnancy-induced hypertension (SIPIH). The diagnosis is based on significant worsening of hypertension, increasing proteinuria, and progressive edema. Serial assessment of proteinuria by 24-hour urine collection is beneficial in making this diagnosis. SIPIH may present with a sudden and dramatic increase in blood pressure and accompanying proteinuria. This situation is of concern for both mother and fetus, and delivery should be expedited once the emergent hypertensive crisis has been controlled.

Pre-eclampsia

Among the variety of related disorders collectively known as pregnancy-induced hypertension (PIH), pre-eclampsia typically refers to the variant that is accompanied by proteinuria and eclampsia and that involves the central nervous system and seizures. The NTPR database indicates that pre-eclampsia was reported in 28% of patients treated with Sandimmune-based therapy, and among 15 and 17% of the limited number of patients treated with Neoral or TRL, respectively (Armenti et al 1997). The diagnosis of pre-eclampsia was not associated with an increased risk of graft loss after pregnancy (Armenti et al 1998). These findings are consistent with the 20-fold- and 10-fold-increased incidences of PIH among patients with underlying renal disease and chronic hypertension, respectively. Although increasing proteinuria near term has been reported in 40% of transplant patients, in the absence of hypertension, it generally regresses postpartum.

While delivery remains the only definitive 'therapy' for PIH, in most circumstances, nontransplant patients with a mild syndrome, namely, blood pressures exceeding 140 mmHg systolic or 90 mmHg diastolic, proteinuria of over 3 g/24 hours, and a premature fetus, can be managed conservatively. However, renal transplant patients frequently display abnormal parameters, thus confounding the diagnosis and requiring close monitoring of blood pressure, proteinuria, liver transaminase levels, serum creatinine, complete blood count with peripheral smear to evaluate hemolysis, and fetal growth and well-being.

Delivery should be strongly considered, despite the prematurity of the fetus, for patients with severe PIH, namely, systolic blood pressure between 160–180 mmHg or diastolic blood pressure greater than 110 mmHg, proteinuria exceeding 4–5 g/24 hours, eclampsia, pulmonary edema, oliguria less than 500 ml/24 hours, microangiopathic hemolysis, thrombocytopenia, elevated liver enzymes (AST/ALT), IUGR, and oligo-hydramnios, as well as symptoms suggesting end-organ damage, such as headache, scotomata, or right upper quadrant pain.

Once a decision is made to proceed with delivery, magnesium sulfate (4 g bolus/20 min followed by a continuous infusion at a rate of 2 g/hour) is initiated for seizure prophylaxis, even in the presence of mild or severe disease, to achieve the preferred therapeutic level of 4–8 mg/dl and is continued for 24 hours after delivery. Respiratory arrest may occur with high magnesium levels; if a symptomatic overdose is suspected, 1 g calcium gluconate is administered over 2 min as a 10 ml solution of 10%. The dose may require adjustment in the transplant patient, especially in the presence of deterioration of either renal function or urine output. Drug-induced toxicity is also suggested by a loss of deep tendon reflexes, a decreased mental status, or a respiratory rate under 14 breaths per min, and is confirmed by elevated levels.

Magnesium therapy does not reduce the elevated blood pressure, which may require hydralazine or labetalol. However, drastic declines in blood pressure are to be avoided, since they may adversely affect maternal status in addition to causing uteroplacental insufficiency and potential fetal distress, as well as adversely affect the renal transplant. Thus, the target blood pressure for therapy is below 140 mmHg systolic and below 100 mmHg diastolic.

The obstetric anesthesia for patients experiencing PIH is a general agent; the blood pressure should be closely monitored. Continuous conduction anesthesia (i.e. epidural) requires extreme caution, not only to maintain appropriate fluid preload to avoid hypertension, but also to avoid the risk of bleeding due to thrombocytopenia. Cesarean delivery is not indicated based solely on the diagnosis of severe PIH or eclampsia; indeed, it may be even less desirable in patients with hemolysis, elevated liver enzymes, and low platelets (HELLP syndrome), since control of hemorrhage is more difficult than with a vaginal delivery.

Infections

Cytomegalovirus (CMV) represents the most common etiology of congenital infections in the US, affecting up to 2% of infants at birth. The congenital problems associated with this infection include low birthweight, microcephaly, intracranial calcifications, chorioretinitis, mental and motor retardation, sensorineural deficits, hepato-splenomegaly, hemolytic anemia, and thrombocytopenia. Unlike many other congenital infections, prior CMV infestation does not assure immunity; reactivation can result in fetal or neonatal disease. Thus, CMV status should be assessed prior to pregnancy if possible.

Primary CMV infection during pregnancy results in an approximately 40% risk of transplacental passage of the virus. The diagnosis is established by a four-fold increase in IgG titers on paired acute and convalescent titers or by an elevated IgM titer. However, only a small percentage of these pregnancies exhibit intrauterine abnormalities suggestive of damage, such as IUGR, hepatosplenomegaly, echogenic bowel, hydrocephaly, microcephaly, or intracranial calcifications. About 10–15% of infected infants will have clinically apparent disease at birth. Some infants infected in utero who appear normal at birth will go on to develop deafness or developmental delay (5–15%).

In the general population, the risk of reactivation of CMV is approximately 0.5–1%. With reactivation, an elevation of IgM may not occur. Among those with reactivation of the virus, only 0–1% show clinical evidence of fetal infection or sequelae. Theoretically, gancyclovir may be useful in preventing or ameliorating effects of fetal CMV exposure, but limited information is available on the efficacy or safety of the drug during pregnancy.

The severity of primary infection with genital herpes simplex virus (HSV) of either type 1 or type 2, as diagnosed by culture of the unroofed lesion, may be affected by presence of crossreacting antibodies from prior episodes with the other virus. Typically, first-episode disease in a pregnant patient lacking antibody results in severe systemic symptoms that, because of the additional immunocompromise accompanying pregnancy, require acyclovir regardless of gestational status.

Vaginal delivery in the presence of an active genital (particularly primary) HSV outbreak can produce serious consequences for the infant. The presence of perineal or cervical lesions or of prodromal symptoms demands a Cesarean delivery. To decrease the likelihood of an outbreak during labor, patients with a history of genital HSV can be offered acyclovir suppression (400 mg thrice daily) beginning at 36 weeks gestation. Although studies using this approach suggest a decreased rate of Cesarean deliveries, the numbers are insufficient to ascertain any difference in neonatal infection rates.

Intrapartum management

Continuous fetal monitoring is advisable during labor. Cesarean section is indicated primarily for obstetric indications. The renal transplant itself is an extremely rare cause of obstruction of labor. Pelvic osteodystrophy is another rare possibility that can result from renal failure or prolonged use of corticosteroids. It is impossible to accurately predict the adequacy of the maternal pelvis for vaginal delivery prior to attempting labor. Cesarean delivery is reported in approximately 50% of renal transplant patients. Although the indications for this high rate are not elucidated in the literature, the cause is theoretically related to the increased incidence of prematurity and growth restriction, as well as the need for induction of labor for associated conditions.

Other considerations demand specific novel therapies during delivery. First, chronic steroid therapy necessitates administration of stress doses during labor, delivery, and the first 24 hours postpartum. Second, antibiotic prophylaxis for group B streptococcus (GBS) should be given during labor for all infants under 37 weeks, for a positive GBS culture, for a history of GBS urinary infection during the pregnancy, or for risk factors such as rupture of the membranes more than 18 hours or fever above 38°C (101°F).

If Cesarean section is indicated, cephalosporin antibiotic coverage (2 g cefoxitin or 1 g cefazolin) as well as anaerobic coverage for the surgical procedure should be given at delivery after the umbilical cord is clamped. To avoid injury to the transplanted kidney, a midline vertical incision should be employed instead of a Pfannenstiel incision. Despite the vertical skin incision, a lower uterine segment incision is usually feasible unless severe adhesions or fetal indications dictate otherwise. A Smead–Jones closure of the abdominal incision should be employed. Delayed removal of staples is also recommended. Postoperative temperature elevations over 38°C are generally attributed to postpartum endomyometritis and treated with a broader-spectrum penicillin, such as ampicillin with sulbactam and clindamycin, avoiding nephrotoxic drugs such as gentamycin. Ticarcillin with clavulinic acid represents an alternative.

Breast-feeding

Although breast-feeding offers many recognized benefits, there is little or no information available on the risks associated with immunosuppression in human milk. Although small amounts of Pred are secreted in breast milk, low doses of steroids do not represent a contraindication to breast-feeding. However, breast-feeding is probably best delayed for 4 hours after dosing. The risk should not be ignored, given that the pediatric literature suggests that high doses and/or a prolonged duration of exposure to steroids may be associated with inhibited bone growth, gastrointestinal ulcers, and glaucoma (Hale 1999).

Because CsA is excreted in breast milk and raises the possibility of immunosuppression of the infant, the American Academy of Pediatrics (AAP) considers the agent to represent a contraindication to breast-feeding. Azathioprine raises similar concerns and, additionally, the possibility of neutropenia.

GYNECOLOGIC CONSIDERATIONS

Disorders of menstruation

Amenorrhea

Delay in menarche is common in young women with ESRD; resumption of more normal pubertal development often follows transplantation. Secondary amenorrhea is defined as the absence of menstruation for more than 6 months in a previously menstruating female. The differential diagnosis of secondary amenorrhea is extensive (Figure 19.3). After excluding pregnancy, the history should evaluate the presence of galactorrhea, the use of medications that could result in amenorrhea (especially psychiatric medications), strenuous exercise regimes, or excessive weight changes. The patient is given a progesterone 'challenge' (10 mg of medroxyprogesterone acetate) daily for 10 consecutive days. Provided the patient has endogenous estrogen and a patent genital tract, this therapy should result in withdrawal bleeding a few days after discontinuing the

735

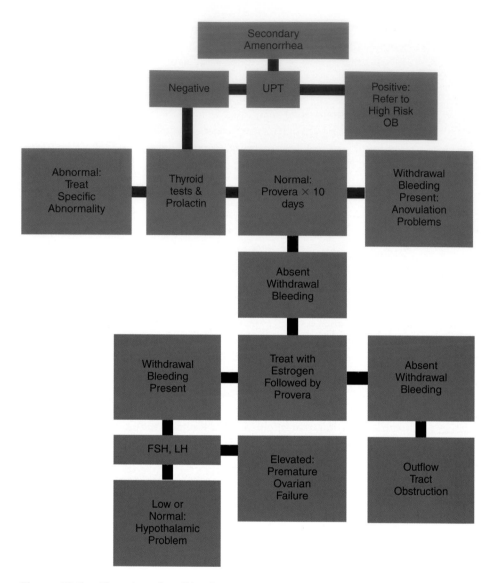

Figure 19.3. Flow chart describing basic evaluation of secondary amenorrhea.

medication. Patients who do experience bleeding may warrant further testing. Thyroid testing and a prolactin level will exclude these easily treatable causes of amenorrhea.

The differential diagnosis for primary amenorrhea in the patient with normal breast development and a uterus includes the same etiologies as secondary amenorrhea. Additional possibilities for primary amenorrhea include congenital obstruction of the outflow tract, such as an imperforate hymen or a transverse vaginal septum. A frequent diagnosis in all patients with primary amenorrhea and normal anatomy without renal disease is pituitary adenoma; prolactin levels should therefore be evaluated. Prolactin levels are frequently elevated in patients with ESRD, which may complicate the diagnosis of pituitary adenoma. Among patients with androgen insensitivity, as well as among all patients possessing intra-abdominal gonads with Y chromosomes, the gonads should be removed to prevent malignant transformation.

Patients with polycystic ovarian syndrome (PCOS) will frequently be anovulatory, display either dysfunctional uterine bleeding or amenorrhea, and have a luteinizing hormone (LH) to follicle stimulating hormone (FSH) ratio greater than 3. Patients with hypothalamic dysfunction may also experience withdrawal bleeding to progesterone challenge. This experience may be brought about by eating disorders, drugs, stress, and/or exercise. Regardless of the etiology, these patients should be treated to avoid excessive proliferation that could then result in hemorrhage or increased risk of hyperplasia or malignancy, and to ensure endometrial shedding by using oral contraceptive pills (OCPs), depomedroxyprogesterone acetate, or continued 10-day medroxyprogesterone acetate on a monthly basis. Depomedroxyprogesterone acetate has a frequent side-effect of amenorrhea, but prevents endometrial thickening. Monthly 10-day treatment with medroxyprogesterone is noncontraceptive and is therefore a poor choice for patients who are not pursuing pregnancy.

All patients who do not experience withdrawal bleeding after progesterone challenge require further evaluation. History should be reviewed with attention to surgical procedures immediately prior to the beginning of amenorrhea, such as dilation and curettage (D&C) or cryotherapy of the cervix. The endometrium can be 'primed' with unopposed estrogen prior to the 10-day treatment with medroxyprogesterone acetate. If this measure elicits bleeding, the amenorrhea may be related to insufficient estrogen, such as with menopause; premature ovarian failure (POF); or other hypothalamic–pituitary failure, namely, severe weight loss, anorexia, Sheehan's syndrome, or pituitary adenoma. Autoimmune disorders may result in POF and are common among patients with chronic renal disease. Premature ovarian failure can be confirmed by an elevated FSH. If the patient fails to experience bleeding despite estrogen priming and the withdrawal of progesterone, evaluation should focus on the outflow tract. It is important to ensure that an adequate Pap smear has been obtained, including endocervical cells, as a malignancy can obstruct the outflow tract. The possibility of cervical stenosis caused by cryotherapy or excision procedures to treat dysplasia can be evaluated by confirming the patency of the internal cervical os with a uterine sound. Patients who have recently undergone a D&C may have Asherman's syndrome of interuterine synechia, particularly after obstetric procedures performed in the presence of infection. The diagnosis may be confirmed by a hysterosalpingogram (HSG) or hysteroscopy, the latter providing the possibility of a simultaneous attempt at treatment. Uterine or endometrial malignancies may also obstruct the outflow tract, generally resulting in hematometra, which is diagnosed upon ultrasound as an enlarged uterine cavity filled with thickened endometrium or fluid.

Patients with chronic renal failure very frequently experience menstrual disturbances, such as amenorrhea or oligomenorrhea; elevated prolactin levels are commonly present

(Morley et al 1979; Cochran and Regan 1997; Holley et al 1997; Kim et al 1998). Normal menstrual cycles often resume after transplantation, occurring approximately 6.9 months posttransplant (Back et al 1991). A normal menstrual pattern is noted in about 60% of patients (Geurts et al 1993; Bierman and Nolan 1977).

Dysfunctional uterine bleeding

Abnormal vaginal bleeding, a common occurrence among renal transplant patients, should be evaluated with Pap smear, examination of vaginal discharge, bimanual examination, pelvic ultrasound, and pregnancy test when applicable. Whereas all patients over the age of 35 should undergo an endometrial biopsy to rule out carcinoma, younger patients requiring the procedure include obese women with a long history of anovulatory cycles. In some cases, a hystersonogram, which combines an ultrasound with instillation of fluid in the uterine cavity, is used to evaluate lesions producing distortions such as polyps and rarely causes infection.

While hormonal manipulation is often employed as an initial treatment, renal transplant patients frequently have coexisting hypertension, a relative contraindication to combination OCPs, as well as an increased risk for development of thromboembolism owing to the hypercoagulability produced by CsA. Furthermore, OCPs compete with CsA for cytochrome P450 3A4 isozymes and thus may increase the concentrations of immunosuppressants. Patients with compromised renal function may display anemia, requiring treatment with iron therapy. To reduce menstrual flow and regulate bleeding, hormonal manipulation with combination OCPs may be curative in patients with irregular and heavy menstruation (menometrorrhagia) who lack other pelvic pathology. In patients with a contraindication to estrogen-containing compounds, therapy with progestagens (medroxyprogesterone acetate 10 mg daily for 10 days each month; for instance, calendar days 16 through 25) should produce regular menstruation but does not prevent pregnancy. Alternatively, depomedroxyprogesterone acetate can be given intramuscularly every 3 months in an attempt to produce amenorrhea. Danazol, an anabolic steroid that suppresses ovulation by inhibiting gonadotropins, has undesirable side-effects, interferes with CsA metabolism, alters fluid balance, and is not a good choice for renal transplant recipients. Another therapeutic option is the use of a gonadotropin-releasing hormone (GnRH) analog, such as leuprolide acetate, to create a biochemical menopause. These analogs are degraded by peptidase rather than by the cytochrome P450 system and thus do not display an interaction with immunosuppressive agents. However, these analogs have a period of usefulness limited to 6 months and may exacerbate the already elevated potential for osteoporosis in renal transplant patients. This therapy produces side-effects similar to those of menopause, including hot flashes.

Failure of hormonal treatment requires surgical therapy. Dysfunctional uterine bleeding (DUB) is the indication for hysterectomy in approximately 20–30% of cases; the procedure provides a definitive cure but represents a major surgical operation. An abdominal approach is preferable in renal transplant patients, except in the presence of a significant uterine prolapse. Endometrial ablation represents a potential alternative for patients who are poor candidates for major surgery. Although the success rate in managing menorrhagia in the general population may be as high as 93%, there is no published literature on endometrial ablation in the renal transplant patient. Not all patients will experience amenorrhea following endometrial ablation; however, most will experience a significant improvement in their symptoms. The potential advantages of this therapy include the ability to perform the procedure in an outpatient setting and the short recovery time. Potential risks of the procedure include the possibility of fluid overload, which may be exacerbated in patients with compromised renal function, failure to resolve the bleeding abnormality, risk of infection, and the unknown risk of the long-term effect on identification of subsequent uterine pathology. Although endometrial ablation was previously a time-consuming procedure performed using hysteroscopic instruments, such as a roller ball or wire loop, a recently developed technique using a thermal balloon is rapid and well-tolerated, and requires minimal operator expertise. It is recommended that the endometrium be evaluated by biopsy prior to the procedure to rule out malignancy. At the time of thermal balloon ablation, a hysteroscopy is frequently performed to further evaluate the endometrial cavity. A D&C is performed to remove excess endometrium. The balloon device is inserted, filled with solution, and heated. The thermal ablation procedure lasts approximately 8 min and is best performed under general anesthesia, since any increase in intraabdominal pressure will cause the device to abate the therapy cycle.

Drug interactions with hormonal agents

Since potential drug interactions occur with various hormonal agents, the physician must assess the potential benefits of their use versus the availability of other therapeutic options. Estrogens and progestagens are capable of inhibiting liver microsome cytochrome P450 3A4 activity (Back et al 1991; Geurts et al 1993); this enzyme inhibition requires protein synthesis and may take 2–3 weeks to become apparent. Corticosteroids can interact with hormones via two mechanisms. First, corticosteroids are metabolized by the cytochrome P450 3A4 oxidative pathway; thus, metabolism could be impaired. Second, estrogen induces corticosteroid binding globulin (CBG), thus lowering free plasma corticosteroid levels (Gustavson and Benet 1985). While this altered metabolism implies the possibility of an increased elimination half-life for corticosteroids with the use of estrogens and progestagens, there are no data demonstrating clinically significant interactions.

Cyclosporine is metabolized via cytochrome P450 3A4. Studies suggest that both ethinylestradiol and progestagens are competitive inhibitors of CsA metabolism (Henricsson et al 1990; Watkins 1990). Interactions between CsA and OCPs may produce alterations in liver enzymes and cholestasis. Although the changes reported are reversible, no controlled studies have addressed this issue. It would therefore appear prudent to follow liver function tests periodically and to monitor CsA levels 2–3 weeks after initiating OCPs.

Vaginal infections

Vaginitis

Vaginal discharge with vulvovaginal irritation is a common gynecologic complaint. With the onset of puberty, the vagina becomes estrogenized and colonized by multiple aerobic and anaerobic organisms. Maintaining a normal vaginal pH of 3.5–4.2 is important in maintaining homeostasis. As pH rises, it inhibits the growth of the normal lactobacilli that are important in controlling the growth of pathogens.

Trichomonas

Trichomonas vaginalis is a flagellated protozoan that causes a fishlike odor and a frothy-appearing gray or green vaginal discharge. It is easily diagnosed by identification of the mobile flagellates on wet mount evaluation of the vaginal discharge. Approximately 25% of patients with this condition are asymptomatic. It can also cause punctate lesions on the cervix, described as 'strawberry cervix'. Pap smear can detect up to 70% of cases of the presence of *Trichomonas vaginalis*. *T. vaginalis* is generally sexually transmitted, and both partners should be treated. Treatment is oral metronidazole given either in a one-time 2-g dosage or as 500 mg twice daily for 7 days. A common side-effect includes a metallic taste, with nausea occurring in less than 10% of patients. The drug should not be taken in combination with alcohol, as it possesses a disulfiram effect. Metronidazole is contraindicated in the first trimester of pregnancy.

Candida

Candidal vulvovaginitis is predominantly caused by *Candida albicans*, although *C. glabrata* and *C. tropicalis* have increased in frequency. Common risk factors for the development of candidal infections in the transplant patient include diabetes, recent antibiotic use, immunosuppressive therapy, OCPs, and pregnancy. The incidence of candidal infections after antibiotic usage ranges from 25 to 70%. Symptoms include exquisite pruritus, burning, dyspareunia, and tenderness. A thick, white, non-malodorous 'cottage cheese'-like discharge is frequently described. Diagnosis is made by identification of budding hyphae on a slide of the discharge prepared with potassium hydroxide (KOH) solution. Since over-the-counter medications provide treatments, their prior use (or other home remedies) should be ascertained. First-line therapy includes the night-time use for 3–7 days of cream or suppository topical agents, namely, terconazole, miconazole, clotrimazole, or butoconazole. Oral therapy is available using fluconazole as a single 150 mg dose. Liver toxicity previously reported with oral ketoconazole is believed to be a much lower risk with fluconazole, but caution should be taken in its use in patients with abnormal liver function tests. The transplant physician should be consulted prior to the use of these agents and CsA levels monitored, as they may be increased by administration of oral antifungal agents. Resistant infections may also be treated using boric acid capsules daily for 14 days.

Bacterial vaginosis

Bacterial vaginosis is the present term used to describe a polymicrobial infection previously referred to as nonspecific vaginitis. The condition is caused by *Gardnerella vaginalis* and *Haemophilus vaginalis*, but commonly includes overgrowth with organisms such as *Bacteroides* species, *Mycoplasma hominis*, *Enterobacteriaceae*, and *Peptostreptococcus* species. Although 50% of patients with the condition are asymptomatic, the other patients tend to complain of a fishy, malodorous vaginal discharge that is thin and grayish in appearance. The discharge displays an elevated pH greater than 4.5, the presence of clue cells on wet mount evaluation, and an amine odor following addition of KOH—the 'whiff test'. When Pap smears reveal the presence of cue cells, particularly in a pregnant patient, the physician must be aware of the association between bacterial vaginosis and premature labor. Topical treatments include intravaginal 0.75% metronidazole gel twice daily for 5 days or 2% clindamycin cream daily for 7 days. Oral metronidazole can be given as 500 mg twice daily for 7 days. Treatment of the partner remains controversial, but may be warranted in the symptomatic patient with recurrent infections. Douching has been implicated in altering the vaginal flora and predisposing to infection. Bacterial vaginosis has recently been associated with an increased incidence of pelvic inflammatory disease (PID), posthysterectomy infections such as cuff cellulitis, and infectious complications related to pregnancy. There is a single case report of a male recipient of a kidney transplant who displayed a perinephric abscess containing *Gardnerella vaginalis* and whose partner was noted to have an asymptomatic vaginal infection (Finkelhor et al 1981).

Chlamydia trachomatis

Chlamydia trachomatis, the most frequently sexually transmitted disease in the US, is associated with multiple complications, including PID, infertility, pregnancy complications, and chronic pelvic pain. Routine cervical testing of sexually active patients who are not monogamous, especially in those under age 30, may prevent future morbidity. DNA probe technology allows adequate testing from swabs sampled from the endocervix. Treatment of asymptomatic patients can be accomplished with 1 g oral azithromycin administered as a single dose, or doxycycline 100 mg twice daily for 7 days. Both patient and partner should be treated simultaneously.

Neisserea gonorrhoeae

Neisserea gonorrhoeae is another common sexually transmitted disease that may be diagnosed using the technique described above for chlamydia. There has been increasing difficulty with resistance to therapy; therefore, current acceptable treatment includes ceftriaxone 125 mg intramuscularly, cefixime 400 mg orally, or ciprofloxacin 500 mg orally. The importance of simultaneous partner referral and treatment cannot be overestimated.

Vulvar infections

Bartholin's cyst and abscess

Bartholin's glands, which are located at the introitus (5 and 7 o'clock positions), become obstructed and enlarged in about 2% of reproductive-age women. Many women bear a cyst of this gland, which may be noted on routine examination as asymptomatic, non-painful, unilateral, and ranging from 1 to 8 cm in diameter. Asymptomatic women under 40 years of age may be managed by sitz baths to encourage drainage of the blocked duct. When abscess formation occurs as a result of polymicrobial infections in these cysts, they become painful and may require drainage by incision at the more vaginally directed portion of the wall. Under coverage of broad-spectrum antibiotics, a small Word catheter is left in place to permit epithelization of the tract in an attempt to avoid recurrences. If this procedure fails, the gland may be marsupialized. Excision of the duct and gland is rarely required and in fact has been associated with significant morbidity, including hemorrhage, hematoma formation, scarring, and dyspareunia. The possibility of adenocarcinoma of this gland should be entertained for patients who have a solid component to the cyst, who have frequent recurrences, or who are over the age of 40.

Molluscum contagiosum

Molluscum contagiosum is an asymptomatic viral disease of the vulvar skin. Owing to immunosuppression, this condition may occur more frequently in transplant patients, although no documentation exists to support this theory. It is caused by a poxvirus, is spread by close contact, and may be transmitted by nonsexual contact. The incubation period ranges from several weeks to many months. It causes dome-shaped lesions that are typically 1–5 mm in diameter, with a center that may appear umbilicated. The nodules may persist for months to years; treatment involves removal of the papules.

Human papilloma virus

Condyloma acuminatum, which involves the vulva, vagina, and cervix, is a sexually transmitted disease caused by human papilloma virus (HPV). Symptomatic infections that are persistent and recurrent and involve more than one genital site occur more commonly in renal transplant patients, due to the use of immunosuppressants (Halpert et al 1986). Diabetes, pregnancy, and local trauma also predispose to clinical infection. The pedunculated wart lesions are usually multiple and frequently clustered, and vary greatly in size. Perianal warts occur in approximately 20% of patients. Any unusual appearance warrants a biopsy in the immunocompromised patient to exclude vulvar dysplasia, or malignancy such as verrucous carcinoma. Complete evaluation includes a Pap smear to exclude cervical disease. Depending on the clinical scenario, vulvar condylomata may be treated using topical concentrated trichloroacetic acid (50–85%), podophyllin solution, immune modulating therapy such as imiquimod cream, or 5-fluorouracil (5-FU). Treatment seeks to destroy the visible lesions, realizing that eradication of the virus is impossible. Podophyllin and 5-FU are contraindicated in pregnancy. Other treatment options involve surgical therapy with simple excision, laser vaporization, cryotherapy, or electrical loop excision.

Genital herpes

Genital herpes is a highly contagious, recurrent, sexually transmitted disease caused by either HSV-1 or -2. The typical incubation period is 2–7 days with the formation of exquisitely tender vesicles that may be single or multiple and that may coalesce. During the first episode of disease, severe symptoms typically last 14 days and are commonly accompanied by bilaterally tender inguinal adenopathy. Systemic symptoms, including fever and malaise, are present in 70% of primary infections. Patients commonly present with complaints of tender 'blisters' or ulcers, but may also experience severe dysuria or urinary retention and, rarely, encephalitis. Although systemic manifestations are not uncommon among immunosuppressed patients who may display a poor outcome (Gomez et al 1999), recurrent disease is local in distribution, with less severe symptoms. The diagnosis is frequently apparent by the presence of tender vesicles, but viral culture as well as an ELISA test for HSV DNA should be performed to confirm the diagnosis. Serologic testing is of limited utility, as it cannot distinguish between oral and genital infection. Treatment consists of oral antiviral therapy (acyclovir, famciclovir, or valacyclovir) for 7–10 days for the initial outbreak. Recurrent disease can be treated with the same medications for 5 days. Prophylactic therapy may be useful in patients with frequent recurrences (Table 19.3). Topical acyclovir cream or topical lidocaine can be used for comfort, in addition to sitz baths and intensified perineal hygiene. Parenteral acyclovir may be required in the immunosuppressed patient with systemic symptoms.

Syphilis

Syphilis is a sexually transmitted infection caused by *Treponema pallidum*, which is a motile anaerobic spirochete (Table 19.4). In the primary stage of syphilis, a chancre appears on the vulva, vagina, or cervix after a 2–12-week incubation period. It is typically firm and nontender, with a clean base and rolled edges. Bilateral adenopathy may be present. Serologic testing for syphilis will be negative at the time of the chancre. Diagnosis is made by dark-field microscopic evaluation for spirochetes from the base of

	First episode	Recurrence	Suppression
Acyclovir	400 mg t.i.d., 7–10 days 200 mg five times per day, 7–10 days	400 mg t.i.d., 5 days 200 mg five times per day, 5 days 800 mg b.i.d., 5 days	400 mg b.i.d.
Famciclovir	250 mg t.i.d., 7–10 days	125 mg b.i.d., 5 days	250 mg b.i.d.
Valacyclovir	1 gm b.i.d., 7–10 days	500 mg b.i.d., 5 days	250 mg b.i.d. 500 mg–1 g per day
t.i.d.: three times daily; b.i.d.: twice daily.			

Table 19.3. Treatment regimes for genital herpes simplex virus (Adapted from Centers for Disease Control and Prevention (1998))

	Syphilis	Herpes	Lymphogranuloma venereum	Chancroid	Granuloma inguinale
Incubation time	1–12 weeks	2–7 days	3 days–6 weeks	1–14 days	1–4 weeks or longer
Organism	*Treponema pallidum*	Herpes simplex virus 1 or 2	*Chlamydia trachomatis* L1, L2, or L3	*Haemophilus ducreyi*	*Calymmatobacterium granulomatis*
Pain	–	+	+/–	+	–
Adenopathy	Firm, nontender, bilateral	Firm, tender, bilateral	+/– Suppurative, tender, unilateral	+/– Suppurative, tender, unilateral	Not present
Diagnostic testing	Dark field microscopy, RPR or VDRL FTA-ABS or MHA-TP	Culture of lesion	Serologic testing of antibody titers	Culture on sensitive media (80% sensitive)	Donovan bodies on biopsy
Therapeutic agents	Benzathine penicillin G	Acyclovir, famciclovir, valacyclovir	Doxycycline, azithromycin	Azithromycin, ceftriaxone, ciprofloxacin	Trimethopamethoprim–sulfamethoxazole or doxycycline

Table 19.4. Evaluation of genital ulcers (Adapted from Centers for Disease and Control and Prevention (1998) and Mischell et al (1997))

the lesion. Regardless of treatment, the chancre will heal in 3–9 weeks. Between 6 weeks and 6 months after infection, systemic symptoms may develop, including malaise, headache, anorexia, and a classic rash that includes erythematous macules on the palms and soles. Condylomata lata may develop on the vulva and upper thighs, and appear as contagious excrescences that may ulcerate and become velvet-like in appearance. Symptoms resolve after 2–6 weeks. The latent stage of syphilis then occurs, during which time patients are frequently diagnosed by routine serologic testing. Tertiary syphilis may develop 2–20 years later in approximately one-third of untreated patients. Manifestations include optic atrophy, tabes dorsalis, gummas, and aortic aneurysm. Treatment for syphilis includes penicillin given as 2.4 million units of benzathine penicillin G intramuscularly. Primary or secondary syphilis can be treated with a single injection, while that of unknown duration or exceeding 1 year requires three weekly injections. A specific antitreponemal antibody test (RPR) should be performed to confirm the diagnosis, but will remain positive indefinitely. Patients should be followed with serial RPR testing every 3 months for the first year after treatment to ensure adequate response to therapy.

Granuloma inguinale

Granuloma inguinale, a chronic ulcerative disease caused by the Gram-negative, nomotile rod *Calymmatobacterium granulomatis*, is spread by close contact, but is not highly contagious and occurs most commonly in tropical regions. The incubation period ranges from 1 to 12 weeks; relapses after effective therapy may occur 6–18 months later. The ulceration is usually nontender and may be beefy red and friable in appearance. Adenopathy is not prominent. The diagnosis is made from a specimen taken from the base and edge of the ulcer, which shows the presence of Donovan bodies, clusters of dark staining bacteria with a safety-pin appearance found in the cytoplasm of mononuclear cells. Treatment includes doxycycline orally 100 mg twice daily for a minimum of 3 weeks and until the lesions have completely healed.

Lymphogranuloma venereum

Lymphogranuloma venereum (LGV) is a chronic infection caused by *Chlamydia trachomatis* serotype L1, L2, or L3. The incubation period ranges from 3 days to 6 weeks. The lesion is usually single. Pain is variable, but tender adenopathy is frequently a predominate feature. Systemic symptoms may be present, including fever and malaise. Although the most frequent location is in the inguinal region, involvement of the perineal and perirectal areas may occur. If untreated, the nodes will enlarge and become matted, forming bubos, and then may spontaneously rupture and form draining sinus tracts and fistulas. Tissue destruction may result in scarring and fibrosis. The diagnosis is usually made by titers greater than 1:64 on complement fixation antibody tests. Identification of *Chlamydia* from cultures of pus or inguinal aspirates may also be useful. The treatment is oral doxycycline 100 mg twice daily for 21 days.

Chancroid

Chancroid is an acute ulcerative sexually transmitted disease caused by *Haemophilus ducreyi*, a highly contagious nonmotile Gram-negative rod that causes a soft but painful ulceration with ragged edges. The incubation period is short, usually 3–6 days. The diagnosis is made by Gram stain and culture of the purulent material, although the organism may be difficult to grow. Treatment options include ceftriaxone 250 mg intramuscularly as a single dose, or azithromycin 1 g orally or ciprofloxacin 500 mg orally twice daily for 3 days. Quinolones are contraindicated in pregnancy.

Pelvic inflammatory disease

Pelvic inflammatory disease (PID) is usually the result of a sexually transmitted disease (STD) affecting the upper genital tract. Owing to the immunocompromised status of renal transplant patients, the incidence of PID is likely to be higher. Typically, PID presents as endometritis (especially following instrumentation), salpingitis, pelvic peritonitis, or as a tubo-ovarian abscess. Any procedure that introduces lower genital tract organisms to the upper tract also raises the risk of PID. Other factors that have been implicated in the development of PID include menstruation, prior episodes of disease, uterine instrumentation, alteration in normal vaginal flora such as bacterial vaginosis, and douching. Pelvic inflammatory disease patients should be educated in STD prevention and contraception.

Diagnosis

The symptoms, which include lower abdominal pain, adnexal tenderness, and cervical motion tenderness, are nonspecific and may be blunted in patients using immunosuppressants. Because PID may present in an atypical fashion, additional criteria to support the diagnosis include oral temperature greater than 38°C, leukocytosis greater than 10 000/mm^2, abnormal cervical or vaginal discharge, elevated C-reactive protein and/or erythrocyte sedimentation rate, as well as laboratory tests that provide evidence of *Neisseria gonorrhea* and/or *Chlamydia trachomatis* upon endocervical sampling.

Because these criteria may be less reliable in transplant patients, ultrasound should be used to detect a pelvic mass, tubo-ovarian abscess, or pyosalpinx; culdocentesis or laparoscopy to aspirate purulent material from the peritoneal cavity (Fornara et al 1997); and endometrial biopsy to detect histopathologic evidence of a plasma cell infiltrate of endometritis.

Pelvic inflammatory disease is usually caused by polymicrobial infections that include facultative aerobes, such as *Escherichia coli* and *Gardnerella vaginalis*; streptococci, such as *Enterococcus* species and *Haemophilus influenzae*; anaerobes, such as *Bacteroides* species, *Peptostreptococcus*, and *Actinomyces*; and mycoplasmas, such as *Mycoplasma hominis* and *Ureaplasma urealyticum*. In up to 25% of cases, neither gonorrhea nor chlamydia is isolated. Pelvic inflammatory disease initiated by gonorrhea typically has a more abrupt and dramatic onset, while that initiated by chlamydia is typically more indolent and more likely to go undiagnosed.

Treatment

Treatment of PID depends on the clinical scenario. Guidelines for inpatient care include immunosuppressant medications, adolescent age, inability to tolerate oral medication, suspected pelvic abscess, severe illness (temperature $\geq 38°C$, WBC > 15 000, and/or sepsis), uncertain diagnosis, pregnancy, HIV, intrauterine device (IUD), uterine instrumentation, failed outpatient therapy, or suspected noncompliance. Inpatient therapy (intravenous cefoxitin or cefotetan, and oral doxycycline unless intravenous therapy is indicated by gastrointestinal symptoms) is continued for 48 hours after resolution of fever and clinical improvement. Following hospital discharge, the patient is treated for a total of 14 days with oral doxycycline therapy. In cases in which a tubo-ovarian abscess is suspected, broad-spectrum antibiotics with abscess penetration and excellent anaerobic coverage are used. If inpatient therapy has not resulted in significant improvement by 48–72 hours, surgical therapy should be considered. Diagnostic laparoscopy can be used to confirm the diagnosis. Operative laparoscopy may be used to lyse adhesions, as well as to irrigate and drain abscesses. Laparotomy is recommended for suspected ruptured tubo-ovarian abscess or severe PID unresponsive to conservative management. At laparotomy, consideration should be given to total abdominal hysterectomy and bilateral salpingo-oophorectomy, depending on desires for future fertility as well as the severity of disease.

Long-term sequelae from PID are estimated to occur in one-quarter of patients. Possible sequelae include infertility, increased risk for ectopic pregnancy, chronic pelvic pain, perihepatic adhesions (Fitz Hugh Curtis syndrome), recurrent PID, dysmenorrhea, and dyspareunia. All patients with PID should be tested for other STDs, including HIV, syphilis, and hepatitis B. Partners should be referred for further evaluation and treatment.

Contraception

No well-controlled studies of contraceptive options are available in renal transplant patients. Nevertheless, contraceptive management of the transplant patient is an important topic and should be addressed prior to hospital discharge after transplantation. If future fertility is not desired, the patient should be counseled on permanent sterilization with tubal ligation, possibly performed at the time of transplantation. Vasectomy of the male partner is an option and lacks the increased risk of ectopic pregnancy associated with tubal ligation.

Contraceptive methods appear to affect the risk of PID. Barrier methods of contraception, such as condoms and diaphragms, reduce the incidence of STDs. Owing to its bactericidal properties, spermicide also reduces transmission. Condoms remain the only contraceptive method potentially reducing transmission of HIV. Oral contraceptive pills reduce the risk of STDs by altering the cervical mucus and reducing the organism's ability to ascend and cause an upper genital tract infection. They also typically reduce menstrual flow and therefore decrease available culture medium for bacterial growth. The IUD appears to increase the incidence of PID primarily around the time of insertion and is likely associated with the introduction of causative organisms during the insertion procedure. Owing to this association, the IUD is contraindicated in the transplant patient.

Oral contraceptive pills

Although low-dose combined OCPs containing estrogen and progesterone are highly effective when taken as prescribed, the potential for a drug interaction with CsA requires periodic monitoring of liver and renal function. Absolute contraindications to the use of OCPs include previous thromboembolism, deep venous thrombosis, estrogen-dependent malignancy, pregnancy, and severe liver disease. Relative contraindications include hypertension, diabetes, smoking at age 35 and over, migraine headaches, and depression. Many of these disorders are present in transplant patients.

Barrier contraceptives

Barrier methods, such as diaphragm, condom, contraceptive sponge, spermicide, or cervical cap, display the lowest risk of side-effects and offer the added advantage of reducing transmission of sexually transmitted diseases. However, these methods may produce local irritation and unfortunately provide the least reliability for contraception, with failure rates for the 'perfect' user as high as 2–9%. They also require a highly motivated user.

Progesterone-only contraception

To avoid the risks associated with estrogen, progestational contraceptive options are available. The progesterone-only 'minipill' must be taken at the same time daily, has a higher failure rate than combination OCPs, and may produce menstrual irregularities. Depomedroxyprogesterone acetate injections, which are administered at 3-month intervals, require a low degree of user motivation. However, because ovulation may be delayed after discontinuing the depomedroxyprogesterone acetate, this method is a poor choice for a patient planning a pregnancy in the near future.

The Norplant (Wyet-Ayerst Laboratories, Philadelphia, PA, USA) device also requires low user motivation. Because these subdermal implants require an office surgical procedure for insertion and removal, as well as remaining effective for 5 years, they should be used with the intention of long-term contraception.

The side-effects frequently reported with progesterone-only methods of contraception include irregular bleeding or amenorrhea, weight gain, altered lipid metabolism, hair loss, vaginal atrophy and depression. Progestational agents may also interfere with CsA metabolism via the cytochrome P450 system; therefore, monitoring must be performed as described above for OCP patients.

Intrauterine device

Two IUDs are commercially available: a copper-containing device that may be left in place for 10 years, and a progesterone-containing device that is replaced yearly. Because the risk of infection is higher near the time of IUD placement, the longer-acting alternative is theoretically more appealing. Prophylactic antibiotics must be used. There are two published case reports of IUD failures in renal transplant patients that have been speculated to be related to immunosuppression (Zerner et al 1981). Because of the increased risk of infection, this form of contraception should be strongly discouraged for the transplant patient.

Menopause

Hormone replacement therapy

Hormone replacement therapy (HRT) is recommended at menopause, owing to many documented benefits, particularly in transplant patients who have an increased risk of osteoporosis (Boot et al 1995; Pichette et al 1997; Table 19.5). The increased risk of osteoporosis among transplant recipients owes to multiple factors, including a history of ESRD, corticosteroid therapy, and the use of calcineurin–calmodulin phosphatase inhibitors, such as CsA and TRL (Rich et al 1992; Wolpaw et al 1994; Thiebaud et al 1995; Stein et al 1996; Rodino and Shane 1998). Glucocorticoids induce bone loss by both reducing bone formation and increasing bone resorption (Hung et al 1996; Reid 1997; Cueto-Manzano et al 1999). Glucocorticoid dose is closely related to the rate of bone loss in the transplant patient, with the most rapid rate of bone loss occurring in the first 6 months of therapy (Epstein et al 1995; Shane et al 1997; Lane and Lukert 1998; Rodino and Shane 1998). Therefore, attention to preventative therapy against additional bone loss is extremely important. Baseline assessment of bone mineral density and subsequent follow-up evaluation is probably warranted in this patient population. The diabetic transplant patient may be at even greater risk of osteoporosis, with a 40% fracture rate at 3 years posttransplant, compared to 11% in nondiabetic transplant patients (Nisbeth et al 1999). Osteoporosis is more prevalent in the Caucasian population, which accounts for the greater ethnic proportion of transplant patients. Furthermore, HRT produces benefits in controlling vasomotor symptoms and mitigating genitourinary atrophy. Estrogen therapy may, in addition, protect against coronary heart disease (Writing Group for the PEPI Trial 1995), possibly by lowering low-density lipid (LDL) cholesterol and increasing high-density lipid (HDL) cholesterol.

While 0.625 mg of conjugated estrogen daily has been proven to provide protection against osteoporosis and cardiovascular disease, higher doses are occasionally required to

Agent	Effect on bone	Effect on breast	Effect on endometrium	Effect on lipids
Calcium	Deficiency causes loss; supplements reduce loss	Absent	Absent	Absent
Vitamin D	Increased bone mass in combination with calcium	Absent	Absent	Absent
Estrogen	Slowed bone loss, increased bone mass	Slightly increased with prolonged use	(Increased endometrial cancer with unopposed estrogen, progesterone required if uterus)	Increased HDL; decreased LDL
Alendronate	Slowed bone loss, increased bone mass	Absent	Absent	Absent
Calcitonin	Inhibited bone resorption	Absent	Absent	Absent
Raloxifene	Slightly increased bone mass	Reduced breast cancer	Similar to placebo	Unchanged HDL; decreased LDL
Fluoride	Increased bone mass but abnormal bone	Absent	Absent	Absent
Tamoxifen	Reduced bone loss	Reduced breast cancer	Increased endometrial cancer	Decreased LDL

Table 19.5. Therapeutic options available for the treatment of osteoporosis

control vasomotor symptoms in younger patients. The potency of the conjugated estrogen in 0.625 mg HRT does not carry the same potency or relative risks as OCPs. Hormone replacement therapy does not alter blood pressure or glucose tolerance. However, studies suggest that HRT does produce a 2–4-fold increased risk of venous thromboembolism, a factor that should be considered among patients with an increased risk of clotting disorders or prior history of venous thromboembolism. If the patient has a uterus, progesterone must be added to estrogen to avoid the risk of unopposed estrogen causing endometrial cancer (Grady et al 1995). Although studies are not conclusive, therapy has been associated with a possible increased risk of breast cancer. Furthermore, routine mammography should be performed, and patients with a history of endometrial or breast cancer should receive extensive counseling on the potential risks and benefits of HRT.

HRT may be administered as either a cyclic or a continuous regimen. Cyclic HRT is useful during the perimenopause period, as it is most likely to result in regulated bleeding. Estrogen (0.625 mg of conjugated estrogen) is given for 25 days, and progesterone (5 or 10 mg medroxyprogesterone) is added for the last 10–12 of these days. The patient then has time off HRT, during which she usually experiences withdrawal bleeding. Alternatively, both hormones can be given simultaneously (0.625 mg of conjugated estrogens and 2.5–5 mg of medroxyprogesterone). While unpredictable bleeding may occur during the first 4 months of therapy, amenorrhea is frequent thereafter. A patient who experiences persistent bleeding may require evaluation by endometrial biopsy, ultrasound, or D&C with hysteroscopy. Transdermal estrogens may also be used as an alternative to oral estrogen in order to bypass the first pass metabolism of oral estrogen through the liver.

Selective estrogen receptor modulators

Selective estrogen receptor modulators (SERMs) are compounds that produce an estrogen-like effect in select tissues while remaining inactive or even antagonistic in other tissues. Ideally, the compound would stimulate bone deposition and cardiovascular health, but remain inactive in the breast and endometrium. For example, tamoxifen, an agent used in cancer patients, displays an antiestrogen effect on breast tissue, but maintains bone mass density in postmenopausal women (Grey et al 1995; Poles et al 1996); the agent reduces total and LDL cholesterol with a similar risk of thromboembolism as estrogen. Tamoxifen, however, has a stimulatory effect on the endometrial lining, producing an increased risk for endometrial cancer.

Raloxifene is a SERM that has estrogen-like effects on bone and serum lipids, but lacks a concomitant stimulatory effect on endometrial or breast tissue (Draper et al 1994, 1996; Turner et al 1994). At a dosage of 30–60 mg daily, the drug is approved for prevention of osteoporosis. It causes less breast tenderness than estrogens and has been demonstrated to reduce the incidence of breast cancer. Since endometrial stimulation does not occur, a progestin is not required (Black et al 1994). Raloxifen does not eliminate symptoms of hot flashes and therefore may not be the therapy of choice for symptomatic patients. Although the drug reduces total and LDL cholesterol, it does not affect HDL or triglycerides. Similar to estrogen, raloxifen is associated with thromboembolic events. Since long-term studies of this compound (as for most drugs in this category) are lacking, information on outcomes such as coronary artery disease is limited. Raloxifen may represent a better alternative for patients with a history of breast cancer than traditional HRT, unless the control of vasomotor symptoms is a prominent patient concern.

Bisphosphonates

Bisphosphonates, which are inhibitors of bone resorption (Table 19.5), work by impairing the resorptive function of osteoclasts and are bone-specific. These agents do not affect the other aspects of menopause. Alendronate is an aminobisphosphonate that is effective in the treatment of osteoporosis regardless of baseline bone marrow density or age (Adami et al 1995; Hosking et al 1996). The dosage is either 5 mg daily for prevention or 10 g daily for treatment. The drug has low oral bioavailability and produces gastrointestinal irritation. It must be taken on an empty stomach with 8 ounces (240 ml) of water; the patient must then remain in an upright position for 30 min. Because of effects on its absorption, alendronate must not be taken simultaneously with transplant medications and is a concern for patient compliance. Owing to their lack of significant gastrointestinal concerns, other oral bisphosphonates, such as etidronate and tiludronate, have been approved for treatment of Paget's disease; a recent report described improved bone density using clodronate in transplant patients (Grotz et al 1998).

Other osteoporosis therapies

At menopause, calcium supplementation is recommended at a dosage of 1000–1250 mg daily for patients on HRT and 1500 mg daily for those not on HRT (NIH Consensus Development Panel on Optimal Calcium Intake 1994; Council on Scientific Affairs, American Medical Association 1997). The efficiency of calcium absorption in the gastrointestinal tract decreases with age, but can be enhanced by vitamin D. The recommended dietary allowance for vitamin D is 200–400 IU daily, but 600–800 IU daily has been shown to improve calcium balance and reduce fracture risk in elderly patients. Dosages above 1000 IU daily may be toxic and should be avoided. A recent study in transplant recipients suggested reduced bone loss and prevention of new vertebral crush fractures using a daily regimen of 3 g calcium carbonate and calcium and with 25-OH-D_3 (Talalaj et al 1996).

Calcitonin inhibits bone resorption by inhibiting osteoclastic activity. The prior limitations of administration have been mitigated by the daily delivery of synthetic salmon calcitonin as a nasal spray (200–400 IU); this treatment is the only osteoporosis therapy shown to decrease fracture-associated pain (Adami et al 1995). Side-effects are minimal, except for possible rhinitis-like symptoms. Cost may be a consideration. A recent study has suggested calcitonin to be effective in the transplant population (Grotz et al 1998).

Although fluoride appears to increase bone mass by osteoblast-mediated new bone growth, studies suggest that the bone may be of suboptimal quality and fracture risk may not be reduced. Additionally, side-effects including gastrointestinal irritation and pain limit the usefulness of fluoride.

GYNECOLOGIC PATHOLOGY

Malignant and premalignant disease

There is a well-known association between immunosuppressive agents and an increased incidence of malignancy in renal transplant patients, with an overall incidence of 4–18% and a younger age of onset (Penn 1993). A significantly increased incidence of carcinoma of the vulva and perineum has been reported in this population (Blohme and Brynger 1985); the average time of presentation was 112 months after transplantation. Carcinoma of the cervix accounted for 12% of neoplasms noted in transplant patients, although the majority (73%) of these were in situ lesions. Rates of HPV infection and cervical neoplasia are significantly increased among immunocompromised and transplant patients (Halpert et al 1986; Brunner et al 1995). Reported genital malignancies in transplant patients, in decreasing order of frequency, include uterus, breast, vulva and perineum, and ovary. These findings suggest that the transplant patient on immunosuppressive therapy should undergo routine cancer screening on a more rigorous schedule than the average patient, including routine Pap smears at 6-month intervals rather than yearly. If HPV or dysplasia is noted at one site, evaluation for premalignant changes at other genital sites should be undertaken; atypical changes should be aggressively investigated.

Cervical dysplasia

A patient with cervical dysplasia should undergo colposcopically directed biopsies using acetic acid to identify abnormalities. In addition, endocervical curettage should be performed to exclude the presence of dysplastic cells high in the canal that may not be visualized on examination. According to the severity of dysplasia, the adequacy of colposcopy, and the presence of endocervical disease, the treatment regimen may include cryotherapy, laser ablation, loop electrosurgical excision procedure (LEEP) or cold knife cone biopsy of the cervix. Regardless of the regimen, close follow-up evaluation of transplant patients must be pursued for persistent or recurrent dysplasia.

Pelvic masses

The presence of the transplanted kidney in the iliac fossa may obfuscate the evaluation of pelvic masses, particularly the palpation of the adnexa. Unsuspected adnexal masses have been noted in 7% of renal transplant patients undergoing ultrasonography (Vaughan et al 1982). Ultrasound, a method of low cost compared to other imaging techniques, provides good visualization of the uterus and ovaries and allows the possibility of Doppler flow studies, which may provide further diagnostic information. Computed tomography (CT) or magnetic resonance (MR) imaging is rarely required in the evaluation of nonmalignant gynecologic masses (Figures 19.4 and 19.5).

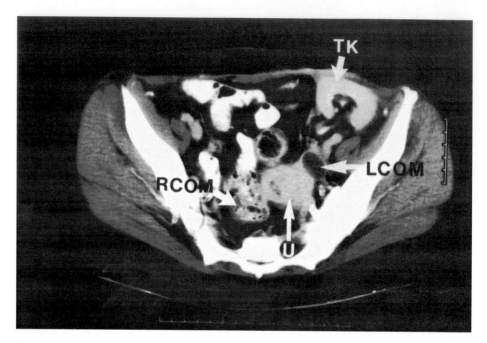

Figure 19.4. MRI evaluation of a female renal transplant patient with bilateral ovarian masses. TK; transplanted kidney; U: uterus; RCOM: right cystic ovarian mass; LCOM: left cystic ovarian mass.

Adnexa

Adnexal masses may involve the ovary, fallopian tube, round ligament, or masses extending into the broad ligament from other sources. The differential diagnosis of benign versus malignant adnexal masses is complex. Many masses in reproductive-aged women are related to functional ovarian cysts. Hydrosalpinx and paratubal cysts may also be mistaken for ovarian pathology. Testing using tumor markers for CA-125 is not unequivocal, since not all malignancies display the marker and since infectious or endometrial causes of peritoneal irritation may elevate the test. Thus, routine screening of CA-125 for early detection of ovarian malignancy is not indicated. Adnexal masses that are large, that occur in menopausal women, or that present with signs suggestive of an acute abdomen or persist should be considered for surgical therapy. If the suspicion for malignancy is low, a laparoscopic procedure can be considered. Cases in which there

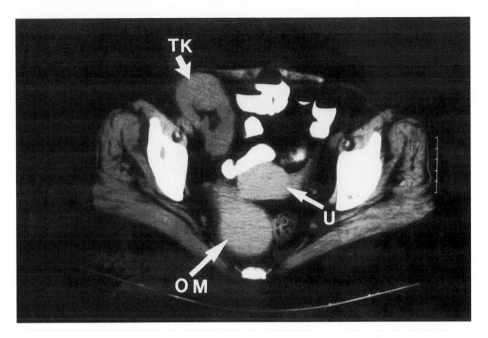

Figure 19.5. MRI of the pelvis in a female transplant patient revealing an ovarian mass. TK: transplanted kidney; U: uterus; OM: ovarian mass.

is a suspicion of malignancy, a history of prior surgeries, or a large mass are best explored via a vertical midline lower abdominal incision. Depending on the presence of malignancy, patient age, specific pathology, and desire for future fertility, ovarian cystectomy, oophorectomy or total abdominal hysterectomy with bilateral salpingo-oophorectomy may be indicated.

Endometrial polyps

Pelvic masses may also be uterine, including the benign disorders, adenomyosis, uterine fibroids, and endometrial polyps that result from estrogen-driven overgrowth of endometrial glands and stroma with core vasculature. The majority of polyps are asymptomatic, may be diagnosed incidentally on an imaging study, and occur between the ages of 40 and 49 years. The symptoms commonly include bleeding abnormalities; indeed, up to 25% of perimenopausal women with an abnormality in the timing of uterine bleeding have polyps. Prolapse of the polyp through the cervix into the vagina may occur. Malignancy is rare. Hysteroscopy and D&C are potentially curative.

Adenomyosis

Adenomyosis refers to the presence of endometrial glands deep in the uterine wall below the basal layer of the endometrium. Although frequently asymptomatic, some patients, particularly multiparous women, experience increasingly severe dysmenorrhea, deep dyspareunia, and menorrhagia. Although the uterus is usually diffusely enlarged, it is rarely more than two to three times the normal size. Diagnosis may be suggested by ultrasound, but a definitive diagnosis is only possible by tissue evaluation. Up to two-thirds of women with adenomyosis have a coexistent uterine process. Management is directed at symptom control, typically using nonsteroidal pain medications or hormonal therapy. Hysterectomy is definitive therapy.

Uterine fibroids

Fibroids are the most common pelvic tumor, occurring in as many as one of four women, depending on the specific ethnic population. In most cases, fibroids appear asymptomatic and usually do not warrant surgical therapy. Fibroids are monoclonal smooth muscle cell tumors that arise from the myometrium. They may grow to become subserosal or submucosal, and may even detach from the uterus and gain vascular supply from another source. Growth of fibroids is estrogen-mediated; thus, they frequently enlarge with pregnancy and regress after menopause. Degeneration commonly occurs and may result in calcification. Occasionally, acute degeneration will result in pain and peritoneal irritation. Many women are asymptomatic, but complaints may include pelvic pressure, worsening dysmenorrhea, and abnormal bleeding. Torsion of a pedunculated fibroid or prolapse of a submucosal fibroid may cause acute pain and require surgical therapy. Growth of presumed fibroids in a postmenopausal woman or rapid growth in any woman requires evaluation to rule out the possibility of leiomyosarcoma.

The majority of fibroids can be adequately evaluated by ultrasound. If the fibroids are asymptomatic and small, no therapy is required. Large fibroids may require surgical therapy on the basis of size alone. Medical therapy may be directed towards controlling symptoms. Heavy bleeding can be treated using the hormonal agents described above for management of abnormal uterine bleeding. Gonadotropin-releasing hormone (GnRH) analogs are effective in decreasing the size of uterine fibroids in most women. The result is temporary, however, with the majority of fibroids returning to pretreatment size by 6 months following therapy, making the use of this medication largely impractical. Gonadotropin-releasing hormone analogs may be useful in causing amenorrhea to resolve anemia prior to surgical therapy. Surgical treatment options include myomectomy or hysterectomy. In rare cases, submucosal fibroids causing bleeding difficulties can be successfully treated using hysteroscopic resection. Myomectomy is a major surgical procedure that is complicated by significant risk of hemorrhage. Additionally, up to one-quarter of women undergoing myomectomy will require future hysterectomy. Therefore, myomectomy should only be recommended for patients desiring future fertility. Hysterectomy provides definitive therapy (Hillis et al 1995). Uterine fibroids account for the indication for hysterectomy in approximately 30% of cases.

Symptomatic pelvic relaxation

Normal pelvic support is provided by the pelvic viscera, ligaments, musculature, and bones. Pelvic ligaments form as condensation of loose areolar connective tissue (endopelvic connective tissue) between the pelvic viscera, bony pelvis, and pelvic floor. These condensations form the cardinal ligaments laterally, uterosacral ligaments posteriorly, and the pubovesicocervical ligaments anteriorly. These ligaments in turn support the uterus, cervix, and upper vagina. Failure of this ligamentous support causes uterovaginal prolapse. The pelvic diaphragm or levator ani musculature is composed of the pubococcygeus, iliococcygeus, puborectalis, and coccygeus. The urethra, vagina, and rectum pass through a potential space centrally in the levator ani. Failure of this muscular support results in cystocele and/or rectocele. In the standing position, the upper third of the vagina lies at an almost horizontal angle, resting on the levator plate (Nichols et al 1970; DeLancey 1994).

The bony pelvis contains the bladder and urethra anteriorly, the uterus and vagina in the midcompartment, and the rectum and anus posteriorly. The support of any of these structures may be damaged by increased abdominal pressure, obesity, childbirth, trauma, or estrogen depletion (Brincat et al 1983). Pelvic floor denervation damaging the pudendal nerve has been shown to correlate with loss of pelvic floor muscle function and stress urinary incontinence (Gilpin et al 1989; Snooks et al 1990). Pelvic floor denervation leading to stress urinary incontinence is more common after prolonged second-stage labor, multiple deliveries, large infant, and perineal trauma during delivery (Snooks et al 1990).

If a patient who is a poor surgical candidate wishes to retain fertility or desires temporary symptom relief until surgery, nonsurgical treatment can be obtained using a pessary. Success with pessary use is limited by difficulty with retention of the pessary in the vagina, owing to the enlarged hiatus and poor pelvic musculature. Prolonged pessary use can result in ulceration and incarceration of the pessary. Frequent removal and cleaning of the pessary, and often estrogen therapy, are required to avoid this problem.

Symptomatic uterine prolapse, the indication accounting for approximately 15% of hysterectomies, is frequently treated by vaginal hysterectomy with restoration of normal anatomy and proper support of the vaginal outlet, walls, and vault. Disorders of support of the genital and urinary tract frequently coexist (Beck 1983). Other pelvic floor dysfunction should be excluded prior to surgical therapy, such as stress urinary incontinence or rectocele, as these problems may be repaired during the same anesthetic.

Standard treatment of anterior vaginal wall prolapse or cystocele is anterior colporrhaphy. This procedure involves plication of the pubocervical fascia under the bladder and urethra. Lateral defects can be repaired by reattaching the vaginal fascia to the arcus tendinis of the lateral pelvic wall (Richardson 1992). The reported success rate for this procedure to remedy prolapse and stress urinary incontinence is 95%.

SURGICAL TECHNIQUE FOR HYSTERECTOMY IN TRANSPLANT PATIENTS

Vaginal hysterectomy

The feasibility of vaginal hysterectomy depends on the clinical situation. Vaginal hysterectomy in the well-suited patient offers advantages to the patient in the postoperative period (Nezhat et al 1994). The procedure is almost entirely an extraperitoneal operation; thus, intestinal manipulation is minimal and return of bowel function is rarely delayed. Patients are frequently ambulatory on the day of surgery, and absence of an abdominal scar may minimize postoperative pain. For patients with other vaginal wall relaxation, combination of vaginal hysterectomy with anterior and posterior colporrhaphy facilitates treatment of these multiple defects. In contrast, large uterine masses, multiple prior abdominal procedures, suspected adnexal masses, and absence of uterine descensus all suggest that an abdominal procedure may be preferable (Hoffman et al 1955; Dorsey et al 1995).

When performing a vaginal hysterectomy, it is important that the gynecologist be aware of the specific location of the transplant ureter (Figures 19.6 and 19.7). The

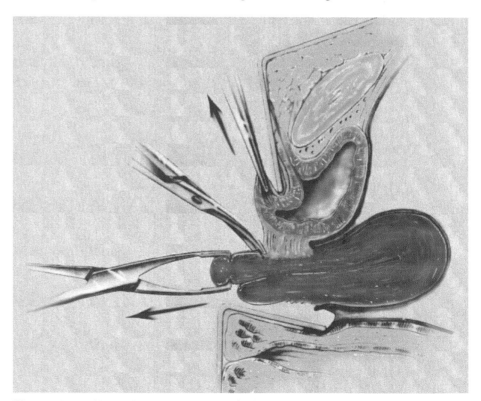

Figure 19.6. Sharp dissection of the bladder fascia upon approach of the anterior cul de sac during vaginal hysterectomy (Thompson JD, Warshaw J. *TeLinde's Operative Gynecology*, 8th edn. Rock JA, Thompson JD (eds). © 1997 Lippincott-Raven Publishers. Used by permission).

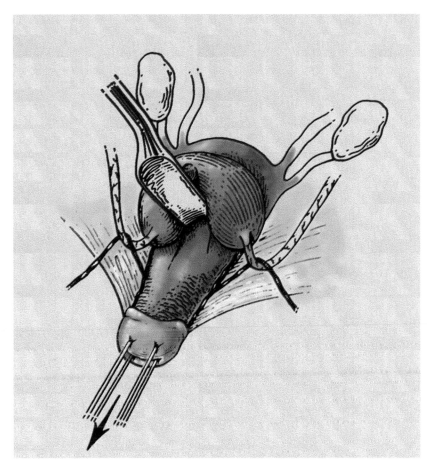

Figure 19.7. Retraction of the bladder after opening the anterior cul de sac during vaginal hysterectomy. This technique helps avoid ureteric injury during the remainder of the procedure (Thompson JD. *TeLinde's Operative Gynecology*, 8th edn. Rock JA, Thompson JD (eds). © 1997 Lippincott-Raven Publishers. Used by permission).

transplant surgeon should be immediately available and the operative report from the transplant should be reviewed preoperatively. In the Lich type of ureteral implantation, the new ureter will be high in the dome of the bladder, minimizing the possibility of surgical injury. With the Leadbetter–Politano procedure, however, the new ureter may be lower on the latter bladder wall, thus increasing the possibility of ureteral injury during attempts to enter the anterior peritoneal space.

Abdominal hysterectomy

Owing to the anatomical location of the transplanted kidney and ureter, a midline vertical skin incision is preferable for abdominal hysterectomy. A Pfannenstiel incision could lead to inadvertent injury to the ureter, especially by the gynecologist unfamiliar with the anatomy specific to kidney transplantation.

Gynecologists are conscious to avoid normal ureters in the retroperitoneal space while dividing the infundibulopelvic ligaments and uterosacral ligaments. Less caution to avoid clamping of the original ureters during hysterectomy is required in the transplant patient, as these ureters are no longer functional. Dissection of the retroperitoneum to identify the original ureters is not beneficial. In the transplant patient, the ureter may be implanted at the dome of the bladder. Caution should be used when dissecting the bladder off the lower uterus and cervix (Figure 19.8). Small pedicles should be taken when securing the uterosacral and cardinal ligaments to avoid clamping the transplanted ureter. Subtotal hysterectomy should be considered if difficulty is encountered, as this procedure may leave the transplanted ureter undisturbed.

Supracervical hysterectomy can be performed using several different techniques (Drife 1994). The cervix can be 'coned out', the uterine vessels can be ligated and the cervix sutured, or the cervix can be suspended and peritonealization performed. Regard-

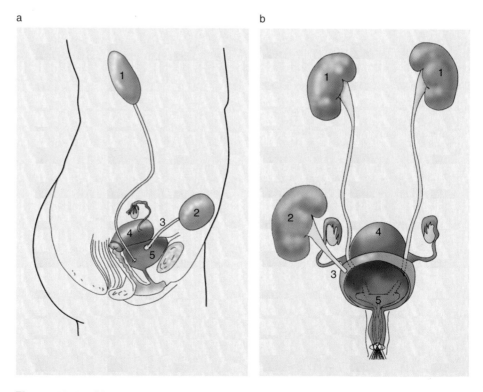

Figure 19.8. Diagram illustrating the relation of the transplanted kidney and ureter to the uterus and bladder. (a) 1: Original kidneys; 2: transplanted kidney; 3: transplanted ureter; 4: uterus; 5: trigone of the bladder. (b) AP view: 1: Original kidney; 2: transplanted kidney; 3: transplanted ureter; 4: uterus; 5: trigone of the bladder.

less of the method employed, if subtotal hysterectomy is performed, the patient must be instructed about the importance of continued Pap smears, as cervical dysplasia or cancer in the cervical stump occurs rarely, namely, in less than 1% in the general population (Tervila 1963; Barillot et al 1993). Theoretically, this risk would be higher in the transplant patient for reasons previously discussed. In addition, it is important to inform the patient that some vaginal bleeding may occur under hormonal influences.

The prolonged use of self-retaining metallic retractors may compress the transplanted kidney and ureter. Therefore, it is advisable to use intermittent retraction by a Richardson retractor held by an assistant, with care being taken to avoid the kidney. A new retractor, the 'protractor', may be advantageous, since it provides retraction by a circular latex ring that allows better exposure. Maintaining perfusion of the kidney is essential during the procedure. Hypotension should be aggressively treated because it may adversely affect the function of the transplanted kidney. Cystoscopy should be considered at the completion of the procedure, possibly using indigo carmine intravenously, to evaluate ureteral patency. Closure of the abdominal incision should be performed using a nonabsorbable suture, preferably employing the Smead–Jones technique to avoid fascial dehiscence. Staples should be removed approximately 7 days postoperatively unless indicated earlier.

The decision to perform an elective bilateral salpingo-oophorectomy at the time of hysterectomy should be thoroughly discussed with the patient preoperatively (Hollenbeck 1955; Terz et al 1967; Jacobs and Oram 1989; Kerlikourske et al 1992). The removal of ovaries lacking pathology is discouraged for patients under age 40 years. In patients nearing menopause, removal of normal ovaries to prevent the risk of subsequent ovarian cancer is frequently preformed. If ovaries are left behind, they likely function at a normal or near-normal level. When bilateral salpingo-oophorectomy is performed, the importance of postoperative estrogen replacement should not be neglected (Weinstein 1990).

CONCLUSION

Common gynecologic concerns are potentially complicated in the renal transplant patient, owing to potential confounding medical conditions and immunosuppressive agents. These concerns must be addressed, ensuring adequate communication between the gynecologist and the transplant physician. As the number of patients who have undergone transplantation and the length of patient survival following the procedure continue to increase, additional information regarding gynecologic concerns will become available and treatment options will become better delineated.

REFERENCES

Abramovici J, Brandes M, Better OS et al (1971) Menstrual cycle and reproductive potential after kidney transplantation. *Obstet Gynecol* 37:121–125.

Adami S, Passeri M, Ortolani S et al (1995) Effects of oral alendronate and intranasal calcitonin on bone mass and biochemical markers of bone turnover in postmenopausal women with osteoporosis. *Bone* 17:383–390.

Armenti VT, Ahlswede KM, Ahlswede BA et al (1994) National Transplantation Pregnancy Registry: outcomes of 154 pregnancies in cyclosporine-treated female kidney transplant recipients. *Transplantation* 57:502–506.

Armenti VT, Radomski JS, Moritz MJ et al (1997) Report from the National Transplantation Pregnancy Registry (NTPR): outcomes of pregnancy after transplantation. In: Cecka MJ, Terasaki PI (eds). *Clinical Transplants*. Los Angeles: UCLA Tissue Typing Laboratory, pp. 101–112.

Armenti VT, McGrory CH, Carter JR et al (1998) Pregnancy outcomes in female renal transplant recipients. *Transplant Proc* 30:1732–1734.

Back DJ, Houlgrave R, Tjia JF et al (1991) Effect of the progestogens, gestodene, 3-keto desogestrel, levonorgestrel, norethisterone and norgestimate on the oxidation of ethinyloestradiol and other substrates by human liver microsomes. *J Steroid Biochem Molec Biol* 38:219–225.

Bailey RR, Rolleston GL (1971) Kidney length and ureteric dilatation in the puerperium. *J Obstet Gynaecol* 78:55–61.

Bar J, Fisch B, Wittenberg C et al (1997) Prednisone dosage and pregnancy outcome in renal allograft recipients. *Nephrol Dial Transplant* 12:760–763.

Barillot I, Horoiot JC, Cuisenier J et al (1993) Carcinoma of the cervical stump. A review of 213 cases. *Eur J Cancer* 29A:1231–1236.

Baylis C (1999) Glomerular filtration rate in normal and abnormal pregnancies. *Semin Nephrol* 19:133–139.

Beck RP (1983) Pelvic relaxation prolapse. In: Kase NG, Weingold AB (eds). *Principles and Practice of Clinical Gynecology*. New York: John Wiley, pp. 677–685.

Bierman M, Nolan GH (1977) Menstrual function and renal transplantation. *Obstet Gynecol* 29:186–189.

Black LJ, Sato M, Rowley ER et al (1994) Raloxifene (LY139481HCl) prevents bone loss and reduces serum cholesterol without causing uterine hypertrophy in ovariectomized rats. *J Clin Invest* 93:63–69.

Blohme I, Brynger H (1985) Malignant disease in renal transplant patients. *Transplantation* 39:23–25.

Boot AM, Nauta J, Hokken-Koelega ACS et al (1995) Renal transplantation and osteoporosis. *Arch Dis Child* 72:502–506.

Briggs GG, Freeman RK, Yaffe SJ (eds) (1998) *Drugs in Pregnancy and Lactation*. Baltimore: Williams & Wilkins.

Brincat M, Moniz CF, Studd JWW et al (1983) Sex hormones and skin collagen content in postmenopausal women. *BMJ* 287:1337–1338.

Brunner FP, Landais P, Selwood NH (1995) Malignancies after renal transplantation: the EDTA-ERA registry experience. *Nephrol Dial Transplant* 10(Suppl 1):74–80.

Cecka MJ, Terasaki PI (1993) *Clinical Transplants*. Los Angeles: UCLA Tissue Typing Laboratory.

Cederqvist LL, Merkatz IR, Litwin SD (1977) Fetal immunoglobulin synthesis following maternal immunosuppression. In: Briggs GG, Freeman RK, Yaffe SJ (eds). *Drugs in Pregnancy Lactation*, 5th edn. Baltimore: Williams & Wilkins, pp. 687–690.

Centers for Disease Control and Prevention (1998) *Guidelines for Treatment of Sexually Transmitted Diseases*. MMWR. Atlanta: Epidemiology Program Office, Centers for Disease Control,

Public Health Service, US Department of Health and Human Services, pp. 47(RR-1).

Christensen T, Klebe JG, Bertelsen V, Hansen HE (1989) Changes in renal volume during normal pregnancy. *Acta Obstet Gynecol Scand* **68**:541–543.

Cochrane R, Regan L (1997) Undetected gynaecological disorders in women with renal disease. *Hum Reprod* **12**:667–670.

Cote CJ, Meuwissen HJ, Pickering RJ (1974) Effects on the neonate of prednisone and azathioprine administered to the mother during pregnancy. In: Briggs GG, Freeman RK, Yaffe SJ (eds). *Drugs in Pregnancy and Lactation*, 5th edn. Baltimore: Williams & Wilkins, pp. 324–328.

Council on Scientific Affairs, American Medical Association (1997) Intake of dietary calcium to reduce the incidence of osteoporosis. *Arch Fam Med* **6**: 495–499.

Cueto-Manzano AM, Konel S, Hutchison AJ et al (1999) Bone loss in long-term renal transplantation: histopathology and densitometry analysis. *Kidney Int* **55**: 2021–2029.

Cunningham FG, MacDonald PC, Gant NF et al (1997) *Williams' Obstetrics*, 20th edn. Stamford: Appleton & Lange, pp. 1125–1144.

Davison JM (1995) Towards long-term graft survival in renal transplantation: pregnancy. *Nephrol Dial Transplant* **10**(Suppl 1):85–89.

Davison JM, Lind T, Uldall PR (1976) Planned pregnancy in renal transplant recipient. *Br J Obstet Gynaecol* **83**:518–527.

Davison JM, Redman CWG (1997) Pregnancy post-transplant: the establishment of a UK Registry. *Br J Obstet Gynaecol* **104**:1106–1107.

Davison JM, Lindheimer MD (1999) Renal Disorders. In: Creasy RK, Resnik R (eds). *Maternal-Fetal Medicine*, 4th edn. Philadelphia: WB Saunders, pp. 873–894.

DeLancey JOL (1994) Vaginographic examination of the pelvic floor. *Int Urogyn J* 5:19.

DeWitte DB, Buick MK, Cyran SE, Maisels MJ (1984) Neonatal pancytopenia and severe combined immunodeficiency associated with antenatal administration of asathioprine and prednisone. In: Briggs GG, Freeman RK, Yaffe SJ (eds). *Drugs in Pregnancy and Lactation*, 5th edn. Baltimore: Williams & Wilkins, pp. 625–628.

Dorsey J, Steinberg E, Holtz P (1995) Clinical indications for hysterectomy route: patient characteristics or physician preferences. *Am J Obstet Gynecol* **173**:1452–1460.

Draper MW, Boss SM, Huster WJ, Neild JS (1994) Effects of raloxifene hydrochloride on serum markers of bone and lipid metabolism: dose response relationships (abst). *Calcif Tissue Int* **54**:339.

Draper MW, Flowers DE, Huster WJ et al (1996) A controlled trial of raloxifene (LY139481) HC1: impact on bone turnover and serum lipid profile in healthy postmenopausal women. *J Bone Miner Res* **11**:835–842.

Drife J (1994) Conserving the cervix at hysterectomy. *Br J Obstet Gynaecol* **101**:563.

Ehrich JHH, Loirat C, Davison JM et al (1996) Repeated successful pregnancies after kidney transplantation in 102 women (Report by the EDTA Registry). *Nephrol Dial Transplant* **11**:1314–1317.

Epstein S, Shane E, Bilezikian JP (1995) Organ transplantation and osteoporosis. *Curr Opin Rheumatol* **7**:255–261.

Finkelhor RS, Wolinsky E, Kim CH et al (1981) *Gardnerella vaginalis* perinephric abscess in a transplanted kidney. *N Engl J Med* **304**:846.

First RM, Combs CA, Weiskittel P, Miodovnik M (1995) Lack of effect of pregnancy on renal allograft survival or function. *Transplantation* **59**:472–476.

Fornara P, Doehn C, Fricke L et al (1997) Laparoscopy in renal transplant patients. *Urology* **49**:521–527.

Framarino di Malatesta ML, Poli L, Pierucci F et al (1993) Pregnancy and kidney transplantation: clinical problems and experience. *Transplant Proc* **25**:2188–2189.

Gaughan WJ, Moritz MJ, Radomski JS et al (1996) National Transplantation Pregnancy Registry: report on outcomes in cyclosporine-treated female kidney transplant recipients with an interval from transplant to pregnancy of greater than 5 years. *Am J Kidney Dis* **28**:266–269.

Geurts TBP, Goorissen EM, Sitsen JMA (1993) *Summary of Drug Interactions with Oral Contraceptives*. New York: Parthenon Publishing Group.

Gilpin SA, Gosling JA, Smith ARB, Warrell DW (1989) The pathogenesis of genitourinary prolapse and stress incontinence of urine. *Br J Obstet Gynaecol* **96**:15–23.

Gomez E, Melon S, de Ona M et al (1999) Disseminated herpes simplex virus infection in a renal transplant patient as possible cause of repeated urinary extravasations. *Nephron* **82**:59–64.

Grady D, Gebretsadik T, Kerlikowske K et al (1995) Hormone replacement therapy and endometrial cancer risk: a meta-analysis. *Obstet Gynecol* **85**:304–313.

Grey AB, Stapleton JP, Evans MC et al (1995) The effect of the anti-estrogen tamoxifen on bone mineral density in normal late postmenopausal women. *Am J Med* **99**:636–641.

Grimes DA (1997) Management of abortion. In: Rock JA, Thompson JD (eds). *TeLinde's Operative Gynecology*, 8th edn. Philadelphia: Lippincott-Raven, pp. 477–499.

Grotz WH, Rump LC, Niessen A et al (1998) Treatment of osteopenia and osteoporosis after kidney transplantation. *Transplantation* **66**:1004–1008.

Gustavson LE, Benet LZ (1985) The macromolecular binding of prednisone in plasma of healthy volunteers including pregnant women and oral contraceptive users. *J Pharmacokinet Biopharm* **13**:561–569.

Hale T (1999) *Medications and Mother's Milk*. Amarillo: Pharmasoft Medical Publishing.

Halpert R, Boyce JG, Butt K, Sillman FH (1986) Human papillomavirus and lower genital neoplasia in renal transplant patients. *Obstet Gynecol* **68**:251–258.

Haugen G, Fauchald P, Sodal G et al (1994) Pregnancy outcome in renal allograft recipients in Norway. *Acta Obstet Gynecol Scand* **73**:541–546.

Henricsson S, Lindholm A, Aravoglou M (1990) Cyclosporin metabolism in human liver microsomes and its inhibition by other drugs. *Pharmacol Toxicol* **66**:49–52.

Hillis S, Marchbanks P, Peterson H (1995) Uterine size and risks of complications among women undergoing abdominal hysterectomy for leiomyomas. *Obstet Gynecol* **876**:539–543.

Hoffman MS, DeCesare S, Kalter C (1955) Abdominal hysterectomy versus transvaginal morcellation for the removal of enlarged uteri. *Am J Obstet Gynecol* **171**:309–313.

Hollenbeck ZJR (1955) Ovarian cancer: prophylactic oophorectomy. *Am J Obstet Gynecol* **21**:442.

Holley JL, Schmidt RJ, Bender FH et al (1997) Gynecologic and reproductive issues in women on dialysis. *Am J Kidney Dis* **29**:685–690.

Hosking DJ, McClung MR, Ravn P et al (1996) Alendronate in the prevention of osteoporosis: EPIC study 2-year results. *J Bone Miner Res* **11**(Suppl 1):S133 (abst).

Hung CJ, Lee PC, Song CM et al (1996) Clinical implication of hormone treatment in postmenopausal kidney transplants. *Transplant Proc* **28**:1548–1550.

Jacobs I, Oram D (1989) Prevention of ovarian cancer: a survey of the practice of prophylactic oophorectomy by fellows and members of the Royal College of Obstetricians and Gynaecologists. *Br J Obstet Gynaecol* **96**:510–515.

Kerlikourske K, Brown J, Grady D (1992) Should women with familial ovarian cancer undergo prophylactic oophorectomy. *Obstet Gynecol* **80**:700–707.

Kim JH, Chun CJ, Kang CM, Kwak JY (1998) Kidney transplantation and menstrual changes. *Transplant Proc* **30**:3057–3059.

Lane NE, Lukert B (1998) The science and therapy of glucocorticoid-induced bone loss: increased risk osteoporosis and fracture. *Endocrinol Metab Clin North Am* **27**:465–483.

Makowski EL, Penn I (1976) Parenthood following renal transplantation. In: DeAlvarez R (ed.). *The Kidney in Pregnancy*. New York: John Wiley.

Meyer S, Schreyer A, De Grandi P, Hohlfeld P (1998) The effects of birth on urinary continence mechanisms and other pelvic-floor characteristics. *Obstet Gynecol* **92**:613–618.

Mischell DR, Stenchever MA, Droegemueller W, Herbst AL (1997) *Comprehensive Gynecology*. St. Louis: Mosby.

Morley JE, Distiller LA, Epstein S et al (1979) Menstrual disturbances in chronic renal failure. *Horm Metab Res* 11:68–72.

National Institutes of Health (1999) Renal transplantation: access and outcome. In: *USRDS 1999 Annual Data Report*. Bethesda, MD: National Institutes of Health, pp. 101–112.

Nezhat C, Bess O, Admon D et al (1994) Hospital cost comparison between abdominal, vaginal, and laparoscopy assisted vaginal hysterectomies. *Obstet Gynecol* 83:713–716.

Nichols DH, Milley PS, Randall CL (1970) Significance of restoration of normal vaginal depth and axis. *Obstet Gynecol* 36:251–256.

NIH Consensus Development Panel on Optimal Calcium Intake (1994) Optimal calcium intake. *JAMA* 272:1942–1948.

Nisbeth U, Lindh E, Ljunghall S et al (1999) Increased fracture rate in diabetes mellitus and females after renal transplantation. *Transplantation* 67:1218–1222.

Penn I (1993) Tumors after renal and cardiac transplantation. *Hematol Oncol Clin North Am* 7:431–445.

Pichette V, Bonnardeaux A, Prudhomme L et al (1997) Long-term bone loss in kidney transplant recipients: a cross-sectional and longitudinal study. *Am J Kidney Dis* 28:105–114.

Poles TJ, Hicks T, Kansa JA et al (1996) Effect of tamoxifen on bone mineral density measured by dual energy's X-ray absorptiometry in healthy premenopausal and postmenopausal women. *J Clin Oncol* 14:78–84.

Reid IR (1997) Glucocorticoids osteoporosis: metabolisms and management. *Eur J Endocrinol* 137:209–217.

Rich GM, Mudge GH, Laffel GL, LeBoff MS (1992) Cyclosporine A- and prednisone-associated osteoporosis in heart transplant recipients. *J Heart Lung Transplant* 11:950–958.

Rock JA, Thompson JD (eds) (1997) *TeLinde's Operative Gynecology*, 8th edn. Philadelphia: Lippincott-Raven.

Rodino MA, Shane E (1998) Osteoporosis after organ transplantation. *Am J Med* 104:459–469.

Rubi RA, Sala NL (1968) Ureteral function in pregnant women. *Am J Obstet Gynecol* 101:230–237.

Shane E, Rivas M, McMahon DJ et al (1997) Bone loss and turnover after cardiac transplantation. *J Clin Endocrinol Metab* 82:1497–1506.

Sims AH, Krantz KE (1958) Serial studies of renal function during pregnancy and the puerperium in normal women. *J Clin Invest* 37:1764–1774.

Snooks SJ, Swash M, Mathers SE, Henry MM (1990) Effect of vaginal delivery on the pelvic floor. *Br J Surg* 77:1358–1360.

Speroff L, Glass RH, Kase NG (1994) *Clinical Gynecologic Endocrinology and Infertility*, 5th edn. Baltimore: Williams & Wilkins.

Stein MS, Packham DK, Ebeling PR et al (1996) Prevalence and risk factors for osteopenia in dialysis patients. *Am J Kidney Dis* 28:515–522.

Sturgiss SN, Davison JM (1991) Perinatal outcome in renal allograft recipients: prognostic significance of hypertension and renal function before and during pregnancy. *Obstet Gynecol* 78:573–577.

Sturgiss SN, Davison JM (1995) Effect of pregnancy on the long-term function of renal allografts: an update. *Am J Kidney Dis* 26:54–56.

Talalaj M, Gradowska L, Marcinowska-Suchowierska E et al (1996) Efficiency of preventive treatment of glucocorticoid-induced osteoporosis with 25-hydroxyvitamin D3 and calcium in kidney transplant patients. *Transplant Proc* 28:3485–3487.

Tervila L (1963) Carcinoma of the cervical stump. *Acta Obstet Gynecol Scand* 42:200.

Terz JJ, Barber HRK, Brunschwig A (1967) The incidence of carcinoma in the retained ovary. *Am J Surg* 113:511–515.

Thiebaud MA, Krieg D, Gillard-Berguer AF, Jacquet JJ (1995) Cyclosporine induces high bone turnover and may contribute to bone loss after heart transplantation. *Eur J Clin Invest* **26**:549–555.

Thompson JD (1997) Surgical correction of defects in pelvic support. In: Rock JA, Thompson JD (eds). *TeLinde's Operative Gynecology*, 8th edn. Philadelphia: Lippincott-Raven, pp. 951–1085.

Thompson JD (1997) Operative injuries to the ureter: prevention, recognition, and management. In: Rock JA, Thompson JD (eds). *TeLinde's Operative Gynecology*, 8th edn. Philadephia: Lippincott-Raven, pp. 1135–1173.

Turner CH, Sato M, Bryant HU (1994) Raloxifene preserves bone strength and bone mass in ovariectomized rats. *Endocrinology* **135**:2001–2005.

Vaughan R, Henderson SC, Rahatzad M, Barry J (1982) Unsuspected adnexal masses in renal transplant recipients. *J Urol* **128**:1017–1019.

Watkins PB (1990) The role of cytochromes P-450 in cyclosporine metabolism. *J Am Acad Dermatol* **23**:1301–1311.

Weinstein L (1990) Hormonal therapy in the patient with surgical menopause. *Obstet Gynecol* **75**:47S–50S.

Whitelaw A (1981) Maternal methyldopa treatment and neonatal blood pressure. In: Briggs GG, Freeman RK, Yaffe SJ (eds). *Drugs in Pregnancy and Lactation*, 5th edn. Baltimore: Williams & Wilkins, p. 471.

Wolpaw T, Deal CL, Fleming-Brooks S et al (1994) Factors influencing vertebral bone density after renal transplantation. *Transplantation* **58**:1186–1189.

Writing Group for the PEPI Trial (1995) Effects of estrogen or estrogen/progestin regimens on heart risk factors in postmenopausal women: the Postmenopausal Estrogen/Progestin Interventions (PEPI) Trial. *JAMA* **273**:199–208. [Erratum, *JAMA* (1995) 274:1676.]

Zerner J, Doil KL, Drewry J, Leeber R (1981) Intrauterine contraceptive device failures in renal transplant patients. *J Reprod Med* **26**:99–102.

20 PSYCHIATRIC CONSIDERATIONS

*In collaboration with K Kahan**

Transplantation poses unique issues for psychiatrists in the subspecialty of consultation–liaison. Psychiatrists may offer assistance during all phases of the transplantation process, from the time of diagnosis to the posttransplant period. Since patients with end-stage renal disease (ESRD) are particularly vulnerable to psychosocial problems, selection of potential transplant candidates requires an intricate analysis of pre-existing stressors, an estimate of potential improvements in quality of life as a result of the procedure, and a prediction of the patient's proclivity to noncompliance, based upon his psychosocial and demographic characteristics (Wolcott 1990).

During the waiting period, transplant candidates may require assistance in coping with the unique psychological stresses of simultaneously preparing to live and preparing to die. After transplant, recipients may experience psychosocial issues related to unfulfilled expectations, medication side-effects, and physiological disturbances. Throughout these periods, physicians may need to prescribe psychotropic medications, adjusting dosages according to the degree of renal insufficiency.

The needs of donors and of the hospital staff constitute other important facets of transplant psychiatry. Reactions to organ donation may include depression, resentment, and avoidance. The hospital staff may also experience stress during the harvesting process; moreover, staff members may feel helpless when they are unable to provide an ailing ESRD patient with a cadaveric donor transplant. Ultimately, psychiatrists may treat recipients, donors, and staff with individual or group therapy in an effort to elicit discussion and resolution of these transplant-related issues.

PSYCHIATRIC ISSUES OF END-STAGE RENAL DISEASE

Initial diagnosis

The diagnosis of end-stage renal disease (ESRD) is usually both emotionally and physi-

---

* *Medical student, Department of Psychiatry, University of Texas Medical School, Houston*

cally devastating to a patient. During the period after initial diagnosis of ESRD, patients must cope with their illness and its treatment; the acceptance of the diagnosis and the commitment to adhere to a rigorous treatment plan of dialysis constitute major obstacles. The psychiatric disturbances during this period of adjustment include depression, anxiety, and mental status changes. However, mood disorders may be difficult to assess, since the somatic symptoms characteristic of endogenous psychiatric disorders—including changes in appetite, sleep, energy, and concentration—may also be caused by uremia, antihypertensive therapy, or steroid treatment, as well as by endogenous psychiatric disorders.

Among 60 ESRD patients, 15 of whom were treated with home hemodialysis (HD), 15 with center HD, 15 with a renal transplant, and 15 with a combination, 30% reported at least one episode of major depression in their lifetimes and, except for one individual, all patients experienced at least one episode after the diagnosis of ESRD (Hong et al 1987). Fifty-five percent of patients noted that coping with ESRD had been the most difficult emotional experience of their lives (Hong et al 1987). These coping stresses are compounded by the neuropsychiatric sequelae of ESRD, which result in impaired judgment, depression, and irritability. During this period, the patient generally relies on a physician to determine the most appropriate treatment modality. Frequently, a decision about the possibility of a transplant is deferred for fear that it may increase the patient's level of apprehension.

Physical functions

Two physical functions are of particular concern. First, limited use of the limb bearing the graft or fistula creates feelings of decreased physical ability. Second, sexual disabilities commonly present at the time of and/or prior to ESRD diagnosis include decreased desire, partial-to-complete impotence, and difficulty with lubrication or ejaculation (Degen et al 1981), resulting from decreased production of testosterone that causes decreases in testicular size as well as sperm quantity and quality. Concomitant vascular disease resulting from diabetes and/or hypertension (Degen et al 1981), disease-exacerbated depression, decreased plasma zinc, and impaired penile blood flow (Gulledge et al 1983) may exacerbate the problem of sexual dysfunction. In addition to physiologic causes, certain antihypertensive drugs may contribute to the psychological conditions. In a study of 94 posttransplant patients, 66% reported successful intercourse at least once a week prior to diagnosis, but only 22% after diagnosis of ESRD ($P < 0.001$; Salvatierra et al 1975). While 85% of patients rated their pre-ESRD sexual desire as 'good', only 28% reported this rating after onset of ESRD.

New physical complaints secondary to renal disease may disturb patients' lives: namely, fractures, peptic ulcers, graft clotting, or graft infection. Dietary restrictions on fluid and salt intake present persistent limitations as well. Furthermore, most ESRD patients undergo at least an initial period of hemodialysis. The dependence on a machine for survival represents a loss of control that is upsetting to many patients; additional stresses of HD treatment include loss of physical functioning, decreased social functioning, and restricted dietary intake (Wright et al 1966), as well as an increase in somatic symptoms.

Psychological responses

Physical causes

Uremia and the initiation of dialysis cause slowed mentation and a decreased attention span. With the progression of uremia, patients may become disoriented and experience visual or auditory hallucinations. During this period, a patient may appear to have depression with psychotic symptoms or a schizophreniform disorder. Indeed, some uremic patients may progress to coma with decerebrate posturing (Glaser 1974). The organic brain syndrome is caused by central nervous system dysfunction from accumulation of toxic metabolites, anemia, hypertension, or cardiovascular insufficiency (Surman 1989). Patients who experience an organic brain syndrome during ESRD are at increased risk to develop delirium posttransplant (House and Thompson 1988). Another syndrome that affects mentation is dialysis dysequilibrium, a phenomenon that results from a rapid decrease in the plasma concentration of urea, which thereby draws plasma into the more concentrated cerebrospinal fluid (Glaser 1974). In addition, chronic dialysis patients are at risk for dialysis dementia (Glaser 1974), which has been attributed to aluminum toxicity.

Emotional causes

The anxiety experienced due both to the illness and to its treatments, as well as their possible complications, leads to overuse of psychological defense mechanisms such as denial, sublimation, projection, and displacement (Levy and Wynbrandt 1975). Using projection, dialysis patients deny that they feel unwell and comment that other patients appear to be much sicker (Wright et al 1966). Displacement of feelings of anger may lead to strained familial relationships as the patient vents his frustrations at home. Most importantly, denial can lead to noncompliance with the treatment regimen, thus endangering the patient's life.

Interestingly, however, ESRD patients have no more difficulty adjusting to their disease than other chronically ill patients. Cassileth et al (1984) evaluated the psychological status of 758 patients affected with any one of six chronic illnesses: arthritis, cancer, renal disease, dermatological disorders, diabetes, and depression. All groups (except the previously depressed patients) showed similar scores on psychological measures of anxiety, depression, loss of control, positive affect, emotional ties, and global mental health; moreover, the results were similar to those of the general public. These data refute the assumption that ESRD produces a disease-specific set of psychosocial changes. The authors maintain that, due to their prolonged course, chronic illnesses produce a similar constellation of problems, and that the individual's intrinsic strength (rather than the specific nature of the disease) determines his psychological outcome. Another study found that renal transplant candidates displayed a decreased incidence of dementia, delirium, and psychiatric disorders compared with other medical and surgical inpatients (Rundell and Hall 1997). The only problem found to be more prevalent among renal patients was hypoactive sexual desire disorder.

It is critical to assess a patient's capacity to cope with ESRD, as this adjustment correlates with chances for survival. A study of 147 dialysis patients suggested that survival was determined more by demographic and psychosocial factors than by physiological factors (Burton et al 1986), and that the occurrence of psychiatric dysfunction served as a greater adverse prognostic factor than medical dysfunction, including the degree of uremia. In a study of 241 home HD patients followed for 18 months, including 204 surviving and 37 deceased patients, the significant factors differentiating survivors were younger age ($P < 0.001$), less depression ($P < 0.04$), and more stress related to dialysis procedures and dietary restrictions ($P < 0.01$; Wai et al 1981).

PSYCHIATRIC IMPLICATIONS OF TREATMENT MODALITIES

The options for ESRD treatment, including HD, continuous ambulatory peritoneal dialysis (CAPD), and renal transplantation, each place unique demands on a patient. Because of the multiple treatment alternatives, studies of quality-of-life issues are meaningful to determine the relative improvements that each treatment offers the patient.

Hemodialysis

HD patients require tight adherence to treatment schedules and must adapt to an unpredictable course that includes fluctuating levels of energy and comfort. Decreased social functioning among ESRD patients includes termination of leisure activities and lack of employment. Decreases in energy and in the ability to concentrate may curtail previously enjoyed leisure activities. Patients on HD also experience difficulty in making long-term plans, since they may be unsure when they will feel well enough to participate in activities. The combination of a lack of energy with the restrictions on time, inherent particularly within center HD, results in unemployment for many patients.

Due to the rigorous schedule of clinic appointments, in addition to the inflexible dietary restrictions, HD seems to be the least tolerable method of treatment. Levy and Wynbrandt (1975) assessed the extent to which 18 HD patients were able to resume life activities such as employment and social outings, rating the patients' quality of life as 'good', 'fair', or 'poor'. The ratings included six 'good', five 'fair', and seven 'poor'. Patients also experience unpleasant body alterations such as fluid retention, needle marks, and graft scarring. To identify disturbances in body image, investigators had 16 HD patients perform the house–person–tree drawing test (Basch et al 1981). Compelling details from the drawings included overuse of the color red, likely due to a preoccupation with blood; trees drawn with prominent roots, displaying an interest in external nourishment; and distorted, incomplete people, signifying losses in physical function.

Other concerns for HD patients include worries about shunt complications and side-effects of treatment (Koch and Muthny 1990). In a study comparing quality of life in HD patients versus CAPD patients, center HD patients reported stress over headaches, bone pain, fluid restriction, dietary restriction, difficulty traveling, and hospitalizations at a significantly higher rate than CAPD patients (Wolcott and Nissenson 1988). Home HD, however, may confer similar benefits to CAPD by allowing the patient control over scheduling treatments (Campbell and Campbell 1978).

Continuous ambulatory peritoneal dialysis

In contrast to HD patients, who must accept a passive role in their therapy, CAPD patients are directly responsible for their own care. CAPD seems to offer a 'middle ground' quality of life between HD and transplantation (Koch and Muthny 1990). Because CAPD patients control their own dialysis, they avoid strict schedules necessitated by center HD. Thus, patients can plan treatments around employment and activities. In a study of 33 matched pairs of patients, CAPD patients had significantly higher ($P = 0.01$) quality of life scores on standard measures compared to center HD patients (Wolcott and Nissenson 1988). However, CAPD patients worry about potential complications such as peritonitis, which can result in hospitalization and, ultimately, peritoneal catheter replacement.

Renal transplantation

The majority of studies conclude that, compared with other modes of treatment, transplantation offers patients the best quality of life (Evans et al 1985; Koch and Muthny 1990; Simmons and Abress 1990). Koch and Muthny (1990) found that 30% of HD patients were dissatisfied with their lives, in comparison with 17% of CAPD patients and only 5% of transplant recipients. In a study of 766 ESRD patients undergoing HD, CAPD, or transplant, the last group of patients scored significantly higher ($P < 0.05$) on measures of physical, emotional, and social well being, as well as satisfaction with treatment (Simmons and Abress 1990). Moreover, Dubovsky and Penn (1980) stated that suicide was less common after transplant than during ongoing dialysis therapy. Freedom from concern over dialysis, coupled with increased energy and vigor, portends an improved functioning. Indeed, the only area in which transplant patients admit to decreased satisfaction with treatment outcome is the fear of medical complications, including rejection of their graft, infection, and side-effects of the immunosuppressive medications (Koch and Muthny 1990).

The most frequently cited study refuting the conclusion that transplantation offers the best quality of life is the study by Kalman et al (1983), in which 57 transplant recipients and 44 HD patients answered health questionnaires at least 5 years after the initiation of either treatment. While HD patients as a group were older and more likely to have undergone three or more hospitalizations in the last 5 years ($P < 0.01$), rates of psychiatric impairment, based upon questioning and past psychiatric history, were comparable between the groups: namely, 46% of transplant and 48% of HD patients. However, since an estimated 10% of HD patients die each year, patients who survive 5 years probably represent a subset with characteristics distinct from those of other HD patients.

One theory that explains the differences in quality of life among the treatment modes is that satisfaction correlates with a patient's perceptions of the intrusiveness of the treatment and his own sense of control, respectively defined as 'the extent to which the illness and/or its treatment interfere with life' and 'one's ability to obtain positive valued outcomes and avoid negative ones' (Devins et al 1984). Among 35 HD patients, 10 CAPD patients, and 25 posttransplant patients at least 1 year after initiation of treatment, HD was believed to be the most intrusive, CAPD less intrusive, and transplant the least intrusive. During periods of rejection, however, transplant patients changed their ratings to most intrusive. Not surprisingly, the likelihood of negative mood symptoms increased with a more intrusive evaluation of therapy and with a decreased level of control (Devins et al 1984).

PSYCHIATRIC ISSUES IN TRANSPLANT CANDIDATE SELECTION

General criteria for selection of candidates

Overall, transplantation provides the best opportunity for an improved quality of life in ESRD patients. Due to the scarcity of donor organs, however, physicians must decide how to allocate this resource among a growing population of patients. The current method of allocation is based upon 'accepted notion of benefit': namely, medical need, time to death, and predicted posttransplant quality of life (Freeman et al 1995).

Four other ethical approaches have been espoused to guide recipient selection. First, the 'physician's duty' theory proposes that physicians preserve life and decrease suffering with the goal of an active, prolonged patient survival. Thus, physicians consider all patients with clear potential for benefit as candidates for transplant, with the possibility to broaden candidacy in selected cases. Second, the 'patient's rights' theory establishes that every patient is a rightful recipient if he has a preference for transplantation. However, this theory likely expends valuable organ resources on recipients with little likelihood for positive outcomes. Third, the 'cost-effectiveness' theory promotes recipient selection based upon projections of which patients will experience the best outcomes at the least expense. Fourth, the 'scientific progress' theory suggests that patients be selected on the basis of whether their treatment may lead to medical progress (Surman and Purtillo 1992). In practice, each transplant center employs a combination of these theories in its decision-making process.

The dilemma over candidate selection raises concern over which psychosocial factors should guide the choice of potential recipients. Olbrisch and Levenson (1995) propose two goals of psychosocial assessment: first, assessment of compliance, family support, and psychiatric disorders, and second, patient understanding of the procedure and its risks. Greenberg et al (1973) also note that a good psychological evaluation should identify intellectual deficits that may interfere with compliance to posttransplant medical regimens.

Frequent relative contraindications to transplantation include a history of suicide attempts, recent or past drug or alcohol abuse, prior medical noncompliance, psychosis, inadequate neurocognitive functioning, and inadequate social and financial support (Freeman et al 1995). Relative 'soft criteria' contraindications include smoking, obesity, legal history, past or current mood disorder, and personality disorders (Olbrisch and Levenson 1995). Transplant centers vary in the importance assigned to each criterion; cardiac programs tend to employ the strictest criteria and renal programs the most lenient, based upon the disparity between patient demand and organ supply.

The organization of these psychosocial contraindications into a standardized method for the assessment of patients remains a goal of organ transplant psychiatry. A study of 154 renal transplant programs showed only 7% had formal psychosocial criteria for the selection of patients (Levenson and Olbrisch 1993). Absolute contraindications used by renal programs included active schizophrenia (72.9%), current suicidal ideation (56.8%), history of multiple suicide attempts (38.7%), dementia (43.2%), and mental retardation with IQ <50 (24%; Levenson and Olbrisch 1993). Only 1% of renal programs excluded patients for psychosocial reasons (Levenson and Olbrisch 1993).

Predictors of patient compliance

One meaningful psychosocial criterion that predicts positive posttransplant outcome is evidence of compliance to the medical regimen. Due to improvements in immunosuppression and anti-infective agents, graft survival rates have increased, while patient morbidity and mortality have decreased. However, an emerging cause of graft failure is patient noncompliance, a preventable reason why previously healthy patients suffer rejection episodes. Among 531 cyclosporine–prednisone- (CsA–Pred-) treated patients, noncompliance accounted for 11.9% of graft losses over a 5-year period and represented (after rejection and systemic infection) the most common reason for graft loss (Didlake et al 1988). In a retrospective study of 260 patients, 18% were noncompliant to their medication regimen (Schweizer et al 1990). The incidences of noncompliance were not significantly different between recipients of cadaveric versus living-related donor transplants. The demographic features associated with noncompliance were recipient age less than 20 years (57% of these patients were noncompliant with medications and clinic followup) and African-American race (37% of these patients were medication-noncompliant). A reanalysis of noncompliance, based upon stratification by socioeconomic level, revealed no difference among ethnic groups (Rovelli et al 1989).

The reasons for patient noncompliance include denial of disease, belief in transplant as a cure, hostility toward doctors, desire to return to the hospital for secondary gain, and concern over Cushingoid appearance secondary to steroid use (Dubovsky and Penn 1980). In addition, some patients react to an initial rejection episode with a belief that graft loss is inevitable and thus become noncompliant in an attempt to exert control over their fate (Gulledge et al 1983). Another explanation for noncompliance is complacency toward treatment, an attitude that progresses with increasing time posttransplant. Ironically, it seems that after the critical period—when rejection episodes and complications are most likely—the patient's decreased fear and anxiety may lead to apathy toward the treatment regimen (DeLone et al 1989). Thus, the major approaches to prevent noncompliance include identification of psychosocial factors that contribute to behavior, simplification of treatment regimens, and continuing education on the need for lifelong immunosuppression (Rovelli et al 1989).

One major issue is the association between pretransplant Axis 1 or Axis 2 psychiatric diagnoses and posttransplant noncompliance (Table 20.1). Among 311 transplant candidates, 60% met criteria for Axis 1 and 31.5% for Axis 2 disorders (Chacko et al 1996). However, the only Axis 1 diagnosis that was associated with past or current noncompliance was past or current drug or alcohol abuse ($P = 0.0001$). Pre-existing Axis 2 disorders correlated to noncompliance in the areas of diet, appointment attendance, and use of medication. In fact, Axis 2 disorders may be more worrisome than Axis 1 disorders, since the former illnesses are more pervasive and difficult to treat (Freeman et al 1995). Further, a family history of psychiatric disorders was significantly related to global noncompliance and drug abuse (Chacko et al 1996).

Three questionnaires used to evaluate the impact of psychosocial factors in transplant candidate selection are the Psychosocial Assessment of Candidates for Transplantation (PACT), the Psychosocial Levels System (PLS), and the Transplant Evaluation Rating Scale (TERS). The PACT studies the correlation between decisions to accept or exclude potential recipients among different evaluators (Olbrisch et al 1989), using psychosocial factors such as drug and alcohol abuse, compliance, social support, psychopathology, lifestyle factors, and transplant knowledge. However, this tool does not predict transplant outcomes. The PLS, which shows good interrater reliability, discriminates three levels of psychosocial adjustment, based on past psychiatric history, prior coping skills, affect, mental status, support, and proneness to anxiety (Futterman et al 1991). Level 1 candidates are defined as patients with no psychiatric history, with appropriate emotional reactions at diagnosis, and with good social support. Level 2 candidates may have a history of depression, emotional reactions of agitation or dysphoria at diagnosis, and fair social support. Level 3 candidates display a significant psychiatric history of substance abuse or major depression in combination with active suicidal ideation.

The TERS evaluation uses 10 psychosocial aspects of functioning to expand the three

Axis 1:   Psychiatric clinical disorders including
Mood disorders
Psychotic disorders
Anxiety disorders
Substance-related disorders
Cognitive disorders
Mental disorders secondary to general medical condition
Sexual disorders

Axis 2:   Personality disorders
Mental retardation

Axis 3:   General medical conditions causing, resulting from, or unrelated to
medical illness, including (but not limited to)
Epilepsy
Cardiovascular disease
Hypertension
Renal disease
Hypothyroidism

Axis 4:   Psychosocial and environmental problems relevant to illness,
including (but not limited to) stressors
Divorce
Crying
Deaths

Axis 5:   Global Assessment of Functioning (GAF) score (evaluates social,
occupational, and psychological functioning)
Scale: 100 (superior) to 1 (grossly impaired)

Table 20.1. Multiaxial classification system for psychiatric diagnosis

levels of the PLS (Twillman et al 1993). These aspects include prior psychiatric history of Axis 1 or Axis 2 disorders, substance abuse, compliance, health behaviors, family support, and prior history of coping with disease. The TERS amends the aforementioned levels of the PLS with several additions. Level 1 candidates may display symptoms of cluster C traits (Table 20.2). Correspondingly, the cluster C trait of obsessive–compulsiveness correlated with a better posttransplant outcome resulting from greater treatment compliance (House and Thompson 1988). Level 2 candidates have a cluster C diagnosis, or symptoms of clusters A and B. Level 3 patients have cluster A and B diagnoses. Upon retrospective analysis, TERS ratings accurately predicted the out

	Cluster A	Cluster B	Cluster C
General characteristics Onset	Odd, eccentric Beginning by early adulthood	Dramatic, erratic, emotional Beginning by early adulthood (except Antisocial; see below)	Anxious, fearful Beginning by early adulthood
Diagnoses	**Paranoid personality disorder:** a pervasive pattern of distrust and suspiciousness of others that their motives are interpreted as malevolent. **Schizoid personality disorder:** a pervasive pattern of detachment from social relationships and a restricted range of expression of emotions in interpersonal settings. **Schizotypal personality disorder:** a pervasive pattern of social and interpersonal deficits marked by acute discomfort with, and reduced capacity for, close relationships as well as by cognitive or perceptual distortions and eccentricities of behavior.	**Antisocial personality disorder:** a pervasive pattern of disregard for and violation of the rights of others, occurring since age 15 years. **Borderline personality disorder:** a pervasive pattern of instability of interpersonal relationships, self-image, and affects, and marked impulsivity. **Histrionic personality disorder:** a pervasive pattern of excessive emotionality and attention seeking. **Narcissistic personality disorder:** a pervasive pattern of grandiosity (in fantasy or behavior), need for admiration, and lack of empathy.	**Avoidant personality disorder:** a pervasive pattern of social inhibition, feelings of inadequacy, and hypersensitivity to negative evaluation. **Dependent personality disorder:** a pervasive and excessive need to be taken care of that leads to submissive and clinging behavior and fears of separation. **Obsessive–compulsive personality disorder:** a pervasive pattern of preoccupation with orderliness, perfectionism, and mental and interpersonal control, at the expense of flexibility, openness, and efficiency.

Table 20.2. Summary of personality disorders (Reprinted with permission from the *Diagnostic and Statistical Manual of Mental Disorders*, 4th edn. © 1994 American Psychiatric Association)

comes of 35 posttransplant liver patients in the areas of compliance, health behaviors, and substance abuse.

Much controversy remains over which psychosocial criteria best predict posttransplant outcomes. First, what relative weight should physicians place on each psychosocial factor? Do some criteria, such as active psychosis, substance abuse, and suicidal ideation, constitute absolute contraindications, while others, such as a history of psychiatric disorders, a lack of family support, and Axis 2 disorders, represent additive prohibitors? Second, what is the usefulness of strict, empirically derived criteria to predict noncompliance (Olbrisch and Levenson 1995)? Some clinicians argue that previous actions do not predict posttransplant behavior, believing that the unique situation of transplantation changes the patient's outlook to such an extent that his future conduct has no relation to previous attitudes. Furthermore, these investigators suggest that psychosocial criteria may be misused and exploited by physicians making value judgments about a patient's social worth (Surman 1989; Olbrisch and Levenson 1995). For instance, while there are no data that correlate legal history to noncompliance, many programs reject felony prisoners (Levenson and Olbrisch 1993).

The term 'good outcome' raises additional controversy. Many investigators consider improvements in psychosocial factors, such as employment, income, and marital happiness, to signify a good outcome. Other physicians argue that a more powerful measure of good outcome is a patient's opinion of his quality of life (Wolcott 1991; Freeman et al 1995).

PSYCHIATRIC ISSUES DURING THE WAITING PERIOD

Patients awaiting cadaveric donor transplantation may experience anxiety due to anticipation of the procedure or, worse, of death while awaiting the procedure. The patient must cope with the realization that his transplant depends on another person's death (Levenson and Olbrisch 1987). Some patients respond to protracted delays with noncompliance, hoping that worsening illness will necessitate earlier transplantation (Levenson and Olbrisch 1987). Because the evaluation of the patient has been completed, contact between the patient and the transplant team is minimal during the waiting period. Additionally, feelings of guilt over the inability to provide an organ may cause team members to avoid the patient (Levenson and Olbrisch 1987).

Individual and group therapy may be useful to the patient coping with psychological stress during the waiting period (Wolcott 1993). Frequent follow-up with expectant patients may be useful to explain donor allocation protocol and to dispel feelings of abandonment, thereby minimizing patient anxiety and reducing the possibility of noncompliance (Levenson and Olbrisch 1987). Group therapy also offers educational opportunities and emotional support for transplant candidates (Abbey 1998). Pretransplant education groups discuss the surgical procedure, as well as its emotional and physical implications. Meetings of potential recipients with posttransplant patients facilitate discussion of the process, suggesting means for coping with ESRD while awaiting the procedure (Surman 1989; Abbey 1998).

PSYCHIATRIC ISSUES AFTER TRANSPLANTATION

Intrapsychic integration of the graft

The posttransplant period poses new psychiatric and psychological problems as the patient copes with his new organ and the treatments that are mandatory to ensure its survival. Changes in body image occur as the patient psychologically accepts the new organ as part of himself. Increases in energy level and sexual function contribute to an improved quality of life, yet patients must accept that they will never fully return to their premorbid state. Furthermore, immunosuppressive agents may create psychiatric disturbances that cause the patient distress and may predispose to noncompliance.

Recognition of the processes necessary to cope with losses of external body parts—such as those that occur with congenital defects or amputations—led to the description of the body image phenomenon (Castelnuovo-Tedesco 1971). In transplantation, however, the recipient must contend with the psychic integration of an added organ into his body image. Muslin (1971) proposed three stages of this internalization. During the 'foreign body stage', a patient views his new organ as a separate entity within his body and experiences 'graft traumatic anxiety'—excessive concern about damaging the organ (Cramond 1967). Recipients protect the graft site against injury in crowds and, for this reason, refuse to engage in sexual intercourse. During this phase, the recipient may identify with the donor and assume he has inherited donor attributes (Muslin 1971). Some recipients feel the need to manifest traits of their donors; for instance, one patient decided to learn Spanish after learning his donor's name was Jaime (Basch 1973). The second stage, 'partial incorporation', includes a decreased investment of psychic energy in discussions about the organ (Muslin 1971). Finally, in the stage of 'complete incorporation', the recipient accepts the new organ, no longer viewing it as a distinct part. However, episodes of rejection and procedures such as biopsies may lead to regression to the 'foreign body stage' (Muslin 1971).

Another common reaction during the posttransplant period is an unconscious belief that the new organ is an introjection of the donor. Difficulties in the relationship between the living donor and the recipient may result in noncompliance and rejection as the patient attempts to rid himself of the introject. Male patients who have underlying fears of feminization experience psychological difficulty after being transplanted with organs from females and may become preoccupied with the notion that some part of their identity is now feminine. For this reason, Cramond (1967) suggested that 'passive, effeminate males' not receive female-donor organs. Similarly, females who have received organs from male donors may worry about their ability to bear children (Basch 1973).

Thus, patients with tenuous gender identity may become confused after cross-gender transplants (Levey et al 1986).

Transplant recipients may experience conscious and unconscious guilt over the acquisition of the graft. If the transplant results from a living-related or -unrelated donor, the recipient feels remorse for having placed the donor's life in danger (Kemph 1970). Recipients of cadaveric donor organs may feel accountable for either causing or benefiting from the donor's death. Projective psychological testing of recipients reveals themes of robbing or stealing from others (Kemph et al 1969) and a need to repay the donor for his sacrifice (Muslin 1971). On the other hand, when the recipient manifests a rejection episode, he may experience resentment toward the donor (Kemph et al 1969).

Improved quality of life

Despite these difficult psychic processes, transplant patients tend ultimately to experience vast improvements in their quality of life. One factor supporting these improvements is the more efficacious immunosuppressive agents. Although cyclosporine–prednisone (CsA–Pred) treatment yielded statistically equivalent rates of survival compared with antilymphocyte globulin–Pred–azathioprine treatment (86% graft and 95% patient versus 84% graft and 98% patient survival, respectively), the CsA–Pred treated patients reported significantly greater feelings of physical and emotional well being ($P < 0.05$; Simmons and Abress 1987). Better-perceived health with CsA probably owes to the reduced occurrence of rejection and infection episodes (Simmons et al 1988).

Sexual functioning also improves posttransplantation. Sixty-nine percent of posttransplant patients deny difficulty with impotence, compared with only 19% of pretransplant patients ($P < 0.05$; Simmons et al 1981). Salvatierra et al (1975) questioned 94 patients with functioning kidney grafts concerning sexual desire and frequency of intercourse. The percentage of patients reporting intercourse at least once a week was 22% among ESRD patients and 47% among transplant patients ($P < 0.001$). In addition, 66% of transplant patients rated their sexual desire as 'good', compared with only 28% of ESRD patients. Self-esteem also increases after transplantation: among nondiabetic individuals, 66% of transplant recipients at 5–9 years posttransplant displayed high scores on self-esteem measures, compared with only 35% of pretransplant patients ($P < 0.01$; Simmons et al 1981).

Unfortunately, the improvement in employment rate after transplant is not as great as expected, although it is better than the rate for HD patients. Koch and Muthny (1990) reported that the average rate of full-time employment posttransplant (28%) is only slightly higher than that of either HD (27%) or CAPD (23%) patients. In another study, 74% of transplant patients were able to work, compared to 37% of center HD, 59% of home HD, and 24% of CAPD patients (Evans et al 1985). Employment posttransplant seems to correlate best with employment pretransplant. Despite vigorous attempts at occupational rehabilitation to increase these percentages, many posttransplant patients possess neither the skills nor the energy required for long-term work.

Despite improvements posttransplant, most recipients cannot duplicate their premorbid existence. The uncertainty of graft survival, the side-effects of medications, and the fear of infection inevitably contribute to an altered situation (Dubovsky and Penn 1980). Even after a successful transplant, some pre-existing diseases, such as systemic lupus erythematosus and diabetes, continue to progress, producing other complications (Gulledge et al 1983). Two observers rated the quality of life among 237 recipients at 5–9 years posttransplant. Investigators rated 32% of the 192 nondiabetic patients to be in excellent condition; 50%, moderately good; and 8%, poor. In contrast, none of the 45 diabetic patients were rated as being in excellent condition, 56% were moderately good, and 44% were poor (Simmons et al 1981). During the previous year, 61% of diabetics required hospitalization, compared to 28% of nondiabetic recipients ($P < 0.01$). Thus, concurrent systemic diseases hamper improvement in quality of life after transplantation.

Psychiatric manifestations

Psychiatric manifestations likely to occur after transplant include anxiety, depression, and delirium. Likely causes of these problems include altered body image, imbalanced electrolytes, or administered steroids (Blazer et al 1976). Uncertainties about graft function and survival, which are prominent in the immediate postoperative course, create anxiety. The patient is most likely to experience depression when the realities of the posttransplant course do not fulfill pretransplant expectations (Dubovsky and Penn 1980). Infections, such as with cytomegalovirus, may also result in depressive symptoms (Surman 1989). Anxiety and depression may manifest as agitation, regression, or noncompliance. Central nervous system infections may present as delirium, seizures, or coma (Conti and Rubin 1988).

Two psychiatric emergencies may occur. First, rejection encephalopathy, a syndrome of confusion, hypertension, irritability, headache, papilledema, disorientation, and generalized seizures, may occur following rapid increases in serum creatinine levels associated with severe rejection episodes (Gross et al 1981). Treatment includes increased amounts of immunosuppression to control the rejection episode, coupled with intravenous diazepam to prevent seizures. A second serious problem is delirium—the most common posttransplant organic mental disorder—resulting from electrolyte imbalances, renal failure, central nervous system hemorrhage, rejection, and drug toxicity (Trzepacz et al 1991). In particular, delirium may result from CsA whole blood trough levels greater than 1000 ng/ml, or particularly adverse reactions to tacrolimus (TRL) at any concentration. Although resolution of the underlying disturbance generally cures the delirium among patients without agitation, haloperidol provides the best treatment for agitated patients (House and Thompson 1988).

NEUROTOXIC EFFECTS OF MEDICATIONS

Some medications necessary for immunosuppressive and infection prophylaxis may produce psychiatric disturbances. Fortuitously, most of these symptoms disappear upon drug discontinuation (Anonymous 1989).

Steroids

Steroids cause multiple psychiatric complications. First, they alter body image by causing 'moon face', acne, truncal obesity, and hirsutism—alterations that are particularly devastating for narcissistic patients (Levy 1986) and for adolescents (Stuber 1993). Second, 6% of steroid-treated patients experience psychiatric symptoms as a direct result of the medication, including emotional lability, anxiety, pressured speech, insomnia, depression, auditory or visual hallucinations, agitation, and distractibility (Hall et al 1979). These symptoms may suggest multiple diagnoses, including depression, mania, psychosis, and delirium (Ling et al 1981; Kershner and Wang-Cheng 1989). Contrary to previous belief, depression seems to be more common than mania (Ismail and Wessely 1995). These manifestations have an average onset of 6 days after treatment initiation and are more likely to occur at doses greater than 40 mg/day (Hall et al 1979). Women appear to be more prone to these complications than men (Ling et al 1981; Kershner and Wang-Cheng 1989; Ismail and Wessely 1995). Interestingly, patients with previous or current mental illness seem not to be at risk for exacerbated or initiated psychiatric symptoms due to steroid therapy. While some studies show that patients with previous episodes of steroid-induced psychiatric symptoms do not have an increased likelihood of psychiatric symptoms upon repeated treatment (Ling et al 1981; Kershner and Wang-Cheng 1989), most physicians exercise caution with steroid therapy in the presence of a history of psychiatric disturbances. Decreasing dosage or discontinuing steroids usually terminates the problem. However, patients with persistent symptoms should be treated with low doses of an antipsychotic medication such as haloperidol. Physicians should avoid the use of tricyclic antidepressants, which appear to exacerbate symptomatology of steroid-induced psychiatric problems (Hall et al 1979; Kershner and Wang-Cheng 1989).

Cyclosporine

Like steroids, the cosmetic effects consequent to high doses of CsA—gingival hyperplasia and hypertrichosis—can lead to a disturbed body image and resultant noncompliance. In addition, a few patients report anxiety, mania, and visual hallucinations. Katirji (1987) reported that two patients experienced visual hallucinations at CsA trough levels of 747 and 1212 ng/ml. These hallucinations reversed as the drug serum level decreased to the therapeutic range. TRL produces not only minor side-effects, such as mood and sleep disturbances, but also, more importantly, major neurological complications of seizure and encephalopathy (Eidelman et al 1991), particularly upon intravenous administration producing high drug concentrations. Compared with patients treated with CsA, patients treated with TRL show lower scores on certain tests assessing concentration, visual-motor coordination, and cognitive flexibility—a finding that indicates a higher incidence of organic brain damage with TRL (DiMartini et al 1997).

Anti-infection agents

Several agents used to treat infections also produce psychiatric syndromes in transplant recipients. Acyclovir administered intravenously in large doses may cause insomnia, hallucinations, depersonalization, and major depression with psychotic features (Sirota et al 1988; Trzepacz et al 1993a). Amphotericin B may lead to confusion and delirium among recipients with fungal infections (Trzepacz et al 1993a). Metronidazole has been associated with both depression (Voth 1969) and hallucinations (Trzepacz et al 1993a).

Beta-blockers

The relationship between beta-blockers and depressive symptomatology is controversial. Although physicians generally believe that beta-blocker therapy predisposes to depression, the current literature does not definitively support this correlation (Ried et al 1998). A study of 77 patients with suspected coronary artery disease undergoing cardiac catheterization failed to show an increased rate of depression among patients treated with beta-blockers as compared with patients on calcium channel blockers, diuretics, or vasodilators (Carney et al 1987). Conversely, a meta-analysis of nine studies totaling 1175 subjects found that propranolol did produce depression at a higher rate than control medications (Patten 1990). The research on this topic raises two main concerns. First, the meta-analysis showed that propranolol produces fatigue, decreased energy, decreased libido, anorexia, and decreased concentration. Because both propranolol and depression cause similar neurovegetative symptoms, it is difficult to separate these etiologies in patients on these drugs. Second, despite the many case reports, controlled, randomized studies have not been performed, nor have consistent measures for diagnosis of depression been developed (Ried et al 1998).

TREATMENT OF PSYCHIATRIC DISORDERS IN PATIENTS WITH RENAL INSUFFICIENCY

Psychopharmacotherapy for patients with renal insufficiency constitutes a growing area of research, as the lifelong immunosuppressive treatment of patients continues to raise new issues on drug dosing and interactions. The kidney is responsible for the elimination of many psychiatric drugs, including lithium, benzodiazepines, and metabolites of tricyclic antidepressants. Renal insufficiency especially affects drugs that circulate by binding to plasma proteins. Because renal dysfunction decreases the amounts of plasma proteins, the proportion of drug that is unbound increases, potentially producing toxicity at seemingly therapeutic serum drug levels. Two methods are utilized to adjust drug dosages in these patients. The interval extension method recommends administration of usual amounts of drug at increased dosing intervals, while the dosage reduction method recommends administration of decreased amounts of drug at usual dosing intervals. The latter method achieves a more constant serum drug level (Bennett et al 1983). As a general rule, reducing drug dosage to two-thirds of the normally recommended value is acceptable in cases of renal insufficiency, but more specific recommendations do exist (Trzepacz et al 1993a).

Multiple antidepressant medications are available for use, including tricyclic antidepressants, serotonin-specific re-uptake inhibitors (SSRIs), monoamine oxidase inhibitors (MAOIs), psychostimulants, bupropion, and trazodone. Tricyclic antidepressants undergo primary hepatic metabolism, creating active metabolites that undergo renal excretion and thus accumulate during kidney failure (Lieberman et al 1985). Further, HD, administration of diuretics, or fluid restriction can abruptly increase or decrease drug serum levels by altering the drug's volume of distribution. In addition, the side-effect profiles of tricyclics to blockade (cholinergic and alpha-1 adrenergic stimuli) may exacerbate pre-existing hypotension or urinary retention in renal patients.

Among the tricyclics, nortriptyline offers two prominent advantages. First, it has a known therapeutic window (50–150 mg/ml) toward which physicians may target drug dosages using serum levels. Second, it is the least anticholinergic and antiadrenergic among this class of drugs. Desipramine and imipramine are also reasonable therapeutic choices, since the serum levels of these drugs can also be monitored.

SSRIs offer the advantages of not causing alpha-1 adrenergic blockade and of having only a minimal effect on cholinergic receptors. Therefore, these drugs show reduced risks of the hypotension and urinary retention seen with tricyclics. Further, the kidneys only minimally participate in the excretion of SSRIs. However, SSRIs interact to varying degrees with the cytochrome P450 (CYP) enzymes responsible for metabolizing the immunosuppressive drugs. Fluoxetine (Prozac) strongly inhibits CYP3A4, the liver enzyme that metabolizes CsA (Fuller et al 1976; Albers et al 1999). SSRIs also inhibit CYP2D6 and CYP2C19, which metabolize propranolol, metoprolol, and codeine. In contrast, sertraline and paroxetine have insignificant effects on cytochrome P450. Therefore, these SSRIs represent better choices for patients on cytochrome P450-metabolized drugs. Physicians must monitor for serotonergic effects, such as gastrointestinal upset, anxiety, insomnia, and sexual dysfunction.

Among the other antidepressants, physicians should avoid MAOIs, which may cause a hypertensive crisis that can lead to cardiac arrhythmias (Tollefson 1983; Trzepacz et al 1993b). Moreover, restrictions on tyramine-containing foods such as wine and cheese compound the already stringent dietary restrictions necessary for HD patients—a combination of limitations that is likely to increase the chances of non-compliance to either regimen. Psychostimulants have been shown to be effective in treating depression in medically ill patients, in some cases within 2 days after initiation (Woods et al 1986). Little research has been conducted to determine the effects of renal insufficiency on bupropion and trazodone (Trzepacz et al 1993b). Because antidepressants generally display similar efficacy in the treatment of depression, a medication should be chosen to avoid or exploit its side-effect profile (Table 20.3). All dosing of antidepressants should be performed according to the dosage reduction method. Finally, if other treatments fail, electroconvulsive therapy has shown positive results in several case reports of affective psychoses (Blazer et al 1976; Franco-Bronson 1996).

Lithium has been used to treat both endogenous and steroid-induced mania. Since renal excretion is the primary route for lithium elimination, and since low-sodium diets or the use of diuretics may increase lithium levels due to competition for reabsorption within the kidney, this agent must be used with caution. Furthermore, CsA increases reabsorption of lithium by the proximal tubule, thus producing higher serum levels (Vincent et al 1987)—an effect that is potentially dangerous, given the narrow therapeutic range of lithium (0.6–1.2 meq/l). At 1.5 meq/l concentration of lithium, the toxic effects include nausea, vomiting, and coarse tremor. Severe toxicity occurs at levels over 2.5 meq/l, and death is possible at levels exceeding 4.0 meq/l (Albers et al 1999). As with the antidepressants, lithium dosing in patients with renal failure should follow the dosage reduction method of management (Bennett et al 1983).

Neuroleptic drugs are used to treat delirium, psychosis, agitation, and acute mania. These drugs also undergo renal elimination; therefore, renal insufficiency leads to increased serum levels of hepatic metabolites. Low-potency neuroleptics, such as chlorpromazine and thioridazine, display anticholinergic, antihistaminic, and anti-alpha-1 adrenergic effects. As is the case with antidepressants, hypotension due to alpha-1 blockade may be compounded by diuretic administration or sodium and fluid restriction in patients treated with neuroleptics. The hypotensive effect is most prominent with intramuscular administration of these drugs. Physicians must avoid treatment of hypotension with epinephrine, since the resultant unopposed beta activity can lead to severe depression of the blood pressure (Trzepacz et al 1993b). Bennett et al (1983) suggest dosage reduction of these drugs. Due to its lack of significant cholinergic, adrenergic, or histaminic blockade, haloperidol is the drug of choice. Dystonic reactions resulting from haloperidol are best treated with benztropine, while akathisia demands beta-blockers or benzodiazepines for resolution.

Benzodiazepines, which are metabolized by the cytochrome P450 system, are used to treat anxiety disorders and insomnia. If administered at doses that produce toxic levels, these drugs may cause paranoia, hallucinations, and anterograde amnesia. Unfortunately, no standards are available to monitor serum levels. Although Bennett et al (1983) state that no drug adjustment is necessary in cases of renal failure, Trzepacz et al (1993b) suggest that physicians prescribe low doses of short-acting benzodiazepines and observe for toxicity.

Another potential treatment for anxiety disorders, particularly generalized anxiety disorder, is buspirone. Among 25 patients suffering gastrointestinal disorders and/or hypertension, most patients reported improvements in their level of anxiety at a mean dose of 23–33 mg/day (McGowan et al 1988). Furthermore, no adverse effects were reported upon combined therapy with antihypertensive agents, such as propranolol and hydrochlorothiazide. However, this study excluded patients with 'uncontrolled or serious medical problems'—a criterion that seems contradictory to the main purpose and, therefore, limits the value of the study.

PSYCHIATRIC ISSUES OF DONATION

Initially, physicians did not recognize the psychological benefits of organ donation for the living donor, assuming that the donor either was coerced or was suffering from psychopathology (Fellner and Schwartz 1971). Because of these early concerns, pretransplant evaluation of living donors became necessary. Today, these interviews are used to detect whether the donor is experiencing psychological pressure from the potential recipient (Kasiske 1988) and whether the potential donor has a normal decision-making capacity (Colomb and Hamburger 1967). However, in general, individuals who truly wish to be donors, by report, do not require a period of active deliberation (Levy 1986).

Recent research has revealed psychological benefits of organ donation, such as improved self-esteem and increased sense of self-worth. When the operation is successful, the donor often experiences a sense of rebirth, as he is responsible for this 'gift of life' (Abram and Buchanan 1976–1977). Interviews of 10 donors 8–10 years after the procedure revealed that all individuals felt content with their decision (Marshall and Fellner 1977).

Although physicians have recently accepted the potential benefits of donation after positive transplant outcomes, they continue to doubt whether these advantages exist for donors of organs that have been rejected by the recipients. However, in a study of 14 donors, none expressed regret over the decision, despite the fact that six of these donations resulted in unsuccessful transplants (Sharma and Enoch 1987). In addition, the incidence of negative psychological effects was not greater among donors of successful versus rejected organs (Sharma and Enoch 1987). In another study, 96% of donors reaffirmed their decision, regardless of the success of the graft (Smith et al 1986). Thus, the positive psychological effects of organ donation seem to be independent of transplant outcome. These arguments are used to support the contention that incompetent persons, such as minors and mentally retarded individuals, are capable of deciding to become donors.

Class	Side-effects	Specific agents	P450 effects	Other specific drug adverse effects
Serotonin-specific reuptake inhibitors (SSRIs)	• Minimal effect on muscarinic, histaminic, adrenergic receptors • Serotonergic effects: GI effects (nausea, vomiting), decreased appetite, insomnia, headache, sexual dysfunction, serotonin syndrome (nausea, confusion, hyperthermia, autonomic instability, rigidity)	Fluoxetine	Inhibits CYP2D6, CYP3A4, CYP2C9, CYP2C19	—
		Paroxetine	Inhibits CYP2D6, CYP2C9	Sedation
		Sertraline	Inhibits CYP2D6, CYP2C9	Lowest overall effect on P450 of SSRIs
		Fluvoxamine	Inhibits CYP1A2, CYP3A4, CYP2C19, CYP2C9	Sedation
Tertiary amine tricyclic antidepressants (TCAs)	• Anticholinergic: dry mouth, blurry vision, constipation, urinary retention, tachycardia • Alpha-1-adrenergic blockade: orthostatic hypotension • Antihistaminic sedation, weight gain • Cardiotoxicity: slowed conduction • Seizures • Neurotoxicity: tremor, ataxia		Many are metabolized by the CYP2D6	All should have decreased dosage in hepatic/renal disease
		Amitriptyline		—
		Clomipramine		Most serotonergic; thus, may cause sexual dysfunction
		Doxepin		Strong antihistaminic agent
		Imipramine Trimipramine		—
Secondary amine tricyclic antidepressants	Same		Same	
		Desipramine		Least sedating, least anticholinergic
		Nortriptyline		Least likely to cause orthostasis Only antidepressant with known therapeutic serum levels (50–150 ng/ml)
		Protriptyline		Least sedating, most activating

		Metabolized by liver	Higher incidence of weight gain, drowsiness, dry mouth, sexual dysfunction
Monoamine oxidase inhibitors (MAOIs)	Phenelzine		
	Tranylcypromine		More likely to cause insomnia
Atypical agents	Bupropion	Metabolized by liver, metabolites excreted by kidney	Insomnia, CNS stimulation, headache, constipation, dry mouth, nausea, tremor, seizures (doses should be ≤450 mg/day)
	Trazodone	Metabolized by liver, metabolites excreted by kidney	Antihistaminic: sedation, weight gain, alpha-1-adrenergic blockade; orthostatic hypotension; minimal anti-cholinergic effects; priapism

- Alpha-1-adrenergic blockade: orthostatic hypotension
- Antihistaminic: sedation, weight gain
- Hypertensive crisis from consuming tyramine: hypertension, headache, sweating, nausea, vomiting, autonomic instability, cardiac arrhythmias

Table 20.3.   The side-effect profiles and P450 effects of commonly used antidepressants (Adapted from Albers et al 1999)

Living-related donors

Reactions to organ donation vary, depending upon the closeness of the relationship between the potential donor and the recipient. Mothers are most willing to donate organs, followed by fathers and, lastly, by siblings (Kemph et al 1969). In a study of 536 living-related donors, 93% of parental donations were unsolicited (Smith et al 1986). One hypothesis for the large percentage of mothers who volunteer to donate is that they feel responsible for the child's defective organ and thus wish to compensate them (Levy 1986). In contrast, siblings express the highest degree of hostility toward the potential recipient. Another scenario occurs when the 'black sheep' of the family offers to donate to garner favor, seeking to regain active status in the family by undergoing the 'punishment' of surgery (Levy 1986). Differences in organ donation also occur along gender lines: females are 28% more likely to donate an organ, while remaining 10% less likely than males to receive a living-related organ ($P < 0.001$; Bloembergen et al 1996).

Family members who do not wish to donate may avoid visiting the prospective recipient. They may also miss appointments for evaluation and not reschedule. If they attend their appointments, they may hope for a 'medical discharge' to avoid the surgery (Abram and Buchanan 1976–1977). Often the spouse of a potential donor opposes the surgery because of perceived risk to his immediate family (Abram and Buchanan 1976–1977). Donor families may worry that someone closer to the donor may eventually need the organ (House and Thompson 1988). These concerns are especially prominent among families with hereditary causes of ESRD, such as polycystic kidney disease.

Other reasons why potential donors may refuse living donation include fears of pain, financial loss, and death. Recognizing the burden of this ordeal, potenial recipients often feel uncomfortable asking a relative directly and instead wait for him to volunteer. Instead of direct confrontation, recipients prefer to use humor and indirect methods to request donation. Similarly, individuals who wish to avoid donation may use indirect methods to inform the family, such as refusing to commit to a date, or evading of contact with other members. Although this 'noncommunication' may postpone the decision to place the recipient on a cadaveric donor waiting list, the lack of formal confrontation does result in better family relations posttransplant (Simmons and Klein 1972). Furthermore, by preserving their relationship with the recipient, family members who do not wish to donate may later offer other services to the recovering relative.

Although the donor's initial motivations may be altruistic, surgery can later cause resentment and depression (Abram and Buchanan 1976–1977). Donors experience a period of sadness and mourning, usually lasting a week. Following the initial convalescence, the donor may feel abandoned as the family's attention returns to the recipient. Donors may become annoyed by a perceived lack of gratitude from the recipient, even though any apparent lack of attention from the recipient probably owes to his preoccupation with both the new treatment regimen and the possibility of rejection (Levy 1986). While emotional reinvestment by the donor may intensify his relationship with the recipient initially, this renewed closeness may also reactivate unresolved conflicts and feelings of resentment (Cramond 1967).

Living-unrelated donors

With advances in immunosuppression, the importance of HLA matching has decreased, thus increasing the chances of success of living-unrelated donor transplants (Levey et al 1986). Living-unrelated-donor transplants offer several advantages over cadaveric donor transplants. First, because it is possible to schedule the operation in advance, recipients may take immunosuppression before transplant, thereby producing a better outcome. Second, advance scheduling allows recipients to choose a time when they are in optimal condition for surgery. Living-unrelated-donor organs have decreased renal ischemia and damage secondary to donor hypotension and shorter cold storage times compared to cadaveric organs. Because coercion is a much greater concern when utilizing living-unrelated donors, psychological evaluation prior to the procedure is mandatory.

Cadaveric donors

Cadaveric transplants create unique psychological problems for both the recipient and the hospital staff. Recipients often feel guilty for surviving while the cadaver has, in effect, died so that they can live (Levy 1986). In one case, a hospitalized transplant candidate learned that a man down the hall was terminally ill and that, when he died, the candidate would get his kidney (Basch 1973). Some recipients avoid all knowledge of the donor; others seek out facts in an attempt to incorporate the donor into their 'new' life (Levy 1986). Since the donor is unknown, the recipient may have fantasies, which are colored by his own feelings and perceptions about death (Basch 1973). In addition, donor families may wish to establish a relationship with the recipient in an effort to retain some contact with their loved one (House and Thompson 1988).

The removal of organs psychologically affects the hospital staff as well (Youngner et al 1985). Nurses may become upset while taking care of young ICU patients in an effort to keep them 'healthy' for harvesting (House and Thompson 1988). Anesthesiologists, along with scrub nurses, expect that the goal of any operation is the patient's successful treatment and resuscitation. With a 'brain-dead' or 'heart-beating' donor, these goals change: the patient leaves the operating room, after the ventilator is disconnected, to be taken to the morgue. The term 'brain death', which signifies 'irreversible loss of brain function while cells, tissues, and organs with support of ventilators remain alive' may not be acceptable to all staff members (Youngner et al 1985). Further complications occur when staff members feel awkward raising the issue of donation to families suffering the unexpected loss of loved ones (Caplan 1984). Although current legislation in the United States mandates that staff discuss this option before disconnecting life support, not even a legal obligation can remove the anxiety over this topic; hence, the policy is not uniformly implemented.

CONCLUSION

Ultimately, the transplant process generates stress for recipients, donors, their families, and the hospital staff. Several types of therapy may serve these needs. Individual psychotherapy is especially helpful for patients with underlying psychiatric disorders. Insight-oriented psychotherapy may explore issues of noncompliance. Group therapy provides an opportunity for discussing body image disturbances, sexual problems, and financial worries. Physical and occupational rehabilitation may improve the disappointing posttransplant employment rates. Staff meetings with psychiatrists or social workers allow members of the team a forum in which to verbalize their anxieties over current patients and situations. Thus, the organ transplant field represents a complex branch of consultation–liaison psychiatry that serves to improve patient outcomes by treating psychiatric and psychological derangements.

REFERENCES

Abbey S, Farrow S (1998) Group therapy and organ transplantation. *Int J Group Psychother* **48**:163–185.

Abram HS, Buchanan DC (1976–1977) The gift of life: a review of the psychological aspects of kidney transplantation. *Int J Psychiatry Med* **7**:153–164.

Albers LJ, Hahn RK, Reist C (1999) *Handbook of Psychiatric Drugs,* 1998–1999 edn. New York: Current Clinical Strategies Publishing.

American Psychiatric Association (1994) *Diagnostic and Statistical Manual of Mental Disorders (DSM-IV),* 4th edn. Washington, DC: American Psychiatric Association.

Anonymous (1989) Medical letter: drugs that cause psychiatric symptoms. *Med Lett Drugs Ther* **31**:113–118.

Basch SH (1973) The intrapsychic integration of a new organ: a clinical study of kidney transplantation, *Psychiatr Q* **42**:364–384.

Basch S, Brown F, Cantor W (1981) Observations on body image in renal patients in psychonephrology. In: Levy NB (ed.). *Psychological Factors in Hemodialysis and Transplantation,* Vol. 1. New York: Plenum, pp. 93–100.

Bennett WM, Aronoff GR, Morrison G et al (1983) Drug prescribing in renal failure: dosing guidelines for adults. *Am J Kidney Dis* **3**:155–193.

Blazer DG, Petrie WM, Wilson WP (1976) Affective psychoses following renal transplant. *Dis Nerv Syst* **37**:663–667.

Bloembergen WE, Port FK, Mauger EA et al (1996) Gender discrepancies in living related renal transplant donors and recipients. *J Am Soc Nephrol* **7**:1139–1144.

Burton HJ, Kline SA, Lindsay RM, Heidenheim AP (1986) The relationship of depression to survival in chronic renal failure. *Psychosom Med* **48**:261–268.

Campbell JD, Campbell AR (1978) The social and economic costs of end-stage renal disease. *N Engl J Med* **299**:386–392.

Caplan AL (1984) Ethical and policy issues in the procurement of cadaver organs for transplantation. *N Engl J Med* **311**:981–983.

Carney RM, Rich MW, teVelde A et al (1987) Prevalence of major depressive disorder in patients receiving beta-blocker therapy versus other medications. *Am J Med* **83**:223–226.

Cassileth BR, Lusk EJ, Strouse TB et al (1984) Psychosocial status in chronic illness: a comparative analysis of six diagnostic groups. *N Engl J Med* **311**:506–511.

Castelnuovo-Tedesco P (1971) Organ transplant, body image psychosis. *Psychoanal Q* **42**:349–363.

Chacko RC, Harper RG, Kunik M, Young J (1996) Relationship of psychiatric morbidity and psychosocial factors in organ transplant candidates. *Psychosomatics* **37**:100–107.

Colomb G, Hamburger J (1967) Psychological and moral problems of renal transplantation. *Int Psychiatr Clin* **4**:157–177.

Conti DJ, Rubin RH (1988) Infection of the central nervous system in organ transplant recipients. *Neurol Clin* **6**:241–260.

Cramond WA (1967) Renal homotransplantation: some observations on recipients and donors. *Br J Psychiatry* **113**:1223–1230.

Degen K, Strain JJ, Zumoff B (1981) Biopsychosocial evaluation of sexual function in end-stage renal disease. In: Levy N (ed.). *Psychonephrology 2: Psychological Problems in Kidney Failure and Their Treatment.* New York: Plenum, pp. 223–233.

DeLone P, Trollinger JH, Fox N, Light J (1989) Noncompliance in renal transplant recipients: methods for recognition and intervention. *Transplant Proc* **21**:3982–3984.

Devins GM, Binik YM, Hutchinson TA et al (1984) The emotional impact of end-stage renal disease: importance of patients' perceptions of intrusiveness and control. *Int J Psychiatry Med* **13**:327–343.

Didlake RH, Dreyfus K, Kerman RH et al (1988) Noncompliance: a major cause of late graft failure in cyclosporine-treated renal transplants. *Transplant Proc* **20**:63–69.

DiMartini AF, Trzepacz PT, Pajer KA et al (1997) Neuropsychiatric side effects of FK506 vs. cyclosporine A. *Psychosomatics* **38**:565–569.

Dubovsky SL, Penn I (1980) Psychiatric considerations in renal transplant surgery. *Psychosomatics* **21**:481–491.

Eidelman BH, Abu-Elmagd K, Wilson J et al (1991) Neurologic complications of FK 506. *Transplant Proc* **23**:3175–3178.

Evans RW, Manninen DL, Garrison LP et al (1985) The quality of life of patients with end-stage renal disease. *N Engl J Med* **312**:553–559.

Fellner CH, Schwartz SH (1971) Altruism in disrepute: medical versus public attitudes toward the living organ donor. *N Engl J Med* **284**:582–585.

Franco-Bronson K (1996) The management of treatment-resistant depression in the medically ill. *Psychiatr Clin North Am* **19**:329–350.

Freeman AM, Westphal JR, Davis LL (1995) The future of organ transplant psychiatry. *Psychosomatics* **36**:429–437.

Fuller RW, Rathbun RC, Parli CJ (1976) Inhibition of drug metabolism by fluoxetine. *Res Commun Chem Pathol Pharmacol* **13**:353–356.

Futterman AD, Wellisch DK, Bond G, Carr CR (1991) The psychosocial levels system: a new rating scale to identify and assess emotional difficulties during bone marrow transplantation. *Psychosomatics* **32**:177–186.

Glaser GH (1974) Brain dysfunction in uremia. *Res Publ Assoc Nerv Ment Dis* **53**:173–197.

Greenberg RP, Davis G, Massey R (1973) The psychological evaluation of patients for a kidney transplant and hemodialysis program. *Am J Psychiatry* **130**:274–277.

Gross MLP, Pearson R, Sweny P et al (1981) Rejection encephalopathy. *Proc Eur Dial Transplant Assoc* **18**:461–464.

Gulledge AD, Buszta C, Montague DK (1983) Psychosocial aspects of renal transplantation. *Urol Clin North Am* **10**:327–335.

Hall RC, Popkin MK, Stickney SK, Gardner ER (1979) Presentation of the steroid psychoses. *J Nerv Ment Dis* **167**:229–236.

Hong BA, Smith MD, Robson AM, Wetzel RD (1987) Depressive symptomatology and treatment in patients with end-stage renal disease. *Psychol Med* 17:185–190.

House RM, Thompson TL II (1988) Psychiatric aspects of organ transplantation. *JAMA* 260:535–539.

Ismail K, Wessely S (1995) Psychiatric complications of corticosteroid therapy. *Br J Hosp Med* 53:495–499.

Kalman TP, Wilson PG, Kalman CM (1983) Psychiatric morbidity in long-term renal transplant recipients and patients undergoing hemodialysis. *JAMA* 250:55–58.

Kasiske BL (1998) Renal transplantation—the evaluation of prospective renal transplant recipients and living donors. *Surg Clin North Am* 78:27–39.

Katirji MB (1987) Visual hallucinations and cyclosporine. *Transplantation* 43:768–769.

Kemph JP (1970) Observations of the effects of kidney transplant on donors and recipients. *Dis Nerv Syst* 31:323–325.

Kemph JP, Bermann EA, Coppolillo HP (1969) Kidney transplant and shifts in family dynamics. *Am J Psychiatry* 125:1485–1490.

Kershner P, Wang-Cheng R (1989) Psychiatric side effects of steroid therapy. *Psychosomatics* 30:135–139.

Koch U, Muthny FA (1990) Quality of life in patients with end-stage renal disease in relation to the method of treatment. *Psychother Psychosom* 54:161–171.

Levenson JL, Olbrisch ME (1987) Shortage of donor organs and long waits. *Psychosomatics* 28:399–403.

Levenson JL, Olbrisch ME (1993) Psychosocial evaluation of organ transplant candidates: a comparative survey of process, criteria, and outcomes in heart, liver, and kidney transplantation. *Psychosomatics* 34:314–323.

Levey AS, Hou S, Bush HL (1986) Kidney transplantation from unrelated living donors: time to reclaim a discarded opportunity. *N Engl J Med* 314:914–916.

Levy NB (1986) Renal transplantation and the new medical era. *Adv Psychosom Med* 15:167–179.

Levy NB, Wynbrandt GD (1975) The quality of life on maintenance haemodialysis. *Lancet* i:1328–1330.

Lieberman JA, Cooper TB, Suckow RF et al (1985) Tricyclic antidepressant and metabolite levels in chronic renal failure. *Clin Pharmacol Ther* 37:301–307.

Ling MH, Perry PJ, Tsuang MT (1981) Side effects of corticosteroid therapy: psychiatric aspects. *Arch Gen Psychiatry* 38:471–477.

Marshall JR, Fellner CH (1977) Kidney donors revisited. *Am J Psychiatry* 134:575–576.

McGowan G, Napoliello M, Alms D (1988) Buspirone for the management of anxiety in patients with concomitant medical conditions: a retrospective preliminary evaluation. *Curr Ther Res* 43:481–486.

Muslin HL (1971) On acquiring a kidney. *Am J Psychiatry* 127:105–108.

Olbrisch ME, Levenson JL (1995) Psychosocial assessment of organ transplant candidates: current status of methodological and philosophical issues. *Psychosomatics* 36:236–243.

Olbrisch ME, Levenson JL, Hamer R (1989) The PACT: a rating scale for the study of clinical decision-making in psychosocial screening of organ transplant candidates. *Clin Transplant* 3:164–169.

Patten SB (1990) Propranolol and depression: evidence from the antihypertensive trials. *Can J Psychiatry* 35:257–259.

Ried LD, McFarland BH, Johnson RE, Brody KK (1998) Beta-blockers and depression: the more the murkier? *Ann Pharmacother* 32:699–708.

Rovelli M, Palmeri D, Vossler E et al (1989) Noncompliance in renal transplant recipients: evaluation by socioeconomic groups. *Transplant Proc* 21:3979–3981.

Rundell JR, Hall CW (1997) Psychiatric characteristics of consecutively evaluated outpatient renal transplant candidates and comparisons with consultation–liaison inpatients. *Psychosomatics* 38:269–276.

Salvatierra O, Fortman JL, Belzer FO (1975) Sexual function in males before and after renal transplantation. *Urology* 5:64–66.

Schweizer RT, Rovelli M, Palmeri D et al (1991) Noncompliance in organ transplant recipients. *Transplantation* 49:374–377.

Sharma VK, Enoch MD (1987) Psychological sequelae of kidney donation. A 5–10 year follow up study. *Acta Psychiatr Scand* 75:264–267.

Simmons RG, Abress LK (1987) Quality of life on cyclosporine versus conventional therapy. *Transplant Proc* 14:1860–1861.

Simmons RG, Abress L (1990) Quality-of-life issues for end-stage renal disease patients. *Am J Kidney Dis* 15:201–208.

Simmons RG, Klein SD (1972) Family noncommunication: the search for kidney donors. *Am J Psychiatry* 129:687–692.

Simmons RG, Kamstra-Hennen L, Thompson CR (1981) Psychosocial adjustment five to nine years posttransplant. *Transplant Proc* 13:40–43.

Simmons RG, Abress L, Anderson CR (1988) Quality of life after kidney transplantation: a prospective, randomized comparison of cyclosporine and conventional immunosuppressive therapy. *Transplantation* 45:415–421.

Sirota P, Stoler M, Meshulam B (1988) Major depression with psychotic features associated with acyclovir therapy. *Drug Intell Clin Pharm* 22:306–308.

Smith MD, Kappell DF, Province MA et al (1986) Living-related kidney donors: a multicenter study of donor education, socioeconomic adjustment, and rehabilitation. *Am J Kidney Dis* 8:223–233

Stuber ML (1993) Psychiatric aspects of organ transplantation in children and adolescents. *Psychosomatics* 34:379–387.

Surman OS (1989) Psychiatric aspects of organ transplantation. *Am J Psychiatry* 146:972–982.

Surman OS, Purtillo R (1992) Reevaluation of organ transplantation criteria: allocation of scarce resources to borderline candidates. *Psychosomatics* 33:202–212.

Tollefson GD (1983) Monoamine oxidase inhibitors: a review. *J Clin Psychiatry* 44:280–288.

Trzepacz PT, Levenson JL, Tringali RA (1991) Psychopharmacology and neuropsychiatric syndromes in organ transplantation. *Gen Hosp Psychiatry* 13:233–245.

Trzepacz PT, DiMartini A, Tringali RD (1993a) Psychopharmacologic issues in organ transplantation. Part 1: Pharmacokinetics in organ failure and psychiatric aspects of immunosuppressants and anti-infectious agents. *Psychosomatics* 34:199–207.

Trzepacz PT, DiMartini A, Tringali RD (1993b) Psychopharmacologic issues in organ transplantation. Part 2: Psychopharmacologic medications. *Psychosomatics* 34:290–298.

Twillman RK, Manetto C, Wellisch DK, Wolcott DL (1993) The transplant evaluation rating scale—a revision of the psychosocial levels system for evaluating organ transplant candidates. *Psychosomatics* 34:144–153.

Vincent HH, Wenting GJ, Schalekamp MADH et al (1987) Impaired fractional excretion of lithium: a very early marker of cyclosporine nephrotoxicity. *Transplant Proc* 19:4147–4148.

Voth AJ (1969) Possible association between metronidazole and agitated depression. *Can Med Assoc J* 100:1012–1013.

Wai L, Burton H, Richmond J, Lindsay RM (1981) Influence of psychosocial factors on survival of home-dialysis patients. *Lancet* ii:1155–1156.

Wolcott DL (1990) Organ transplant psychiatry: psychiatry's role in the second gift of life. *Psychosomatics* 31:91–97.

Wolcott DL (1991) Psychiatric aspects of renal dialysis and organ transplantation. *Psychiatry Med* 9:623–640.

Wolcott DL (1993) Organ transplantation psychiatry. *Psychosomatics* 34:112–113.

Wolcott DL, Nissenson AR (1988) Quality of life in chronic dialysis patients: a critical comparison of continuous ambulatory peritoneal dialysis and hemodialysis. *Am J Kidney Dis* 11:402–412.

Woods SW, Tesar GE, Murray GB, Cassem NH (1986) Psychostimulant treatment of depressive disorders secondary to medical illness. *J Clin Psychiatry* 47:12–15.

Wright RG, Sand P, Livingston G (1966) Psychological stress during hemodialysis for chronic renal failure. *Ann Intern Med* 64:611–621.

Youngner SJ, Allen M, Bartlett ET et al (1985) Psychosocial and ethical implications of organ retrieval. *N Engl J Med* 313:321–323.

21 CURRENT RESULTS AND PROSPECTS ARISING FROM COMPUTERIZATION

INTRODUCTION

The last 30 years have witnessed enormous progress in kidney transplantation. Patient and graft survival rates have improved considerably, and most patients now achieve a high level of rehabilitation. Although several factors have enabled these advances, the major contribution has been the introduction of more effective immunosuppressive drugs, particularly those directed at specific molecular targets. Other improvements have resulted from refinements in the diagnosis and treatment of renal and extrarenal complications. Once viewed as a highly experimental therapy, transplantation is today the treatment of choice for patients afflicted with irreversible renal failure, including those who until a few years ago were considered too frail to undergo either the surgery or the chronic immunosuppressive therapy required following the procedure.

As we project beyond the turn of the millennium, we can reasonably expect a 'third wave' of intellectual development in our information-age society—a wave driven by computerization. Undoubtedly, computer technology in the twenty-first century will open vistas for application in all fields of healthcare—particularly in transplantation, since the recent development of integrated-circuit microelectronics provides computers with the requisite speed and power. One application, computerized data management, provides a means to meet the societal imperative of high-quality, low-cost care. A second application, decision-support devices based on artificial intelligence (AI) programs, may provide efficient analysis of vast amounts of patient and disease data. A third application, analysis of the crystallographic structure of critical target molecules involved in immunological processes, may allow computer-aided design of more effective immunosuppressive drugs. Finally, 'nanomachines' may be used to construct stable atomic structures that perform specialized diagnostic and therapeutic tasks. This chapter describes the current state of renal transplantation, as well as the potential computer-based strategies currently being explored to meet the imperatives of the future.

PATIENT SURVIVAL

During the initial period of renal transplant activity in the 1960s, high mortality rates were particularly prevalent within the first few months after surgery. Improvements in clinical care and immunosuppressive therapy progressively increased patient survival rates. In the US, the mortality rates for cadaveric renal transplant recipients at 1 year fell from 20% in 1980 to 12.5% in 1985 and 8.7% in 1990 (Agodoa and Eggers 1995). The most recent data indicate a 1-year mortality rate of 6%. Present data suggest a 5-year patient survival rate of 81% for cadaveric and 90% for living renal transplant recipients, with patient half-lives of 21 and 30 years, respectively (Cecka 1999).

Causes of death

In addition to the declines in the mortality rates of transplant recipients, the causes of death have changed. During the initial period of renal transplantation, deaths were caused mainly by infection resulting from the nonselective immunosuppressive regimen that was used to prevent and treat acute rejection. The prevalence of infection has diminished over time, while cardiovascular disease has emerged as the primary cause of death. The European Registry reported that in 1991 cardiovascular disease accounted for 46% of deaths of renal transplant recipients, infection 23%, liver disease 4%, and other causes the remaining 27% (Mallick et al 1995). Based on the UNOS data of renal transplants performed between 1991 and 1998, Gjertson (1999) reported that, in the first year, approximately 32% of deaths were caused by infection, 32% by cardiovascular disease, 9% by cancer, and 26% by other complications. At 5 years, 39% of deaths owed to cardiovascular disease, 16% to infection, 14% to cancer, and 31% to other causes.

Cardiovascular risk factors are usually acquired prior to transplantation, particularly during the period of dialysis (Ritz and Koch 1991; Foley et al 1996). Following transplantation, the patient's cardiovascular risk profile may be exacerbated by the comorbidities of elevated blood pressure (Ponticelli et al 1993; Kasiske et al 1996; Opelz et al 1998), hyperlipidemia (Ross 1999), diabetes mellitus (Aakus et al 1999), and/or the administration of corticosteroids (Ponticelli et al 1997). Excess body weight, physical inactivity, and smoking may further contribute to cardiovascular mortality among renal transplant recipients. Useful strategies to maximize patient survival include careful selection and preparation of the transplant candidate, combined with vigorous antihypertensive and lipid countermeasure treatment, physical activity, appropriate diet, cessation of smoking, and reduction or withdrawal of corticosteroids.

Prevention of posttransplant infections is also a primary goal of immunosuppression. While pre-emptive antibacterial and antiviral prophylaxis represent obvious approaches, it also must be recognized that many dialysis patients are malnourished (Bergström 1995) and that uremia itself may depress the immune status (Descamps-Latscha et al 1994). Optimal timing of transplantation following careful preparation of the recipient can minimize the risk of life-threatening infections.

The choice of the immunosuppressive regimen represents a second strategy to minimize infections. The intensity of the immunosuppressive therapy may be excessive, thus dampening the host's ability to respond against micro-organisms. Clearly, the more selective the mechanism of action of the immunosuppressive drug regimen, the lower the risk of infection. Corticosteroids and other agents dampen multiple elements of the immune and inflammatory systems (Ponticelli 1997) and thus may expose patients to frequent and severe infections. In contrast, agents such as the anti-CD25 monoclonal antibodies (MAbs), which interfere with a target highly specific for T cells, do not increase the risk of infection (Nashan et al 1997; Vincenti et al 1998; Kahan et al 1999b).

Liver failure represents a third and relatively frequent cause of death of transplant recipients, particularly in the long-term. Most transplant patients who die of liver failure are carriers of the hepatitis B or C virus (HBV or HCV). Although these patients often remain asymptomatic for years, their mortality rate increases at 10–20 years posttransplant compared with HBV- and HCV-negative counterparts (Aroldi et al 1998; Mathurin et al 1999). Alcohol consumption, as well as the presence of both HCV genotypes (1a and 1b), increases the risk of death. Studies are under way to assess whether lamivudine in HBV or ribavirin plus interferon-α in HCV patients reduces the impact of this important risk factor, as has been suggested by preliminary data.

Cancer has emerged as a fourth major cause of long-term mortality, accounting for 26% of deaths among patients who survived for at least 10 years with a functioning renal allograft (Sheil et al 1993). The most common neoplasms are lymphoproliferative disorders, Kaposi's sarcoma, as well as carcinomas of the skin and lips, kidney, vulva, perineum, and hepatobiliary tree (Penn 1999). The incidence of neoplastic disease may be reduced by prevention of viral infections, avoidance of excessive exposure to sunlight, and regular monitoring of potential and actual premalignant lesions. Because antilymphocyte antibodies increase the risk of lymphoproliferative disorders (Opelz and Henderson 1993), their use should be weighed against the increased risk of lymphoma. In the setting of induction therapy, milder forms of immunosuppression, anti-CD25 antibodies, such as basiliximab and daclizumab, are preferable to the potent antilymphocyte reagents, such as OKT3. Although some types of neoplasia, such as Kaposi's sarcoma or lymphoproliferative disorders, may in some cases respond to withdrawal or reduction of immunosuppression, most show continued progression despite the combination of these maneuvers with intense chemotherapy.

Risk factors for death

In selecting the modality of renal replacement therapy, both the clinician and the patient should consider the pros and cons of the available treatments, particularly as they affect life expectancy (Table 21.1). Although dialysis once offered a greater chance of survival than transplantation, particularly in the short term, several national registries have recently reported a lower risk of mortality among renal transplant recipients versus

Age (very young or older patients)
Long-term dialysis
Smoking
Loss of primary renal allograft

Table 21.1. Pretransplant risk factors for death of renal transplant recipients

dialysis patients (Agodoa and Eggers 1995; Disney 1995; Mallick et al 1995; Teraoka et al 1995). Death occurred within 90 days after starting renal replacement therapy in 1.3% of patients undergoing pre-emptive transplantation, in 3.7% of patients undergoing peritoneal dialysis, and in 4.0% undergoing hemodialysis (Tsakiris et al 1999). These findings are obviously limited by selection bias, since it is likely that dialysis patients with severe morbidity were not accepted for transplantation. However, other studies comparing patient survival rates show that engrafted individuals display less mortality than those remaining on the waiting list. UNOS data reveal that, despite the increased risk of death in the early posttransplant period, the 1-year mortality rate of transplant recipients was 59–67% lower, depending on the degree of HLA compatibility, than that of dialysis patients remaining on the waiting list (Edwards et al 1997). A long-term follow-up study also confirmed the lower mortality rate associated with transplantation versus dialysis: adopting a hazard rate of 1.0 for age, gender, and underlying disease for patients on the waiting list, the relative risk of mortality at 8 years posttransplant was 0.31 for transplanted patients (Schnuelle et al 1998).

Even among elderly patients, transplantation offers better results than dialysis. The US Renal Data System (USRDS) showed that, among patients aged above 65 years, renal transplantation reduced the risk of death by more than three-fold compared with dialysis (Becker et al 1996). Although case selection may bias these data, other studies strikingly confirm the findings, even after correction for comorbid factors. A Canadian study revealed an 80% 5-year survival rate for transplant patients above 60 years of age, compared with 50% for patients on the waiting list and remaining on dialysis (Schaubel et al 1995). Another study found a better 1-year survival rate among patients on dialysis, but a better 5-year survival rate among transplanted (86%) versus dialysis patients (77%; Bonal et al 1997). Similarly, an Italian study showed an 85% 5-year survival rate for transplanted patients above 55 years of age, compared with 72% of patients from the same age group selected for transplantation but remaining on the waiting list (Segoloni et al 1998). Thus, for patients deemed suitable for the procedure, transplantation may offer a better life expectancy than dialysis.

Several pretransplant variables may influence patient survival after transplantation. A multivariate analysis suggested that reduced survival of cadaveric renal transplant recipients correlated with older age, longer duration of pretransplant dialysis treatments, diabetes, and/or smoking, but not with any specific posttransplant variables (Cosio et al 1998).

The incidence of deaths per year per 1000 transplant recipients, as reported to the UNOS Scientific Registry, revealed 25 among pediatric, 10 among adults under age 75 years, and 80 among adults at or above age 75 years (Gjertson 1999). An increased time on dialysis prior to transplantation and both left-ventricular hypertrophy and cardiomegaly among older patients were associated with reduced patient survival. Diabetic patients are also at greater risk of death, namely, 20 deaths per year per 1000 transplant patients at or under age 30 years versus 92 deaths for patients at or above 75 years (Gjertson 1999). Cardiovascular disease and infections account for most deaths among transplanted diabetics. Despite evidence that smoking represents an independent variable associated with increased mortality, a single-center study of smokers versus nonsmokers failed to reveal a significant difference between the rates of any particular cause of death (Cosio et al 1999). However, the prevalence of strokes and malignancy was numerically but not statistically significantly higher among smokers.

Although recipients of living-related donor kidneys are at a lower risk of death than cadaveric kidney recipients, the risks among living-unrelated and cadaveric kidney recipients are similar. However, the mortality rates do not differ substantially between HLA-matched and -mismatched recipients, nor between African-American and non-African-American recipients. The risk of death for retransplanted children is higher than that of pediatric recipients of a primary allograft; however, this difference is not observed in adults (Gjertson 1999). Prior renal allograft loss significantly correlates with increased recipient mortality rates. Ojo (1998) reported that 34.5% of patients who experienced transplant failures died during follow-up. Most deaths occurred among patients who had not undergone retransplantation; only 5% of deaths occurred in retransplanted patients.

Graft survival

The introduction of cyclosporine (CsA) in the early 1980s improved the 1-year cadaveric graft survival rate from 50–60% to 80%, a percentage that has improved progressively over the years. UNOS data indicate that the mean 1-year renal allograft survival rate, as calculated by the Kaplan–Meier survival estimate, was 88% for cadaveric renal transplants performed in 1997 (Cecka 1999).

Another modality to assess the probability of graft survival is graft half-life, a measure that is calculated based upon the long-term outcome of grafts that were functioning at 1 year posttransplant. The half-life corresponds to the time necessary to halve the number of grafts that were functioning at 1 year. From 1988 to 1996 the half-life for grafts from living donors increased in the USA from 12.7 to 21.6 years and that for cadaveric donors increased from 7.9 to 13.8 years (Hariharan et al 2000). An analysis of the data of the Collaborative Transplant Study showed a 10-year graft survival of 82% for patients on CsA monotherapy, 80% for those treated with CsA and azathioprine (AZA), 71% for those treated with CsA plus steroids, and 71% for patients treated with CsA, AZA, and steroids. The respective half-lives were 30.0, 25.6, 17.4, and 17.6 years, respectively (Opelz 1995).

Causes of graft failure

Although acute rejection was once by far the leading cause of graft failure, the advent of recent immunosuppressive regimens has reduced both the incidence and the severity of acute rejection episodes (Table 21.2). Recent multicenter randomized trials report that only a small minority of cadaveric renal transplant recipients lose their graft to acute rejection (Halloran et al 1997; Lodge and Pollard 1997; Mayer et al 1997; Nashan et al 1997; Pirsch et al 1997; Ponticelli et al 1997; Vincenti et al 1998; Kahan et al 1999b).

With the decline of acute rejection as a cause of graft failure, chronic rejection now represents the leading cause of long-term graft failure. Many failures attributed to chronic rejection actually represent the consequence of ongoing subclinical immunological aggression. However, other cases of graft loss labeled 'chronic rejection' in fact owe to nonimmunological factors, such as poor quality of the donated kidney and/or the nephrotoxicity of the calcineurin inhibitor.

Death has become an increasing cause of graft failure. UNOS data indicate that death accounted for 22% of 1-year graft failures over the period from 1987 to 1988 and for 39% of failures from 1997 to 1998. A similar trend was observed for the 4–5-year posttransplant followup. Between 1987 and 1988, death accounted for 26% of graft failures at 4–5 years posttransplant, compared with 48% from 1993 to 1994 (Gjertson 1999). In one series, patient death represented the most common cause of renal transplant failure among smokers, diabetics, and patients above age 40 years (Cosio et al 1999). The importance of death as a cause of graft failure has been pointed out by a recent analysis of the UNOS data (Hariharan et al 2000). The half-life for cadaveric grafts transplanted in 1995 was 13.8 years. After censoring of data for patients who died with functioning grafts, the half-life increased to 19.5 years.

Short- or long-term graft failure may be caused by recurrence of the original disease, such as type 1 primary hyperoxaluria (Marangella 1999), hemolytic–uremic syndrome (Muller et al 1998), or focal segmental glomerulosclerosis (Ehrich et al 1992). In the long term, recurrence of membranoproliferative glomerulonephritis (Andresdottir et al 1998), immunoglobulin A (IgA) nephritis (Bumgardner et al 1998), and diabetic nephropathy (Hariharan et al 1996) frequently account for cases of graft failure. Furthermore, graft survival is lower among patients whose pretransplant renal failure was caused by analgesic nephropathy, amyloidosis, and polyarteritis, owing mainly to higher mortality rates (Briggs and Jones 1999).

Acute rejection
Death
Recurrence of primary disease
Chronic rejection
Nonimmunological allograft nephropathy
Vascular thrombosis
Urologic complications

Table 21.2. Primary causes of graft failure

Surgical complications represent yet another cause of graft loss. Renal allograft thrombosis occurs in 2–7% of renal grafts early after transplantation (Irish 1999). Technical problems are not infrequently associated with dense arteriosclerotic lesions in the recipient or donor vessels, particularly in the presence of a hypercoagulable state (such as one owing to antiphospholipid antibodies) and/or a genetic predisposition to thrombosis. Urologic complications may also contribute to short-term graft loss, particularly in the case of a severe urinary leak with concomitant sepsis. Ureteral obstruction only rarely produces allograft loss in the early postoperative period, since the diagnosis is readily established and appropriate treatment promptly instituted. However, progressive stenosis of the distal ureter secondary to fibrosis or chronic ischemia may cause renal failure in the long term. Minimizing this risk factor demands that the physician consider this possibility when performing a differential diagnosis of deteriorating graft function, since surgical complications are frequently diagnosed using noninvasive tools and remedied by operative intervention.

Factors influencing graft survival (Table 21.3)

ABO incompatibility

Small numbers of transplants have been performed across an ABO incompatibility between donor and recipient. Among 113 cases, the 3-year cadaveric graft survival was 40%. Grafts with zero or one HLA mismatch had a 20% better success rate than grafts with two mismatches (Opelz 1993). As expected, most grafts were lost immediately after transplantation, but the subsequent courses of ABO-compatible and -incompatible transplants were remarkably similar. Recently, good results have been obtained across ABO-incompatible living-donor renal transplants using the combination of pretransplant splenectomy, plasmapheresis to eliminate anti-A or -B antibodies, and powerful immunosuppression (Uchida et al 1998), particularly when the disparity is A_2 subgroup donors to blood group O recipients.

Immunosuppression	Repeat transplantation
ABO incompatibility	Source of donor (living or cadaveric)
HLA incompatibility	Gender of donor
Preformed antibodies	Age of donor
Center effect	Diseases of donor
Age of the recipient	Non-heart-beating donor
Pretransplant blood transfusions	Delayed graft function
Race of the recipient	Acute rejection
Comorbidity of the recipient	Degree of compliance
Duration of dialysis	

Table 21.3. Factors influencing graft survival

HLA compatibility

Even in the era of modern immunosuppression, HLA matching seems to influence the results of renal transplantation. UNOS data indicate a graft half-life of 24.8 years for living-donor transplants with two, 13.9 years for one, and 14.1 years for zero identical haplotype matches. Among cadaveric transplant recipients, zero mismatches resulted in a graft half-life of 12.7 years—a value that progressively declined with an increasing number of mismatches, reaching only 8 years for six mismatches (Cecka 1999).

Preformed humoral antibodies

The higher the content of preformed lymphocytotoxic antibodies, the greater the risk of graft failure. This risk is minimal among patients having antibodies that produce cytotoxic effects against less than 10%, intermediate if 11–50%, and elevated if above 50% panel reactive antibodies (PRA)—namely, the fraction of members of a panel of lymphocytes from unrelated individuals that are susceptible to lysis by patient serum. The degree of HLA compatibility particularly influences the chance of graft survival in a hyperimmunized patient (Feucht and Opelz 1996).

Transplant center effect

One strong influence on the outcome of renal transplantation is the variation in the patient cohorts and physician practices among different centers—the 'center effect'. A retrospective evaluation of cadaveric renal transplants in the US reveals that the 1-year graft survival rates span from 52 to 100%, and the graft half-lives from 3 to 25 years. The only circumstance that has been shown to overcome the center effect is transplantation between HLA-identical siblings (Gjertson et al 1993).

Age of the recipient

Very young children have a high incidence of perioperative complications that can reduce graft survival. For example, renal vessel thrombosis occurs frequently among children weighing less than 10 kg (Arbus et al 1986). Furthermore, the results among patients aged 6–18 years are inferior to those observed among patients aged 19–60 years (Ehrich et al 1992; Cecka 1999). The lower rate of graft survival among younger recipients has been explained by their stronger immune reactivity and poorer degree of compliance to the immunosuppressive and dietary regimens.

The lower graft survival rate among patients above age 60 years owes mainly to their higher mortality rate. In fact, patients older than 60 years display a better pure graft survival rate (excluding death) than any other age group (Takemoto and Terasaki 1989). Reduced inflammatory and immune responses, as well as better compliance to the medication and dietary regimens, may explain the improved graft survival rates among elderly patients compared with other age groups.

Pretransplant blood transfusion

Prior to the introduction of CsA, Opelz et al (1973) showed that pretransplant blood transfusions produced a marked improvement in graft survival rates. The mechanisms for the beneficial effect of blood transfusions remain speculative (Kahan 1984). More recently, improvements in immunosuppression compensated for the higher immunological reactivity of nontransfused patients (Flechner et al 1984). Nevertheless, a randomized trial of deliberate preoperative transfusions of CsA-treated cadaveric renal transplant recipients suggested a superior graft survival rate compared with nontransfused patients (Opelz et al 1997).

Ethnicity of recipient

Recent UNOS data indicate that Asian recipients display a better 5-year cadaveric graft survival rate (70%) than Caucasians (60%), African-Americans (48%), or any other ethnic group. The corresponding graft half-lives were 16.7, 11.1, and 6.2 years, respectively (Cecka 1999). The higher rates of allograft failure and acute rejection episodes among African-American renal transplant recipients compared to Caucasian recipients have been well documented (Opelz et al 1977; Rostand et al 1982; Ward et al 1987; Diethelm et al 1988; Dunn et al 1989; Opelz et al 1989; Dawidson et al 1990; Kasiske et al 1991; Koyama et al 1994; Cecka and Terasaki 1995) and may result from several factors. First, owing to the predominance of Caucasian donors and to the high degree of polymorphism of antigens among and distinctive for African-Americans, patients in the latter ethnic group tend to receive cadaveric allografts bearing a greater number of mismatched donor–recipient HLA and/or Lewis blood group antigens (Milford et al 1987; Butkus et al 1992; Scantlebury et al 1998). Second, African-Americans display pharmacokinetic and pharmacodynamic risk factors. While the more limited drug absorption (Kahan et al 1986; Lindholm et al 1993a) characteristic of this group has been at least partly mitigated by the new microemulsion formulation of CsA, Neoral® (as opposed to the oil-based version, Sandimmune®; both Novartis, E. Hanover, NJ, USA) (Keown and Niese 1998), the more rapid drug clearance rates of CsA (Lindholm et al 1992) and tacrolimus (FK506; TRL; Neylan 1998) displayed by African-Americans predispose transplant recipients in this ethnic group to the occurrence of rejection episodes. Compared with other ethnic groups, African-Americans exhibit lower clearance rates and smaller volumes of distribution, resulting in higher levels of cortisol (Tornatore et al 1995); however, they display a pharmacodynamic resistance to methylprednisolone in assays of lymphocyte performance both in the resting and activated states (Ward et al 1993). Furthermore, African-Americans rapidly methylate, and thereby inactivate, AZA (Chocair et al 1992). Third, transfusions with Caucasian blood products cause African-Americans to display a greater incidence of presensitization (Kerman et al 1991b). Fourth, African-Americans display an increased alloreactivity in both nonspecific immune assays and donor-specific responses of recipient cells in mixed lymphocyte cultures (Kerman et al 1991a), which may explain why African-Americans require higher doses of antirejection agents, such as steroids, CsA (Diethelm et al 1988; First et al

803

1996), mycophenolate mofetil (MMF; Neylan 1997), TRL (Neylan 1998), and OKT3 (Light et al 1993). A fifth contributing factor to graft loss is the exaggerated vascular reactivity of African-American patients, which leads to a higher incidence and severity of hypertension. Finally, the rate of noncompliance to medication regimens (Didlake et al 1988) is disproportionately higher among African-Americans than among recipients belonging to other ethnic groups of similar socioeconomic status (Butkus et al 1992). While little can be done to mitigate immunological, genealogical/medical, or social/economic risk factors, new, more potent immunosuppressive regimens may improve outcomes for African-American renal transplant recipients.

Comorbid factors

Patients with severe extrarenal diseases are obviously at an increased risk of complications and require reductions in immunosuppression. Unless judiciously executed, these adjustments could result in irreversible rejection of an allograft. Patients with a history of long-term dialysis, diabetes, cardiovascular complications, liver insufficiency, refractory hypertension, or bone marrow hyporesponsiveness often require these adjustments and thus display higher rates of graft failure.

Duration of dialysis

Long duration of dialysis constitutes an independent variable associated with poor long-term graft function (Montagnino et al 1997). This association may reflect the severe comorbidities that are often present in long-term dialysis patients, necessitating reduction of immunosuppression.

Repeat transplants

For many years, it was thought that the risk of graft failure rises with retransplant, particularly if acute rejection was the cause of loss of the primary transplant. However, with improvements in crossmatch techniques, recent UNOS data indicate that the survival rate of second transplants is only 2% lower than that of first transplants, both for cadaveric and for living-donor allografts (Cecka 1999).

Donor source

Despite modern immunosuppression, the 5-year results of renal transplants continue to be superior among living- (76%) versus cadaveric-donor (62%) kidneys, with respective half-lives of 16.7 and 10.4 years. The better results of living-donor transplantation are observed among both African-Americans and Caucasians, for first and repeat transplants, for patients with and without preformed anti-HLA antibodies, and for young and older recipients. Interestingly, transplants from fully HLA-mismatched living-related donors display better 5-year graft survivals (75 versus 69%) and half-lives (14.1 versus 12.7 years) than perfectly matched cadaver kidneys (Cecka 1999).

This higher rate of survival of grafts from living-related donors despite poor HLA matching has been attributed to the fact that the living-donor kidneys are healthy, without the reduction of nephron mass caused by pre-existent disease, organ harvest, or posttransplant acute tubular necrosis commonly found in cadaver organs (Terasaki et al 1995). It has also been observed that brain death is associated with hemodynamic instability and massive release of cytokines and growth factors (Takada et al 1998), which can increase the risk of acute graft failure, upregulate HLA antigen expression on tubular and endothelial cells, and consequently increase the risk of rejection (Goes et al 1995).

Donor factors that influence graft survival include gender, age, disease, and physiologic factors. First, the 3-year graft survival of kidneys from female donors is 5% lower than that of kidneys from males, a difference that might result from the lower nephron mass of female kidneys (Busson et al 1995). Second, UNOS data show that cadaveric donor age profoundly affects transplant survival: the 5-year graft survival for donors aged 19–30 years was 68%; 46–60 years, 55%; and over 60 years, 44%. The effect of age on outcome seems to be less pronounced among living-donor transplants (Cecka 1999). Third, a multivariate analysis by UNOS showed that prolonged donor hypertension had a statistically significant deleterious effect on outcome. The historical features of diabetes, smoking, or cancer in the donor failed to show any relevant impact on graft survival (Cho 1999). Kidneys from donors who died of cranial trauma showed a better 1-year survival rate than did those from donors who died of cerebral hemorrhage (Donnelly et al 1991). Fourth, non-heart-beating donor kidneys displayed a graft survival rate inferior to that of brain-dead donor kidneys, mainly because 4% of kidneys from non-heart-beating donors experienced primary nonfunction. However, kidneys from non-heart-beating donors who died of trauma seem to display the same 3-year graft survival rate as kidneys from brain-dead donors (Cho 1999). Nevertheless, kidneys from non-heart-beating donors clearly have a greater rate of delayed graft function than those from brain-dead donors.

While some studies have reported a poorer graft survival among patients with delayed graft function (Kahan et al 1987; Montagnino et al 1997; Pfaff et al 1998), others failed to find an association between acute tubular necrosis and graft dysfunction (Tejani et al 1996; Lehtonen et al 1997). Owing in part to upregulated immunogenicity and decreased resistance to immune injury, delayed graft function is associated with an increased incidence and severity of acute rejection episodes and is thus a likely predictor of poor graft survival (Cosio et al 1997).

Acute rejection

A shorter half-life of kidney allografts is observed among patients who develop acute rejection than among those that do not develop this complication (Dunn et al 1990; Lindholm et al 1993b). Late rejections are more predictive of a poor outcome than are early episodes (Basadonna et al 1993; Massy et al 1996). Recurrent rejections carry a particularly severe prognosis (Tejani et al 1996; Montagnino et al 1997). However,

Opelz (1997) claimed that a completely reversible rejection episode poses no penalty to the 6-year graft survival rate.

Compliance

Poor compliance with therapy represents the third major cause of long-term graft failure (Didlake et al 1988). Young patients, as well as those with poor graft function, tend to show a lower degree of compliance with the therapeutic regimen (Greenstein and Siegal 1998).

Immunosuppression

Immunosuppressive therapy plays a pivotal role in the success of the renal transplantation enterprise. The main challenge is to tailor the therapy for an individual patient: excessive treatment may increase the risk of severe and even life-threatening complications, while insufficient immunosuppression heightens the risk of irreversible rejection. Moreover, both CsA and TRL, the most commonly used drugs for baseline immunosuppression, may lead to renal toxicity, which can accelerate the progression to graft failure. Unfortunately, no reliable test is available to determine the immune status of a given transplant patient; thus, the choice of immunosuppressive treatment and its modifications must be based on the clinical acumen of the physician.

Although a transplant recipient often requires a tailored immunosuppressive regimen, the choice among the available agents must depend upon the clinician's assessment of benefits based on the results of prospective randomized trials in cohorts of 'ideal', primary transplant recipients who do not display comorbidities. After two large, controlled studies (European Multicentre Trial Group 1983; Canadian Multicentre Transplant Study Group 1986) and two single-center experiences (Rosenthal et al 1983; Kahan et al 1985) showed the superiority of CsA over AZA, most transplant units adopted CsA as the baseline immunosuppressive agent. Concern remains that the renal toxicity of CsA may, in the long term, dissipate the advantage of the drug to more effectively prevent rejection compared to AZA. However, two randomized trials showed that patients receiving CsA displayed significantly better 10-year cadaveric renal allograft survival rates than did those receiving AZA (Beveridge and Calne 1995; Ponticelli et al 1996). Moreover, several groups have reported graft half-lives of about 20 years in CsA-treated patients (Opelz 1995; Montagnino et al 1997; Vanrenterghem 1998).

The optimal schedule and dosage for CsA are still being debated. A meta-analysis of the randomized studies reported that induction therapy with antilymphocyte antibodies improved the 2-year graft survival by only 5% in CsA-treated patients; however, the small size of the studies and the small number of events limited the power of the analysis (Szczech et al 1997). A recent multicenter randomized trial found no difference among the 4-year graft survival rates of cadaveric renal transplant recipients treated with CsA alone versus CsA plus steroids versus CsA plus steroids plus AZA (Ponticelli et al 1997). A retrospective analysis of other databases showed that a daily dose of CsA 3–6 mg/kg resulted in the best long-term kidney graft outcome at 1 year (Opelz 1998).

The new microemulsion formulation of CsA (Neoral) has been shown to significantly reduce the risk of acute rejection to a greater degree than the original, oil-based formulation (Sandimmune; Lodge and Pollard 1997; Keown and Niese 1998). Two large, randomized trials showed that, compared to CsA Sandimmune, TRL also significantly reduced the incidence of acute rejection episodes but not of graft failure (Mayer et al 1997; Pirsch et al 1997). Used in combination with CsA, MMF also reduced the rate of acute rejection episodes compared to AZA (Halloran et al 1997).

Recent multicenter trials showed that adjunctive administration of daclizumab and basiliximab, two MAbs directed against the α-chain of the interleukin-2 (IL-2) receptor, significantly reduced the rate of acute rejection episodes without increasing the incidence of side-effects of a CsA-steroid regimen (Nashan et al 1997, 1999; Vincenti et al 1998; Kahan et al 1999b).

Sirolimus (SRL) also significantly reduces the incidence of acute rejection: a 7.5% acute rejection was reported among patients treated with SRL and CsA, compared with 32% among patients treated with Pred plus concentration-controlled doses of CsA (Kahan et al 1998). Among non-African-American patients, addition of SRL to a CsA-based regimen permitted marked dose reduction of the latter drug (Kahan et al 1999a).

Whether the beneficial effects of these new immunosuppressive drugs on the occurrence of acute rejection episodes, as reported by various trials, will translate to improved long-term graft survival is still unknown, since each of the studies had short follow-up periods. One multicenter trial, reporting 3-year results, compared the effects of MMF with those of placebo in CsA-treated cadaveric renal transplant recipients and showed a significant reduction in the rate of 'pure' graft loss (i.e. excluding death) among patients treated with MMF (European Mycophenolate Mofetil Cooperative Study Group 1999).

REHABILITATION AND QUALITY OF LIFE

Many physical symptoms improve soon after successful renal transplantation. A Canadian study of 168 patients reported that fatigue, bone aches, sleep disturbances, gastrointestinal complaints, pruritus, headache, cramps, and dizziness improved within 1 month following transplantation (Laupacis et al 1996). At 3 months following transplantation, many patients complained of side-effects of immunosuppressive therapy, such as cosmetic problems, weight gain, and tremors. However, these symptoms improved between 3 months and 2 years after transplantation (Laupacis et al 1996). An elegant study by Kramer et al (1996) demonstrated a beneficial effect of renal transplantation on cognitive brain function.

Dew et al (1997) analyzed 218 independent studies of the quality of life (QOL) of organ transplant recipients, including 66 on renal replacement. Renal transplantation significantly improved physical function QOL, mental health/cognitive status, social functioning, and overall QOL perceptions. Although the QOL of transplant recipients did not equal that of healthy individuals, the majority of studies documented physical, functional, and global QOL advantages for transplant recipients compared with candidates who did not undergo the procedure.

A further advantage of transplantation is the increased rate of employment, even in the short term. Laupacis et al (1996) reported that 30% of graft recipients were employed prior to transplantation, whereas 45% of patients were employed 2 years after the procedure. The long-term results are even better: in a study of 150 patients bearing a functioning cadaveric graft for at least 10 years, 57.3% were employed full-time, and another 5.3%, part-time. Another 25 patients (16.7%) believed they were able to work but could not find suitable employment opportunities, and 18.7% were retired. Only three patients (2%) were physically unable to work (Ponticelli et al 1999).

Some transplant patients remain depressed, anxious, and unsatisfied with their appearance; others, suffering from clinical complications acquired before or after transplantation, may realize only incomplete physical rehabilitation. Nevertheless, the evidence suggests distinct benefits of transplantation to improve both rehabilitation and QOL (Table 21.4).

Physical activity	Mental state	Social interaction
Ambulation	Depression	Employment capacity
Fatigue	Anxiety	Social interrelation
Mobility	Psychiatric disorders	Family interrelation
Pain	Sleep and rest	
Sports	Concentration	

Table 21.4. Quality-of-life (QOL) parameters that usually improve after successful renal transplantation

CURRENT PROBLEMS OF RENAL TRANSPLANTATION

Despite the improving results of renal transplantation, many challenges lie ahead. The most urgent issues include the ongoing shortage of donor organs, as well as chronic graft dysfunction and other complications caused by immunosuppressive therapy.

Shortage of donor organs

Throughout the world, the gap between the number of patients awaiting a transplant and the number of available organs continues to widen. In 1995, the annual incidence of new patients requiring renal replacement therapy in Europe was 120 per million population, while the incidence of new transplants was only 30 per million population (Berthoux et al 1999). In the US, where the yearly incidence of new end-stage renal disease (ESRD) patients is 262 per million population, the projected number of patients awaiting transplantation in the year 2000 should increase by more than 200%, with only a 30% rise in the number of available cadaver renal organs (Braun 1994). In Japan, the number of patients entering dialysis is similar to that of the US, but the number of transplants performed is considerably lower (Teraoka et al 1995). An estimated 40 000 patients in Western Europe and more than 56 000 in the US are currently awaiting transplantation (Miranda and González-Posada 1998). It is likely that the recent improvements in the results of transplantation will expand the spectrum of potential candidates, thus increasing the number of patients on the waiting lists. Although efforts to increase the number of organ donations are under way in several countries (Table 21.5), it is unlikely that they will be sufficient to meet the enormous increase in potential transplant candidates.

Campaigns to sensitize politicians, mass media, physicians, and the general population
Donor action
Use of 'marginal' donors
Use of non-heart-beating donors
Increased use of living-unrelated donors

Table 21.5. Primary approaches to increase number of donor organs

Chronic allograft dysfunction

Among the main challenges for the transplant community is the need to reduce the rates of chronic allograft attrition, a complex phenomenon involving immunological and nonimmunological factors (Table 21.3). Although the allocation of kidneys to HLA-matched recipients can improve the results, immunosuppressive therapy remains key to long-term allograft function. Unfortunately, the calcineurin inhibitors that represent the most widely used agents may themselves compromise long-term function of the kidney allograft. This risk may be minimized by careful monitoring of the patient. Although new immunosuppressive agents such as SRL will likely allow further reductions in the doses of calcineurin inhibitors, thus mitigating the nephrotoxicity associated with CsA and TRL, it remains unclear whether new agents will improve the *long-term* results of renal transplantation.

Drug-induced toxicity

Many of the life-threatening hazards of immunosuppressive drugs occur in dose-dependent fashion. Because corticosteroids can promote the progression of infectious and cardiovascular complications, they should be administered only at minimal doses. Several studies are currently under way to investigate the long-term outcome of renal transplant recipients treated with steroid-free regimens. Moreover, reduced doses of CsA and TRL may prevent the development of diabetes, hyperlipidemia, and hypertension. Avoidance of the use of antilymphocyte antibodies may reduce the risk of viral infection and posttransplant lymphoproliferative disease (PTLD).

Presently, maintenance immunosuppression is based on three main therapeutic strategies. First, combinations of various drugs at relatively low doses seek to prevent not only rejection but also drug-related toxicity. However, the combination of agents interfering with various cascades within the immune response might produce, theoretically, an increased risk of lymphoma. Second, the use of a single drug, such as CsA or TRL, may yield good results, but with a penalty of side-effects and a necessity for adjunctive corticosteroids in a number of patients. Third, a double- or triple-drug regimen of MMF-steroids or SRL-steroids or AZA-SRL-steroids may be employed to limit the use of calcineurin inhibitors, reserving the latter agents only for patients undergoing acute rejection episodes. Preliminary studies suggest promising results of the last strategy, but long-term data are not yet available.

THE FUTURE: INFORMATION SYSTEMS

The challenges of the coming millennium are to minimize the comorbidity, improve the convenience, and reduce the cost of the transplant effort. To achieve these goals, the enterprise requires more efficient information management, better analysis of clinical data, and new modes of strategic decision-making. Computerization proffers the opportunity to meet these imperatives. For instance, combinations of donor and recipient characteristics discussed above, such as gender, age, ethnicity, and HLA match, may be assessed by computer algorithm to provide a probable scenario for transplantation outcome. Although databases have long been used to match candidates to cadaveric donor organs (Mishelevich et al 1976; Offermann 1988), increasingly more sophisticated database systems have been refined to reduce waiting periods and improve HLA matching (Wujciak and Opelz 1993; MacQueen et al 1997; Sirchia et al 1998).

Computer programs encode information systems that seek to convert complex, real-world situations into idealized models that can be experimentally validated and then used to generate new information for diagnosis or treatment. Many transplant centers already utilize computerized information storage, such as in 'seamless' data management systems that organize, maintain, and store data from a variety of laboratory, office, pharmacy, and hospital environments (Figure 21.1). These uses demand human input: the expertise of the physician is required to gauge the significance of the information. However, current computer technologies to improve transplant practice exploit physician experience via programs that distinguish relevant from irrelevant facts by first stratifying the importance of data that reflect the physician's observations, as well as the patient's laboratory parameters and clinical course.

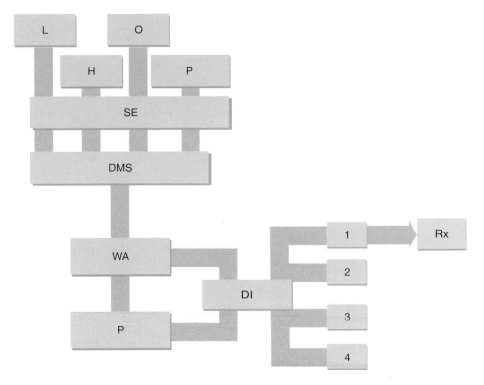

Figure 21.1. Schematic representation of the medical informatics technology. Information from the laboratory (L), hospital (H), office (O), and pharmacy (P) is integrated into a seamless environment (SE) that feeds a database management system (DMS) that, with appropriate weighting, can provide a warning alert (WA) or even a panic (P) that triggers diagnostic interventions (DI) to exclude unlikely alternates that can potentially lead to specific therapy (Rx).

A second type of computer program, based on artificial intelligence (AI), utilizes procedural knowledge to determine the diagnostic interventions likely to yield the additional information required for selecting an appropriate treatment. Artificial intelligence programs describe a validated theory to account for a large class of observations and/or measurements (Figure 21.2). The AI decision-support device permits inductive reasoning about a conceptual model of transplantation outcome that is readily integrated with a global knowledge base of outcomes in a large number of patients to permit analysis of individual patient courses (Figure 21.3). This medical informatics technology translates real-world situations to an 'idealized model' that is verified by testing and evaluation. A robust, user-friendly, and portable decision-support device could provide insights into diagnosis and disease management. This tool would forecast an adverse outcome and reduce the possibility of clinical progression of a complication or disease. Currently available decision-support systems may be based on any of three decision-making strategies: statistical tools, hierarchical structures, or neural networks.

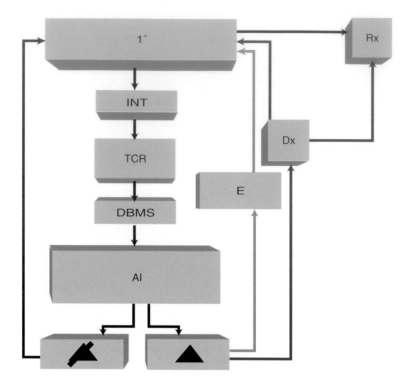

Figure 21.2. Cyberspace applications in transplantation. Primary information sites distant from the transplant center (1°) utilize the Internet (INT) to the transplant center (TCR) for integration in the database management system (DBMS), which suggests the need for change, no change (▲) or change (▲), which is evaluated by artificial intelligence programs (AI) suggesting the need for evaluation on site at the center (E), for diagnostic studies (Dx) or for a treatment intervention (Rx).

Statistical tools

The usual statistical methods for making decisions employ probability techniques, particularly Bayes's theorem. Standard statistical methods, such as logistic regression analysis, are applied to identify the most likely diagnosis or clinical outcome that is consistent with the clinical findings. Two drawbacks limit the use of statistically based programs: first, these methods consider only a relatively few independent variables; second, these programs cannot account for an unusual presentation of a disease or for the presence of conflicting pathological signs. To address these limitations, weighting factors must be introduced.

Hierarchical strategies for artificial intelligence

Unlike statistical methods, AI systems are based on either hierarchical or neural network decision-making strategies that mimic human thought patterns and accommodate mul-

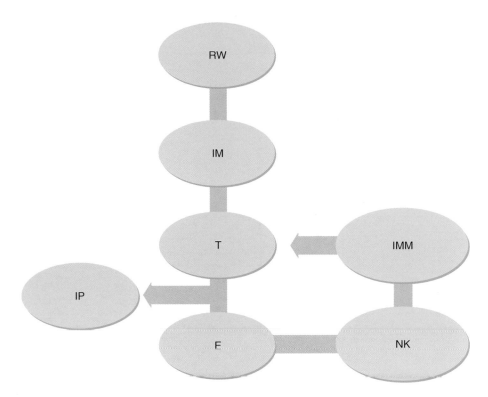

Figure 21.3. Schematic representation of Medical Informatics Technology. The complex real world situation (RW) is conceptualized as an 'idealized model' (IM) that can be subjected to testing (T) and evaluation (E) to generate new knowledge (NK) and an improved model (IMM), leading to improved performance (IP).

tiple independent variables (Figure 21.4). These systems translate medical data into symbolic form. A program guides the computer to analyze the data by making simple, straightforward deductions based upon reasoning that is clear to the user. Artificial intelligence systems seek to understand and to react 'intelligently' to a problem (Kassirer and Gorry 1978). Whereas statistically based programs may make unjustified assumptions about the underlying distribution of data, AI systems based on a decision-tree hierarchical strategy can analyze, preprocess, and transform data collected from a representative population, the outcome of which has been verified by the gold standard of experience. To establish a diagnosis for a new set of circumstances, the hierarchical strategy identifies a limited number of active hypotheses and then progressively discards those that are inconsistent with the patient's condition, in the same fashion as the usual course of human thinking.

The heart of a hierarchical strategy is a production system, in which sets of facts, states, and/or clinical/laboratory values are organized into 'domains', namely, collections of rules that describe the interactions between the elements of the knowledge base. An 'inference engine' or computational scheme interprets the rules and links knowledge in

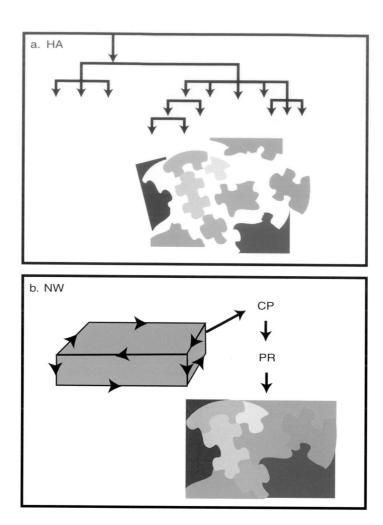

Figure 21.4. Comparison of two processes of discovery in artificial intelligence. (a) Hierarchical algorithm (HA)-driven schemes attempt to order bits and pieces of the picture. (b) Networking (NW) solves combinational problems (CP), leading to pattern recognition (PR) and generation of the 'total picture'.

the domain to the reasoning program that seeks to derive the correct answer. Within each domain are 'frames', namely, data structures that represent situation types. In a medical decision-support system, each frame contains slots, such as the patient or family history, the results of a physical examination, or the laboratory tests of a patient. For any given problem, each attribute in the frame is assigned a value that is weighted according to the specific rules of that domain.

Frames form the core of the diagnostic tools INTERNIST and CADUCEUS (Pople 1982), which draw from databases of 3000–4000 manifestations of some 500 diseases. A possible diagnosis (D) is defined by associations between that disease and a set of manifestations (M), namely, signs, symptoms, or laboratory results. Hierarchical reasoning derives a score that weights the possibility of a given disease based on the degree to which the patient's manifold manifestations, M_j, are linked with a given diagnosis, D_i. As new facts are garnered, the system can also identify a complementary diagnosis that is, a diagnosis that together with the primary diagnosis explains the patient's manifestations better than either one alone or a competitive diagnosis—that is, an alternate diagnosis to the primary computer-selected diagnosis.

The Present Illness Program (Pauker and Szolovits 1977), which includes 70 frames pertaining to renal disease, emulates the decision-making process of an expert physician. The system assesses the probability of a given diagnosis based upon the association between observed and predicted signs. The 'matching' or 'finding' score is the total number of signs that are consistent with the hypothesis. In another program, the Centaur system (Aikins 1980), frames are combined with 142 production rules that analyze 59 clinical parameters, such as age or total pulmonary capacity. A rules program assigns a value between 1 and 5 as a measure of the relative importance of that parameter to describe the condition indicated by the frame. The system assigns a score that evaluates the match of the subject to the frame. Using a hierarchical algorithm that weighs the significance of each measured component, Centaur discards inconsistent or incorrect facts and confirms or rejects a given hypothesis.

The CADUCEUS, Present Illness Program, and Centaur systems are based on a decision-tree, hierarchical, decision-making strategy, whereby objects within a domain are conceptually displayed as nodes that are either linked or not linked by a binary relation. For example, the CASNET system (Figure 21.5) for the management of glaucoma derives a diagnosis or treatment decision based on four levels or planes that are connected by causal links (Kulikowski and Weiss 1982). The plane of observation includes symptoms and signs. A second type of semantic structure achieves a higher level of reasoning by assembling pathophysiological knowledge into five representational levels, each of which is a semantic structure. A third type of semantic structure utilizes first-order predicate calculus to express the causal relationships between data based upon no more than 10 axioms or 'inference' rules.

At least four obstacles limit the utility of hierarchical strategies. First, it is doubtful that real-life situations can be reduced to stereotypical forms. Second, a hierarchically structured decision-making strategy (tree structure) does not accurately mimic human reasoning. Third, the links between signs and precise pathophysiology have not been clearly defined by present medical knowledge. Fourth, a well-recognized causal relationship between two disease states and a third does not necessarily indicate that the original two states are related.

Network strategies for artificial intelligence

Hierarchically based AI systems derive decisions through deductive reasoning processes, such as analyses, mathematical models, and inferences, whereas AI systems based on

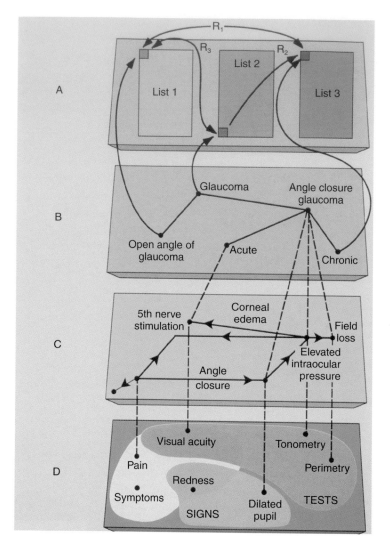

Figure 21.5. The levels of description of disease in CASNET. The hierarchical system links treatment categories (plane A) to disease entities (plane B) to pathophysiological states (plane C) to clinical observations (plane D).

neural networks derive decisions through inductive reasoning processes by selecting rules or procedures that are known to work for the problem—in other words, based on collective clinical experience. Neural networks seek to exploit the intrinsic properties of the term 'intelligence', which may be defined as the ability to act rightly in a given situation. Intelligence implies not merely the ability to think logically, but also the capacity to discard large amounts of information in an effort to focus on relevant data. Artificial intelligence systems based on neural networks use a mode of reasoning, the limited rationality principle, that addresses only a portion of the complexity of an issue, and deals with an incomplete knowledge base and information that is of insufficient quality because it is characterized by vagueness and uncertainty. Artificial intelligence neural networks are trained through the study of a large number of well-documented cases. Therefore, these systems 'learn' to solve problems, understand concepts, process knowledge, and behave like a human expert in that they adapt to particular situations according to the circumstances (Fieschi 1990).

The general operational structure of an AI system uses attributes or semantic variables, namely, extent, intensity, and circumstances, as modifiers of the medical terms (or elementary facts), which are the 'entities' or atoms, namely, the symptoms, signs, or laboratory results. The processing mechanism of an AI system is the program or 'inference engine' by which it runs, consisting of a set of interpretation, unification, and matching procedures that is used to determine the connections between 'working space' of facts and the agenda of rules and actions. The inference engine also includes a knowledge database of rules related to domain knowledge, to the use of heuristics, to definitions of and inferences from concepts, as well as to pattern recognition and meta-rules for resolution. This program, which should have a user-friendly, human–machine interface, is based on symbolic logic, whereby calculus techniques allow it to reason and to derive new facts or properties consistent with the evidence.

The simplest form of symbolic logic is propositional logic, or logic based on declarative phrases, assertions, or atoms, which may be true or false (Figure 21.6). Phrases are constructed by joining logical connectors of negation ('no'), conjunction ('and'), disjunction ('or'), implication ('if . . . then'), and equivalence ('if and only if'). However, the representation of knowledge as true/false propositional logic is 'idealized'; most evaluations require logic that is based on a finer scale to account for imprecise concepts (Zadeh 1965), such as 'fuzzy logic', which assigns a range of probability. A fuzzy subset A of reference E (the study field) is characterized by its membership function, M_A, which indicates whether an element 'e' of 'E' belongs more or less to 'A'. Transition between membership and nonmembership in a fuzzy subset is not abrupt, but gradual. Fuzzy subsets are assigned a value across a range of 0 to 1 (equivalent to false/true in propositional logic). A fuzzy inference rule called a 'meta-implication' interprets the compatibility of the connections between observations and diagnoses as a possibilities distribution, which reflects the distributions and measures the possibility as the basis of fuzzy propositions.

The 'general problem-solver' of AI systems discriminates elements of a problem that are partially as opposed to completely specified descriptions of objects (or situations) and actions. Data structures are represented conceptually in AI neural networks as collections of 'processing units' (nodes) and 'operators' (arcs) that describe pathways toward the solution (Figure 21.7). All connections between the nodes are given small arbitrary weights, which are changed as the system is 'trained' by input of actual case data and outcomes. The arcs that connect nodes are 'weighted' by flexible, nonlinear models that reflect the experience represented by a large set of known cases in order to achieve the most probable prediction pathway (Cross et al 1995). A mathematical model sums the weighted signals from input connections to the nodes, producing an output signal that

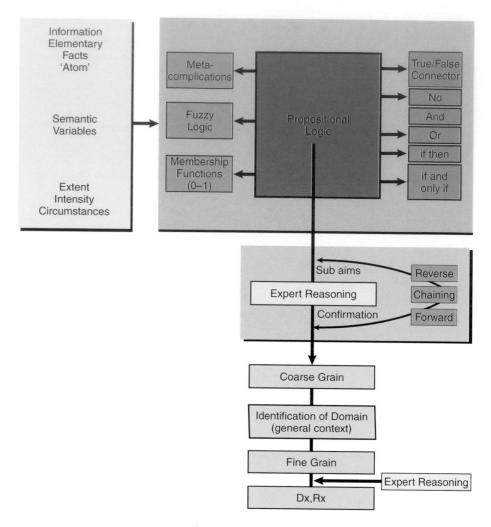

Figure 21.6. Schematic representation of symbolic logic for medical decision-making. See text for description.

is a nonlinear function of the 'net' input. Thus, the system empirically learns the required input/output conditions; there are no individual rules. The power of the neural network is derived not from the properties of each node, but from the density and complexity of the interactions between the nodes (like the human brain). Artificial intelligence neural networks express combinatorial problems as patterns, thereby recognizing the total picture. Thus, they work best for solving problems with multiple acceptable solutions, such as those that are common in medicine. Inference engines defer to experience; they do not make an inference if there is evidence that refutes it. Furthermore, if the evidence is self-contradictory, the computer proposes increasingly better

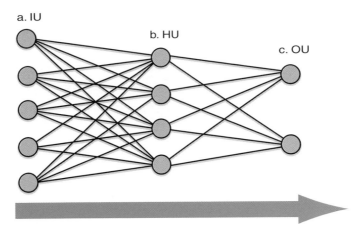

Figure 21.7. Schematic diagram of multi-layer perception type neural network. (a) The input units (IU) include data that are weighted in (b) as hidden units (HU) to yield output units (OU). Each yellow circle represents a node or connection. The solid blue arrow shows the flow of information.

solutions. This learning process encodes knowledge to link initial objects with goals, in other words, via a means-ends analysis.

Once a system is in place, the expert reasoning program addresses a new problem by identifying the most probable framework. Given a set of new data structures for analysis, the computer performs a search procedure that generates a graph that consumes a relatively small portion (less than 100 nodes) of the possible graphic space, which may easily contain 10^9 nodes. The problem-solver uses a generation process to check whether the graph contains a path that connects prespecified sets of nodes, namely, a solution to the problem. Because the procedure is usually not initially successful, the search must use a strategy that is heuristic—that is, one that serves to discover or approximate—rather than an algorithmic procedure that searches the entire database. Heuristic reasoning employs 'rules of thumb,' namely, intuition, educated guessing, and application of experience. The heuristic search procedure estimates the value of each node as part of the solution, using reasoning program language that expresses causality, temporality, ability, relevance and plausibility, possibility and probability, knowledge and certainty, desirability and undesirability, equivalence and denotation, existence, as well as suppositionality or hypotheticalness (weighted signals; Figure 21.8). Heuristic search strategies are syntax-oriented; they search selectively by using 'generator functions' to visualize portions of the levels below an initial set of clauses in a depth-first manner, looking for a refutation by using ordering strategies that contain 'evaluator functions'.

Whereas some hierarchical generation processes proceed breadth-first, the generation process of an AI neural network system proceeds depth-first. Because depth-first

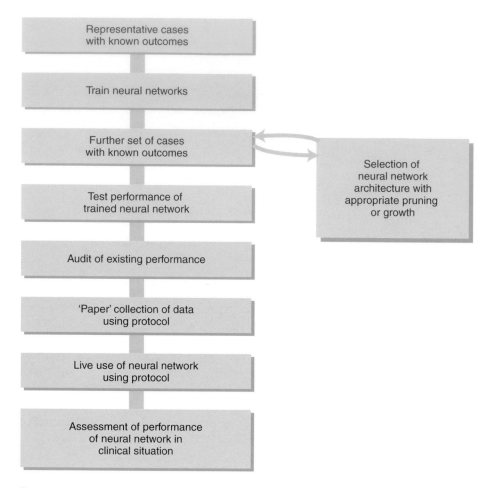

Figure 21.8. Schematic representation of the flow diagram of the training process for neural networks. See text for description.

procedures may search forever in the wrong direction, most programs use a 'bounded' search procedure which, if unsuccessful, backs up and generates more nodes in a different direction. Heuristic reasoning directs the generator function to be systematically oriented toward the most promising portions of the state space, and the evaluator function estimates the value of each node, meaning the likelihood that the node lies on a path to a goal node. The process continues until a solution path is achieved, that is, one reaches a goal node. The AI neural network system uses parallel architecture to find a 'best fit' to an answer. In a parallel architecture structure, the elements work as an aggregate; individual processing elements function independently and in parallel with other processing systems.

To prevent the network from being overwritten with new information or noise, a feedback mechanism, based upon adaptive resonance theory, determines whether new information fed into the net is congruent with the stored information. If it is a member of the same class, the knowledge about that diagnosis is updated; if it is not a member, a new class is established. A vigilance parameter defines the closeness with which the information stored must match the input to be included as a member of the same class. The estimate of the error of the process is serially assessed using receiver operating characteristic (ROC) functions that compare the effects of differing thresholds on the accuracy, sensitivity, and specificity of the network.

The AI neural network converts expert knowledge to a domain of medical language in the form of production rules. This knowledge operates through replets that combine entities into single premises. The heuristic process begins with 'coarse-grain' knowledge that places the patient's case within a general context, that is, a list of diagnostic hypotheses that should be considered before looking for more specific data to affirm or reject each one. If the AI program cannot solve the problem using coarse-grain knowledge, it seeks to discover facts about the representations from their interactions, that is, 'meta-knowledge'. In contrast to 'object' knowledge, the set of observations and their relations that describes the real world, meta-knowledge describes the necessary conditions of objects and the relations between the actions, namely, knowledge about the representation itself. The meta-architecture database management system includes a resource dictionary and a meta-database, which includes directories and constraints of the data units. Thus, meta-logic mimics the complexity of a person's cognitive skills, values, and beliefs.

In the AI network SPHINX system (Fieschi 1990), a project geared to provide physicians with an information system aid to diagnostic decision-making, the original problem is decomposed in a step by step fashion into better-defined sub-aims by 'reverse chaining'. Then, by application of 'forward chaining', one can identify the extent to which an observation confirms an hypothesis. Penny and Frost (1996) report that the decisions made by neural networks are as accurate as a clinician's diagnosis. Indeed, Shoskes et al (1998) report that back-propagating neural networks could be used to predict both the occurrence and quality of early graft function among cadaveric renal transplant recipients. In a recent, retrospective trial of 27 renal allograft recipients, Simic-Ogrizovic et al (1999) found that a neural network accurately predicted the variables most closely associated with the occurrence of chronic rejection.

Neural networks are limited by three generic drawbacks. First, they are imprecise. Second, they have difficulty representing procedural operations. Third, they often fail to derive the correct diagnosis because of the fundamental differences between human understanding of concepts and computer-based symbol manipulation. On the one hand, human thought is holistic, is indivisible into sub-processes, and copes with infinite exceptions and ambiguities. On the other hand, AI neural networks require that 'states' and 'operators' be finitely describable, a requirement inconsistent with certain problems of the real world. Thus, Baxt (1995) described the limitations of neural networks to diagnose appendicitis, back pain, dementia, myocardial infarction, and skin disorders, as well as to evaluate imaging studies, analyze wave forms, and predict outcomes.

COMPUTER-BASED DRUG DESIGN

A second potential application of computers is to design new drugs based upon steric representations of the active site of critical enzyme targets. The ability of computers to process X-ray crystallographic data rapidly allows scientists to predict molecular conformations that most precisely fit, or to indirectly modify the active sites on, critical targets more quickly. Recent progress in the development of immunosuppressive drugs for transplantation has depended upon identifying targets of drug action, such as calcineurin inhibition by CsA and TRL. Over 10 years ago, it was discovered that these drugs bind to intracellular proteins. Cyclosporine binds to cyclophilin (CyP) (Handschumacher et al 1984), and TRL to FK binding proteins (FKBPs) (Harding et al 1989; Siekierka et al 1989).

A protein nuclear magnetic resonance (NMR) method revealed that CsA (Loosli et al 1985; Fesik et al 1991; Weber et al 1991) and TRL (Michnick et al 1991; Moore et al 1991) bind to an array of highly conserved aromatic residues on, and produce major conformational changes in, the corresponding immunophilins, CyP and FKBP, respectively. For example, X-ray analysis of decameric CyP–CsA crystalline complexes revealed that the binding process everts the biologically active position 1-hydroxyl group of docked CsA (Pflügl et al 1993). Indeed, deletion of the CyP immunophilin gene of yeast DNA produces resistance to CsA (Tropschug et al 1989); deletion of FKBP causes resistance to TRL (Heitman et al 1991) and to the structurally related macrocyclic lactone SRL (Koltin et al 1991). Although drug binding inhibits the rotamase enzymatic properties of the immunophilins CyP and/or FKBP, this inhibition per se does not mediate the immunosuppressive effect (Bierer et al 1990a, b; Dumont et al 1990; Hultsch et al 1991). Rather, immunosuppression depends upon the binding of the drug–immunophilin complex to an effector molecule, calcineurin A, a 77-kDa Ca^{2+} calmodulin-dependent serine–threonine protein phosphatase. Affinity chromatography of cytoplasmic extracts of CsA–CyP or TRL–FKBP complexes documents binding of calcineurin A (Liu et al 1991). Furthermore, the two drug–immunophilin complexes (CsA–CyP and TRL–FKBP) competitively inhibit the phosphatase activity of calcineurin A, which indicates that they share similar or overlapping binding sites. In contrast, neither the drug alone nor the immunophilin alone binds to calcineurin A.

Recent studies using computer techniques revealed the nature of the interaction between frozen crystals of isolated bovine calcineurin A combined with its regulatory calcineurin B subunit and TRL–FKBP12 complexes. Griffith et al (1995) utilized the techniques of heavy atom parameters, phase combination, histogram matching, electron density molecular simulations, and solvent flattening to reconstruct phase extension images of oscillation photographs on a phosphor detector. The computer analysis was based on atomic diffraction of some of the powerful X-rays that were passed through the crystal. The diffraction scatter patterns identified each atom in the molecule. The analysis documented that the site of interaction of the TRL–FKBP complex is distinct from the catalytic site of calcineurin A. Indeed, its inhibitory effect owes not to steric hindrance of the access of macromolecules to the active site, but rather to an 'allosteric' effect that mimics the action of natural inhibitors, such as an anchoring protein (Kissinger et al 1995). These studies are likely to lead to the design of drugs with enhanced avidities for the allosteric or for the active site of target molecules.

A recent advance in this field, the Advanced Photon Source (APS), the world's brightest X-ray source, produces 10 000 times the illumination of current technology and enables biologists to study complex structures by capturing molecular interactions in microseconds. The computer analyzes interactions by gathering, storing, analyzing, and archiving data in a massive parallel system of 128 separate processors that decompose the problem into many smaller problems that can be solved simultaneously.

Thus, the inefficient process of serendipitous drug discovery is being replaced by structure-based drug design. Powerful X-ray machines easily and rapidly capture the structure of crystallized molecules, and supercomputers quickly analyze the vast amount of data generated by X-ray crystallography to produce three-dimensional images of the molecules, which can be viewed from various angles. The objective of computer-based drug design is to create chemicals that 'fit' molecular locks in the same fashion as critical enzymes, not to open or stimulate them, but rather to jam or inhibit these locks, perhaps by making the chemicals so tight-fitting that the complex cannot dissociate. The inhibitor may bind to the active site itself or to another site that is capable of affecting the structure and/or activity of the active site. Unfortunately, the molecular flexibility of targets in vivo complicates present crystallographic approaches that only predict rigid structures.

A major challenge to rational drug design is the difficulty in distinguishing potent inhibitor designs from those that do not bind; thus, this technology awaits development of a computational approach to synthesizing only active drug designs (Jackson 1995). However, recent experiments have shown significant advances in computer-assisted design of immunosuppressive agents. Rather than relying on the three-dimensional structure of the target receptor to design ligands, Grassy et al (1998) employed a computer-aided 'in silico screening' approach, based on various topological and shape descriptors in combination with an analysis of molecular dynamics trajectories, to design a potent immunosuppressive peptide that prolonged skin and heart allograft survival times in mice.

COMPUTER-AIDED MANUFACTURING

Currently, biochemists can only assemble complex molecules by using cellular machines. The gene machines of cells encode DNA messages, which can be rewritten and edited by transfection techniques that cut and paste DNA fragments generated by the actions of restriction enzymes. On a second level, cellular molecular machines translate DNA messages onto RNA tapes that direct ribosomes to build enzymatic, signaling, mechanical, or adhesive proteins. However, for any stipulated shape or function, we currently do not know how to write a DNA tape that builds that protein. In mechanical engineering, this technique was employed in 1800 by Joseph Marie Jacquard, who built a loom that wove complex patterns according to instructions determined by a chain of punched cards. Similarly, chemists now assemble complex molecules by adding individual components to linear chains one binding site at a time.

Cellular machines primarily build protein scaffolds. However, proteins may not be the optimal molecules to guarantee stipulated shapes or functions for two reasons. First, proteins display an astronomical array of folding patterns that are controlled by weak forces. Second, proteins lose their structure when dried, chilled, or cooled. These considerations suggest the need for molecular machines capable of fabricating materials more durable than proteins. Molecular manufacturing is based on the proposition that it is possible to improve the evolutionary process; for example, graphite composites are stronger than bone, and copper is more conductive than axonal cytoplasm. Because in nanomechanical systems production of an unwanted thermomechanical ionization disrupts chemical function, diamondoid structures have been selected for several reasons. First, it is relatively difficult to produce an electron-hole pair in them. Second, they represent the strongest, stiffest structure presently known at ordinary pressure. Third, they do not undergo surface reconstruction by reaction with ions in the medium. Fourth, they show stronger binding, resulting in greater strength and better modulus (strain versus stress) relations than biologic structures. Diamondoid structures can function as bearings, gears, motors, and computers in a fashion quite different from the bacterial flagellar or actin–myosin motors.

Ribosomes represent natural analogs of molecular manufacturing; they follow a series of instructions to produce a complex product. In molecular machines, phase conditions are eutectic: that is, the paths of atoms during the synthesis seldom deviate from a nominal trajectory by more than an atomic diameter while executing complex motions in an extended region from which freely diffusing molecules are rigorously excluded. Just as enzymes assemble large molecules by grabbing small molecules from the water around them, a flexible programmable protein machine grasps a large molecule (the work piece) while bringing a small molecule up against it in just the right place to band the molecules together. For instance, Freitas (1999) suggests that a scanning probe microscope could be used to position DNA-tagged molecular building blocks. Molecular manufacturing systems synthesize an array of compounds and therefore differ from biologic systems that only synthesize a stereotyped set of polymer structures that acquire their shapes through the action of weak forces, namely, hydrogen bonds, salt bridges, van der Waal's attraction, or hydrophobic forces. Second-generation nanomachines—assemblers—will use tools of almost any of the reactive molecules employed by chemists under the control of a swift flow of instructions from molecular computers. These instructions will be derived by reversing the information obtained from disassemblers that analyze the structures, namely, a nanomachine that pries groups of atoms free while recording what it removes layer by layer. The disassembler program then controls an assembler through a nanocomputer. Thus, molecular manufacturing is likely to produce stable molecules for diagnostic or therapeutic purposes in biologic systems (Drexler 1987).

PROSPECTS

In the coming years, transplant specialists must harness the possibilities that computerization offers, rather than clinging to the established methodologies of an out-of-step industrial society. Knowledge in the form of data information, images, symbols, processes and meta-architecture is the currency of the third wave. The information age brain-based society of the new millennium must create and exploit knowledge. Although computer hardware, software programs, and telecommunications represent a significant initial investment, the compilation of a seamless database, and particularly the application of AI tools, may result in substantial long-term savings as well as improved health care.

In the new millennium, economies of speed will replace economies of scale. Because each transplant case generates an overwhelming amount of data, and because of the increasing requirement that clinical decisions be made in 'real time', the new millennium requires an information-based transplant team that contributes added value, particularly in the form of symbolic processing. Exploitation of the third wave demands more sophisticated integration and knowledge processing to understand the behavior of systems in turbulence—that is, how order evolves out of a chaotic condition and how systems must be developed to understand higher levels of diversity. Rather than backward chaining to break a process into its smallest constituent parts, this wave demands forward chaining of a synthesized, symbolic integrative unit. Cyberspace will be employed to provide efficient systems for patient management, improve the armamentarium of new drugs, and introduce new diagnostic/therapeutic tools fabricated by nanomachines.

REFERENCES

Aakhus S, Dahl K, Wideroe TE (1999) Cardiovascular morbidity and risk factors in renal transplant patients. *Nephrol Dial Transplant* 14:648–654.

Agodoa LY, Eggers PW (1995) Renal replacement therapy in the United States: data from the United States Renal Data System. *Am J Kidney Dis* 25:119–133.

Aikins JS (1980) Prototypes and production rules: a knowledge representation for computer consultations, Stanford Heuristic Project. Memo HPP-80–17, Department of Computer Science, Report No. STAN-CS-80–814.

Andresdottir MB, Assmann KJ, Hoitsma AJ et al (1997) Recurrence of type I membranoproliferative glomerulonephritis after renal transplantation: analysis of the incidence, risk factors, and impact on graft survival. *Transplantation* 63:1628–1633.

Arbus GS, Geary DF, McLorie GA et al (1986) Pediatric renal transplants: a Canadian perspective. *Kidney Int Suppl* 19:S31–S34.

Aroldi A, Lampertico P, Elli A et al (1998) Long-term evolution of anti-HCV-positive renal transplant recipients. *Transplant Proc* 30:2076–2078.

Basadonna GP, Matas AJ, Gillingham KJ et al (1993) Early versus late acute renal allograft rejection: impact on chronic rejection. *Transplantation* 55:993–995.

Baxt WG (1995) Application of artificial neural networks to clinical medicine. *Lancet* **346**:1135–1138.

Becker BN, Ismail N, Becker YT et al (1996) Renal transplantation in the older end stage renal disease patient. *Semin Nephrol* **16**:353–362.

Bergström J (1995) Nutrition and mortality in hemodialysis. *J Am Soc Nephrol* **6**:1329–1341.

Berthoux F, Jones E, Gellert R et al (1999) Epidemiological data of treated end-stage renal failure in the European Union (EU) during the year 1995: report of the European Renal Association Registry and the National Registries. *Nephrol Dial Transplant* **14**:2332–2342.

Beveridge T, Calne RY (1995) Cyclosporine (Sandimmune) in cadaveric renal transplantation: 10-year follow-up of a multicenter trial. European Multicentre Trial Group. *Transplantation* **59**:1568–1570.

Bierer BE, Mattila PS, Standaert RF et al (1990a) Two distinct signal transmission pathways in T lymphocytes are inhibited by complexes formed between an immunophilin and either FK506 or rapamycin. *Proc Natl Acad Sci USA* **87**:9231–9235.

Bierer BE, Somers PK, Wandless TJ et al (1990b) Probing immunosuppressant action with a nonnatural immunophilin ligand. *Science* **250**:556–559.

Bonal J, Clèries M, Vela E (1997) Transplantation versus haemodialysis in elderly patients. Renal Registry Committee. *Nephrol Dial Transplant* **12**:261–264.

Braun WE (1994) Allocation of cadaver kidneys: new pressures, new solutions. *Am J Kidney Dis* **24**:526–530.

Briggs JD, Jones E (1999) Renal transplantation for uncommon diseases. Scientific Advisory Board of the ERA-EDTA Registry. European Renal Association–European Dialysis and Transplant Association. *Nephrol Dial Transplant* **14**:570–575.

Bumgardner GL, Amend WC, Ascher NL, Vincenti FG (1998) Single-center long-term results of renal transplantation for IgA nephropathy. *Transplantation* **65**:1053–1060.

Busson M, Benoit G, N'Doye P, Hors J (1995) Analysis of cadaver donor criteria on the kidney transplant survival rate in 5129 transplantations. *J Urol* **154**:356–360.

Butkus DE, Meydrech EF, Raju SS (1992) Racial differences in the survival of cadaveric renal allograft: overriding effects of HLA matching and socioeconomic factors. *N Engl J Med* **327**:840–845.

Canadian Multicentre Transplant Study Group (1986) A randomized clinical trial of cyclosporine in cadaveric renal transplantation. Analysis at 3 years. *N Engl J Med* **314**:1219–1225.

Cecka JM (1999) The UNOS Scientific Renal Transplant Registry. In: Cecka JM, Terasaki PI (eds). *Clinical Transplants 1998*. Los Angeles: UCLA Tissue Typing Laboratory, pp. 421–436.

Cecka MJ, Terasaki PI (1995) The UNOS scientific renal transplant registry. In: Terasaki PI, Cecka JM (eds). *Clinical Transplants 1994*. Los Angeles: UCLA Tissue Typing Laboratory, pp. 1–18.

Cho YW (1999) Expanded criteria donors. In: Cecka JM, Terasaki PI (eds). *Clinical Transplants 1998*. Los Angeles: UCLA Tissue Typing Laboratory, pp. 767–772.

Chocair PR, Duley JA, Simmonds HA, Cameron JS (1992) The importance of thiopurine methyltransferase activity for the use of azathioprine in transplant recipients. *Transplantation* **53**:1051–1056.

Cosio FG, Pelletier RP, Falkenhain ME et al (1997) Impact of acute rejection and early allograft function on renal allograft survival. *Transplantation* **63**:1611–1615.

Cosio FG, Alamir A, Yim S et al (1998) Patient survival after renal transplantation: I. The impact of dialysis pre-transplant. *Kidney Int* **53**:767–772.

Cosio FG, Falkenhain MF, Pesavento TE et al (1999) Patient survival after renal transplantation. II. The impact of smoking. *Clin Transplant* **13**:336–341.

Cross SS, Harrison RF, Kennedy RL (1995) Introduction to neural networks. *Lancet* **346**:1075–1079.

Dawidson IJ, Coorpender L, Fisher D et al (1990) Impact of race on renal transplant outcome. *Transplantation* 49:63–67.

Descamps-Latscha B, Herbelin A, Nguyen AT et al (1994) Immune system dysregulation in uremia. *Semin Nephrol* 14:253–260.

Dew MA, Switzer GE, Goycoolea JM et al (1997) Does transplantation produce quality of life benefits? A quantitative analysis of the literature. *Transplantation* 64:1261–1273.

Didlake RH, Dreyfus K, Kerman RH et al (1988) Patient noncompliance: a major cause of late graft failure in cyclosporine-treated renal transplants. *Transplant Proc* 20:63–69.

Diethelm AG, Blackstone EH, Naftel DC et al (1988) Important risk factors of allograft survival in cadaveric renal transplantation: a study of 426 patients. *Ann Surg* 207:538–548.

Disney AP (1995) Demography and survival of patients receiving treatment for chronic renal failure in Australia and New Zealand: report on dialysis and renal transplantation treatment from the Australia and New Zealand Dialysis and Transplant Registry. *Am J Kidney Dis* 25:165–175.

Donnelly P, Veitch P, Bell P et al (1991) Donor–recipient age difference: an independent risk factor in cyclosporin-treated renal transplant recipients. *Transplant Int* 4:88–91.

Drexler KE (1987) *Engines of Creation: The Coming Era of Nanotechnology.* New York: Doubleday.

Dumont FJ, Staruch MJ, Koprak SL et al (1990) Distinct mechanisms of suppression of murine T cell activation by the related macrolides FK-506 and rapamycin. *J Immunol* 144:251–258.

Dunn J, Vathsala A, Golden D et al (1989) Impact of race on the outcome of renal transplantation under cyclosporine–prednisone. *Transplant Proc* 21:3946–3948.

Dunn J, Golden D, Van Buren CT et al (1990) Causes of graft loss beyond 2 years in the cyclosporine era. *Transplantation* 49:349–353.

Edwards EB, Bennett LE, Cecka JM (1997) Effect of HLA matching on the relative risk of mortality for kidney recipients: a comparison of the mortality risk after transplant to the mortality risk of remaining on the waiting list. *Transplantation* 64:1274–1277.

Ehrich JH, Loirat C, Brunner FP et al (1992) Report on management of renal failure in children in Europe, XXII, 1991. *Nephrol Dial Transplant* 7(Suppl 2):36–48.

European Multicentre Trial Group (1983) Cyclosporin in cadaveric renal transplantation: 1-year follow-up of a multicentre trial. *Lancet* 2:986–989.

European Mycophenolate Mofetil Cooperative Study Group (1999) Mycophenolate mofetil in renal transplantation: 3-year results from the placebo-controlled trial. *Transplantation* 68:391–396.

Fesik SW, Gampe RT, Eaton HL et al (1991) NMR studies of [U-13C]cyclosporin A bound to cyclophilin: bound conformation and portions of cyclosporin involved in binding. *Biochemistry* 30:6574–6583.

Feucht HE, Opelz G (1996) The humoral immune response towards HLA class II determinants in renal transplantation. *Kidney Int* 50:1464–1475.

Fieschi M (1990) *Artificial Intelligence in Medicine: Expert Systems* (Cramp D, translator). New York: Chapman and Hall.

First MR, Schroeder TJ, Monaco AP et al (1996) Cyclosporine bioavailability: dosing implications and impact on clinical outcomes in select transplantation subpopulations. *Clin Transplant* 10:55–59.

Flechner SM, Kerman RH, Van Buren CT, Kahan BD (1984) Successful transplantation of cyclosporine-treated haplo-identical living-related renal recipients without blood transfusions. *Transplantation* 37:73–76.

Foley RN, Parfrey PS, Harnett JD et al (1996) Impact of hypertension on cardiomyopathy, morbidity and mortality in end-stage renal disease. *Kidney Int* 49:1379–1385.

Freitas RA Jr. (1999) Pathways to molecular manufacturing. In: Freitas RA Jr. (ed). *Nanomedicine, Vol. I: Basic Capabilities.* Austin, TX: Landes Bioscience, pp. 39–69.

Gjertson DW (1999) The role of death in kidney graft failure. In: Cecka JM, Terasaki PI (eds). *Clinical Transplants 1998*. Los Angeles: UCLA Tissue Typing Laboratory, pp. 399–412.

Gjertson DW, Terasaki PI, Cecka JM, Takemoto S (1993) Reduction of the center effect by HLA matching. *Transplant Proc* 25:215–216.

Goes N, Urmson J, Ramassar V, Halloran PF (1995) Ischemic acute tubular necrosis induces an extensive local cytokine response. Evidence for induction of interferon-gamma, transforming growth factor-beta 1, granulocyte-macrophage colony-stimulating factor, interleukin-2, and inter-leukin-10. *Transplantation* 59:565–572.

Grassy G, Calas B, Yasri A et al (1998) Computer-assisted rational design of immunosuppressive compounds. *Nat Biotechnol* 16:748–752.

Greenstein S, Siegal B (1998) Compliance and noncompliance in patients with a functioning renal transplant: a multicenter study. *Transplantation* 66:1718–1726.

Griffith JP, Kim JL, Kim EE et al (1995) X-ray structure of calcineurin inhibited by the immunophilin–immunosuppressant FKBP12-FK506 complex. *Cell* 82:507–522.

Halloran PF (1998) Designing studies to measure the benefit of low-toxicity regimens. *Transplant Proc* 30(Suppl 8A):25S-29S.

Halloran P, Mathew T, Tomlanovich S et al (1997) Mycophenolate mofetil in renal allograft recipients: a pooled efficacy analysis of three randomized, double-blind, clinical studies in preven-tion of rejection. The International Mycophenolate Mofetil Renal Transplant Study Groups. *Transplantation* 63:39–47 (Erratum, *Transplantation* 63:618).

Handschumacher RE, Harding MW, Rice J et al (1984) Cyclophilin: a specific cytosolic binding protein for cyclosporin A. *Science* 226:544–547.

Harding MW, Galat A, Uehling DE, Schreiber SL (1989) A receptor for the immunosuppressant FK506 is a cis-trans peptidyl-prolyl isomerase. *Nature* 341:758–760.

Hariharan S, Smith RD, Viero R, First MR (1996) Diabetic nephropathy after renal transplanta-tion. Clinical and pathologic features. *Transplantation* 62:632–635.

Hariharan S, Johnson CP, Bresnahan BA et al (2000) Improved graft survival after renal trans-plantation in the United States. *New Engl J Med* 342:605–612.

Heitman J, Movva NR, Hiestand PC, Hall MN (1991) FK 506-binding protein proline rotamase is a target for the immunosuppressive agent FK 506 in *Saccharomyces cerevisiae*. *Proc Natl Acad Sci USA* 88:1948–1952.

Hultsch T, Albers MW, Schreiber SL, Hohman RJ (1991) Immunophilin ligands demonstrate common features of signal transduction leading to exocytosis or transcription. *Proc Natl Acad Sci USA* 88:6229–6233.

Irish A (1999) Renal allograft thrombosis: can thrombophilia explain the inexplicable? *Nephrol Dial Transplant* 14:2297–2303.

Jackson RC (1995) Update on computer-aided drug design. *Curr Opin Biotechnol* 6:646–651.

Kahan BD (1984) Donor-specific transfusions—a balanced view. In: Morris P, Tilney N (eds). *Progress in Organ Transplantation*, Vol. 1. London: Blackwell, pp. 115–148.

Kahan BD, Van Buren CT, Flechner SM et al (1985) Clinical and experimental studies with cyclosporine in renal transplantation. *Surgery* 97:125–140.

Kahan BD, Kramer WG, Wideman C et al (1986) Demographic factors affecting the pharmaco-kinetics of cyclosporine estimated by radioimmunoassay. *Transplantation* 41:459–464.

Kahan BD, Mickey R, Flechner SM et al (1987) Multivariate analysis of risk factors impacting on immediate and eventual cadaver allograft survival in cyclosporine-treated recipients. *Transplanta-tion* 43:65–78.

Kahan BD, Podbielski J, Napoli KL et al (1998) Immunosuppressive effects and safety of a sirolimus/cyclosporine combination regimen for renal transplantation. *Transplantation* 66:1040–1046.

Kahan BD, Julian BA, Pescovitz MD et al (1999a) Sirolimus reduces the incidence of acute rejection episodes despite lower cyclosporine doses in Caucasian recipients of mismatched primary renal allografts: a phase II trial. Rapamune Study Group. *Transplantation* **68**:1526–1532.

Kahan BD, Rajagopalan PR, Hall M (1999b) Reduction of the occurrence of acute cellular rejection among renal allograft recipients treated with basiliximab, a chimeric anti-interleukin-2-receptor monoclonal antibody. United States Simulect Renal Study Group. *Transplantation* **67**:276–284.

Kasiske BL, Neylan JF, Riggio RR, et al (1991) The effect of race on access and outcome in transplantation. *N Engl J Med* **324**:302–307.

Kasiske BL, Guijarro C, Massy ZA et al (1996) Cardiovascular disease after renal transplantation. *J Am Soc Nephrol* **7**:158–165.

Kassirer JP, Gorry A (1978) Clinical problem solving: a behavioral analysis. *Ann Int Med* **89**:245–255.

Keown P, Niese D (1998) Cyclosporine microemulsion increases drug exposure and reduces acute rejection without incremental toxicity in de novo renal transplantation. International Sandimmune/Neoral Study Group. *Kidney Int* **54**:938–944.

Kerman RH, Kimball PM, Van Buren CT et al (1991a) Possible contribution of pretransplant immune responder status to renal allograft survival differences of black versus white recipients. *Transplantation* **51**:338–342.

Kerman RH, Kimball PM, Van Buren CT et al (1991b) Stronger immune responsiveness of blacks vs whites may account for renal allograft survival differences. *Transplant Proc* **23**:380–381.

Kissinger CR, Parge HE, Knighton DR et al (1995) Crystal structures of human calcineurin and the human FKBP12-FK506-calcineurin complex (Letter). *Nature* **378**:641–644.

Koltin Y, Faucette L, Bergsma DJ et al (1991) Rapamycin sensitivity in *Saccharomyces cerevisiae* is mediated by a peptidyl-prolyl cis-trans isomerase related to human FK506-binding protein. *Mol Cell Biol* **11**:1718–1723.

Koyama H, Cecka JM, Terasaki PI (1994) Kidney transplant in blacks. *Transplantation* **57**:1064–1068.

Kramer L, Madl C, Stockenhuber F et al (1996) Beneficial effect of renal transplantation on cognitive brain function. *Kidney Int* **49**:833–838.

Kulikowski CA, Weiss SM (1982) Representation of expert knowledge for consultation: The Casnet and Expert projects. In: Szolovits P (ed). *Artificial Intelligence in Medicine*. Boulder, CO: Westview Press, p. 21.

Laupacis A, Keown P, Pus N et al (1996) A study of the quality of life and cost-utility of renal transplantation. *Kidney Int* **50**:235–242.

Lehtonen SR, Isoniemi HM, Salmela KT et al (1997) Long-term graft outcome is not necessarily affected by delayed onset of graft function and early acute rejection. *Transplantation* **64**:103–107 (Erratum, *Transplantation* **66**:678).

Light JA, Kelly JL, Aquino A et al (1993) Improving renal transplant outcomes in African Americans with OKT3 induction therapy. *Transplant Proc* **25**:2436–2438.

Lindholm A, Welsh M, Alton C, Kahan BD (1992) Demographic factors influencing cyclosporine pharmacokinetic parameters in patients with uremia: racial differences in bioavailability. *Clin Pharmacol Ther* **54**:359–371.

Lindholm A, Welsh M, Rutzky L, Kahan BD (1993a) The adverse impact of high cyclosporine clearance rates on the incidences of acute rejection and graft loss. *Transplantation* **55**:985–993.

Lindholm A, Ohlman S, Albrechtsen D et al (1993b) The impact of acute rejection episodes on long-term graft function and outcome in 1347 primary renal transplants treated by 3 cyclosporine regimens. *Transplantation* **56**:307–315.

Liu J, Farmer JD, Lane WS et al (1991) Calcineurin is a common target of cyclophilin-cyclosporin A and FKBP-FK506 complexes. *Cell* **66**:807–815.

Lodge JP, Pollard SG (1997) Neoral vs Sandimmune: interim results of a randomized trial of efficacy and safety in preventing acute rejection in new renal transplant recipients. The UK Neoral Study Group. *Transplant Proc* 29:272–273.

Loosli H-R, Kessler H, Oschkinat H et al (1985) Peptide conformations 31. The conformation of cyclosporin A in the crystal and in solution. *Helv Chim Acta* 68:682–704.

MacQueen JM, Sanfilippo FP, Thacker L, Ward FE (1997) Regional organ procurement (ROP) trays in renal allograft distribution and outcome. *Clin Transplant* 11:488–492.

Mallick NP, Jones E, Selwood N (1995) The European (European Dialysis and Transplantation Association–European Renal Association) Registry. *Am J Kidney Dis* 25:176–187.

Marangella M (1999) Transplantation strategies in type 1 primary hyperoxaluria: the issue of pyridoxine responsiveness. *Nephrol Dial Transplant* 14:301–303.

Massy ZA, Guijarro C, Wiederkehr MR et al (1996) Chronic renal allograft rejection: immunologic and nonimmunologic risk factors. *Kidney Int* 49:518–524.

Mathurin P, Mouquet C, Poynard T et al (1999) Impact of hepatitis B and C virus on kidney transplantation outcome. *Hepatology* 29:257–263.

Mayer AD, Dmitrewski J, Squifflet JP et al (1997) Multicenter randomized trial comparing tacrolimus (FK506) and cyclosporine in the prevention of renal allograft rejection: a report of the European Tacrolimus Multicenter Renal Study Group. *Transplantation* 64:436–443.

Michnick SW, Rosen MK, Wandless TJ et al (1991) Solution structure of FKBP, a rotamase enzyme and receptor for FK506 and rapamycin. *Science* 251:836–839.

Milford EL, Ratner L, Yunis E (1987) Will transplant immunogenetics lead to better graft survival in blacks? *Transplant Proc* 19(Suppl 2):30–32.

Miranda B, González-Posada JM (1998) Cadaver kidney procurement. *Curr Opin Organ Transplant* 3:197–204.

Mishelevich DJ, Stastny P, Ellis RG, Mize SG (1976) Rentran. An on-line computer-based regional kidney transplant matching system. *Transplantation* 22:223–228.

Montagnino G, Tarantino A, Cesana B et al (1997) Prognostic factors of long-term allograft survival in 632 CyA-treated recipients of a primary renal transplant. *Transplant Int* 10:268–275.

Moore JM, Peattie DA, Fitzgibbon MJ, Thomas JA (1991) Solution structure of the major binding protein for the immunosuppressant FK506. *Nature* 351:248–250.

Muller T, Sikora P, Offner G et al (1998) Recurrence of renal disease after kidney transplantation in children: 24 years of experience in a single center. *Clin Nephrol* 49:82–90.

Nashan B, Moore R, Amlot P et al (1997) Randomised trial of basiliximab versus placebo for control of acute cellular rejection in renal allograft recipients. CHIB 201 International Study Group. *Lancet* 350:1193–1198 (Erratum, *Lancet* 350:1484).

Nashan B, Light S, Hardie IR et al (1999) Reduction of acute renal allograft rejection by daclizumab. Daclizumab Double Therapy Study Group. *Transplantation* 67:110–115.

Neylan JF (1997) Immunosuppressive therapy in high-risk transplant patients. *Transplantation* 64:1277–1282.

Neylan JF (1998) Racial differences in renal transplantation after immunosuppression with tacrolimus versus cyclosporine. *Transplantation* 65:515–523.

Offermann G (1988) HLA-based local donor/recipient matching in renal transplantation: a microcomputer program. *Int J Biomed Comput* 22:251–257.

Ojo A, Wolfe RA, Agodoa LY et al (1998) Prognosis after primary renal transplant failure and the beneficial effects of repeat transplantation: multivariate analyses from the United States Renal Data System. *Transplantation* 66:1651–1659.

Opelz G (1993) *CTS Collaborative Transplant Study Newsletter* 3.

Opelz G (1995) Influence of treatment with cyclosporine, azathioprine and steroids on chronic allograft failure. The Collaborative Transplant Study. *Kidney Int Suppl* 52:S89–S92.

Opelz G (1997) Critical evaluation of the association of acute with chronic graft rejection in kidney and heart transplant recipients. The Collaborative Transplant Study. *Transplant Proc* 29:73–76.

Opelz G for the Collaborative Transplant Study (1998) Relationship between maintenance dose of cyclosporine and long-term kidney graft survival. *Transplant Proc* **30**:1716–1717.

Opelz G, Henderson R (1993) Incidence of non-Hodgkin lymphoma in kidney and heart transplant recipients. *Lancet* **342**:1514–1516.

Opelz G, Mickey MR, Terasaki PI (1973) Blood transfusions and unresponsiveness to HL-A. *Transplantation* **16**:649–654.

Opelz G, Mickey MR, Terasaki PI (1977) Influence of race on kidney transplant survival. *Transplant Proc* **9**:137–142.

Opelz G, Pfarr E, Engelmann A, Kepel E (1989) Kidney graft survival rates in black cyclosporine-treated recipients. *Transplant Proc* **21**:3918–3920.

Opelz G, Vanrenterghem Y, Kirste G et al (1997) Prospective evaluation of pretransplant blood transfusions in cadaver kidney recipients. *Transplantation* **63**:964–967.

Opelz G, Wujciak T, Ritz E (1998) Association of chronic kidney graft failure with recipient blood pressure. Collaborative Transplant Study. *Kidney Int* **53**:217–222.

Pauker SG, Szolovits P (1977) Decision tree analysis. In: Schneider, Sagwall-Hein (eds). *Computational Linguistics in Medicine*, Amsterdam: North Holland.

Penn I (1999) Posttransplant malignancies. *Transplant Proc* **31**:1260–1262.

Penny W, Frost D (1996) Neural networks in clinical medicine. *Med Decis Making* **16**:386–398.

Pfaff WW, Howard RJ, Patton PR et al (1998) Delayed graft function after renal transplantation. *Transplantation* **65**:219–223.

Pflügl G, Kallen J, Schirmer T et al (1993) X-ray structure of a decameric cyclophilin–cyclosporin crystal complex (Letter). *Nature* **361**:91–94.

Pirsch JD, Miller J, Deierhoi MH et al (1997) A comparison of tacrolimus (FK506) and cyclosporine for immunosuppression after cadaveric renal transplantation. FK506 Kidney Transplant Study Group. *Transplantation* **63**:977–983.

Ponticelli C (1997) Glucocorticoids and immunomodulating agents. In: Ponticelli C, Glassock RJ (eds). *Treatment of Primary Glomerulonephritis*. Oxford: Oxford Medical Publishers, pp. 25–77.

Ponticelli C, Montagnino G, Aroldi A et al (1993) Hypertension after renal transplantation. *Am J Kidney Dis* **21**(Suppl 2):73–78.

Ponticelli C, Civati G, Tarantino A et al (1996) Randomized study with cyclosporine in kidney transplantation: 10-year follow-up. *J Am Soc Nephrol* **7**:792–797.

Ponticelli C, Tarantino A, Segoloni GP et al (1997) A randomized study comparing three cyclosporine-based regimens in cadaveric renal transplantation. Italian Multicentre Study Group for Renal Transplantation (SIMTRe). *J Am Soc Nephrol* **8**:638–646.

Ponticelli C, Aroldi A, Elli A et al (1999) The clinical status of cadaveric renal transplant patients treated for 10 years with cyclosporine therapy. *Clin Transplant* **13**:324–329.

Pople HE Jr (1982) Heuristic methods for imposing structure on ill-structured problems: the structuring of medical diagnostics. In: Szolovits P (ed). *Artificial Intelligence in Medicine*. Boulder, CO: Westview Press, pp. 119–189.

Ritz E, Koch M (1993) Morbidity and mortality due to hypertension in patients with renal failure. *Am J Kidney Dis* **21**(Suppl 2):113–118.

Rosenthal JT, Hakala TR, Iwatsuki S et al (1983) Cadaveric renal transplantation under cyclosporine-steroid therapy. *Surg Gynecol Obstet* **157**:309–315.

Ross R (1999) Atherosclerosis: an inflammatory disease. *N Engl J Med* **340**:115–126.

Rostand SG, Kirk KA, Rutsley EA, Pate BA (1982) Racial differences on the incidence of treatment for end stage renal disease. *N Engl J Med* **306**:1276–1279.

Scantlebury V, Gjertson D, Eliasziw M et al (1998) Effect of HLA mismatch in African Americans. *Transplantation* **65**:586–588.

Schaubel D, Desmeules M, Mao Y et al (1995) Survival experience among elderly end-stage renal disease patients. A controlled comparison of transplantation and dialysis. *Transplantation* **60**:1389–1394.

Schnuelle P, Lorenz D, Trede M, Van Der Woude FJ (1998) Impact of renal cadaveric transplantation on survival in end-stage renal failure: evidence for reduced mortality risk compared with hemodialysis during long-term follow-up. *J Am Soc Nephrol* **9**:2135–2141.

Segoloni GP, Messina M, Tognarelli G et al (1998) Survival probabilities for renal transplant recipients and dialytic patients: a single center prospective study. *Transplant Proc* **30**:1739–1741.

Sheil AG, Disney AP, Mathew TH, Amiss N (1993) De novo malignancy emerges as a major cause of morbidity and late failure in renal transplantation. *Transplant Proc* **25**:1383–1384.

Shoskes DA, Ty R, Barba L, Sender M (1998) Prediction of early graft function in renal transplantation using a computer neural network. *Transplant Proc* **30**:1316–1317.

Siekierka JJ, Hung SHY, Poe M et al (1989) A cytosolic binding protein for the immunosuppressant FK506 has peptidyl-prolyl isomerase activity but is distinct from cyclophilin. *Nature* **341**:755–757.

Simic-Ogrizovic S, Furuncic D, Lezaic V et al (1999) Using ANN in selection of the most important variables in prediction of chronic renal allograft rejection progression. *Transplant Proc* **31**:368.

Sirchia G, Poli F, Cardillo M et al (1998) Cadaver kidney allocation in the north Italy transplant program on the eve of the new millennium. *Clin Transplant* 133–145.

Szczech LA, Berlin JA, Aradhye S et al (1997) Effect of anti-lymphocyte induction therapy on renal allograft survival: a meta-analysis. *J Am Soc Nephrol* **8**:1771–1777.

Takada M, Nadeau KC, Hancock WW et al (1998) Effects of explosive brain death on cytokine activation of peripheral organs in the rat. *Transplantation* **65**:1533–1542.

Takemoto S, Terasaki PI (1989) Donor and recipient age. In: Terasaki PI (ed). *Clinical Transplants 1988*. Los Angeles: UCLA Tissue Typing Laboratory, pp. 345–356.

Tejani A, Cortes L, Stablein D (1996) Clinical correlates of chronic rejection in pediatric renal transplantation. A report of the North American Pediatric Renal Transplant Cooperative Study. *Transplantation* **61**:1054–1058.

Teraoka S, Toma H, Nihei H et al (1995) Current status of renal replacement therapy in Japan. *Am J Kidney Dis* **25**:151–164.

Terasaki PI, Cecka JM, Gjertson DW, Takemoto S (1995) High survival rates of kidney transplants from spousal and living unrelated donors. *N Engl J Med* **333**:333–336.

Tornatore KM, Biocevich DM, Reed KA et al (1995) Post-transplant diabetes mellitus and methylprednisolone pharmacokinetics in African-American and Caucasian renal transplant recipients. *Clin Transplant* **9**:289–296.

Tropschug M, Barthelmess IB, Neupert W (1989) Sensitivity to cyclosporin A is mediated by cyclophilin in *Neurospora crassa* and *Saccharomyces cerevisiae*. *Nature* **342**:953–955.

Tsakiris D, Jones EH, Briggs JD et al (1999) Deaths within 90 days from starting renal replacement therapy in the ERA-EDTA Registry between 1990 and 1992. *Nephrol Dial Transplant* **14**:2343–2350.

Uchida K, Tominaga Y, Haba T et al (1998) ABO-incompatible renal transplantation: dissociation of ABO antibodies. *Transplant Proc* **30**:2302–2303.

Vanrenterghem YF (1998) Approaches to improving long-term allograft outcome. *Transplant Proc* **30**(Suppl 8A):S2–S6.

Vincenti F, Kirkman R, Light S et al (1998) Interleukin-2-receptor blockade with daclizumab to prevent acute rejection in renal transplantation. Daclizumab Triple Therapy Study Group. *N Engl J Med* **338**:161–165.

Ward HJ, Koyle M, Terasaki PI, Cecka JM (1987) Outcome of renal transplantation in blacks. *Transplant Proc* **19**:1546–1548.

Ward M, Lazda VA, Gaddis PJ et al (1993) In vitro response to immunosuppressive agents in blacks. *Transplant Proc* 25:2470–2471.

Weber C, Wider G, von Freyberg B et al (1991) The NMR structure of cyclosporin A bound to cyclophilin in aqueous solution. *Biochemistry* 30:6563–6574.

Wujciak T, Opelz G (1993) Computer analysis of cadaver kidney allocation procedures. *Transplantation* 55:516–521.

Zadeh LA (1965) Fuzzy sets. *Information and Control* 8:338–353.

INDEX

Note: page numbers in **bold** refer to figures and those in *italics* to tables. Abbreviations used in subheadings are: AI = artificial intelligence; CNA = calcineurin antagonist; HLA = human leukocyte antigen; MHC = major histocompatibility complex.